SPORTS MEDICINE FOR PRIMARY CARE

EDITED BY

JOHN C. RICHMOND, M.D.

Associate Professor of Orthopaedic Surgery
Tufts University School of Medicine
Director of Sports Medicine
New England Medical Center
Boston, Massachusetts

EDWARD J. SHAHADY, M.D.

Professor of Family Medicine
Director of Medical Education and
Family Practice Residency
University of Florida/North Broward Hospital District
Ft. Lauderdale, Florida

**Blackwell
Science**

To all of our students, residents,
fellows, and trainers

BLACKWELL SCIENCE
Editorial offices:
238 Main Street, Cambridge, Massachusetts 02142,
  USA
Osney Mead, Oxford OX2 0EL, England
25 John Street, London WC1N 2BL, England
23 Ainslie Place, Edinburgh EH3 6AJ, Scotland
54 University Street, Carlton, Victoria 3053, Australia
Arnette Blackwell SA, 1 rue de Lille, 75007 Paris,
  France
Blackwell Wissenschafts-Verlag GmbH
  Kurfürstendamm 57, 10707 Berlin, Germany
  Feldgasse 13, A-1238 Vienna, Austria

DISTRIBUTORS:

North America
  Blackwell Science, Inc.
  238 Main Street
  Cambridge, Massachusetts 02142
  (Telephone orders: 800-215-1000 or 617-876-7000)

Australia
  Blackwell Science Pty Ltd
  54 University Street
  Carlton, Victoria 3053
  (Telephone orders: 03-347-5552)

Outside North America and Australia
  Blackwell Science, Ltd.
  c/o Marston Book Services, Ltd.
  P.O. Box 87
  Oxford OX2 0DT
  England
  (Telephone orders: 441-865-791155)

Notice: The indications and dosages of all drugs in
this book have been recommended in the medical
literature and conform to the practices of the general
medical community. The medications described do
not necessarily have specific approval by the Food
and Drug Administration for use in the diseases and
dosages for which they are recommended. The
package insert for each drug should be consulted for
use and dosage as approved by the FDA. Because
standards of usage change, it is advisable to keep
abreast of revised recommendations, particularly
those concerning new drugs.

Acquisitions: Michael Snider
Development: Debra Lance
Production: Karen Feeney
Manufacturing: Kathleen Grimes

Printed and bound by Braun-Brumfield,
  Ann Arbor, MI
© 1996 by Blackwell Science, Inc.
Printed in the United States of America
96 97 98 99 5 4 3 2 1

Library of Congress Cataloging in Publication Data
Sports medicine for primary care / edited by
  John C. Richmond, Edward J. Shahady.
      p.   cm.
      Includes bibliographical references and index.

    1. Sports medicine.   I. Richmond, John C.
  II. Shahady, Edward J.
    [DNLM: 1. Athletic Injuries.   2. Primary Health
  Care.   3. Sports Medicine.   QT 281 S765 1986]
  RC1210.S688   1996
  617.1'027—dc20
  DNLM/DLC
  for Library of Congress   95-32073
                                           CIP

CONTENTS

Contributors, v

Foreword, ix

Preface, xi

1 Exercise Physiology and Exercise
Benefits, 1
Edward J. Shahady

2 The Role of the Sports Medicine Physician
in the Community, 31
John F. Duff

3 Preparticipation Evaluation of the School
Athlete, 53
Karl B. Fields

4 Head Injuries in Sports, 73
*Abraham Mintz and Zev David
Nijensohn*

5 Neck Injuries in Sports, 95
Stuart C. Belkin

6 On-Site Assessment of Eye Injuries:
Can the Athlete Return to Play?, 123
Michael Easterbrook

7 The Chest and Thorax, 135
Gregory Tuttle

8 The Abdomen, 149
Gregory Tuttle

9 Back Injuries in Sports, 177
Larry B. Lipscomb

10 Shoulder Injuries in Sports, 209
Timothy N. Taft

11 Elbow Injuries in Sports, 285
Louis C. Almekinders

12 The Wrist, 317
Donald K. Bynum, Jr.

13 The Hand and Fingers, 333
Donald K. Bynum, Jr.

14 Pelvis, Hip, and Thigh Injuries in Sports, 361
Eric T. Shapiro

15 The Knee, 387
John C. Richmond

16 Ankle Injuries in Sports, 445
M. Patrice Eiff

17 Injuries of the Lower Leg, Between the
    Knee and Ankle, 469
    Richard M. Wilk

18 The Foot, 499
    Michael Petrizzi

19 Heat Illness, 525
    Karl Watts and Gertjan Mulder

20 Three Common Medical Problems in
    Sports, 541
    Karl B. Fields

21 Exercise in Persons with Cardiovascular
    Disease, 555
    Randal J. Thomas and Richard Wei

22 Nutritional Concerns in Sports
    Medicine, 583
    Judy Goffi, Johanna Dwyer, and Miriam Nelson

23 Women Athletes: Unique Issues, 609
    Donna I. Meltzer

24 Wilderness Medicine, 631
    *James S. Kramer and
    Richard R. Ehinger*

25 Drug Abuse in Sports, 653
    William E. Moats

26 Sports Psychology and the Injured
    Athlete, 667
    R. Kelly Crace and Charles J. Hardy

27 Nonsteroidal Anti-inflammatory
    Drugs, 681
    Timothy J. Ives

Index, 693

CONTRIBUTORS

Louis C. Almekinders, M.D.
Associate Professor of Orthopaedic
Surgery and Sports Medicine
Division of Orthopaedic Surgery
Sports Medicine Section
University of North Carolina at Chapel Hill
  School of Medicine
Chapel Hill, North Carolina

Stuart C. Belkin, M.D.
Associate Team Physician
University of Bridgeport and
Sacred Heart University Athletic Teams
Trumbull, Connecticut

Donald K. Bynum, Jr., M.D.
Associate Professor of Orthopaedic Surgery
Division of Orthopaedic Surgery
University of North Carolina at Chapel Hill
  School of Medicine
Chapel Hill, North Carolina

R. Kelly Crace, Ph.D.
Counseling Center
College of William and Mary
Williamsburg, Virginia

John F. Duff, M.D.
Medical Director

North Shore Sports Medical Center
Danvers, Massachusetts

Johanna Dwyer, D.Sc.,R.D.
Professor of Medicine and Community Health
Tufts University School of Medicine
Director
Frances Stern Nutrition Center
New England Medical Center
Boston, Massachusetts

Michael Easterbrook, M.D., FRCS(C), FACS
Associate Professor
University of Toronto Faculty of Medicine
Chief of Ophthalmology
Wellesley Hospital
Staff
Toronto General and Toronto Western
  Hospitals
Team Physician
Toronto Maple Leaf Hockey Club
Toronto, Canada

Richard R. Ehringer, M.D.
Village Family Practice
Greensboro, North Carolina

M. Patrice Eiff, M.D.
Assistant Professor of Family Medicine

Oregon Health Sciences University School of
  Medicine
Portland, Oregon

John A. Feagin, Jr., M.D.
Associate Professor of Orthopaedic
  Surgery
Department of Surgery
Duke University School of Medicine
Associate Professor of Biomedical
  Engineering
Duke University School of Engineering
Chief of Orthopaedic Surgery
Veterans Administration Medical Center
Durham, North Carolina
Clinical Professor of Surgery
Uniformed Services University of the Health
  Sciences
F. Edward Hebert School of Medicine
Bethesda, Maryland

Karl B. Fields, M.D.
Associate Professor of Family Medicine
Director of the Sports Medicine Fellowship
  Program
Moses H. Cone Family Practice Residency
  Program
University of North Carolina at Chapel Hill
  School of Medicine
Diplomate
American Board of Family Practice with CAQ
  in Sports Medicine
Greensboro, North Carolina

Judy Goffi, M.S., R.D.
Nutritionist
Frances Stern Nutrition Center
New England Medical Center
Boston, Massachusetts

Charles J. Hardy, Ph.D.
Professor and Chair of Sport Science and
  Physical Education
Georgia Southern University
Statesboro, Georgia

Timothy J. Ives, Pharm.D., M.P.H.
Associate Professor of Pharmacy and Family
  Medicine
University of North Carolina at Chapel Hill
  School of Medicine
Chapel Hill, North Carolina

James S. Kramer, M.D., ABFP
Sports Medicine Center
Murphy Wainer Orthopedic Specialists
Greensboro, North Carolina

Larry B. Lipscomb, M.D.
Assistant Professor of Family Practice and
  Community Medicine
University of Texas Medical School at
  Houston
Assistant Medical Director
Harris County Sheriffs Department
Houston, Texas

Donna I. Meltzer, M.D.
Clinical Assistant Professor of Family
  Medicine
University Medical Center
State University of New York at Stony Brook
Stony Brook, New York

Abraham Mintz, MD
Diplomate
American Board of Neurological Surgery
Bridgeport, Connecticut

William E. Moats, M.D.
Assistant Professor of Family Practice
Northeastern Ohio Universities College of
  Medicine
Diplomate
American Board of Family Practice with CAQ
  in Sports Medicine
Akron, Ohio

Gertjan Mulder, M.D.
Clinical Professor of Family Medicine
University of Washington School of Medicine

Associate Director
Family Practice Residency of Idaho
Boise, Idaho

Miriam Nelson, Ph.D.
Scientist II
Human Physiology Laboratory
USDA Human Nutrition Research Center on
  Aging
Tufts University School of Medicine
Boston, Massachusetts

Zev David Nijensohn, B.A.
Dartmouth College
Hanover, New Hampshire

Michael Petrizzi, M.D.
Associate Professor of Family Medicine
Medical College of Virginia
Residency Director
Hanover Family Physicians Family Practice
  Residency Program
Diplomate
American Board of Family Practice with CAQ
  in Sports Medicine
Mechanicsville, Virginia

John C. Richmond, M.D.
Associate Professor of Orthopaedic
  Surgery
Tufts University School of Medicine
Director of Sports Medicine
New England Medical Center
Boston, Massachusetts

Edward J. Shahady, M.D.
Professor of Family Medicine
Director of Medical Education and Family
  Practice Residency Program
University of Florida/North Broward Hospital
  District
Diplomate
American Board of Family Practice with CAQ
  in Sports Medicine
Ft. Lauderdale, Florida

Eric T. Shapiro, M.D.
Orthopaedic Surgery Associates
Boca Raton, Florida

Timothy N. Taft, M.D.
Max M. Novich Professor and Director of
  Sports Medicine
Orthopaedic Surgery
University of North Carolina at Chapel Hill
  School of Medicine
Chapel Hill, North Carolina

Randal J. Thomas, M.D., M.S.
Assistant Professor of Preventive Medicine
Northwestern University Medical School
Chicago, Illinois

Gregory Tuttle, M.D.
Team Physician/University Physician
University of North Carolina at Chapel Hill
Clinical Assistant Professor of Emergency
  Medicine
Adjunct Assistant Professor of Family Medicine
Adjunct Clinical Assistant Professor of
  Orthopaedics and Surgery
University of North Carolina at Chapel Hill
  School of Medicine
Diplomate
American Board of Family Practice with CAQ
  in Sports Medicine
Chapel Hill, North Carolina

Karl Watts, M.D.
Clinical Assistant Professor of Family Medicine
University of Washington School of Medicine
Faculty
Family Residency of Idaho
Director
Primary Care Sports Medicine Fellowship and
  Boise Center for Sports and Excercise
  Medicine
Boise, Idaho

Richard Wei, M.D.
Fellow

Occupational Medicine
University of Illinois College of Medicine
Chicago, Illinois

Richard M. Wilk, M.D.
Clinical Instructor of Orthopedic Surgery
Boston University School of Medicine
Staff Surgeon
Department of Orthopedic Surgery
Lahey Clinic Hospital
Burlington, Massachusetts

FOREWORD

Sports and sports medicine are vital parts of our lives. As affluence and leisure have afforded us the privileges of spirited competition at all levels of ability and every age, so have these privileges created an epidemic of injuries, resulting from both trauma and overuse.

Who should treat this epidemic of injuries?

Regardless of a patient's health care choice, the challenge of treating these injuries rightfully falls to his or her primary care physician. With challenge comes responsibility and thus comes *Sports Medicine for Primary Care*. The primary care physician who chooses to care for recreational, high school, and college athletes must be qualified—through choice, study, experience, and apprenticeship. This book is a splendid reference/study manual for the sports medicine practitioner who has chosen to match the athlete's dedication, discipline, and quest for excellence.

Sports Medicine for Primary Care will be a joy to any practioner because of its extensive coverage and lucid presentation of the science of sports medicine

John A. Feagin, Jr., M.D.

PREFACE

The field of sports medicine has developed at an accelerated rate over the past few years. This development has been stimulated by a variety of changes in our society. Television has brought many athletic events into our living rooms. Injuries to athletes are now considered news. Team physicians and team trainers are part of this news, and thus sports medicine has increasingly become a part of the everyday language of the average American. Coupled with the public awareness of elite athletes and their health is the increased public focus on exercise as a means of preventing health problems such as hypertension, heart disease, and cancer. Exercise is an inexpensive and effective means of preventing and treating many of the health problems that face us today.

Sports medicine is a field that has expanded from the care of the elite athlete to the care of the average everyday athlete, the weekend athlete, the college athlete, and the high school athlete. In the past this care was provided by any physician, coach, or volunteer trainer. We have seen a dramatic change whereby trainers are now certified by a national organization and the specialty of sports medicine has been created. Al-though orthopedic physicians and primary care physicians are both involved in the care of athletes, a certificate of added qualification in sports medicine is available to physicians who are board certified in family practice, pediatrics, internal medicine, and emergency medicine.

Sports medicine is practiced by many physicians. The leader of the health care team is the primary care physician, so it is important that this person receive certification in sports medicine. There are also many subspecialists who have an interest in sports medicine, including ophthalmologists and neurosurgeons. These two specialties have a special interest because of the mortality and morbidity seen in sports related injuries in these two specialties. For example, one of the leading causes of blindness is sports related trauma. Sports related injuries are also a major cause of trauma induced paralysis.

Sports Medicine for Primary Care is intended to help primary care physicians better understand all the ramifications of practicing sports medicine and help them become better practitioners of sports medicine. The book covers both the medical and musculoskeletal aspects of sports medicine. The medical portions include a chapter on exercise medicine, which discusses some of the new concepts of benefits of exercise and how exercise influences many of the body systems. Other chapters include a discussion of heart disease and participation in athletic events, psychology of sports, wilderness medicine, drug abuse, and proper drug use. There is also a discussion of some of the unique medical problems such as asthma, diabetes, and mononucleosis that occur in athletes. Another excellent chapter also discusses the basis of good nutrition and preparation of pre- and post-game meals. A chapter on preparticipation evaluation discusses some of the keys to an appropriate preparticipation evaluation of athletes.

The chapters on musculoskeletal medicine are written specifically for the primary care physician. Each chapter begins with the discussion of the epidemiology of that injury in primary care and in particular sports. Although rare problems are mentioned, the emphasis is on common problems. The history and physical are the critical portions of each chapter. Case histories are utilized when appropriate and line art drawings are scattered throughout the text to help the physician better understand the anatomy as well as the mechanism of injury. Diagnostic testing such as radiography is discussed, especially from the perspective of "is the x-ray really needed?" Treatment options stress nonsurgical therapy.

In addition to the usual chapters on injury to the neck, shoulder, knee, and so on, there is also an emphasis placed on injuries to the eye, the chest, the thorax, and the abdomen, areas that are sometimes neglected in sports medicine books.

As one will quickly note, another unique aspect of this book is that it is written both by primary care physicians and physicians in other specialties; adding a distinctive flavor to the book and increasing its credibility. The fact that it is edited by both a family physician and an orthopedic surgeon gives the reader assurances that both the general and specific issues of each injury receive appropriate consideration. We recommend *Sports Medicine for Primary Care* to you as a book that can be used as both a textbook and reference. It covers the majority of problems that the primary physician will see in sports medicine.

John C. Richmond
Edward J. Shahady

EXERCISE PHYSIOLOGY AND EXERCISE BENEFITS

1

EDWARD J. SHAHADY

Inactivity
The Body's Response to Exercise
Exercise Prescription
Benefits of Exercise
Confusing Health Issues with Exercise
Issues in Training
Pregnancy and Exercise
Nutrition

"The human body becomes more efficient with increased use. Unfortunately, with disuse, the body quickly becomes an inefficient organism."

INACTIVITY

There are probably 40 million adults in the United States whose sedentary habits place them at increased risk of morbidity and mortality from several diseases (1). It is now clear that regular physical activity reduces the risk of morbidity and mortality from several chronic diseases and increases physical fitness, which leads to improved function (2). Inactivity and sedentary lifestyle begin in adolescence. Continuous observation of the physical activity of 56 children, 5 to 11 years of age, in England was conducted by Sleap and Warburton (3). Children were noted to spend 32% of their time engaged in moderate to vigorous physical activity. They were more active during school breaks and less active during free time at home. Only 8 of the 56 children (14%) were observed to have participated for sustained exercise periods of 20 minutes or longer. A random sample of 55 physical education classes was observed and only 6 children engaged in sustained periods of physical activity of 5 minutes or longer, and no children participated in a sustained period of 10 minutes or longer (3).

Adolescent males are 25% more fit and 15% to 25% more active than females over the school-age years. However, there is a constant decline in physical activity in both genders—males decreasing by about 2.7% per year and females decreasing by about 7.4% per year—during the teenage years (4).

Race is also a predictor of fitness. Desmond administered a modified Harvard step test and a 70-item questionnaire to 257 high school students (mean age, 16 yr). Fifty-one percent of black females, 27% of black males, 35% of white females, and 16% of white males were in poor physical condition. White students were more knowledgeable than black students based on the exercise knowledge scale (5).

What are the characteristics of an inactive individual? Bauman and colleagues reviewed recent trends in sociodemographic determinants of exercise in Australia. They used population surveys for their data collection instruments. Over the survey period, there was a slight increase in the number of Australians who participated in a regular physical activity and a significant decline in the number who reported being totally sedentary, from 32.9% in 1984 to 25% in 1987. Women, older people, less educated people, and those with lower incomes were less likely to perform regular physical activities. The inequalities in the social distribution in exercise participation paralleled those found for other health risk factors (5). Owen and Bauman, using pooled data from 17,000 participants, identified over 5000 people (approximately 30%) who could be classified as sedentary in their recreational exercise habits. The main reasons given for not exercising were: lack of time (33%), physical inability (23%), and a lack of desire to exercise (13%). Women were more likely to report being physically unable to exercise, and lower income was associated with a physical disability and not wanting to exercise (6). Bonheur and Young conducted a survey of 105 university students and found that significant differences existed between exercisers and nonexercisers on scales regarding self-esteem, perceived benefits of exercise, and perceived barriers to exercise. These three variables accounted for 32% of the variation in exercisers versus nonexercisers (7).

Although regular exercise has been associated with numerous health benefits, not all physicians are enthusiastic about recommending exercise. One survey of 126 primary care physicians found that physicians who follow up on their patients, who have been in practice for over 10 years, who exercise themselves, and who estimate that more than 10% of their patients exercise, encourage exercise with at least 50% of their patients (8).

Knowledge about exercise and its benefits in the prevention and treatment of disease has increased over the past few years. This chapter reviews some of this knowledge. The primary care physician can use this information to help motivate patients and to better understand how to use exercise as a therapeutic agent.

THE BODY'S RESPONSE TO EXERCISE

Fitness or conditioning is measured by the maximum amount of oxygen uptake with exercise. This is also known as the $\dot{V}O_2max$, a commonly used term in exercise physiology. $\dot{V}O_2max$ is an index of total body fitness, as well as a measure of the body's ability to extract oxygen from the air and transport that oxygen to muscles.

Dynamic exercise that involves contraction of the body's large muscle groups stimulates the cardiorespiratory system. Cardiorespiratory adaptations occur throughout the whole body, primarily in the heart centrally and the muscle peripherally. These changes can occur in all populations: the young, the old, the sick, and the healthy. Of course, there will be degrees of change depending on the health of the organs involved and the age of the patient.

Exercise produces significant physical changes in the heart. The normal training adaptation is characterized by greater left ventricular chamber size with corresponding large end-diastolic volumes at rest and during exercise. Left ventricular mass has also been found to be increased in athletically trained individuals compared to sedentary individuals. There are accompanying increases in cardiac dimension and stroke volume at rest and during exercise as well as an increase in the maximal cardiac output. The nonconditioned heart has an end-diastolic volume less than that of the well-conditioned heart. For example, as noted in Figure 1.1, the nonconditioned heart has an end-diastolic volume of 120 mL and an end-systolic volume of 50 mL. The stroke volume is therefore 70 mL per beat and the ejection fraction 58%. In the conditioned heart, the end-diastolic volume is 160 mL, whereas the end-systolic volume is 30 mL, making the stroke volume 130 mL and the ejection fraction 84%. The conditioned heart is larger at the end of diastole and smaller at the end of systole. It is not only larger but more efficient. Exercise, therefore, improves the efficiency of the cardiorespiratory system.

In addition to an increased cardiac output, there is a redistribution of the blood

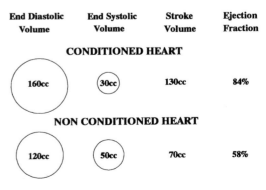

End Diastolic Volume	End Systolic Volume	Stroke Volume	Ejection Fraction
CONDITIONED HEART			
160cc	30cc	130cc	84%
NON CONDITIONED HEART			
120cc	50cc	70cc	58%

Figure 1.1. Comparison of the conditioned vs nonconditioned heart.

flow in exercise. As noted in Table 1.1, for example, the cardiac output at rest was 5900 mL; it increases with exercise to 24,000 mL and the blood flow is redistributed. Coronary blood flow increases from 240 mL at rest to 1000 mL during exercise. Brain flow stays the same at 750 mL both at rest and during exercise. Flow to the kidneys, gastrointestinal tract, and liver decreases from 3100 mL at rest to 600 mL at maximum exercise. There is marked shunting of blood away from these organs to muscle. Muscle flow increases from 1300 mL at rest to over 20,000 mL at maximum exercise. Blood volume also increases as an outcome of aerobic training, thus enhancing the oxygen delivery capacity of the cardiorespiratory system. The resting heart rate and the exercise heart rate at submaximal workloads decrease as a result of endurance training. This slowing of the heart rate is probably a reflection of the enhanced vagal tone that accompanies endurance training. Heart rate is decreased at rest and during submaximal exercise because of increased parasympathetic tone and the effect of increased stroke volume on reflex sympathetic tone.

At the onset of exercise, signals from the central nervous system result in immediate vagal withdrawal and increases in heart rate and arterial blood pressure (9).

Aerobic exercise training induces an increase in coronary vascular transport capacity. This increased transport capacity is the result of increases in both blood flow capacity and capillary exchange capacity. The changes are due first to a structural vascular adaptation and second to control of vascular resistance. There is a change in the cross-sectional area of the proximal coronary arteries and angiogenesis. In animal studies, training-induced changes in coronary vascular control have been shown to include altered coronary responses to vasoactive substances, changes in endothelium-mediated vasoregulation, and alterations in the cellular molecular control of intercellular free calcium in both the endothelial and vascular smooth muscle cells (10). Static or isotonic exercise sports such as weight lifting or other high-resistance activities are used by athletes to gain strength and skeletal muscle bulk. However, static exercise does cause significant increases in blood pressure, heart rate, myocardial contractility, and cardiac output. Static exercise is characterized by a pressure load to the heart and can be differentiated from dynamic isotonic exercise, which involves a volume load to the heart. Physical training with static exercise leads to concentric left ventricular hypertrophy, whereas training with dynamic exercise leads to eccentric hypertrophy. The magnitude of cardiac hypertrophy is less with static exercise than with dynamic exercise. Peripheral cardiovascular adaptation can occur in response to static exercise training. Although controversial, these adaptations include modest decreases in resting blood pressure and smaller increases in blood pressure during a given workload. These responses are greater when the training involves frequent repetitions of moderate weight rather than training that involves fewer repetitions of larger weight (11). Systemic exercise increases maximal cardiac

Table 1.1. Cardiovascular responses

	At Rest (mL)	During Exercise (mL)
Cardiac output	5900	24,000
Coronary flow	250	1000
Brain flow	750	750
Renal, gastrointestinal tract, liver	3100	600
Muscle flow	1300	20,850

output because of the increase in maximal stroke volume.

Lungs also become conditioned. The tidal volume and minute volume are increased as the individual becomes fit. The muscles of respiration become more efficient and tidal volumes will increase from 500 mL at rest to 2000 mL with exercise. This increased ability to deliver air to the pulmonary capillary bed, coupled with increased cardiac output, enables a large amount of oxygen to be delivered to muscle.

The drive to breathe in exercise is thought to result from a combination of neural and humoral factors, but the exact nature of the controlling factors is controversial. A recent review suggests that potassium could be the signal that drives ventilation in exercise. Potassium is lost from working muscle during exercise, and there is a resultant increase in plasma potassium. This rise in potassium is directly proportional to the increase in carbon dioxide production during exercise and is strongly correlated with ventilation in normal subjects and also in subjects who do not produce lactic acid (McArdle's disease) (12).

Specific cellular changes occur in the muscle as a result of training. There is an increase in both the size and number of mitochondria, enabling muscle cells to extract and use oxygen more efficiently. These specific cellular changes improve the ability of muscles to oxidize both fat and carbohydrate. Trained muscles also have high concentrations of myoglobin, which improves the oxygen diffusing capacity (13).

Incremental graded and short-term anaerobic exercise may lead to an increase in β-endorphin levels. The extent correlates with lactate concentration during incremental graded exercise. β-Endorphin levels increase when the anaerobic or lactate threshold has been reached. In endurance exercise performed at a steady state between lactate production and elimination, β-endorphin levels in the blood did not increase until exercise duration exceeded approximately 1 hour (14).

When body temperature rises, skin blood flow increases by transfer of metabolic heat from the core to the skin. This convective heat transfer is never more important than during dynamic exercise. Control of skin blood flow involves complex interactions in the regulatory system, that is, body temperature, blood pressure, metabolism, passive withdrawal of constrictive tone, and vasodilation (15).

Expansion of plasma volume, called *hypervolemia*, has been well documented in many studies as a consequence of endurance exercise training. Plasma volume expansion can account for nearly all of the exercise-induced hypervolemia for up to 2 to 4 weeks. After this time, expansion may be distributed equally between plasma and red cell volumes. The net increase of body fluids with exercise training is associated with increased water intake and decreased urine output. The mechanism of reduced urine output appears to be increased renal tubular reabsorption of sodium through more sensitive aldosterone action (16).

EXERCISE PRESCRIPTION

Most studies of exercise suggest a linear dose-response relationship and recommend at least moderate physical activity, e.g., 30 minutes of walking per day or the equivalent energy expenditure in other activities. It does not matter what type of physical activity is performed; sports, planned exercise, household or yard work, and occupational tasks are all beneficial. The key factor is total energy expenditure. If it is constant, improvement in fitness and in health will be comparable.

In 1990, the American College of Sports Medicine revised their 1978 position paper on exercise prescription (17). The new position statement recommended the following quality and quantity of exercise for developing and maintaining cardiorespiratory and muscular fitness in adults. The training frequency should be 3 to 5 days a week. The intensity of exercise should be approximately 60% to 85% of maximum heart rate, which is about 60% to 85% of the $\dot{V}o_2$max. The duration of activity should be 20 to 30 continuous minutes. The mode of activity should use the large muscle groups of the body, such as rowing, cycling, dancing, cross-country skiing, swimming, running, and walking. It is not necessary to run a marathon or become an elite runner to gain benefit from exercise.

Work site exercise programs have proved beneficial. Although their stated objective has been to boost corporate moral or employee health rather than to have a direct economic benefit, suggested benefits include an improvement in corporate image, lower employee turnover, gains of productivity, a reduction in absenteeism, a reduction in medical costs, an improvement in employee life-style, and fewer industrial injuries. In practice, the corporate impact of the program is variable, depending on such factors as the prevalence of need, participation rate, and program response. The cost to the corporation includes promotion facilities, equipment, and professional leadership. These items sometimes require the maximum mobilization of resources by the company involved. For this reason, activities that can be built into the normal day of the employees, such as walking or cycling

to and from work, may prove more acceptable and more cost effective than formal work site classes (18).

For the noncompetitive athlete, training programs should begin with a general progression of low-intensity activities that encourage compliance and reduce risk. Short-term, attainable goals documenting a gradual increase in activity have been shown to be successful in terms of compliance and desired benefits (19). The exercise prescription will more likely be followed if the physician helps the patient to establish realistic goals and to understand that a minimum of exercise can lead to improvement. It can also be extremely helpful if the physician individualizes the program to make it convenient and fun, provides supervision and ample positive reinforcement, and teaches by example (20).

BENEFITS OF EXERCISE

Research studies over the past several decades confirm the health benefits of regular physical activity, a concept with foundations in antiquity. The following statement is attributed to Hippocrates.

> All parts of the body which have a function, if used in moderation, and exercised in labors to which each is accustomed, become thereby healthy and well developed, and age slowly; but if unused and left idle, they become liable to disease, defective in growth and age quickly. This is especially so with joints and ligaments if one does not use them.

Exercise is known to benefit hypertension, diabetes, lipid disorders, obesity, coronary artery disease, arthritis, osteoporosis, chronic diseases, disability, aging, and mental health. Each one of these areas will be discussed.

Hypertension

Physically active and fit individuals with hypertension have lower rates of mortality than sedentary, unfit, hypertensive individuals (21). Numerous published studies state that aerobic exercise prevents hypertension and reduces blood pressure and mortality in hypertensive patients. One meta-analysis reviewed 22 of these studies. A decrease in resting systolic pressure of 0 to 44 mm Hg after exercise was reported in 21 of 22 studies and in all 22 a decrease in resting diastolic pressure of 1 to 21 mm Hg was reported. In 13 of the controlled studies, the decreases in blood pressure with exercise were greater in subjects with higher baseline systolic pressure. Mean decreases in blood pressure with exercise were 11.3 mm Hg systolic and 7.5 mm Hg diastolic. The reduction of blood pressure with exercise was greater when the exercise was performed seven times weekly as compared to only three times weekly. Studies that lasted longer than 13 weeks produced more sustained blood pressure drops than those of a shorter duration. Although the findings of these studies should be interpreted cautiously, they do suggest that physical activity lowers blood pressure, that daily exercise appears to be more effective than less frequent exercise, and that moderate-intensity exercise appears to be as effective as vigorous activity in lowering blood pressure (22). Other studies suggest that the mode of exercise should be large muscle activity with a frequency of 3 to 5 days a week and should last from 20 to 60 minutes. The intensity should be from 50% to 85% of maximal oxygen uptake. Exercise training appears to elicit an even greater reduction in blood pressure in patients with secondary hypertension due to renal dysfunction.

Hypertensive patients have lower cardiac outputs and stroke volumes, higher heart rates, and a higher peripheral resistance than normotensive individuals with the same intensity of exercise. Patients with mildly elevated resting blood pressures have an increased myocardial oxygen demand during exercise. Endurance training offers hypertensive patients a means of lowering exercise heart rate, reducing systolic blood pressure and myocardial oxygen consumption, and improving physical work capacity (23). The decrease in blood pressure and heart rate that accompanies physical training is associated with an increase in vagal tone and a decrease in plasma epinephrine. The blood pressure lowering effect of training programs is probably secondary to a reduction in resting sympathetic nerve activity (24).

Stress is associated with an increased level of blood pressure and sympathetic tone. Work site studies of occupational stress indicate that people in high-stress jobs have increased blood pressure throughout the day and night, which is consistent with the behaviorally mediated theory of hypertension.

Exaggerated blood pressure response to exercise predicts adult-onset essential hypertension. Increases in systolic blood pressure to greater than 180 mm Hg during exercise can indicate future hypertension, especially in groups of normotensive individuals with a family history of hypertension, although left ventricular mass, measured echocardiographically, and resting systolic blood pressure seem to be better predictors (25).

Diabetes

Physical training is associated with lower plasma insulin concentrations and increased sensitivity to insulin in the skeletal muscle and adipose tissue of individuals with non–insulin-dependent (type II) diabetes. Exercise may also benefit pregnant women with gestational diabetes mellitus by preventing excessive weight gain and preventing or decreasing the severity of hypertension and hyperlipidemia during pregnancy (26).

Resistance training may provide the individual with diabetes physiologic benefits that in some cases may equal or exceed those gained through aerobic training. These benefits may include improved blood lipid profiles, increased absolute left ventricular wall contractility, decreased resting blood pressure, improved insulin sensitivity and glucose tolerance, as well as improved muscle strength and endurance. By using a combination of aerobic and resistance training, the individual with diabetes experiences a more comprehensive exercise program; also, more options in the type of exercise may enhance exercise compliance (27).

The positive metabolic benefits of exercise are short lived and of minimal help in controlling glycemia and weight in diabetic individuals unless the exercise is performed on a regular basis. Because of medical problems and chronic diseases, many individuals with diabetes are not good candidates for an exercise program. For this reason, the optimal target population should be those at risk for premature atherosclerosis. The at-risk population should include offspring of patients with these disorders and individuals with impaired glucose tolerance, hyperinsulinemia, gestational diabetes, and an android pattern of fat distribution. Because non–insulin-dependent diabetes is more common in blacks than in the general U.S. population, it is suggested that blacks, particularly black women, be targeted for exercise programs (28).

Metabolic studies suggest that the major

effect of exercise is to change the level of insulin sensitivity and insulin resistance. Experience in the early stage of the disease has its greatest effects. Exercise later in the course of the disease provides help with metabolic control in prevention or delay of chronic complications in non–insulin-dependent diabetic patients (29).

Peripheral resistance to insulin is a prominent feature of both insulin-dependent (type I) and non–insulin-dependent diabetes. Skeletal muscle is the primary site for insulin-induced glucose utilization in diabetic patients. Glucose transport is the rate-limiting step for glucose utilization in muscle; that cellular process is defective in human and animal diabetes (30). Insulin resistance is responsible for decreased glucose utilization. Muscle strips from a group of lean, non–insulin-dependent diabetic patients demonstrated a 50% decrease in insulin responsiveness for glucose transport compared with nondiabetic subjects. Both regular physical exercise and insulin therapy normalize the decreased capacity for glucose transport in diabetic rat muscles (31).

Glucose transport in muscle and adipose tissue is regulated by such factors as insulin and exercise. Glucose transport levels in muscle are increased with exercise training. The adaptive increase in muscle glucose transporters that is found with exercise training has beneficial effects in insulin-resistant states such as non–insulin-dependent diabetes (32).

Lipids

Exercise is widely believed to induce favorable changes in lipid profiles; specifically, it increases the high-density lipoprotein (HDL) fraction. In older women, some research studies fail to demonstrate a rise in the HDL fraction in the absence of other interventions. However, high volumes of exercise may increase HDL levels in younger women. Exercise programs of moderate intensity tend to modify the HDL-lowering effects of a hypocaloric fat-restricted diet (33).

Lipids are metabolized directly by contracting skeletal muscles. The supply of free fatty acids far exceeds what is taken up by the muscle. Seldom is more than 2% to 4% of the amount of free fatty acid delivered to an exercising limb taken up by the muscles, and only part of that percentage is oxidized. Physical training induces changes that enhance the uptake of fatty acids by the contracting muscle (34).

Exercise increases lipoprotein lipase (LPL) activity in muscle. This causes an increase in muscle and cardiac free fatty acid uptake and a decrease in LPL activity in adipose tissue. Control of LPL is coordinated by mechanisms that result from the reduction of insulin resistance and the increase in catecholamines induced by exercise (35).

During intense exercise, large increases in the plasma glucose concentration occur and a state of insulin resistance exists for a few hours following exercise. But increased sensitivity to insulin is found one day after intense exercise. Increased sensitivity to insulin is also found after endurance training, whereas insulin sensitivity is decreased after inactivity. Exercise training increases the ability of muscle to take up and oxidize free fatty acids during exercise and also increases the activity of LPL and muscle. The activity of LPL and muscle correlates with muscle insulin sensitivity. This might explain why insulin resistance is often associated with hypercholesterolemia, hypertriglyceridemia, and low HDL levels (36).

Obesity

Although obesity is traditionally considered a disorder of energy intake, accumulating evidence underscores the importance of energy expenditure in the development and treatment of obesity. Relatively little evidence supports the common belief that obese individuals have significantly more energy intake than nonobese individuals. Current evidence suggests that physical activity may be particularly important in helping sustain initial losses through increased total energy output and preservation of lean body mass (37).

Caloric restriction in overweight persons produces more weight loss than does exercise, although more of the weight loss by dieting is from lean body mass. The addition of exercise to diet produces more weight loss than does dieting alone. Exercise has a favorable effect on body fat distribution with a reduction in the waist-to-hip ratio. Several perspective studies have shown that overweight men and women who are active and fit have lower rates of morbidity and mortality than overweight persons who are sedentary and unfit (38). Acute and chronic exercise has been shown to influence all components of total energy expenditure. Acute endurance exercise at greater than 70% $\dot{V}o_2$max increases postexercise resting metabolic rate. Chronic exercise training may increase resting metabolic rate, thus enhancing weight loss.

Coronary Artery Disease

The influence of exercise on hypertension, diabetes, lipids, obesity, and on the reduction of hyperinsulinemia and insulin resistance in sedentary individuals accounts for the benefit of physical activity in preventing coronary artery disease in the general population. Exercise and diet are most likely to be effective when initiated in the young individual, before the onset of irreversible vascular alterations (39).

Arthritis

Without question, the person with arthritis has a need to develop muscular strength and endurance to maintain functional movement. Arthritis produces deficits in muscular strength, muscular endurance, range of motion, and physical fitness. Research studies have indicated that the results of fitness training in persons with arthritis are promising, but there are some deficits in the literature on the types of specific exercise that are most effective. Nevertheless, resistance exercise programs are an important component of the rehabilitation of individuals with arthritis (40).

Routine and regular exercise is important in patients with inflammatory arthritis. Most patients with stage I or II rheumatoid arthritis are capable of engaging in an exercise program. Benefits of this exercise include increased cardiovascular and muscle endurance, which allows patients to function more independently and with an improved quality of life. These exercise programs are designed to restore range of motion, improve strength and endurance, and at the same time, provide a social outlet and an opportunity for improved self-esteem. An individual's ability to participate in aerobic exercises may be contingent on the ability to maintain a neutral or stabilized spine. An individual who has been unable to jog because it is painful may be able to jog after that individual learns trunk stabilization techniques and is able to keep the spine in a pain-free position.

Some physicians contend that jogging is an inappropriate activity for an individual with low back pain, but others believe that jogging can protect a person from low back pain. Poor biomechanics in running can exacerbate existing low back pain as well as bring about new problems due to compensatory adaptations. For example, poor running technique might lead to an excessive forward lean counterbalanced by contraction of the back extensors, which would then become overused and produce pain. An upright posture with a minimal forward lean is advocated. The biomechanics of running are also important from the perspective of shock absorption, so it is important to cushion the footstroke to "give" at the ankle, knee, and hip joints when running. In addition to good biomechanics, it is important to use quality footwear and to run on a soft track. Patients with back pain should probably avoid hills. In addition to jogging for low back pain, some physicians have suggested backstroke swimming, brisk walking, and stair climbing. Others endorse the cross-country skiing machines because they provide an excellent opportunity to develop aerobic conditioning without impact. The skiing machines incorporate the tenets of stabilization training because the individual uses the abdominal muscles to brace and stabilize the trunk. Not all individuals can adapt readily to skiing machines because of coordination problems (41).

Does weight-bearing exercise cause osteoarthritis? Available data suggest that reasonable recreational exercise carried out within the limits of comfort—putting joints through normal motions without underlying joint abnormality—need not inevitably lead to joint injury, even over many years. Some anecdotal observations suggest a relationship between recreational activities and degenerative joint disease, but there are no controlled studies that prove that exercise has a role in the pathogenesis of osteoarthritis. In fact, the opposite seems to be true, in that exercise is therapeutic. The only caution would be that if osteoarthritis does exist in the major joints such as the knee exercises that put additional stress on that joint are probably not advised.

The Bones and Osteoporosis

The incidence of osteoporotic fractures rises with age and is increasing faster than the aging population demographically. Physical activity has great potential to reduce the risk of osteoporotic fractures. Three factors contribute to the risk of fractures: 1) bone strength, 2) the risk of falling, and 3) the effectiveness of the neuromuscular response that protects the skeleton from injury. Exercise, therefore, not only reduces fracture risk by preventing bone loss, but it decreases the risk of falling and increases the effectiveness of the neuromuscular response. Extreme physical inactivity causes rapid loss of bone—up to 40%—whereas athletic activity results in bone hypertrophy—up to 40%. In both middle-aged and elderly women, weight-bearing physical activity can reduce bone loss and increase bone mass. The mechanism of maintenance of the skeletal integrity relies not only on cellular response, but also on mechanical load. Studies in animal models show that training affects cellular activity. In osteoporotic animals, cellular erosion is increased and mineral apposition rate is decreased compared with normal age-matched controls (42).

Weight-bearing exercise has a positive effect on bone metabolism and can decrease the incidence of osteoporosis. Snow-Harter and colleagues conducted a controlled exercise trial on a group of healthy college women (mean age, 19.9 yr). They measured bone mineral density as well as muscle strength and endurance. Weight training was associated with significant increases in muscle strength in all muscle groups. Bone mineral density increased in both runners and weight trainers (43).

Growing bones respond to low or moderate exercise through significant additions or new bone in both cortical and trabecular areas and result in adaptation through periosteal expansion and endocortical contraction. Young bones have a greater potential for periosteal expansion than do aging bones, allowing them to adapt more rapidly and efficiently to an acute need for increased strength. From cross-sectional studies, differences in bone mass in exercising and nonexercising adults are generally less than 10%. Moderate to intense training can bring about modest increases of about 1% to 3% in bone mineral content of both men and premenopausal women. In young adults, very strenuous training may increase bone mineral content up to 11% and bone density by 7%. Some evidence indicates that exercise can also add bone mass to the postmenopausal skeleton. Increases as high as 5% to 8% can be found after 1 to 2 years of intense exercise, but additions of bone to the femur and radius are generally less than 2%. Detraining or deconditioning reduces any bone mass increase to preexisting values. Long-term benefits are only retained with continuing exercise (44). Aging is associated with changes in body composition, and one of the most prominent of these changes is sarcopenia (age-related loss in skeletal muscle mass). This loss results in decreased strength and aerobic capacity and thus in decreased functional capacity. Bone mineral loss is closely linked to sarcopenia. Physical exercise, especially resistance training, may help to reduce or prevent sarcopenia (45). Treatment of osteoporosis should include both aerobic and resistance training.

Disability

Disability attributed to age or chronic disease is decreased by exercise. Inactivity compounds the effects of disability, which deserves recognition, because it is reversible and not inevitable. Shephard reviewed the benefits of enhanced activity in the disabled and found improvement in mood state with a reduction of anxiety and depression, an increase in self-esteem, and feelings of greater self-efficacy. Sociologic gains included new experiences, new friendships, and a decrease in the stigmatization of disability. Perceived health was improved from a long-term perspective, and the risk of many chronic diseases was reduced. Finally, there was a greater likelihood of employment with less absenteeism and enhanced productivity. Both the health and industrial benefits of exercise in the disabled could make an important contribution toward the expense of physical exercise programs suitably adapted for the disabled (46).

Chronic Disease

Although most patients with chronic obstructive pulmonary disease (COPD) have a ventilatory limitation to exercise in the later stages of their disease, hemodynamic factors may contribute. The main hemodynamic abnormality in COPD is raised pulmonary vascular resistance and pulmonary hypertension. This is particularly evident when the vascular bed is stressed, as in exercise. The absence of reserve collateral vessels prevents the normal reduction in pulmonary vascular resistance and, hence, pressure increases with flow. Studies of the effects of physical training on pulmonary hemodynamics have been few, but none has shown any significant improvement. There is, however, an impressive increase in work tolerance after training in individuals with COPD. The increase in work tolerance may be in part due to an increase in muscular coordination and technique. There may be some increase in $\dot{V}o_2$max because of better cardiac fitness (47).

The effectiveness of lower and upper limb physical training in individuals with chronic airway obstruction has been evaluated. After 6 to 8 weeks of training, a 60% increase in $\dot{V}o_2$max and a reduction in heart rate occurred (48). Training programs as part of pulmonary rehabilitation should be founded on the same principles that are used in exercise training of healthy subjects. Exercise therapy in COPD is directed toward improving ventilatory muscle function. The three goals are: (1) a reduction in load, (2) an increase in intrinsic ventilatory muscle function, and (3) a reduction in dyspnea perception (49,50).

The biochemical and histologic patterns of skeletal muscle change seen in patients with heart failure are consistent with the effects of long-term exercise deconditioning in normal subjects. Recent studies suggest the beneficial effect of training in subjects with moderate or even severe left ventricular dysfunction by showing increased exercise tolerance (51). The pathophysiology of exercise intolerance in patients with chronic heart failure is not fully understood. Peak exercise cardiac output is an important predictor of $\dot{V}o_2$max. It is likely that a reduced cardiac output to work rate relationship and congestive heart failure causes hypoprofusion of both working skeletal muscle and visceral organs, which leads to early anaerobic metabolism and fatigue. Although some patients with severe systolic left ventricular dysfunction can increase their cardiac output with exercise, some patients may be unable to increase stroke volume during exercise due to diastolic left ventricular dysfunction (52).

Mental Health

A study by deGeus and associates reviewed the influence of regular exercise and aerobic fitness in relation to psychological makeup and physiologic stress reactivity. Stress reactivity was measured by cardiovascular and urinary catecholamine response. Psychological makeup did not change as a consequence of exercise training (53). The relationship between exercise and anxiety has been extensively examined. Three separate meta-analyses were conducted to quantitatively review the literature on exercise anxiety. The results substantiate the claim that exercise is associated with a reduction in anxiety, but only with aerobic forms of exercise. Training programs need to exceed 10 weeks before significant changes in anxiety occur. Cardiovascular measures of anxiety, for example, blood pressure and heart rate, yielded significantly fewer effects than did other measures. The only variable that was significant across all three meta-analyses was exercise duration. Exercise for over 20 minutes was necessary to achieve reduction in anxiety (54).

Physical exercise is increasingly advocated as a means of maintaining and advancing good mental health. Exercise is associated with improvements in mental health, including mood state and self-esteem. Research on acute exercise indicates that 20 to 40 minutes of aerobic activity results in improvement that lasts for several hours. These changes occur in individuals with both normal and elevated levels of anxiety. In healthy individuals, the principal psychological benefit of exercise may be the prevention of emotional illness (55).

Juvenile delinquents are usually handicapped with depression and low self-esteem, far more than the population at large. Athletic participation by teenagers imparts desirable educational and social and personal values, and has been included in remedial programs for troubled youngsters. The psychological benefits of aerobic exercise have been investigated in juvenile delinquency, and changes include reduction in anxiety, tension, and depression and increased self-esteem. These effects are thought to be due to a sense of increased self-control and an alteration in neurotransmitter levels (56).

Aging

Despite the loss of exercise capacity with age, the ability to sustain a relatively high intensity of aerobic exercise appears preserved. It has been shown, unequivocally, that cardiorespiratory training of older men and women is effective in increasing $\dot{V}o_2$max and results in obvious benefits (57). There is an approximate 30% decline in muscle strength and a 40% reduction in muscle area between the second and seventh decades of life. Muscle mass is, therefore, the major factor in age-related loss of muscle strength. The loss of muscle mass is due to a significant decline in both type I and type II muscle fibers, plus a decrease in the size of muscle cells.

Progressive resistance training results in muscle hypertrophy and increased strength in the elderly. Advancing age is associated with sarcopenia defined as the age-related loss in skeletal muscle mass. Sarcopenia is also closely linked to age-related decreases in bone and mineral content and basal metabolic rate and increases in body fat. Physical exercise training, especially resistance training, can prevent or delay or minimize the degree of sarcopenia (58).

This training increases the ability to carry out the activities of daily living and exerts a beneficial effect on such age-associated diseases as non–insulin-dependent diabetes, coronary artery disease, hypertension, osteoporosis, and obesity (58).

Both chronically ill and healthy adults benefit from exercise programs. Exercise may produce improvements in gait and balance; arthritic patients experience long-term functional status benefits, including improved mobility and decreased pain symptoms. There also is evidence that exercise improves cognitive function (59). Other issues to consider in terms of exercise for older adults include promoting long-term adherence to exercise and maintaining a low rate of exercise injuries for older adults as well as finding cost-effective interventions that require less supervision.

Frailty is a state of reduced reserve associated with an increased susceptibility to disability and reduced neurologic control, mechanical performance, and energy metabolism. Although being frail is probably secondary to having a disease, being frail is also due to the adaptive effects of a sedentary life-style. This sedentary life-style is often the result of the accumulation of acute insults such as illnesses, injuries, and major life events that result in periods of limited activity and bed rest. To some extent, frailty is preventable. Bed rest, although advisable oftentimes, has its disadvantages. Many times the advice of the physician to "take it easy for a few days" is prolonged into weeks and months. Most hospitalizations are accompanied by prolonged and sometimes unnecessary bed rest. It is important that the physician who cares for older patients with medical or surgical problems realizes that recovery from illnesses such as pneumonia and heart failure includes re-

turn of any loss of neuromuscular strength and control (60).

Walking and low-impact aerobics are excellent exercises for the elderly. Unfortunately, many of the frail elderly are unable to walk or do low-impact aerobics. One of the more attractive alternatives for these individuals is a water-based program that allows the elderly to gain all of the advantages of land-based exercise without the stress or strain on arthritic joints. Water walkers, a buoyancy device that attaches easily around the waist, can be used to allow total freedom of movement without fear of deep water. Heyneman and Premo described a water walker's exercise program for the elderly that includes 45-minute sessions consisting of a warm-up period, stretching, a cardiovascular segment, a cool-down period, strength training, and final stretching. All exercises were conducted with immersion up to the shoulders while wearing the water walkers. This program demonstrated both physical and psychological benefits (61).

Shay and Roth reviewed the association between aerobic fitness and visuospatial performance in healthy, older adults. The study showed significant differences between high- and low-fit subjects only in tasks with heavy visuospatial demands. These findings suggest that participation in aerobic exercise activity selectively preserves some cognitive functions that normally decline with age. The benefits of activity appear to be most evident on tasks that require visuospatial processing (62). Probart's study investigated the benefits of 26 weeks of moderate aerobic exercise for women 70 years or older. The exercise group walked on a treadmill three times per week for 20 minutes at 70% of maximum heart rate. The $\dot{V}o_2$max increased by 8% and the total exercise time on the treadmill increased by 25% (63). Posner and colleagues examined the long-term effects of aerobic exercise on the occurrence and time to onset of cardiovascular diagnoses. They randomized 184 initially healthy, older adults into a long-term exercise group, short-term exercise group, and a control group of no exercise. After 2 years in the study, the occurrence rate for new onset of cardiovascular diagnosis was 13% for the nonexercisers and 3% for exercisers. The average time to onset was the greatest for the long-term exercisers (64).

CONFUSING HEALTH ISSUES WITH EXERCISE

Exercise produces changes in the immune system, heart, blood volume, and gastrointestinal tract that can be confused with disease states; some of these changes, however, are actually disease states. The following discussion helps clarify some of these issues.

Immune Function

Immune function can be examined by charting susceptibility to infections, differential total white cell counts or lymphocyte counts, and measures of cell proliferation and immunoglobulin synthesis in response to external mitogens. Comparisons suggest that under resting conditions, well-conditioned individuals show some lymphocytosis, increased natural killer cell activity, higher levels of interleukin-1, and possibly an enhanced reaction to mitogens. The length of the acute response to exercise is transient and quite variable; it depends on the type of exercise and the intensity of effort relative to the fitness of the individual. Lymphocytosis and a decrease in the number of T and B cells mainly reflect changes of blood volume, margination,

and migration of cells. Prolonged exercise leads to a decrease in serum and salivary immunoglobulin levels.

Moderate training does not greatly change the exercise response, whereas excessive training can suppress immune function, but the changes are slight and difficult to relate to overtraining (65). A tentative trend may be discerned whereby light to moderate exercise may increase immune responsiveness, but highly competitive sports, especially involving extensive endurance training, may lead to a degree of immunosuppression. Such immune malfunction may be part of the overtraining syndrome in which recurrent infections during periods of maximum training or competition stress may occur. Some evidence suggests that such overworked muscles may fail to supply adequate glutamine for normal lymphocyte function (66).

Sports Anemia

One of the major factors influencing oxygen delivery to muscle tissue is red cell mass. A decrease in total hemoglobin can adversely affect exercise capacity, so it is only natural that any decrease in hematocrit or hemoglobin will be of concern in the setting of exercise.

Mean hemoglobin levels in elite athletes are lower than hemoglobin levels found in nonendurance athletes and nonathletes. The change in hemoglobin levels is considered a normal response to exercise. It is a delusional phenomenon secondary to expanded plasma volume. Conserving plasma volume is a normal response to the stress of exercise. Studies show that blood volume increases range from 6% to 25% in endurance athletes. Red cell mass does not increase, and in some people it may actually show small decreases. This expansion of volume with no change in red cell mass is considered a positive adaptation because it decreases viscosity, maximizes stroke volume and cardiac output, and enhances oxygen delivery (67).

The diagnosis of sports anemia is one of exclusion and other causes need to be considered. Iron deficiency anemia is the most common diagnosis to consider in women. Up to 20% of women are iron deficient and half of those are clinically anemic. Serum ferritin is the most sensitive test for evaluating iron deficiency. If men are iron deficient a search for a source of bleeding should be considered. Total iron losses in feces, urine, and sweat in endurance-trained athletes are approximately 1.75 mg/day compared with reference values of 1 mg/day in males and approximately 2.3 mg/day compared with a reference value of 1.4 in women because of the additional iron losses with menses. Therefore, iron deficiency can be a problem in athletes who do not increase their iron intake above that of the general population (68). Intravascular hemolysis caused by intense exercise (march hemoglobinuria) is another diagnosis to consider. Signs of hemolysis include a fall in serum haptoglobin, an increased number of reticulocytes hemoglobinuria, and an increase in mean corpuscular volume. Hemolysis is sometimes associated with running on hard surfaces (69).

The Athletic Heart

Athletic heart syndrome is a benign condition consisting of physiologic adaptations to the increased cardiac workload of exercise. Its primary features are biventricular hypertrophy and bradycardia associated with normal systolic and diastolic function. Due to a number of factors, there is a difference in the pattern of cardiac mechanics encountered in athletes. Some athletes will experience ventricular dilatation with appropriate hypertrophy and preservation of the ventricular mass-to-volume ratio, whereas others manifest concentric hypertrophy with an increased mass-to-volume ratio (70). Endurance-trained athletes experience greater changes in left ventricular diameter and left ventricular mass. These changes are useful in maintaining high levels of exercise because cardiac output and stroke volume are increased.

End-diastolic left ventricular diameter is increased in competitive athletes who perform dynamic or aerobic sports, but not in athletes who only perform strength training or anaerobic sports. This is explained by the different volume load on the heart. In sports with high dynamic and low status demands, wall thickness is usually proportional to the size of the internal diameter so that *relative* wall thickness is not different from that of nonathletes, called *eccentric hypertrophy*. In athletes who concentrate on strength, there is an increase in wall thickness without internal diameter change, called *concentric hypertrophy*, and the changes in cardiac output and stroke volume are minimal (71). Electrocardiographic (ECG), radiographic, and echocardiographic abnormalities can occur. It is important to be aware of these changes so they are not misinterpreted as pathologic states (72).

Physical examination in athletic heart syndrome is characterized by bradycardia and sinus arrhythmia. Systolic ejection murmurs in the aortic area are usual. Valsalva maneuvers usually decrease the intensity of these murmurs. ECG abnormalities include left ventricular hypertrophy by voltage criteria ($SV_1 + RV_5 > 35$), first-degree atrioventricular block, Mobitz type 1 second-degree block, and junctional bradycardia. ST segment abnormalities are noted. The most common is early repolarization, which consists of mild ST segment elevation in the V leads with terminal slurring of the R waves.

Gastrointestinal Tract

Digestion is a process that occurs in the resting condition. Exercise is characterized by a shift in blood flow away from the gastrointestinal tract toward active muscle. Changes in circulating hormones, peptides, and metabolic end products lead to changes in gastrointestinal motility, blood flow, absorption, and secretion. In exhausting endurance events, 30% to 50% of participants may suffer from one or more gastrointestinal symptoms, which have often been interpreted as being a result of maldigestion, malabsorption, changes in small intestinal transient, and improper food and fluid intake. Results of studies have shown that pre-exercise ingestion of foods rich in dietary fiber, fat, and protein, as well as strongly hypertonic drinks, may cause upper gastrointestinal symptoms such as stomachache, vomiting, and reflux or heartburn. There is no evidence that ingestion of nonhypertonic drinks during exercise induces gastrointestinal distress and diarrhea.

Dehydration as a result of insufficient fluid replacement has been shown to increase the frequency of gastrointestinal symptoms. Lower gastrointestinal symptoms such as intestinal cramps, diarrhea, and urge to defecate seem to be more related to changes in gut motility, tone, and secretions. These symptoms are largely induced by a decrease in gastrointestinal blood flow and by secretory substances such as intestinal peptide. Intensive exercise causes considerable reflux, delays small intestinal transit time, reduces absorption, and decreases colonic transit time. The last may reduce whole-gut transient time. The gut is not an athletic organ in the sense that

it adapts to increased exercise-induced stress. However, adequate training leads to a less dramatic decrease in blood flow at submaximal exercise intensities and is important in the prevention of gastrointestinal symptoms (73). Approximately 50% of athletes will develop gastrointestinal symptoms at some stage in their career. Fortunately most of these cases are mild.

Gastrointestinal bleeding can occur with prolonged exercise and is probably mediated by visceral ischemia. It may produce acute hemorrhage or more chronic symptoms with anemia or result in hemepositive stools with no correlated clinical disease. Hemorrhagic colitis and gastritis are some of the rarely recognized lesions, and they are usually transient and reversible. Acid suppression with H_2-blockers may be effective in selected patients with recurrent hemorrhage (74).

ISSUES IN TRAINING

Training effect depends on the frequency, intensity, and duration of exercise. In general, the lower the stimulus, the lower the training effect, and the greater the stimulus, the greater the training effect. Energy expenditure during marathon training and competition is among the highest reported for any endurance activity. Although training intensity for a marathon may vary between 60% to 125% of maximal physical work capacity, elite runners must run consistently at about 80% to 90% of $\dot{V}o_2$max to achieve successful competitive performances (79). A well-rounded training program includes resistance training and flexibility exercises as well as aerobic endurance training. Although age itself is not a limiting factor to exercise training, a more gradual approach in applying the exercise prescription at older ages seems prudent. Endurance training of less than 2 days a week at less than 50% of maximum oxygen uptake and less than 10 min/day is inadequate for developing and maintaining fitness in healthy adults. It is crucial to design a program of physical activity for the individual that provides maximal benefit at the lowest risk. Emphasis should be placed on factors that result in permanent life-style change and encourage a lifetime of physical activity (80).

Many endurance athletes and coaches fear a decrease in physical conditioning and performance if training is reduced for several days or longer. This is largely unfounded. Maximal exercise measures, such as $\dot{V}o_2max$, are maintained for 10 to 28 days with reduction in training volume of up to 70% to 80% of prior levels. Blood measures of training are maintained for up to 5 to 21 days of reduced training, as are glycogen storage and muscle oxidative capacities. These findings suggest that endurance athletes can reduce training prior to competition and not lose their competitive edge. This principle can be helpful following injury, for recovery from periods of intense training, and for preventing staleness (81).

Overtraining, or "Staleness"

Overtraining is an imbalance between training and recovery, exercise and exercise capacity, stress and stress tolerance. *Short-term overtraining* lasting from a few days to 2 weeks is termed *overreaching*. Short-term overtraining is associated with fatigue, stagnation, reduction of maximum performing capacity, and brief competitive incompetence. Recovery is achieved within days, so the prognosis is favorable. *Long-term overtraining* lasting weeks to months causes overtraining syndrome, or "stale-

ness." The symptomatology associated with overtraining syndrome has changed over the last 50 years from excitation and restlessness to phlegmatic behavior and inhibition. Increased volume of training at a high-intensity level is likely the culprit. Accumulation of exercise or nonexercise fatigue, stagnation, reduction in maximum performance capacity, mood state disturbances, muscle soreness, stiffness, and decreased competitiveness and incompetence can be expected. Complete recovery takes weeks to months, so the prognosis is unfavorable (75).

As the athlete becomes more exhausted and frustrated with his or her performance, chronic fatigue and depression are obvious. Symptoms include altered mood states, sleep disturbances, inability to concentrate, loss of interest in other activities, and suicidal thoughts and gestures. Past history or family history of depression can indicate a high risk for depression in the athlete. Suicide is a real risk for athletes, as it is for the general population. Health personnel associated with athletes should be capable of both prevention and recognition of this entity.

Muscle biopsy demonstrates diminished muscle glycogen in some of these athletes with staleness and overtraining. The average American diet consists of about 45% carbohydrates. A high-performance athlete should be consuming a diet of 60% to 70% carbohydrates in order to replenish muscle glycogen. It takes about 20 to 24 hours to replenish muscle glycogen after exhausting exercise (76).

Lactate

Blood lactate is a by-product of muscle metabolism, and it accumulates in the blood during vigorous exercise. High levels are associated with fatigue. Lactate threshold (also called anaerobic capacity and anaerobic threshold) is the speed at which endurance races are won and close to the speed providing optimal aerobic training. Maximal blood lactate is often used in exercise and sports physiology to judge anaerobic capacity or threshold. This threshold is the exercise intensity at which performance is maximal and able to be sustained for at least 50 minutes. Trained subjects have shown a capacity to generate greater levels of lactate in maximum exercise when compared to sedentary subjects. In contrast, trained subjects generate less lactate for any given workload than do untrained cohorts. Higher maximal blood lactate values are observed in sprint and power athletes who demonstrate higher anaerobic capacity, compared to endurance athletes and untrained individuals.

Opinion is divided on the utility of maximal blood lactate as an estimate of anaerobic threshold. Other biochemical and physiologic markers of fitness have not always paralleled changes in maximal blood lactate. Both blood lactate and ventilatory gases have been used to measure anaerobic threshold. However, the relationship between these two methods is not conclusive. With the variety of techniques used in assessing anaerobic threshold, caution should be exercised in interpreting the results using different protocols. It is also important to account for the individual's unique response to such exercise (77). Despite problems interpreting the physiologic meaning of minimal blood lactate levels, this measure is still used in both research and athletic settings to describe anaerobic capacity. Its use is supported by the strong correlation between maximal blood lactate and short duration exercise performance.

Ventilatory break points formally considered to indicate lactate threshold correlate more closely with the accumulation of potassium than lactate (78). The ventilatory threshold does not seem to be dependent on blood lactate.

Strength Training

There are a wide variety of methods and equipment for improving muscular strength and endurance. Training systems can usually be classified as isometric, isotonic, and isokinetic. *Isometric or static training* is performed when the muscle maintains a constant length as resistance is applied; there is no change in the joint position. *Isotonic training* is performed when constant tension is applied to muscle, and contractions occur through a range of motion against resistance. There are two phases in isotonic training: concentric and eccentric. The concentric phase is also called positive work and the eccentric phase, negative work. The concentric phase involves a shortening contraction of the muscle, such as a bicep curl. The muscle shortens as the elbow flexes and the weight is lifted. The eccentric phase involves a lengthening contraction of the involved muscle when the muscle is lowered back to the starting position. For example, following a bicep curl the elbow would extend and the biceps muscle would lengthen. *Isokinetic exercise* is defined as contraction at a constant speed with resistance. The speed of movement is controlled and resistance is proportional to the force exerted at each point through a full range of motion. This usually requires some type of mechanical assistance.

Isometric training has limited applicability in the average individual's training program, primarily because of lack of feedback, difficulty in monitoring progress, and minimal carryover of isometric strength gains to functional activity and athletic performance. Isometric work can also cause significant increases in blood pressure and left ventricular wall stress and can be dangerous in individuals with hypertension and congestive heart failure or other forms of cardiovascular disease. Isotonic training is effective in developing strength and should be considered the mainstay for strengthening normal muscle as well as an integral part of most rehabilitation programs. The variety of equipment that can be used includes free weights as well as fixed resistance stations using cables and pulleys. Isokinetic exercise requires specialized equipment such as a Cybex dynamometer. So, in effect, most training that occurs is of the isotonic type because of the ease of performance and the greater benefit-to-risk ratio.

Progressive resistance exercise results in increased muscular strength and, thus, especially with heavy resistance training, increased muscle size. This hypertrophy occurs primarily because of an increase in the number and size of existing myofibrils. Both men and women are capable of similar relative strength gains with training, although the degree of hypertrophy is not the same in women, unless anabolic steroids are used. Of course, this cannot be medically justified or condoned. There is typically no muscle capillary neoformation with strength training. Therefore, with increased muscle size, there is a relative decrease in capillary density. There is a greater increase of fast-twitch fibers. The cardiovascular effects of resistance training are sometimes confusing. If circuit training is used (i.e., smaller weights with more repetition), an increase in maximal oxygen uptake can be noted. Evidence also supports the notion that resistance isometric training produces sustained hypertension in normotensive individuals. Isotonic exercise is therefore safer than isometric exercise for individuals with hypertension.

The effect of strength training is lost at a rate of 5% to 10% per week after cessation of training. However, moderate levels of muscular strength can be maintained with reduced training protocols. Immobilization results in rapid muscle atrophy. Strength can actually decline at rates of 1% to 3% a day. Joint position is a factor in that a muscle under tension seems to become atrophied less readily. For example, a knee that is immobilized in partial flexion will develop less quadriceps atrophy than a knee immobilized in full extension. Aging also results in a loss of muscle mass. Strength levels remain constant until about 40 to 50 years of age and then decrease rapidly, especially with a sedentary life-style. By age 65, typically 20% has been lost. This may be due more to sedentary life-style than to aging, because active elderly individuals show less change. With strength training, hypertrophy can occur in both type I and type II muscle fibers in individuals in their 70s, and strength gains were reported even in 90-year-old individuals (82).

Vandervoort reviewed the effects of aging on human neuromuscular function. The review focused on age-related declines in muscle mass and strength, including a discussion of the potential for improvement of neuromuscular function following exercise training programs. He found that high-resistance exercise training programs are effective in improving both muscle size and voluntary strength even in very old and frail men and women. These improvements yield significant gains in performance of activities of daily living such as walking. Maintenance exercise programs are advocated to avoid rapid detraining effects seen in elderly people who become sedentary (83).

Resistance training is effective in increasing strength in early pubertal children. Resistance training appears to have little or no effect on muscle size, but it does result in changes in motor skill coordination, increases in levels of neuromuscular activation, and changes in the intrinsic contractual characteristics of muscle (84). The improved motor coordination contributes to increases in strength, especially for more complex strength maneuvers. The risk of injury from prudently prescribed and closely supervised resistance training appears to be low for preadolescents (85).

There is no average formula that should be used for a workout, but it is usually a good idea to do one to three sets for each muscle group with 8 to 12 repetitions per set. Resistance to weight should be chosen in increasing increments of 5% to 10%. There should be a 48-hour rest for each muscle.

An athlete's trained muscles have three to four times higher oxidative enzyme levels and two- to threefold more capillaries per muscle fiber than untrained muscles. The oxidative enzyme increase occurs over 6 to 8 weeks and is lost in 4 to 6 weeks if training is stopped (86). Maximal strength and ability to fully flex the arms show the greatest decrements immediately after exercise with a linear restoration of the functions over the next 10 days. Blood creatine kinase levels increase precipitously 2 days after exercise, which also is the time when spontaneous muscle shortening is most pronounced (87).

Muscle Soreness

There are two types of soreness. One is secondary to temporary ischemia of working muscle and the accumulation of lactic acid and other metabolites. This type of soreness usually occurs shortly after exercise. The other type of soreness typically occurs 24 to 72 hours after exercise. It is more disabling and may last several days. This delayed muscle soreness is not well understood and may be the result of muscle tissue tears and damage resulting in fluid retention and muscle spasm. Eccentric contractions result in significantly higher incidences of delayed-onset muscle soreness than do concentric isometric contractions.

Most exercise results in some skeletal muscle damage. Unaccustomed exercise or eccentric exercise can cause more damage. This type of exercise-induced muscle damage causes a response that can be characterized by a cascade of metabolic events. Delayed-onset muscle soreness and weakness, the most obvious manifestations of the damage, peak within 24 to 48 hours. Increased circulating neutrophils and interleukin-1 levels occur within 24 hours, but skeletal muscle levels remain elevated for much longer. There is also degradation of muscle protein and depletion of muscle glycogen stores. These metabolic alterations may result in the increased need for dietary protein, particularly at the beginning of a program that has a high eccentric component such as strength training (88).

Muscle Fatigue

Muscle fatigue is manifested by a decline in the force or power capacity and may be prominent in both submaximal and maximal contractions. Disturbance in muscle electrolytes plays an important role in the development of muscular fatigue. Intense muscular contraction is accompanied by an increased muscle water content, decreased muscle potassium, and increased muscle sodium and chloride. The net result of this intracellular ionic change is a marked rise in intracellular pH concentration, or acidosis. This acidosis is linked with decreased muscle function.

The concentrations of extracellular and intracellular potassium in skeletal muscle influence muscle cell function and are important determinants of cardiovascular and respiratory function. An increase in localized potassium causes dilatation of the vascular bed within contracting muscle, resulting in increased blood flow to contracting muscle. This exercise hyperemia aids in the delivery of metabolic substrates to, and in the removal of metabolic end products from, contracting and recovering muscle. In contrast to these beneficial aspects, the response of contracting muscle to decreases in intracellular potassium ion and increases in intracellular sodium ion concentrations contribute to a reduction in the strength of muscular contraction. Resting muscle has a higher intracellular potassium concentration and exercise causes a decrease in intracellular potassium and an increase in plasma potassium. Muscle potassium loss is a major factor associated with muscle fatigue, but this fatigue is a safety mechanism. Its purpose is to prevent the muscle cell from self-destruction. Net loss of potassium ion and an associated net gain of sodium ion by contracting muscles may also contribute to the pain, swelling, and degenerative changes seen after prolonged exercise (89).

Adenosine triphosphate (ATP) is the sole fuel for muscle contraction. During near maximal intense exercise, the muscle store of ATP will be depleted. Therefore, to maintain normal contractile function, ATP must be continually resynthesized, which is accomplished principally by oxidation of carbohydrates. With prolonged extensive exercise, glucose derived from skeletal muscle and liver glycogen stores is the primary source of glucose for ATP resynthesis.

The point of exhaustion is closely related to the depletion of muscle and liver glycogen stores. Carbohydrate depletion results in the inability of skeletal muscle to maintain a required rate of ATP resynthesis, and therefore work intensity is reduced (90). A common metabolic denominator of muscle fatigue during these and many other conditions is a reduced capacity to generate ATP, which is expressed by the increased metabolism of the adenine nucleotide pool (91).

Electrolytes and Fluids

Current evidence indicates that adequate fluid ingestion during exercise enhances athletic performance; prevents a fall in plasma volume; and increases stroke volume, cardiac output, and blood flow to the skin. It also maintains serum sodium ion concentration and serum osmolality, lowers rectal temperature, and prevents a progressive rise in heart rate.

The provision of glucose in ingested solution may be necessary to optimize performance. Sweetened drinks containing carbohydrates may also increase fluid intake during exercise, thereby minimizing voluntary dehydration. The optimum solution for ingestion during exercise should probably provide carbohydrates at a rate of 1 g/min and electrolytes in concentrations that, when drunk at the optimum rate, maintain serum osmolality and plasma volume at pre-exercise levels by replacing water and electrolyte loss from the extracellular space. Unfortunately, the composition of the extracellular loss is not always known, and the replacement rate depends on the intensity of the exercise and the rate of loss of sweat. Furthermore, high rates of fluid intake (greater than 1 L/hr) are difficult to achieve during exercise, because this leads to feelings of abdominal discomfort. Practicing regular drinking during training might reduce the severity and frequency of these symptoms, possibly by increasing intestinal absorptive capacity. Most athletes are reluctant to drink during exercise and do not ingest fluid at rates equal to the rates of fluid loss. Fluid consumption is enhanced by ingestion of cold, sweet fluids. Simultaneous food consumption also stimulates fluid ingestion (92,93).

Scientific attitudes toward sports drinks have changed over the past 20 years. Initial caution that the carbohydrate–electrolyte drinks compromise gastric emptying during exercise has now been shown to be unjustified. Numerous studies have shown that 5% to 10% solutions of glucose and other simple sugars have suitable gastric-emptying characteristics for the delivery of fluid and moderate amount of carbohydrates. The optimum concentration of electrolytes, particularly sodium, remains unknown. Most currently available sports drinks provide low levels of sodium, 10 to 15 mmol/L. The sodium level of sports drinks will probably be more influenced by the palatability of the drink. Low sodium levels are more palatable. Whatever is provided, it must be refreshing and palatable for athletes to accept and drink appropriate amounts of fluid (94). The ideal solution usually depends on duration and intensity of exercise, environmental conditions, and the characteristics of the individual. Variation among individuals is broad, and optimum strategy can only be established through experience (95).

Classic studies conducted in the 1920s and 1930s established that the consumption of a high-carbohydrate diet before exercise and the ingestion of glucose during exercise delayed the onset of fatigue in part by preventing the development of hypoglycemia.

For the next 30 or 40 years, however, interest in carbohydrate ingestion during exercise waned. Unfortunately, it still remains a popular belief that water replacement to prevent dehydration and hyperthermia is more important than carbohydrate replacement during prolonged exercise. This statement was reinforced because studies in the early 1970s showed that ingestion of carbohydrate solutions delayed gastric emptying compared with water alone, and might even exacerbate dehydration. In the early 1980s, with commercial interest in carbohydrate products on the rise, exercise physiologists again began to study the effect of carbohydrate ingestion, and these studies soon established that carbohydrate ingestion during prolonged periods of exercise could delay fatigue. Other studies have shown that significant quantities of ingested glucose can be oxidized during exercise. Peak rates of glucose oxidation occur approximately 75 to 90 minutes after ingestion (96).

PREGNANCY AND EXERCISE

A significant body of evidence exists that supports the idea that healthy women can perform acute exercise of moderate intensity and duration without jeopardizing fetal well-being (97). Women who exercise strenuously throughout gestation have smaller babies than control subjects, with a very mild retardation in asymmetric growth. Their labor starts earlier and is of shorter duration, and they experience less obstetric and surgical intervention (98). Although, theoretically, there is risk to both mother and fetus with exercise, the current literature includes the following consistent finding. Women who exercise before pregnancy and continue to do so during pregnancy tend to weigh less, gain less weight, and deliver smaller babies than controls. There was no increased incidence of fetal or maternal problems. All women, regardless of initial level of physical activity, decrease their activities as pregnancy progresses. No information is available to assess whether active women had better pregnancy outcome than their sedentary counterparts, although physically active women appear to tolerate the pain of labor better.

Pregnancy is not a state of confinement, and cardiovascular and muscular fitness can be reasonably maintained. Physical activity should not be restricted unless definite obstetric or medical problems indicate restriction (99). There are some potential risks to the fetus resulting from maternal exercise, including hypoxia, hyperthermia, and abnormal heart rate changes. The benefits, however, appear to outweigh the risks, which can be minimized by prescribing appropriate exercising and avoiding overheating and dehydration. Swimming, biking, aerobic walking, and moderate aerobic exercise are safe provided that the pregnancy is normal.

Exercise can be used as an alternative and safe therapeutic approach for gestational diabetes. Exercise benefits pregnant women with gestational diabetes mellitus by preventing excessive weight gain and preventing or decreasing the severity of hypertension or hyperlipidemia, or both, during pregnancy (100).

NUTRITION

Increasing the relative amount of protein in the diet of athletes has been suggested to optimize anabolic processes and to improve physiologic response to training and performance. Most sports nutritionists state that as long as athletes ingest 15% of their total caloric intake in the form of protein, additional supplements of protein are not necessary. Recently, amino acids have become popular nutritional supplements. Little scientific evidence seems to support the hypothesis that amino acid supplementation enhances physiologic responses to strength training when athletes consume dietary protein within the recommended guidelines (101).

Carbohydrates are important substrates for contracting muscle during prolonged strenuous exercise, and fatigue is often associated with muscle glycogen depletion or hyperglycemia, or both. Thus, the goals of carbohydrate nutritional strategies before, during, and after exercise are to optimize the availability of muscle and liver glycogen and blood glucose. During heavy training, the carbohydrate requirements of athletes may be as high as 8 to 10 g/kg body weight, or 60% to 70% of total energy intake. Ingestion of a diet high in carbohydrates should be encouraged to maintain carbohydrate reserves and the ability to train intensely. Ingestion of a high-carbohydrate meal 3 to 4 hours prior to exercise ensures adequate carbohydrate availability and enhances exercise performance.

Muscle glycogen and plasma glucose are oxidized by skeletal muscle to supply the carbohydrate energy needed to exercise strenuously for several hours. With increasing duration of exercise, there is a progressive shift from muscle glycogen to blood glucose. Carbohydrate feeding throughout exercise delays fatigue by 30 to 60 minutes, apparently by maintaining blood glucose concentrations and the rate of carbohydrate oxidation necessary to exercise strenuously. Very little muscle glycogen is used for energy during the 3 to 4 hours of prolonged exercise, suggesting that blood glucose is the predominant carbohydrate source. Carbohydrate supplementation during exercise delays fatigue by 30 to 60 minutes but does not prevent fatigue (102).

CONCLUSIONS

Exercise is a good and healthy activity for people of all ages, no matter what their state of health. It prevents as well as treats disease. Supervised exercise, or at least exercise following the advice of a knowledgeable person, will be of benefit to athletes of all ages.

References

1. Blair SN, Kohl HW, Gordon NF, Paffenbarger RS Jr. How much physical activity is good for health? Ann Rev Pub Health 1992;13:99–126.

2. Fentem PH. Exercise in prevention of disease. Br Med Bull 1992;48:630–650.

3. Sleap M, Warburton P. Physical activity levels of 5–11-year-old children in England as determined by continuous observation. Res Q Exer Sport 1992;63:328–345.

4. Sallis JF. Epidemiology of physical activity and fitness in children and adolescents. Crit Rev Food Sci Nutr 1993;33:403–408.

5. Bauman A, Owen N, Rushworth RL. Recent trends and socio-demographic determinants of exercise participation in Australia. Comm Health Stud 1990;14:19–26.

6. Owen N, Bauman A. The descriptive epidemiology of a sedentary lifestyle in adult Australians. Int J Epidemiol 1992;21:305–310.

7. Bonheur B, Young SW. Exercise as a health-promoting lifestyle choice. Appl Nurs Res 1991;4:2–6.

8. Reed BD, Jensen JD, Gorenflo DW. Physicians and exercise promotion. Am J Prev Med 1991;7:410–415.

9. Kjaer M, Secher NH. Neural influences on cardiovascular and endocrine responses to static exercise in humans. Sports Med 1992;13:303–319.

10. Laughlin MH, McAllister RM. Exercise training-induced coronary vascular adaptation. J Appl Physiol 1992;73:2209–2225.

11. Longhurst JC, Stebbins CL. The isometric athlete. Cardiol Clin 1992;10:281–294.

12. Paterson DJ. Potassium and ventilation in exercise. J Appl Physiol 1992;72:811–820.

13. Holloszy JO, Coyle EF. Adaptations of skeletal muscle to endurance exercise and their metabolic consequences. J Appl Physiol 1984;56:831–838.

14. Schwarz L, Kindermann W. Changes in beta-endorphin levels in response to aerobic and anaerobic exercise. Sports Med 1992;13: 25–36.

15. Kenney WL, Johnson JM. Control of skin blood flow during exercise. Med Sci Sports Exerc 1992;24:303–312.

16. Convertino VA. Blood volume: its adaptation to endurance training. Med Sci Sports Exerc 1991;23:1338–1348.

17. American College of Sports Medicine. The recommended quantity and quality of exercise for developing and maintaining cardiorespiratory and muscle fitness in healthy adults. Med Sci Sports Exerc 1990;22:265–271.

18. Shephard RJ. A critical analysis of work-site fitness programs and their postulated economic benefits. Med Sci Sports Exerc 1992;24:354–370.

19. Cox MH. Exercise training programs and cardiorespiratory adaptation. Clin Sports Med 1991;10:19–32.

20. Anthony J. Psychologic aspects of exercise. Clin Sports Med 1991;10:171–180.

21. American College of Sports Medicine. Position Stand. Physical activity, physical fitness, and hypertension. Med Sci Sports Exerc 1993;25:i–x.

22. Arroll B. Does physical activity lower blood pressure: a critical review of the clinical trials. J Clin Epidemiol 1992;45:439.

23. Franz IW. Blood pressure response to exercise in normotensives and hypertensives. Can J Sport Sci 1991;16:296–301.

24. Grassi G, Seravalle G, Calhoun D, Bolla GB, Mancia G. Physical exercise in essential hypertension. Chest 1992;101(5 suppl):312S–314S.

25. Goble MM, Schieken RM. Blood pressure response to exercise: a marker for future hypertension? Am J Hypertens 1991;4:617S–620S.

26. Horton ES. Exercise in the treatment of NIDDM. Diabetes 1991;40(suppl 2):175–178.

27. Soukup JT, Kovaleski JE. A review of the effects of resistance training for individuals with diabetes mellitus. Diabetes Educ 1993;19:307–312.

28. Ruderman N, Apelian AZ, Schneider SH. Exercise in therapy and prevention of type II diabetes. Implications for blacks. Diabetes Care 1990;13:1163–1168.

29. King H, Kirska AM. Prevention of type II diabetes by physical training. Epidemiological considerations and study methods. Diabetes Care 1992;15:1794–1799.

30. Klip A, Marette A, Dimitrakoudis D, et al. Effect of diabetes on glucoregulation. From glucose transporters to glucose metabolism in vivo. Diabetes Care 1992;15:1747–1766.

31. Wallberg-Henriksson H. Interaction of exercise and insulin in type II diabetes mellitus. Diabetes Care 1992;15:1777–1782.

32. Rodnick KJ, Piper RC, Slot JW, James DE. Interaction of insulin and exercise on glucose transport in muscle. Diabetes Care 1992;15:1679–1689.

33. Taylor PA, Ward A. Women, high-density lipoprotein cholesterol, and exercise. Arch Intern Med 1993;153:1178–1184.

34. Saltin B, Astrand PO. Free fatty acids and exercise. Am J Clin Nutr 1993;57(5 suppl):752S–757S.

35. Guezennec CV. Role of lipids on endurance capacity in man. Int J Sports Med 1992;(13 suppl 1):S114–S118.

36. Richter EA, Turcotte L, Hespel P, Kiens B. Metabolic responses to exercise. Effects of endurance training and implications for diabetes. Diabetes Care 1992;15:1767–1776.

37. King AC, Tribble DL. The role of exercise in weight regulation in nonathletes. Sports Med 1991;11:331–349.

38. Blair SN. Evidence for success of exercise in weight loss and control. Ann Intern Med 1993;1998(7 pt 2):702–706.

39. Ruderman NB, Schneider SH. Diabetes, exercise, and atherosclerosis. Diabetes Care 1992;15:1787–1793.

40. McCubbin JA. Resistance exercise training for persons with arthritis. Rheum Dis Clin North Am 1990;16:931–943.

41. Leimohn W. Exercise and arthritis. Exercise and the back. Rheum Dis Clin North Am 1990;16:945–970.

42. Smith EL, Gilligan C. Physical activity effects on bone metabolism. Calcif Tissue Int 1991;49(suppl):S50–S54.

43. Snow-Harter C, Bouxsein ML, Lewis BT, Carter DR, Marcus R. Effects of resistance and endurance exercise on bone mineral status of young women: a randomized exercise intervention trial. J Bone Miner Res 1992;7:761–769.

44. Forwood MR, Burr DB. Physical activity and bone mass: exercises in futility? Bone Miner 1993;21:89–112.

45. Evans WJ, Campbell WW. Sarcopenia and age-related changes in body composition and functional capacity. J Nutr 1993;123(2 suppl):465–468.

46. Shephard RJ. Benefits of sport and physical activity for the disabled: implications for the individual and for society. Scand J Rehabil Med 1991;23:51–59.

47. Rogers TK, Howard P. Pulmonary hemodynamics and physical training in patients with chronic obstructive pulmonary disease. Chest 1992;101(5 suppl):289S–292S.

48. Gimenez M, Predine E, Marchand M, et al. Implications of lower- and upper-limb training procedures in patients with chronic airway obstruction. Chest 1992;101(5 suppl):279S–288S.

49. Belman MJ. Factors limiting exercise performance in lung disease. Ventilatory insufficiency. Chest 1992;101(5 suppl):253S–254S.

50. Mahler DA. The measurement of dyspnea during exercise in patients with lung disease. Chest 1992;101(5 suppl):242S–247S.

51. Rossi P. Physical training in patients with congestive heart failure. Chest 1992;101(5 suppl):350S–353S.

52. Sullivan MJ, Cobb FR. Central hemodynamic response to exercise in patients with chronic heart failure. Chest 1992;101(5 suppl):340S–346S.

53. de Geus EJ, van Doornen LJ, Orlebeke JF.

Regular exercise and aerobic fitness in relation to psychological make-up and physiological stress reactivity. Psychosom Med 1993;55:347–363.

54. Petruzzello SJ, Landers DM, Hatfield BD, Kubitz KA, Salazar W. A meta-analysis on the anxiety-reducing effects of acute and chronic exercise. Outcomes and mechanisms. Sports Med 1991;11:143–182.

55. Raglin JS. Exercise and mental health. Beneficial and detrimental effects. Sports Med 1990;9:323–329.

56. MacMahon JR. The psychological benefits of exercise and the treatment of delinquent adolescents. Sports Med 1990;9:344–351.

57. Paterson DH. Effects of aging on the cardiorespiratory system. Can J Sport Sci 1992;17:171–177.

58. Rogers MA, Evans WJ. Changes in skeletal muscle with aging: effects of exercise training. Exerc Sport Sci Rev 1993;21:65–102.

59. Buchner DM, Beresford SA, Larson EB, LaCroix AZ, Wagner EH. Effects of physical activity on health status in older adults. Ann Rev Publ Health 1992;13:469–488.

60. Buchner DM, Wagner EH. Preventing frail health. Clin Geriatr Med 1992;8:1–17.

61. Heyneman CA, Premo DE. A 'water walkers' exercise program for the elderly. Public Health Rep 1992;107:213–217.

62. Shay KA, Roth DL. Association between aerobic fitness and visuospatial performance in healthy older adults. Psychol Aging 1992;7:15–24.

63. Probart CK, Notelovitz M, Martin D, Kahn FY, Fields C. The effect of moderate aerobic exercise on physical fitness among women 70 years and older. Maturitas 1991;14:49–56.

64. Posner JD, Gorman KM, Gitlin LN, et al. Effects of exercise training in the elderly on the occurrence and time to onset of cardiovascular diagnoses. J Am Geriatr Soc 1990;38:205–210.

65. Shephard RJ, Verde TJ, Thomas SG, Shek P. Physical activity and the immune system. Can J Sport Sci 1991;16:169–185.

66. Sharp NC, Koutedakis Y. Sport and the overtraining syndrome: immunological aspects. Br Med Bull 1992;48:518–533.

67. Pate R. Sports anemia: a review of the current research literature. Physician Sports Med 1983;11:115.

68. Weaver CM, Rajaram S. Exercise and iron status. J Nutr 1992;122(3 suppl):782–787.

69. Balaban EP. Sports anemia. Clin Sports Med 1992;11:313–325.

70. Colan SD. Mechanics of left ventricular systolic and diastolic function in physiologic hypertrophy of the athlete heart. Cardiol Clin 1992;10:227–240.

71. Fagard RH. Impact of different sports and training on cardiac structure and function. Cardiol Clin 1992;10:241–256.

72. Bryan G, Ward A, Rippe JM. Athletic heart syndrome. Clin Sports Med 1992;11:259–272.

73. Brouns F, Beckers E. Is the gut an athletic organ? Digestion, absorption and exercise. Sports Med 1993;15:242–257.

74. Moses FM. Gastrointestinal bleeding and the athlete. Am J Gastroenterol 1993;88:1157–1159.

75. Lehman M, Foster C, Keul J. Overtraining in endurance athletes: a brief review. Med Sci Sports Exerc 1993;25:854–862.

76. Costill DL, Flynn MG, Kirwan JP, et al. Effects of repeated days of intensified training on muscle glycogen and swimming performance. Med Sci Sports Exerc 1988;20:249–254.

77. Loat CE, Rhodes EC. Relationship between the lactate and ventilatory thresholds during prolonged exercise. Sports Med 1993;15:104–115.

78. Spurway NC. Aerobic exercise, anaerobic exercise and the lactate threshold. Br Med Bull 1992;48:569–591.

79. Hagerman FC. Energy metabolism and fuel utilization. Med Sci Sports Exerc 1992;24(9 suppl 10):S39–S44.

80. Schweiz Z. The recommended quantity and quality of exercise for developing and maintaining cardiorespiratory and muscular fitness in healthy adults. Position stand of the American College of Sports Medicine. Sports Med 1993; 14:127–137.

81. Houmard JA. Impact of reduced training on performance in endurance athletes. Sports Med 1991;12:380–393.

82. Fiatarone NA, Marks EC, Ryan ND, et al. High intensity strength nonagenarians: effects on skeletal muscle. JAMA 1990;263: 3029–3034.

83. Vandervoort AA. Effects of aging on human neuromuscular function: implications for exercise. Can J Sport Sci 1992;17:178–184.

84. Blimkie CJ. Resistance training during pre- and early puberty: efficacy, trainability, mechanisms and persistence. Can J Sport Sci 1992;17:264–279.

85. Blimkie CJ. Resistance training during preadolescence. Sports Med 1993;15:389–407.

86. Henriksson J. Effects of physical training on the metabolism of skeletal muscle. Diabetes Care 1992;15:1701–1711.

87. Clarkson PM, Nosaka K, Braun B. Muscle function after exercise-induced muscle damage and rapid adaptation. Med Sci Sports Exerc 1992;24:512–520.

88. Evans WJ. Muscle damage: nutritional considerations. Int J Sport Nutr 1991;1:214–224.

89. Lindinger MI, Sjgaard G. Potassium regulation during exercise and recovery. Sports Med 1991;11:382–401.

90. Hultman E, Greenhaff PL. Skeletal muscle energy metabolism and fatigue during intense exercise in man. Sci Prog 1991;75(298 pt 3–4): 361–370.

91. Sahlin K. Metabolic factors in fatigue. Sports Med 1992;13:99–107.

92. Noakes TD. Fluid replacement during exercise. Exerc Sport Sci Rev 1993;21:297–330.

93. Brouns F, Saris W, Schneider H. Rationale for upper limits of electrolyte replacement during exercise. Int J Sport Nutr 1992;2:229–238.

94. Burke LM, Read RS. Dietary supplements in sport. Sports Med 1993;15:43–65.

95. Maughan RJ. Fluid balance and exercise. Int J Sports Med 1992;13(suppl 1):S132–S135.

96. Hawley JA, Dennis SC, Noakes TD. Oxidation of carbohydrate ingested during prolonged endurance exercise. Sports Med 1992;14:27–42.

97. Wolfe LA, Mottola MF. Aerobic exercise in pregnancy: an update. Can J Appl Physiol 1993;18:119–147.

98. Katz VL. Physiologic changes during normal pregnancy. Curr Opin Obstet Gynecol 1991;3:750–758.

99. Artal R. Exercise and pregnancy. Clin Sports Med 1992;11:363–377.

100. Horton ES. Exercise in the treatment of NIDDM. Diabetes 1991;40(suppl 2):175–178.

101. Kreider RB, Mirial V, Bertun E. Amino acid supplementation and exercise performance. Analysis of the proposed ergogenic value. Sports Med 1993;16:190–209.

102. Coyle EF. Carbohydrate supplementation during exercise. J Nutr 1992;122(3 suppl):788–795.

THE ROLE OF THE SPORTS MEDICINE PHYSICIAN IN THE COMMUNITY

2

JOHN F. DUFF

The Primary Care Sports Medicine
  Physician
The Physician's Contribution to Sports
  Medicine in the Community
Sports Medical Education for the Primary
  Care Physician
The Recreational Athlete
Sports Medicine in the School System
Sports Safety in the Community

Rapidly expanding athletic competition and sports activities in urban, suburban, and rural communities make it crucial for physicians to become more directly involved in sports medicine. More than ever before there is a demand for well-organized sports medical programs guided by a physician. Today's athletic activities, competitions, and numbers of active athletes have far outdistanced the programs designed to prevent injuries and coordinate medical care.

When physicians become involved in sports medicine, their value to the community will depend on the expertise, time, effort, and leadership they offer. In return, physicians who initiate and support a well-organized sports medical program will be strongly appreciated in the community. The personal satisfaction and rewards for their endeavors can be extraordinary.

With the tremendous amount of information available today, many sports injuries can be prevented or greatly reduced by a community health program that includes education and vigilant watchfulness as well as comprehensive medical care. As adult recreational athletes and the parents of young athletes become more aware of the injury risks of sports and learn more about ways to prevent injuries, the demand for good sports medicine physicians will increase sharply.

Many communities now lack any organized system that can provide a young athlete or adult who engages in recreational athleticism with coordinated and simple care by a physician. Such a system requires good coordination among the medical services in the community, plus an educational program and carefully designed communication procedures. Fortunately, it is increasingly practical to put a sports medical program in place and establish a referral and consulting system that meshes with the medical care already available. The emergency room, the primary care physician, the urgent care center, the orthopedist, the school health care office, and the high school trainer may all be involved in the care of young athletes and older recreational athletes.

There are, however, some potential stumbling blocks to developing and organizing an effective sports medical program in the community. One problem is the competitiveness among sports medical centers and individual physicians. In many cases, the hospital clinic, a sports medical center, and a rehabilitation center with certified trainers and physical therapists will all be vying for the care of school athletes and adult recreational athletes. Another obstacle is the bureaucratic structure of some community health care centers, local hospital programs, and private practices of individual physicians. As a result of these problems, a sports medical program may be disorganized and uncoordinated, met with lack of interest, and hampered by a demoralizing competitiveness.

The key to dealing with these problems is leadership by a primary care physician in private practice with hospital privileges and an interest in community sports activities. Good leadership and a small but dedicated group of volunteers can offer a complete, well-balanced sports medical program with minimal cost and minimal interference with private practices, hospitals, clinics, the school system, and youth leagues. This program will bring great benefits to both young athletes and adult recreational athletes.

THE PRIMARY CARE SPORTS MEDICINE PHYSICIAN

The need for leadership, direction, and availability from the primary care physician is essential today for a well-balanced community sports medicine program. Since the early 1980s, a substantial number of physicians have become increasingly involved in the care of athletes. It has become quite noticeable that some physicians, physical therapists, podiatrists, and chiropractors list themselves as sports medicine specialists.

Any physician planning to establish a sports medical practice today should be knowledgeable about preventing and treating sports injuries and should participate in the care of those involved in community athletic activities. The individual should participate as a team physician for a high school or a youth sports team in the community and devote a significant percentage of time to sports and sports medicine.

The physician should take advantage of continuing education programs that focus on sports medicine and join local and national organizations that are shaping the field of sports medicine. Certificates of added qualification in sports medicine can be obtained by physicians who are certified in family practice, internal medicine, pediatrics, and emergency medicine.

Regardless of their specialty, interested physicians can become involved in sports medicine. Their ability to recognize injuries in specific sports and the actions that cause these injuries will help them give a clear picture and enhance the care of the athlete. Knowing the sport helps both in identifying the injury and understanding the athlete.

Knowledge of a sport will also enhance the image of a sports medicine physician who takes care of injured athletes in that sport. This is particularly true with a sport that dominates the community. In some areas, football dominates. In other areas the dominant sports can be soccer, lacrosse, ice hockey, basketball, skiing, horsemanship, gymnastics, swimming, or even hang gliding. The primary care physician will do well to be knowledgeable not only about the injuries of the sport, but also its history, rules and regulations, records, and great names.

It is critical in athletic care to evaluate an injury as soon as it occurs. If possible, you (or a member of your group) should attend the games and evaluate the injured athlete immediately. The golden period before swelling occurs will allow a more exacting diagnosis. Delaying an office appointment for even a day or two can cloud the picture and the diagnosis. In addition, inaccurate evaluation by a physician not aware of the principles of sports medicine can lead to a prolonged recovery for the injured individual. These individuals must be thorough and accurate in their assessments and early initiation of proper treatment. Such an evaluation must include the decision on when the athlete can resume participation in the sport, rehabilitation, and prevention of reinjury. Repeated intermittent visits and care under multiple disciplines can create confusion and may lead to a prolonged disability. Consistency is crucial.

Someone active in a competitive sport may be engaged in that sport every day, and after an injury he or she may feel differently than the occasional recreational athlete about when to return. Understanding the different mind sets of young competitive athletes and adult recreational athletes is essential. A physician must consider the competitiveness that often exists and the drive to get back into the sport as soon as possible; insight into each patient is important.

Care of the injured athlete requires a thorough knowledge of the anatomy, physiology, and pathology involved with injury. Primary care physicians should be aware of when an injury will require further evaluation and consultation. This book helps the primary care physician with that process. Specific recommendations are made for consulting the orthopedic surgeon.

THE PHYSICIAN'S CONTRIBUTION TO SPORTS MEDICINE IN THE COMMUNITY

Sports Medicine in the Hospital

Chances are that a local or regional hospital has a sports medical center with a medical care program including both preventive and primary care for the athlete. Major urban institutions and university hospitals will have the most sophisticated sports medical units.

The primary care physician can readily become a major player in one of these sports medical centers by volunteering to organize the sports physicals in the school system, cover community athletic activities, and develop a community educational program for sports injury prevention. The smaller the sports medical center, the more valuable the physician's leadership will be in helping the physical therapist in the rehabilitation unit, the physician's assistant at the hospital and medical practice, and the emergency medical technician based at the hospital and ambulance center.

The Emergency Room Physician

The emergency room or urgent care physician's role is at the critical point in the care of many sports injuries. Coordination between the sports medicine physician and the emergency room physician is crucial. Good care of the injured athlete is best implemented by a prearranged format for the treatment and referral procedures within

the medical community. The emergency room physician should be responsible for initial evaluation and referral. The referral should be done in concert with the athlete's primary care physician or directly to the orthopedic surgeon.

Follow-up should be within 24 to 48 hours so that proper rehabilitation instructions can be given. Too often, the emergency room physician is frustrated by the lack of follow-up in determining the significance of a sports injury. The treating physician should provide follow-up to the emergency room physician. Some mechanism of communication between the two specialists should exist. Education is key. A program of continuing education can be developed to help emergency room physicians and nurses and urgent care physicians to identify specific sports-related injuries and conditions. Large HMOs should also provide educational programs for physician assistants, nurse practitioners, and physical therapists.

Primary Care Physicians (Family Physicians, Internists, and Pediatricians)

Primary care physicians are ideally suited to practice sports medicine. As the first point of contact, they see the injuries first. They know the families and they have systems for follow-up. They can be involved with teams as well as the weekend athlete.

Orthopedists

Over the past 20 years the orthopedic surgeon has been involved as the team physician in some communities, in others the orthopedist has acted as a consultant to the team physician. Orthopedists and primary care physicians can form an excellent team to care for athletes of all ages. They can work as a team!

Other Specialists

Other specialists, such as neurosurgeons, pulmonologists, and dermatologists, are becoming more involved in sports medicine. Head and neck injuries are common in contact sports and the neurosurgeon may be involved in the more serious or potentially serious injuries. Asthma first discovered with exertion is a common problem in athletes. Some of these athletes require complex evaluation by a pulmonologist. Skin problems are common in adolescents. Acne and bacterial skin infections can become severe and the dermatologist may need to become involved. These specialties should be aware of the different needs of the athletic population.

These physicians care not only for the normal competitive athlete but also for the special needs of youngsters—such as those with cerebral palsy or Down syndrome—who are active in sports but require medical care other than that offered by orthopedists. This would be of tremendous value because of the increase in competition by athletes with disabilities. Understanding the youngster with cerebral palsy in competition and placing the youngster in proper categories require a medical team. Youngsters with mental retardation and other developmental disabilities who are capable of participating in sports need input from a primary care physician as well as a therapist. The Special Olympics, which originated in the United States and is now international, is one of the most outstanding programs a primary care physician can be involved in. Sports medical specialists who specialize in rehabilitation can deal locally with paraplegics and quadriplegics while they continue to be active in available physical programs.

SPORTS MEDICAL EDUCATION FOR THE PRIMARY CARE PHYSICIAN

A primary care physician who wants to promote a sports medical image in the community—including enthusiasm and availability—must have a certain amount of expertise in this field. This would include an in-depth knowledge of specific sports injuries, the rules of various sports prevalent in the community, the regulations, and the equipment. Perhaps the physician coaches Little League baseball or community soccer. Simply attending and supporting the local high school games is a plus.

Where can a young physician in training get the necessary sports medical expertise? Most primary care residency programs will have a sports medical section. By volunteering for this section and devoting time to disciplined reading, the young primary care physician can start out his or her practice with a strong sports medical background.

In addition, a number of primary care sports medical programs are available in the United States. A good source of information about these programs is the American Medical Society for Sports Medicine (see Appendix A).

What if no sports medical education is available in the physician's residency or training program? In that case, look for community sources of sports medical expertise. For example, a local physician who is active as a team physician could be a good information source. There may be a rehabilitation center concentrating on athletes, or a college or university sports medicine program. Other specialists may be sports medical consultants. These are just a few possible sources of useful knowledge outside of formal, documented training.

For the physician who has already established a practice and is interested in sports medicine, a number of organizations can help in gaining the necessary expertise. Among others, the American College of Sports Medicine, the American Medical Society for Sports Medicine, and the American Orthopedic Society for Sports Medicine offer educational programs to the practitioner. An outstanding example is the Team Physician program organized by the American College of Sports Medicine. In addition to such programs, the physician can turn to the libraries and available video programs. Many courses, conferences, and programs that can help the primary care physician gain expertise in sports medicine are offered throughout the country.

The Orthopedic Sports Medicine Specialist

Most orthopedic surgeons in general orthopedic practice consider themselves sports medical experts because orthopedic surgery is directly related to the locomotive system involving the arms, legs, and body. Because millions of sports injuries occur every year, all orthopedic surgeons are necessarily involved, even if they are not particularly interested in sports medical practice.

However, simply treating sports injuries does not make one a sports medical specialist. That designation should only be given if the orthopedist or any physician meets certain requirements:

- Participates in the local sports medicine education program
- Devotes a substantial amount of time to caring for the young athletes of a high school or youth league team
- Is an active member of the American Orthopedic Society for Sports Medicine, if an orthopedist

Over the past 30 years the American Orthopedic Society for sports medicine and the American Medical Association have established a standard of care for the athlete that must be maintained as the primary care physician becomes an integral part of this care.

The Paramedic/Emergency Medical Technician

To strengthen a community's sports prevention and medical care program, training programs for paramedics and emergency medical technicians (EMTs) should include an expanded and sophisticated level of training on sports injuries. A paramedic or EMT who covers any sports event should have an advanced sports injury support certification.

Caring for and making decisions on an injured athlete in the midst of competition calls for a different kind of expertise than dealing with trauma on the highway or cardiac resuscitation. This is particularly true when young athletes are injured. A fractured ankle on the football field can be handled the same way as a fractured ankle anywhere, but a knee injury at the height of competition, for example, calls for a special understanding and a critical decision. Therefore, paramedics and EMTs who care for sports injuries should be highly qualified, especially because they often provide the medical coverage for hockey games, marathons, high school football games, and other sports events.

Today, few paramedics and EMTs are well versed in the sports that they cover or the procedures for understanding, recognizing, and making decisions on particular injuries. To remedy that situation, paramedic and EMT certification programs should include a sports medicine course.

Youth Sports Leagues

Youth sports leagues have done much to improve the health and safety of athletes. Since 1980, the youth leagues, organizations associated with them, parents, and physicians have made tremendous efforts to improve both the emotional and physical well-being of young athletes in the leagues. The National Youth Coaches Association has developed an outstanding national policy for youth sports. It includes 11 elements, all related to young athletes, coaches, and parents. This policy should be incorporated into every community sports medicine program.

One way a physician can get involved with youth sports leagues is by becoming an instructor in the Little League International Sports Medical Prevention Program organized by Little League International Inc and the American Orthopedic Society for Sports Medicine, another way is to assist youth leagues that are registered in the community's parks and recreational department. Physicians who need more information about a particular sport and its safety can consult the director of the youth league for that sport and find out how they can assist in the program. It may take some extra energy and time, but it will be well worth it.

THE RECREATIONAL ATHLETE

There is little opportunity for the primary care physician to be formally involved in adult recreational athletic activities because they are so loosely organized. Many of the activities are informal, spontaneous, and weekend warrior-type activities such as the company picnic competition, volleyball, flag football, and pick-up soccer games.

Any formal sports injury prevention program or medical coverage of events is unlikely. A physician would probably get involved only when called because of an injury or if he or she were a participant in the activity. There are many adult recreational activities that are arranged by municipal governments, civic organizations, and churches. Basketball, softball, soccer, and volleyball are some of the more popular ones. An educational package that included suggestions for conditioning, first aid, and what to do when injured would probably be helpful to this group of athletes.

SPORTS MEDICINE IN THE SCHOOL SYSTEM

High schools have perhaps the most organized of all sports medical programs. All of the 17,000 high schools in the United States are heavily involved in interscholastic sports competitions, and many schools have 16 to 30 different sports activities in their programs. This requires enormous organization, numerous coaches, medical care, and a safety education program. The primary care physician can make a crucial contribution to the education of the student athlete and the prevention of injuries in the school sports system. There are three types of organized school athletic activities: 1) interscholastic competition, 2) intramural competition, and 3) physical education classes.

The school committee in a community initiates, controls, and administers the sports activities within the school system, and thus has the basic responsibility for the health and safety of student athletes. However, the superintendent of the school system designates the individuals directly responsible for the sports education and injury prevention program; for interscholastic competition it is usually the athletic director, with medical care in the hands of the certified trainer and the team physician. For intramural competition and physical education classes, the director of physical education is usually responsible for preventing injuries, making activities safe, and providing immediate care of injuries that occur.

The Team Physician

The team physician can contribute greatly to the physical health as well as the emotional well-being of the team. His or her support of the coaching staff, the trainer, and the competitive young athletes can be the key to a well-balanced athletic program. The team is a family, and the physician should function as a leader in that family. There are several important requirements for a team physician:

- Have personal expertise in the overall sports medical field and in sports injuries
- Be available to support the physical and psychological well-being of the team, educate on preventing injuries, and participate in safety administration, including equipment, facilities, transportation, communication, and environment
- Be directly involved in the medical care of the young athlete from preseason to the time of any injury and in the follow-up care
- Be the one who decides when the young athlete can return to play, either on the field after an injury or after recovery from an injury
- Communicate directly with parents as well as coaches, as part of the family
- Be a major support to the certified trainer

Being actively committed to the care of young team athletes is very time consuming, and there is very little remuneration for the physician. But this activity brings substantial rewards in terms of immeasurable personal satisfaction. The physician will receive high visibility in the community and the appreciation of all those who are involved with the team. In fact, the strong emotions raised by local high school competition frequently elevate the team doctor to a special pedestal. He or she is respected by everyone, including administrators, coaches, parents, players, and cheerleaders (I have even known schools with a special cheer for the team doctor).

But let me repeat, it is no longer acceptable to show up at game time, pat the athletes on the shoulder, and vanish as soon as the game is over. Today, a very specific expertise and a dedicated commitment are demanded. For example, an "okay" to go back into the game should be based on a clinically astute evaluation of the injury, as well as an awareness of the particular youngster involved. Coaches and players will have a secure feeling when a new team physician makes a sharp, clear decision, whether on the sidelines, in the locker room, or later at the office. When the decision is made, whether it's "okay to go" or "no competition," the doctor should give firm, coherent reasons to the young athlete and the parents.

The team physician must be easily contacted, for minor injuries as well as major clinical decisions. The physician's home telephone number should be given out to all those involved with the team. Parents should be made to feel comfortable in calling, speaking to, and taking the advice of the team physician. Psychological support from the physician is essential for the stability of a team and will bring a sense of security to the coaches, the players, and the parents. A friendly, understanding team physician who maintains confidentiality can help solve personal problems and will boost the entire well-being of the school's athletic system.

Education is an important part of the team physician's role. In coordination with the school's athletic director, the team physician and the trainer should provide a preventive sports safety program for all those involved in school sports. Coaches should also be thoroughly educated so they know how to make sure that facilities and equipment are safe.

When youngsters, their parents, and coaches are well educated about sports injuries, the decisions of the team physician at the preseason physical examination are more likely to be accepted. A youngster disqualified by the physician for competition because of a medical condition may be unhappy, but will respect the physician's decision.

Decisions at the playing field should be made by the team physician in coordination with the trainer, without interference from coaches, parents, or anyone else. Permission to return to play after an injury should be fully explained and documented, including any qualifications or restrictions.

A medical emergency preparedness system should be in place that includes equipment, transportation, and communications. The team physician should be able to call readily on specialists, general surgeons, ophthalmologists, neurosurgeons, and urologists for consultations, referrals, and any other requests. The physician should reach a clear understanding with the local hospital emergency room about emergency procedures when team injuries are involved. The local ambulance service should also be familiarized with the needs of the team physician in an emergency. A well-organized triage system should be established along with other preparations for the possibility of injuries.

The physician in a school system should be closely involved in the physical and emotional well-being of the athlete competing at any level, whether varsity, junior varsity, or freshman. This includes the preparation and equipment necessary for good care as well as educating the coaches, athletes, and parents. The physician must play a major role in the educational program, which should not be relegated to the nursing staff or the coaching staff. The physician should monitor all information that is given to coaches, athletes, and parents.

Guidelines for a High School Sports Medicine Program

Many elements go into an effective, well-run sports medical program for high schools. Some of the most important are discussed.

Preparticipation Examination

An annual physical examination is essential for a safe sports program. Physicians must identify medical problems or conditions that can disqualify a student and evaluate the individual athlete and his or her preparation for athletic competition.

Locker Room Medical Facilities

Working with the trainer and the athletic director, the physician should ensure a well-stocked and equipped room set aside for the care of the young athlete. The room should include examining tables, hot and cold running water, scales, and the medical equipment needed for examinations of injuries and standard care of bumps, bruises, and lacerations. In addition, there should be adequate equipment for emergencies (Table 2.1). Very little attention is given to these rooms in many schools. Some basic public health standards should be met. Another locker room item should be the "trainer's

Table 2.1.   The training room—guidelines

A clean room
Good lighting
Examination and "taping" tables
Scales
Sink (running water, hot and cold)
Refrigeration, for ice and medicines
Modalities available, whirlpool, etc.

Emergency Equipment
   Available large equipment, stored in an
      immediately accessible location.
   Spine board (or fracture board)
   Stretcher
   Large fracture splints
   Sand bags
   Crutches
   Blankets

Communications
   Emergency list of names and telephone
      numbers (office and home) and location.
   Ambulance service
   Hospital
   Team physician
   Specialists
      Neurosurgeon
      Ophthalmologist
      Orthopedist
      General surgeon

Emergency Transportation
   Ambulance availability
   Secondary transportation (station wagon,
      etc.)

bag," a bag that is stocked with all the items
needed to care for injuries on the sidelines
during competition (Table 2.2).

Education for Coaches

It is essential for the athletic director
to require the sports safety education of
all coaches. Coaches should have not
only a first aid certification but a basic
cardiopulmonary resuscitation (CPR) certification as well. They should also be certified through one of the available coaching

certification systems (see Appendix A). In
today's sports medical world, the team
physician or primary care physician should
make sure that these certification requirements are mandated. The day in which any
volunteer can be allowed to coach without
the proper education has long gone.

Education for Parents

The Sports Medical Night for Parents
outlined in my book *Youth Sports Injuries*
(Collier Books, 1992) is an ideal way to educate the parents of young athletes on sports
injury prevention and treatment. A sports
medical night should be held at the beginning of the season and should include all
sports played during that season. At least
one parent from each family and all coaches
should be encouraged to attend. The actual
program should be planned and coordinated by the trainer and the team physician.
A comprehensive sports medical night
should include the elements shown in Table
2.3. This annual event is recommended for
any school in which the athletic program is
organized through the athletic director, the
team physician, and the trainer. Both parents and coaches should be encouraged to
attend. Parents will get comprehensive information about the sport in which their
youngster participates, including the rules
and regulations, the necessary equipment
and why it is necessary, the facilities
available in case of an injury, and the communications system for locating parents
and medical personnel when an injury
occurs.

The team physician has the primary role
in the parent's night meeting—his or her
participation is critical to a well-structured
educational evening.

Field Care

The athletic director, team physician, and
trainer should develop a system of primary
field care for varsity competition and field

Table 2.2. The trainer's bag

A. For Resuscitation
Oral airways (small, medium, large)
15-gauge needle
Padded tongue blades

B. For Identifying the Injury
Flashlight (penlight)
Flashlight (standard)
Blood pressure cuff and gauge
Stethoscope
Tongue blades
Safety pins
Thermometer
Reflex hammer
Measuring tape
Tourniquet (possibly an
ophthalmoscope)

C. Treatment—Bumps, Bruises, Cuts
Bandage scissors
Cotton swabs
Slings and triangular bandage
Ace bandages (3", 4", 6")
Bandaids
Steri-strips (butterflies)
Towels (2)
Ice packs
Leather laces
Adhesive tape
Paper tape
Gauze pads
Sterile gloves (possibly)
Alcohol wipes
Betadine wipes
Aerosol adherent

D. Medicines
Sugar or candy
Aspirin, Tylenol
Antibiotic ointment
Pepto-Bismol tablets
Tums
Sucrets (lozenges)
Vaseline
Prescription drugs for any player on
special treatment
Smelling salts
Ben Gay
Nasal decongestant
Tinactin (antifungicide)
Solarcaine

**E. Treatment—Sprains, Ligament Injuries,
and More Serious Hurts**
Finger splints
Fracture splints
Plaster of Paris
Tape
Knee immobilizers
Cervical collars
Webril, padding

F. Eye Care
Mirror for contact lenses
Contact lens kit
Ophthalmic (eye) irrigation solution
Ophthalmic (eye) irrigation cup and syringe
Eye patches and eye dressing kits
Foreign body forceps

G. Allergic Reactions
Antihistamine tablets
Epinephrine
Needle and syringe
Epinephrine autoinjectors

H. Miscellaneous
Tweezers
Swiss Army knife
Cigarette lighter and paper clip
Rubber bands
Belt cutter
Filters, screwdriver
Plastic bags for ice
Prep razor
Scalpel
Superglue
Baby powder
Kotex pads
Tape stripper
Brown paper bags
Mouth guards
Toenail clippers
Chapstick
String
Magnifying glass
Pen, pencil, pad
Marking pencil
Felt padding
Foam sheets
Moleskin
Clear fog (facemasks)
Change for telephone
Ring cutter
Elastoplast

Table 2.3. Guidelines for a parent's sports medical night

1. The meeting leader introduces all officials involved in each sport, with special attention to the trainers and their responsibilities.
2. Coaches hand out the rule books for each sport and review the rules specifically designed to minimize injuries.
3. Coaches explain their own disciplinary rules and regulations concerning such problems as use of alcohol and drugs.
4. Coaches describe their conditioning program and what conditioning exercises the young athletes are expected to do at home.
5. The trainer or coach recommends a home health program, including improved eating and sleeping habits.
6. The athletic director explains the specific plan of action followed when an injury occurs and also describes the medical care available in communities where "away" games are played.
7. Each family receives an information sheet with emergency telephone numbers, health insurance and hospital information, and steps to be used in an emergency.
8. The trainer presents the contents of the trainer's bag and explains how each item is used.
9. The trainer or physician explains the risks of each sport, the typical injuries that occur, and specific care plans for a particular injury.
10. Coaches demonstrate the equipment worn for each sport and explain how it helps to prevent injuries. A good approach is to have a fully equipped player remove each piece of equipment as the coach explains its purpose.

practice in all active sports. Practice sessions in hockey, soccer, cross-country, tennis, football, and other sports should be covered for any unexpected major injury or catastrophe. In some cases the coach may be designated for sports injury care. Whoever is assigned should have a certified education for both first aid and CPR.

Medical Communication

The team physician should take the lead in developing a communication network for handling injuries to student athletes. This network should include the athletic director, coaches, parents, hospitals, and physicians. It is particularly important that the parents be notified in case of injury.

SPORTS SAFETY IN THE COMMUNITY

The Sports Safety Committee

With the surging numbers of young athletes and adult recreational athletes, it is paramount for a community to establish an overall program for sports safety. This would simply be following the preventive approach in health and medicine, such as immunization of babies, sex education, well-balanced diets, and nonsmoking. A sports safety program can minimize significant permanent injuries that occur to young athletes and adult recreational athletes.

An important first step is to establish a sports safety committee made up of responsible leaders involved in sports activities in the community. The committee should be small, limited in its goals, and not cumbersome or overindulgent. It should cover the major sports activities in the community, including activities run by the municipality's parks and recreation department, such as youth leagues and adult recreational leagues; school sports; individual sports activities; and private clubs in private competition.

As shown by the chart in Figure 2.1, the committee should be chaired by a physician

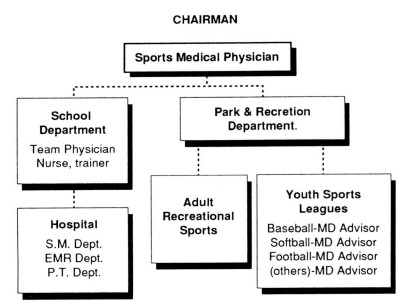

CHAIRMAN

Sports Medical Physician

School Department

Team Physician
Nurse, trainer

Hospital

S.M. Dept.
EMR Dept.
P.T. Dept.

Park & Recretion Department.

Adult Recreational Sports

Youth Sports Leagues

Baseball-MD Advisor
Softball-MD Advisor
Football-MD Advisor
(others)-MD Advisor

Figure 2.1. Community sports safety committee. In a well-established town or city, a YMCA/YWCA member may sit on the committee as well as a member of the special needs organization or a member of an active elderly community.

with expertise in sports medicine. Other members would include the high school team physician, nurse, and certified trainer; a representative of at least one youth league, such as Little League Baseball, Inc, the Youth Soccer League, or the National Youth Hockey Program; the director of parks and recreation; and a representative of the local hospital emergency room or sports clinic.

This small group would assemble useful sports safety information, set up simple monitoring systems, distribute helpful educational material, and assist the community in securing personnel for sports activities when needed (this could be done through the Boy Scouts, Girl Scouts, Demolay, or other youth organizations with adult leadership). Here are some suggestions for how a sports safety committee can carry out its mission successfully.

- Establish a volunteer organization coordinated with each of the sports programs in the community.

- Determine the number of participants in the different sports activities in the community, which would guide the committee in estimating the particular needs of each activity.
- Identify and coordinate available medical care in the community. A reference manual listing hospitals, sports medical clinics, HMOs, and private practitioners available for sports medical care would be helpful.
- Disseminate injury prevention material through the Boy Scouts, Girl Scouts, other voluntary organizations, and the high school.
- Support the education of coaches in first aid, CPR, and sports injury prevention.
- Establish a voluntary system of recording injuries. The figures may be somewhat inaccurate to begin with, but they would help in pinpointing problem areas.
- Coordinate with such programs as Little League Baseball, Inc and the Na-

tional Youth Coaches Association in carrying out sports medical prevention programs.

- With the help of a computer, register every athlete active in the community.

The most costly part of the program—beyond the volunteer's time—would be for educational and promotional literature. However, there are ways to reduce these costs. Such major organizations as the American College of Sports Medicine, the American Orthopedic Society for Sports Medicine, and the American Medical Society for Sports Medicine have a wealth of material at minimal cost. Other sources are private programs concerned with preventing sports injuries and government agencies such as state public health departments and the federal Department of Health and Human Services.

The sports safety committee can make a contribution of immeasurable value to the community by coordinating all youth and adult recreational sports programs with one central sports medical educational program.

Athletic Facilities in the Community

In most communities, athletic facilities are run by one of the following: 1) the school system, 2) the public works or parks departments, and 3) a private owner, or local colleges and universities.

Safety of school facilities is handled by the athletic director and the school maintenance department. Nonschool public playing fields and other sports facilities and usually maintained by the public works department in conjunction with the parks and recreational department and the local administrator of major sports such as baseball and soccer. College and university facilities are maintained by the school athletic department. These facilities are frequently used by community sports leagues in such sports as hockey, gymnastics, and basketball.

The limited availability of funds can adversely affect the maintenance of public sports facilities. Despite this, community pride and the popularity of sports can produce safe facilities. Unfortunately, however, there are often no set standards, regulations, or laws—or sometimes even fixed responsibilities—concerning the safety of community sports facilities. This is particularly true of privately owned facilities such as YMCA facilities, fitness centers, and aquatic schools.

This is a situation that can be changed by a sports medicine primary care physician who is actively involved in community sports programs. The physician can publicize the established safety standards for facilities in such sports as baseball, soccer, and football. If there is a community sports medical committee, the physician can take the lead in making sure that responsibility for the safety of local sports facilities is properly assigned. Just as we see areas in our communities being adopted by business, the various local athletic organizations can adopt community sports facilities.

The Primary Care Physician's Role in Injury Prevention

To significantly reduce the number of sports injuries in a community, the first step is to make the community aware of the problem. A community educational program is critical if safety procedures are to be improved. The primary care physician or the sports medical committee in association with the local hospital should present a safety awareness program for each sports activity in the community. Although statistics on sports injuries within a community may not be accurate or available at all, plenty of facts are available generally to make the community aware of the hazards of various sports. For example, it is unacceptable today to have a death from heat stroke during late summer high school football practice or cases of heat exhaustion in a cross-country running event. The facts about these hazards are well known and so are the procedures for reducing them.

Several publications are available that provide sports safety plans and guidelines for community sports activities. The National Youth Sports Coaches Association has an excellent sports injury prevention program. Communities should also consult their high school athletic department, which usually has a well-organized injury prevention program.

The sooner that community leaders become aware of the value of education in preventing sports injuries, the sooner the high cost of these injuries—in both suffering and money—will be reduced. The overuse of medical facilities will be eased as well. Safe sports are very cost effective.

Of course, awareness is meaningless unless it is followed by action. For example, once the parks and recreation department is made aware of baseball injuries and their prevention, it should supply such items as safety bases and safe fencing to reduce these injuries.

Sports Injury Prevention in Adult Recreational Leagues

One of the most difficult problems in sports injury prevention is to get the message to the massive number of adults actively competing in recreational leagues in a typical community. Most of them lead such busy lives that they are unlikely to attend seminars on the subject. One of the most effective ways to reach them is through a simple pamphlet or flyer distributed through banks, shopping malls, and other organizations. This publication should contain basic tips on such subjects as physical examinations, conditioning, coordinating competition, and plan of care.

Sports and Health

Sports medicine today does not deal only with sports injuries, but with the health benefits of sports. Good health is directly related to physical activity. From weight lifting to jogging, physical action and conditioning give people not only a feeling of well-being but a body that is actually healthier. Proper exercise is reported to lower blood pressure, control weight, and improve our ability to handle stress.

The primary care sports medicine physician (PCSMP) can be active in this area by speaking at weight-control clubs, aerobic groups, golden-age exercise programs, and similar groups. This will not only inform people of the health value of their activities but also enhance the image of the physician as someone who cares and is participating in the community.

The PCSMP can also participate in the referral system within the community for support and advice on drug and alcohol abuse, nutrition, family problems, and weight loss. In addition, the PCSMP should be aware of available visiting nurse programs, the nursing structures and programs for home care, and family organizations, as well as programs organized through churches and synagogues for young and old.

Medical Coverage of Athletic Events in the Community

It is important that athletic events in the community have good medical coverage in case of injuries.

All youth leagues and parks department activities should have an advisory physician, and coaches should be required to have training in first aid and CPR.

A PCSMP available for urgent consultation would be of tremendous value.

Special athletic events—an annual road race, gymnastic competition, swimming meet, trial event in horsemanship—should have an advisory physician and in some cases a physician actually present at the event.

APPENDIX A
RESOURCES ON SPORTS INJURIES AND SAFETY

Amateur Athletic Union
3400 West 86th Street
Indianapolis, IN 46268
317/872-2900

American Academy of Pediatricians
Committee on Sports Medicine
141 North West Point Boulevard
Elk Grove Village, IL 60009
312/228-5055

American Academy of Sports Physicians
7535 Laurel Canyon Boulevard
North Hollywood, CA 91605

American Alliance for Health, Physical
Education, Recreation, and Dance
900 Association Drive
Reston, VA 22091
703/476-3400

American College of Sports Medicine
P.O. Box 1440
Indianapolis, IN 46206
317/637-9200

American Medical Society for Sports
Medicine
P.O. Box 623
Middleton, WI 53562
608/831-4484

American Orthopaedic Society for Sports
Medicine
6300 N. River Road
Rosemont, IL 60018
708/292-4900

American Osteopathic Academy of Sports
Medicine
P.O. Box 623
Middleton, WI 53562
608/831-4484

American Physical Therapy Association
Sports Medical Section
505 King Street, Suite 115
Lacrosse, WI 54601
608/784-5800

Consumer Product Safety Commission
5401 Westband Avenue
Washington, DC 20207
301/504-0580

National Athletic Trainers Association
2952 Stemmons Freeway
Dallas, TX 75247
214/637-6282

National Federation of State High School
Associations
11724 Plaza Circle
Box 20626
Kansas City, MO 64153
816/464-5400

National Operating Committee on Standards
for Athletic Equipment (NOCSAE)
10111 West 87th Street
Shawnee Mission, KS 66212
913/888-1340

National Safety Council
444 North Michigan Avenue
Chicago, IL 60611
800/621-7619

National Youth Sports Foundation for the
Prevention of Sports Injuries
10 Meredith Circle
Needham, MA 02192
617/449-2499

United Sports Academy
124 University Boulevard
P.O. Box 8650
Mobile, AL 36608

United States Olympic Committee
Sports Medicine
1 Olympic Plaza
Colorado Springs, CO 80909
719/632-5551

RESOURCES ON COACHING EDUCATION

American Coaching Effectiveness Program
P.O. Box 5076
Champaign, IL 61825
217/351-5076

Coaching Association of Canada
1600 Prom. James Naismith Drive
Gloucester, Ontario, Canada K1B SN4
613/748-5624

National Youth Sports Coaches Association
2611 Old Okeechobee Road
West Palm Beach, FL 33409
407/684-1141

Youth Sports Institute
Michigan State University
213 I.M. Sports Circle
East Lansing, MI 48824
517/353-6689

RESOURCES ON YOUNG ATHLETES WITH DISABILITIES

National Handicapped Sports and Recreational
    Association
4405 East-West Highway, Suite 603
Bethesda, MD 20814
301/652-7505

National Wheelchair Athletic Association
3595 East Fountain Boulevard
Colorado Springs, CO 80910
719/574-1150

Special Olympics International
1325 G Street, N.W., Suite 500
Washington, DC 20005
202/628-3630

United States Association for Blind Athletes
33 North Institute Drive
Colorado Springs, CO 80903
719/630-0422

United States Cerebral Palsy Athletic
    Association
34518 Warren Road, Suite 264
Westland, MI 48185
313/425-8961

RESOURCES ON SPECIFIC SPORTS

Babe Ruth Baseball

P.O. Box 5000
1770 Brunswich Avenue
Trenton, NJ 08630
609/695-1434

Baseball

Little League International, Inc
P.O. Box 3485
Williamsport, PA 17701
717/326-1921

Basketball

USA Basketball
5465 Mark Dabling Boulevard
Colorado Springs, CO 80918
719/590-4800

Cycling

United States Cycling Federation
1 Olympic Plaza
Colorado Springs, CO 80909
719/632-5551

Dance

National Dance Association
1900 Association Drive
Reston, VA 22091
703/476-3490

Equestrian Sports

American Horse Show Association
220 East 42nd Street
New York, NY 10017
212/972-2472

Fencing

United States Fencing Association
1 Olympic Plaza
Colorado Springs, CO 80909
719/578-4511

Field Hockey

United States Field Hockey Association
1 Olympic Plaza
Colorado Springs, CO 80909
719/578-4567

Football

Pop Warner Football
1315 Walnut Street, Suite 1632
Philadelphia, PA 19107
215/735-1450

Golf

American Junior Golf Association
2415 Steeplechase Lane
Roswell, GA 30076
404/998-4653

Gymnastics

Young American Gymnastic School
10601 Northwest Ambassador Drive
Kansas City, MO 64153
816/891-1077

Hockey

Amateur Hockey Association of the United
  States
2997 Bradmore Valley Road
Colorado Springs, CO 80906
719/578-4990

Lacrosse

U.S. Women's Lacrosse Association
45 Maple Avenue
Hamilton, NY 13346
315/824-8661

Lacrosse Foundation, Inc
Newton H. White Athletic Center
  Baltimore, MD 21218
301/235-6882

Skating

United States Figure Skating Association
20 First Street
Colorado Springs, CO 80906
719/635-5200

Skiing

United States Skiing Educational Foundation
P.O. Box 100
Park City, UT 84060
801/649-9090

Soccer

United States Soccer Federation
1 Olympic Plaza
Colorado Springs, CO 80909
719/578-4779

United States Youth Soccer Association
1835 Union Avenue, Suite 190
Memphis, TN 38104
800/476-2237

Softball

Amateur Softball Association of America
2801 N.E. 50th Street
Oklahoma City, OK 73111
405/424-5266

Squash and Racquetball

United States Squash and Racquet Association
P.O. Box 1216
23 Cynwyd Road
Bala-Cynwyd, PA 19004
215/667-4006

Swimming

United States Swimming, Inc.
1 Olympic Plaza
Colorado Springs, CO 80909
719/578-4578

AAU USA Junior Olympics
3400 West 86th Street
Indianapolis, IN 46268
317/872-2900

Tennis

United States Tennis Association
707 Alexander Road
Princeton, NJ 08540
609/452-2580

Track and Field

A T Congress
P.O. Box 120
Indianapolis, IN 46206
317/261-0500

Volleyball

United States Volleyball Association
1 Olympic Plaza
Colorado Springs, CO 80909
719/632-5551

Weight Lifting

National Strength and Conditioning
    Association
300 Old City Hall Landmark
9160 Street, P.O. Box 81410
Lincoln, NE 68501
402/476-6976

Wrestling

USA Wrestling
6155 Lehman Drive
Colorado Springs, CO 80918
719/598-8181

PREPARTICIPATION EVALUATION OF THE SCHOOL ATHLETE

KARL B. FIELDS

National and State Standards
Goals and Format for the Preparticipation
  Evaluation
Conditions That Limit Participation
Conditions That Increase the Risk of
  Injury
Sports-Specific Physical Evaluation
The Role of Laboratory and Other Testing
Disposition of the Athlete

In the 1960s the American Medical Association's Committee on Medical Aspects of Sports endorsed a "bill of rights for the school and college athlete." The first health provision on this document was the right to a ". . . thorough preseason history and medical examination." The intent of this action was to reduce "sports tragedies" that occurred from "unrecognized health problems" (1). This effort quickly spread to most states and mandatory preparticipation evaluations (PPEs) became the norm before athletes could compete in school organized sports. Although physicians, coaches, and parents agree about the importance of screening athletes, sports medicine research has not determined what constitutes a thorough PPE.

In addition to disagreement concerning the thoroughness of these examinations, no consensus has emerged about who performs the examination, where the examination takes place, how often athletes need examinations, and what legal standing the examinations hold. These unanswered questions have not deterred growing use of this medical visit. Marked increases in the numbers of male and female participants in sports programs have helped push PPEs to the second most frequent health maintenance visit following well baby examinations.

In 1992, five medical organizations concerned with the care of school-aged athletes presented a joint publication entitled *Preparticipation Physical Evaluation* (2). Although this monograph did not resolve the areas of disagreement listed above, certain specific risks and concerns regarding sports participation are clearly discussed (see Appendix B). Consensus has emerged that PPEs must address sports-specific questions and help direct athletes to safe activity in sports and everyday life.

This chapter reviews current thinking about controversial and noncontroversial issues surrounding the prescreening of athletes.

NATIONAL AND STATE STANDARDS

National standards have not been established for PPEs; however, sports medicine committees for state medical associations have generally recommended forms adopted by their high school athletic associations. In a few areas, local school systems mandate the standards for preparticipation evaluation. Four states lack specific guidelines. A majority of states have declared these to be medical examinations that require the clearance of a licensed medical practitioner. A review of current requirements is listed in Tables 3.1 and 3.2 (personal communication, North Carolina High School Athletic Association).

GOALS AND FORMAT FOR THE PREPARTICIPATION EVALUATION

The original intent of the PPE was to screen athletes for conditions that might

Table 3.1. Preparticipation examiner requirements (50 states)

Physicians* only	22
Physician assistants and nurse practitioners	15
Chiropractors	7
Naturopaths	1
Physical therapists	1
Not specified	4

* Physicians can complete these in all 50 states and by law must supervise physicians assistants and in most states nurse practitioners.

Table 3.2. Preparticipation examination
frequency (50 states)

Yearly	37
At entry to high or middle school	2
Every other year	6
Before each sport	1
Left to local school district	4

lead to catastrophic injury. The primary
goals of the examination are thus to detect
potentially lethal or serious medical conditions and to identify problems that place
the athlete at greater risk of serious injury.
Some authors feel that meeting insurance
and legal requirements should be listed
as a primary goal (2). However, these
change from year to year and from state
to state, and it is unclear whether any
examination satisfies legal and insurance
standards.

Secondary goals include general health,
counseling, maturity assessment, and fitness evaluation (2). Whether any secondary
goals can be achieved on a PPE depends on
the format chosen for the examination.
Over the past two decades authors have
suggested three divergent approaches to
the PPE. These include focusing the examination to address sports-specific risks, expanding the examination to better meet
needs of general health care, or changing
the examination to evaluate the common
problems in adolescent medicine. Each of
these approaches has persuasive argu-
ments, but no outcome studies have indicated the superiority of one approach over
another.

Sports medicine physicians who opt for
focused examinations feel that adolescents
seeking clearance for participation are
rarely interested in more medical care. They
cite a 1% disqualification rate as demonstra-
tive of the futility of expending too much
medical attention on a relatively healthy
population. Another factor limiting widespread adoption of comprehensive examinations is limited access—particularly to
primary care physicians. Focused examinations can direct more careful evaluation to
high-risk areas like the musculoskeletal and
the cardiovascular systems, while devoting
minimal attention to any other area of the
physical examination unless patient history
indicates a cause for concern. These examinations can be completed quickly, thus
eliminating some of the stress on the health
care providers, particularly in rural or
underserved areas.

Proponents of a *comprehensive examination*
feel that screening examinations fail to detect important medical conditions and offer
little benefit to the athlete. A more extensive
evaluation also offers the opportunity to
initiate preventive care and health promotion. They argue that the origins of many
serious health problems such as coronary
artery disease, hypertension, and obesity
begin in childhood or adolescence. Failure
to detect these at an early age may delay
effective intervention for years.

Adolescent medicine specialists generally see limited utility in either a sports-
specific or medically oriented examination.
They note that most sports activity occurs
during the formative years when athletes
are more at risk for accidental injury or
suicide than for most medical conditions.
Because adolescents rarely see a physician,
the PPE has been viewed as a window of
opportunity to target *adolescent health care*.
Issues such as sexually transmitted diseases, emotional distress, risk-taking
behavior, and substance abuse become a
core part of the process. They feel these take
precedence over the limited risk that sports
activity entails.

Because sports PPEs are performed by multiple specialties, inherent biases for one type of examination versus another are common. Recommendations from sports medicine committees in neighboring states sometimes lead them to adopt essentially opposite approaches to PPEs. For example, the state of North Carolina adopted a focused examination that reviews a brief history (13 questions) and a core examination consisting of blood pressure, weight, vision, a musculoskeletal examination, and a cardiovascular examination (3) (see Appendices C and D). They recommend performing these in the personal physician's office when possible. The neighboring state of Virginia asks physicians to perform station examinations in which complete physical assessment also includes Tanner stages and body fat analysis.

The ideal PPE would integrate the best components of each format. The athlete's personal physician certainly brings more continuity to medical care but may lack special skills. Unfortunately, few physicians are equally competent in medical, orthopedic, and adolescent health care. A team of evaluators may better perform these multiple aspects of the examination, but the value of this is lost if they fail to communicate a consistent opinion to parents or coaches. Because no one approach consistently achieves a better result, the skills of individual physicians and the setting in which the examination takes place may dictate the format chosen. Regardless of physician preference, parents and athletes ultimately determine whether they feel more comfortable in a private office setting or a station examination. Recognizing this, national organizations have chosen not to endorse either format but to educate physicians about the advantages and disadvantages to each.

CONDITIONS THAT LIMIT PARTICIPATION

Cardiac Problems

Medical conditions that affect the cardiovascular system are the ones that most commonly result in disqualification from sports activity. The most serious cardiac problems increase the risk of sudden cardiac death with exercise. Estimates suggest that 1 in 200,000 athletes will die suddenly from cardiac causes. Autopsy studies identify the most common conditions that cause sudden cardiac death as hypertrophic cardiomyopathy, concentric left ventricular hypertrophy, Marfan's syndrome, congenital coronary artery anomalies, and myocarditis. Arrhythmias may cause death without detectable pathology at autopsy. A variety of conditions including preexcitation syndromes, long QT syndromes, and mitral valve prolapse can trigger potentially dangerous rhythm disturbances. (For a more extensive discussion of cardiac abnormalities, see Chapter 21.) Classic cardiac anomalies such as valvular disease, anomalies of the great vessels, septal defects, and cushion defects generally have been diagnosed before sports participation. An exception to this may be the Special Olympics competitor. Unfortunately, a new class of acquired cardiac disease relates to use of illicit drugs and ergogenic substances. Examples include cocaine with its known tendency to induce cardiac damage and anabolic steroids, which have caused marked hyperlipidemia and subsequent coronary artery thrombosis.

The best method of screening for sudden cardiac death (SCD) seems to be a careful history. Questions of particular importance include: Has anyone in the athlete's immediate family died suddenly before age 50? Has the athlete experienced severe dizziness or passed out during or immediately after exercise? Has the athlete been told he or she has a heart murmur or heart problem?

These sample questions all focus on cardiac symptoms or factors that increase risk for heart problems. Hypertrophic cardiomyopathy is an autosomal dominant condition with variable penetration. A family history of premature death suggests this condition. Dizziness or syncope may occur with outflow obstruction (valvular or subvalvular disease) or arrhythmias. Any of the common conditions that lead to SCD can trigger arrhythmias, and so this question screens for a number of pathologic conditions. An athlete with a prior history of murmur or heart disease needs a more cautious evaluation to be sure no residual cardiac problem is overlooked.

A history of chest pain with exertion helps identify patients with classic angina but is a less useful question for adolescent competitors. Coronary artery disease is the most common cause of SCD for athletes over the age of 35 but remains rare in the school-aged athlete. Chest pain in younger athletes remains a somewhat vague symptom. One series of cardiac evaluations of younger athletes with exertional chest pain demonstrated exercise-induced asthma as the most common cause. Musculoskeletal problems and reflux esophagitis also produce chest pain that may mimic cardiac causes.

Hypertension

Preparticipation studies identify hypertension as one of the most frequent medical disorders detected on screening. This has been the case, although none of the major studies adjusted pressures to conform to lower levels for hypertension established by the Second Task Force on Blood Pressure Control in Children. Research demonstrates that 5% to 10% of children and adolescents may have an exaggerated blood pressure elevation with exercise (e.g., systolic pressure greater than 180 to 200 mmHg depending on age), and these percentages are much higher than the 1% to 2% typically identified on PPEs. Preliminary studies suggest that athletes with a hypertensive response following exercise have a strong likelihood of developing hypertension within 10 years. Echocardiographic evidence of diastolic dysfunction occurs within 10 years of diagnosis in young hypertensives. This raises the question of whether unrecognized severe hypertension may be the etiologic factor responsible for concentric left ventricular hypertrophy, a leading cause of SCD. Asking the athlete if he or she has ever had high blood pressure or if any immediate family members have had hypertension may indicate a need for more careful blood pressure follow-up.

Rather than rely on a fixed number as representative of blood pressure elevation, physicians should adjust blood pressure measures to reflect the age of the athlete. Using the percentile method, athletes classified as severe hypertensives (>99th percentile for age) should be disqualified from strenuous sports activity until they come under adequate control, even though no direct association between hypertension and SCD has been found (Table 3.3). Athletes in the significant hypertension group (>95th percentile) should not be disqualified from participation as long as close monitoring shows that blood pressure is adequately controlled. Mild or borderline hypertensives may participate in all sports activity. They should follow standard non-pharmacologic measures including reduction of sodium intake. They need to balance

Table 3.3. Hypertension in adolescents

	Normal to High (>90th%)	Hypertension (>95th%)	Severe Hypertension (>99th%)
Age 13–15			
Systolic (mm Hg)	130–135	136–143	>143
Diastolic (mm Hg)	80–85	86–91	>91
Age 16–18			
Systolic (mm Hg)	136–141	142–149	>149
Diastolic (mm Hg)	84–91	92–97	>98

resistance and isometric exercise with a minimum of 45 minutes of moderate aerobic exercise weekly. A regimen of resistance exercise only may have a negative rather than positive impact on their blood pressure control. Routine scheduled follow-ups and monitoring of medical therapy should be prerequisites for play.

Neurologic Injury or Illness

Concussion occurs commonly in contact/collision sports. Football statistics reveal 250,000 concussions yearly in the United States. A single concussion increases the risk of a subsequent occurrence by fourfold. In addition, case reports of "second impact catastrophic head injuries" point out that not all clinically minor concussions are benign and that multiple concussions increase risk. In fact, increased use of computed tomography and magnetic resonance imaging scans demonstrates cortical contusions, minor hemorrhages, and pathologic lesions for many athletes who have minimal ongoing neurologic symptoms or signs (see Chapter 4). Asking the athlete, Have you ever been knocked out (had a concussion)? helps select individuals who deserve further questioning. Any ongoing symptoms or a history of multiple concussions merits cautious neurologic clearance.

The implications of *brachial plexus injury* are less clear. Follow-up evaluation of football players reveals a significant number who have recurrent grade 1 brachial plexus injuries commonly referred to as stingers or burners. Follow-up data have not shown that these individuals later experience permanent neurologic injury. However, persistent symptoms or weakness mandate further evaluation. In addition, most physicians would not clear a player with a history of transient quadriplegia to return to contact/collision sports (see Chapter 5).

A history of *epilepsy* does not specifically exclude athletes from sports participation. However, the athlete must have well-controlled seizures before competing in any sport with a risk of collision or contact. In addition, water sports, aerial sports, and riding sports (equipment or equestrian) place these athletes at an unacceptable risk even if their seizures are well controlled. With a rare breakthrough seizure, the chances of a fatal accident are too high.

Asthma

Screenings of the 1984 and 1988 Olympic teams emphasized how commonly athletes experience exercise-induced asthma (EIA). In these tests 9% to 11% had EIA. The author has screened 300 school-aged athletes of whom 17% had peak exercise flow rate (PEFR) drops consistent with EIA following a standard free run challenge of 8 to 10 minutes. Asking the following question identifies a high-risk group: Do you have a history of asthma (wheezing), hay fever, or persistent coughing after exercise? Estimates vary but virtually 100% of athletes with true asthma will wheeze at some point with exercise; approximately 40% of allergic rhinitis patients experience EIA; and one study showed 80% of those with a history of persistent exercise-induced cough showed drops in PEFR consistent with EIA. At least half of the positive individuals identified on testing are unaware of any problem; thus, diagnosis remains elusive unless the physician probes.

The emphasis on diagnosis of EIA patients is to allow them to continue participating in sports. Often these athletes are labeled as "lazy" or "attitude problems." Aggressive treatment allows even severe asthmatics to control symptoms sufficiently to compete. In fact, a higher percentage of asthmatic participants in Olympic games have won medals when compared to nonasthmatic peers.

Heat Illness

Has the athlete ever had heat stroke, severe cramping, or dehydration in hot weather? This type of query allows the doctor to identify individuals who have a serious risk for a potentially fatal condition. Heat problems are avoidable; thus, the continued yearly occurrence of deaths represents a failure to adequately identify or treat susceptible individuals. Risk factors that place athletes at greater risk include poor condition, obesity, lack of acclimatization to environmental conditions, medical illnesses, dehydration, use of certain medications, and prior problems handling heat stress. Certain individuals have

a physiologic difficulty dissipating heat. Careful monitoring of pre- and postpractice weights and even on-field temperature assessments may be needed to protect the athlete's safety (see Chapter 19).

Poor fitness leads the athlete to have a higher caloric expenditure for the same level of work. Burning calories produces heat and higher core temperatures. These athletes will sweat excessively in an effort to lower their body temperatures. These and other factors add to place the "out of shape" person in a special risk group. To try to predict this, some physicians advocate asking about fitness. For example, the doctor may ask, Can you run a mile without stopping? Any athlete not in the poorest fitness level should answer this affirmatively.

Substance Abuse

Substance abuse has been identified in a number of sudden death cases and may replace congenital cardiac anomalies as the leading cause of mortality in athletes (Table 3.4) (4). Cocaine usage causes specific medical problems including arrhythmias, coronary artery vasospasm, myocardial infarction, aortic rupture, cerebrovascular accidents, and increased susceptibility to heat illness. Anabolic steroids have numerous effects, some of which

Table 3.4. Drug use among intercollegiate athletes

Alcohol	88%
Amphetamines	8%
Anabolic steroids	6.5%
Cocaine	17%
Marijuana	36%

SOURCE: Adapted from Mellion MB, Walsh WM, Shelton GL, eds. The team physician's handbook. St. Louis: Mosby–Year Book, 1990:112.

are not clearly understood, but usage has been associated with myocardial infarction, cerebrovascular accidents, psychosis, and hepatic dysfunction. Despite the serious toxicities of cocaine and anabolic steroids, alcohol remains the most commonly abused substance and leads to the greatest morbidity. Amphetamines and marijuana are also used commonly. See Chapter 25 for a more extensive discussion of substance abuse.

Getting the athlete to discuss concerns about substance abuse requires rapport and good interviewing skills. These problems are unlikely to come to light unless the PPE takes place in a private setting and the athlete feels certain that confidential information would not be reported to coaches or parents. Open-ended questions help create the opportunity for the athlete to respond in sensitive areas. For example, Do you have anything you want to talk to me about? Asking questions about the home situation—How are things at home? Does anyone in your household use too much alcohol?—may help initiate discussion about personal stress. Clearly, the continuity of working as a team physician gives the doctor many more chances to detect substance abuse than does the PPE.

General Health Concerns

Many athletes have a chronic medical illness. Fortunately, when treated appropriately most can participate in competitive sports. For example, specific recommendations may be needed for skin disorders before wrestling participation. Diabetic individuals in cross-country sports must adjust their diets or medications because of the increased caloric needs of vigorous activity. In each situation care must be individualized, but team physicians and trainers need to know about each athlete's

specific medical needs. The following questions help obtain this information: Do you take any regular medications? Do you have any chronic illnesses or see a doctor regularly? Other aspects of general medical care include knowledge of the past medical history including concerns about allergies, absence of a paired organ, and previous hospitalizations or surgeries. Current visual status, dental health, and immunization status need to be updated.

CONDITIONS THAT INCREASE THE RISK OF INJURY

One of the classic wisdoms in sports medicine is that the most common injury is reinjury. Prospective studies of knee injuries in particular have documented that an athlete with knee injury in one season has a greatly increased risk of a knee injury during the next season. Additional research shows that muscles around the injured joint rarely recover full strength by the time athletes return to competition. These types of observations imply that rehabilitation is inadequate—whether due to noncompliance by athletes or failure to prescribe by physicians. For this reason physicians should ask about prior musculoskeletal problems. For example: Have you ever broken a bone, had to wear a cast, or had an injury to any joint? Asking specifically about wearing a cast is important because some athletes do not understand that the terms "broken bone" and "fracture" are equivalent. If an athlete has had musculoskeletal trauma, asking about the type of therapy received and the ongoing exercise program gives some idea whether the individual is likely to have done enough to prevent recurrent problems.

SPORTS-SPECIFIC PHYSICAL EVALUATION

Since the history identifies 85% of the problems, this part of the PPE deserves primary emphasis. Nevertheless, certain areas of the physical examination yield a number of pertinent findings. Problems identified during the history may point to which parts of the examination are likely to be abnormal. Sports-specific risks also merit more cautious screening. For example, skin infections have led to major problems in wrestling, so a skin examination is important for this athlete, but less so for a tennis player.

General evaluation includes the overall appearance of the athlete. Extremely thin athletes or obviously obese athletes warrant questioning about dietary habits. The only objective sign of an eating disorder may be the general appearance. The height and weight are essential components of the examination and the physician may choose to list a minimal or maximal safe weight for competition to ensure the athlete's safety. Occasionally a flat affect may suggest depression. Extreme agitation during a routine examination may raise the question of occult substance abuse in an athlete trying to hide this from the doctor.

Vital signs offer important information that too often is cursorily obtained. Elevated pulses may arise from nervousness but could indicate a persistent low-grade infection, use of a stimulant medicine, a myocarditis, or other serious problem. The anxious athlete's pulse returns to normal after a brief period of rest. As noted above, blood pressures deserve careful measurement and when elevated need repeated checks. Many athletes require larger cuffs because of muscular arms. If pressures are high, arm and leg pressures are indi-cated. Elevation of either temperature or respiratory rate needs clarification.

Visual acuity usually can be screened with simple Snellen charts. However, when athletes use contacts or glasses, corrected and uncorrected visions are helpful. The examination should note whether the athlete actually uses the visual aid in competition. One pertinent physical finding concerning the eyes is the presence of anisocoria. This type of finding could be interpreted incorrectly if the athlete experienced a head injury.

Cardiovascular examination seeks to identify murmurs that are pathologic markers. Because many athletes at some time have a benign-sounding flow murmur, determining characteristics that indicate disease is important. The critical murmur to identify is the one suggestive of hypertrophic cardiomyopathy that causes most sudden cardiac death in athletes. Generally this is a systolic murmur that begins shortly after the first heart sound and often is loudest at the left sternal border. Fortunately, certain specific maneuvers accentuate this murmur. Rising to a standing position from a lying one increases the intensity of the murmur because this position change allows blood to pool in the lower extremities, increasing the degree of subvalvular stenosis. Valvular murmurs, regurgitant murmurs, patent ductus aorta, and other classic murmurs have characteristics well described in standard physical diagnosis texts. Fortunately, these conditions are usually detected in childhood. Coarctation of the aorta and atrial septal defect are two additional entities that sometimes escape detection until adolescent years. The athlete with hypertension on arm measurement but lower blood pressures in the thigh and a diminished femoral pulse may have an undiagnosed coarctation. An athlete with a benign-sounding pulmonic flow murmur but a fixed split second heart sound deserves evaluation for an atrial septal defect.

Marfan's syndrome more likely would be suspected because of classic findings including arachnodactyly, long arm span, hypermobile joints, pectus excavatum or carinatum, high arched palate, or ectopic lens. Cardiac changes are variable but include valvular regurgitant murmurs of both the aortic and mitral valves, mitral valve prolapse with a click, or an entirely normal auscultation. Myocarditis, cardiomyopathies, long QT syndrome, Wolff-Parkinson-White syndrome, and other conditions may not have a specific marker on physical examination. Detection or irregular beats or unexplainable tachycardia may be a clue to some of these entities, and diagnosis is established with electrocardiography (ECG) and further work-up.

Musculoskeletal examination detects the greatest number of athletes who have a condition that may limit their ability to compete. For this reason the author does not suggest use of widely publicized shortcuts such as "the 2-minute musculoskeletal examination." No published references clarify that these screens can reliably identify instability of major joints. A careful evaluation of the knee, ankle, and shoulder can be completed quickly. Instability of one of these three joints accounts for the vast majority of disqualifications and identifies a number of athletes who need rehabilitation before participation.

Knee instabilities account for 50% of the disqualifications from sport in a number of the studies that recorded the findings from PPEs. The most common serious problem is a torn anterior cruciate ligament. A positive Lachman test shows that the ligament is severed and will not prevent anterior translation of the knee. An anterior drawer may demonstrate the same finding but less reliably. The athlete with significant knee pathology usually shows atrophy of the quadriceps on the affected side with the vastus medialis obliquus most severely affected. McMurray's test for meniscus injuries and collateral ligament stress tests occasionally reveal injuries to these structures that escape detection until the PPE. Although these serious problems are rare, conditions like patellofemoral stress syndrome (chondromalacia), painful plicas, and inflammation of the iliotibial band insertion commonly occur. Identification can allow the physician to prescribe appropriate therapy. (See Chapter 15 for further discussion.)

Ankle sprains are the most common sports injury that cause athletes to miss practice and competition. An athlete who has laxity to inversion, cannot bear full weight on the outer edge of either inverted foot, and has trouble running zigzag patterns does not have adequate ankle stability to play most running or jumping sports. Functional maneuvers more reliably show the degree of ankle disability than does a simple physical exam.

Shoulder examination focuses on clinical problems that frequently lead to difficulty. For example, an apprehension test stresses the shoulder in a position of abduction and external rotation. This is the most vulnerable position for anterior shoulder dislocation. An athlete who has had a prior shoulder dislocation but has not rehabilitated the shoulder girdle shows fear of a repeat injury when tested in this fashion. Similarly, impingement of the supraspinatus tendon in a limited anatomic space commonly causes shoulder problems in racquet sports, swimming, or throwing sports. Stress applied against the arm as the shoulder is flexed to 90°, internally rotated, and tested in various degrees of abduction (e.g., "empty beer can position") can identify positions in which impingement clinically causes weakness of the supraspinatus mechanism. Careful testing of the rotator cuff, deltoid, bicipital tendon, and other structures around the shoulder girdle may show that an athlete needs specific strengthening before starting sports that require heavy use of the upper extremity. (See Chapter 10 for further discussion.)

The remainder of the musculoskeletal examination including screening the neck, wrist, elbow, hands, and feet; looking at the back for scoliosis; and examining the lower extremity for malalignment can be accomplished through observation and simple maneuvers, without testing strength or specific ligamentous integrity. On rare occasions the history suggests a more in-depth evaluation.

Ear, nose and throat, lungs, abdomen, genitourinary tract, skin, and neurologic review have a minimal role in PPEs. These areas rarely demonstrate significant abnormalities in physically fit athletes. For individuals whose history places them at increased risk of injury additional examination serves a function. Ear, nose and throat and lung evaluations are indicated in an atopic athlete or one with asthma. A recent history of mononucleosis mandates an abdominal examination to detect splenomegaly. In general, the individual physician will exercise judgment about how comprehensive the evaluation should be and which of these components of a physical merit inclusion. Screening for testicular cancer merits consideration but privacy issues make this controversial.

Assessment of Maturity

Theoretically, physically immature athletes who compete in contact and collision sports should experience greater risk and more frequent serious injuries. This makes logical sense when one simply compares the dramatic difference in physical characteristics of two 13-year-olds, one who is Tanner 2 and another Tanner 4 on the maturity scale. Injury statistics in sport have not borne out this logical conclusion. The highest risk for adolescent sports injury is in the 16- and 17-year-old athletes virtually all of whom are Tanner stage 4. Why is this the case? Originally, researchers felt that older athletes had more playing time and thus more injuries. This did not consider that practice time was similar. In fact, when contact hours are the same, the older athletes still experience more injuries. Other explanations include that the older adolescent may be more of a "risk taker" in sports just as they are in other aspects of life. Another possibility is that the greater muscle strength in Tanner 4 athletes actually allows them to develop greater speed and hit with enough impact to increase injury risk.

Tanner classifications for maturity have proven validity in determining the maturational development of adolescents. A major problem in using these is that they rely on the changes of secondary sexual development to estimate maturity. Adequate privacy for athletes, chaperoning needs, and emotional stress for shy, perhaps physically immature athletes are among the drawbacks to incorporating these as a component of routine PPEs. Sensitivity to these issues led to studies of Tanner self-rating by using pictures. This method seems to correlate well with actual examination and many physicians use this approach as a substitute. One other type of screen that does not require disrobing relies on standards for grip strength. Using a hand grip dynamometer, athletes who test above a certain level of grip strength predictably have reached physical maturity.

Despite the development of several reliable maturity screens, the basic question remains—Should maturity assessment be a part of routine PPEs? Currently, no epidemiologic evidence shows a preponderance of physical or other injuries to less mature athletes in standard American sports. Recently, the highest numbers of physical injuries seem to occur in age-matched sports such as youth soccer in which the competitors are well matched, but the intensity may be high for the age groups participating. Until more information emerges, physicians should follow their personal bias as to whether to include maturity assessment as a part of the PPE. Although physicians may advise immature athletes to consider less risky sports, no firm evidence suggests disqualification.

Assessment of Fitness Level

Little debate exists about the value of determining fitness level. Athletes with better strength and cardiovascular fitness have fewer problems adapting to the rigors of sports. From the safety perspective, cardiovascular fitness has protective benefits against heat and altitude illness. Flexibility and muscular strength may play a role in injury prevention. Numerous simple techniques allow the physician to reliably measure both flexibility and strength. Cardiovascular fitness can be estimated by comparing distance run in a given time versus standardized charts (e.g., Cooper 12-minute test). At best, though, these measures, while helpful, generally supplement the core components of a PPE. Only in extreme circumstances would deconditioning be a cause for disqualification. In fact, the "out of shape" athlete may benefit most from consistent sports activity. The limiting factor is that most physicians have minimal

time to complete the basic PPE and though they may wish to assess fitness, can better delegate this task to coaching staffs. Advice from a team physician may influence coaches to devote more attention to the importance of balanced training to develop both musculoskeletal strength and cardiovascular conditioning.

THE ROLE OF LABORATORY AND OTHER TESTING

Historically urinalysis and hematocrit were the core laboratory evaluations on PPEs. Numerous athletes showed proteinuria on dipstick testing. Subsequent follow-up of the utility of this finding in demonstrating significant genitourinary pathology showed that this was not a marker for disease. Nor did the glucose testing find unsuspected diabetics. For these reasons, routine urinalysis was dropped from PPEs as a recommended test.

Hematocrit or hemoglobin measures do detect a reasonable number of athletes with anemia. Female athletes with heavy menstruation or with poor dietary intake often develop iron deficiency anemia. This is important clinical information, but the hemoglobin level does not determine who can safely participate. For this reason the screen for anemia seems most appropriate as a part of ongoing medical follow-up rather than the PPE. If the examining physician is also the athlete's family physician, then the measurement of hemoglobin can be done with plan for appropriate treatment and follow-up.

In special situations additional laboratory testing may arise because of positive responses in the history. For example, if an athlete gave a history of amenorrhea specific tests differentiate medical causes from exercise-induced amenorrhea. The athlete with amenorrhea who also shows anemia deserves special attention. Without menstrual periods excessive iron loss is unlikely, so that assessment of possible eating disorders or extreme diets may be triggered by the abnormal lab value. (See Chapter 23 for further discussion.)

ECG testing is not a routine part of PPEs, but often follows finding of irregular beats on the routine cardiovascular examination. Although some physicians have advocated extensive prescreening of cardiovascular risk for all athletes with ECGs and even echocardiograms, studies to date have not shown sufficient sensitivity of these tests to screen for the rare athlete who may be at risk for SCD. Subgroups of athletes such as those with hypertension or specific murmurs should have an ECG before competition, but until more definitive studies arise routine use is not indicated.

DISPOSITION OF THE ATHLETE

Physicians often fail to use all options when evaluating an athlete for participation. The decision whether an athlete may compete safely may require more information than can be obtained in a brief screening. In this situation the physician should defer clearance until all needed data are collected. For example, an athlete who had knee injury or surgery the previous season may return with some atrophy and strength difference on the affected extremity. If any doubt exists as to whether the muscles will withstand the rigors of competition, quantitative assessment of strength on standardized testing equipment by a physical therapist may objectively assess readiness to play. Appropriate strengthening programs can be prescribed for athletes with an identified strength deficit. For most

orthopedic problems clearance to participate can follow rehabilitation and occasionally corrective surgery. The physician seeks to establish that the athlete has regained at least 90% of expected strength, the full range of motion of any affected joints, and functional use of the anatomic area. Although joint instability is the major cause for disqualification, appropriate treatment returns these athletes to play at a later date in most cases.

The cardiovascular examination disqualifies the second largest number of athletes from participation. Nevertheless, of all competitors referred for full cardiac evaluation because of suspected pathologic problems only 20% truly have cardiac disease. Athletic hearts that cause rhythm disturbances, functional murmurs, and ECG changes are more common than true pathology. A common statistical principle explains this phenomena in that false positive findings are more common than true positive findings in a population with low prevalence of disease. Throughout adolescence organic disease occurs less commonly than changes related to growth and development, psychological adjustment, or risk-taking behavior. Often for suspected organic disease, clearance to participate can follow more extensive work-up.

An example of a conditional clearance would be the athlete with mild to moderate hypertension. As long as blood pressure treatment keeps levels in an acceptable range no restrictions are necessary. Clearance would depend on scheduled follow-up blood pressure checks and acceptable compliance of the athlete with the treatment regimen.

Clearance also varies by sport (see Appendix E). For example, an athlete with a hemoglobinopathy may have splenomegaly. This athlete could not safely be cleared for participation in contact or collision sports. However, as long as the athlete has adequate aerobic capacity, he or she could compete in a sport such as tennis.

SUMMARY

No single format or standardized examination determines clearance for athletic participation. Individual physician bias, local school system requirements, demands of specific sports, availability of professionals, and other factors determine which type of examination best fits a given locale. Nevertheless, attempts to define a core examination that most states will endorse continue. Important problems that merit careful screening have been identified in the history and physical to help detect the rare athlete who may be at undue risk of serious injury or death. The PPE at minimum should address the core areas that allow safe participation. Perhaps in the ideal form, the PPE can occasionally address problems of general prevention and adolescent development.

The physician should always remember that physical activity may be the best predictor of good health and longevity. These examinations should encourage participation and only on rare instances lead to disqualification. In assisting the athlete to compete in the sport the physician may well give the best preventive medicine that exists. In this sense the PPE has a value that far outweighs its utility for detecting medical problems.

References

1. O'Donoghue DH. Treatment of injuries to athletes. Philadelphia: WB Saunders, 1970.
2. American Academy of Family Physicians, American Academy of Pediatrics, American Medical Society for Sports Medicine, American Orthopaedic Society for Sports Medicine, American Osteopathic Academy of Sports Medicine. Preparticipation physical evaluation, 1992.
3. Fields KB. Clearing athletes for participation in sports: the North Carolina Medical Society's recommended examination. NC Med J 1994;55(4):116–121.
4. Mellion MB, Walsh WM, Shelton GL, eds. The team physicians handbook. St. Louis: Mosby–Year Book, 1990.
5. American Academy of Pediatrics—Committee on Sports Medicine: recommendations for participation in competitive sports. Pediatrics 1988;81:737–739.

Bibliography

Fields KB, Delaney MJ. Focusing the preparticipation sports examination. J Fam Pract 1990;30:304–312.

Fields KB. Primary care of the athlete. In: Sloane PD, Slatt LM, Curtis P, eds. Essentials of family medicine, 2nd ed. Baltimore: Williams & Wilkins, 1993:95–102.

Gillette PC. Congenital heart disease. Pediatr Clin North Am 1990;37(1):1–231.

Goldberg B, Saramiti A, Witman P, Gavin M, Nicholas JA. Preparticipation sports assessment: an objective evaluation. Pediatrics 1980;66:736–745.

Hulse E, Strong WB. Preparticipation health evaluation for competitive sports. Pediatr Rev 1987;9:173–182.

Linder CW, Durant RH, et al. Preparticipation health screen of young athletes. Am J Sports Med 1981;9:187–193.

Maron BJ, Roberts WC, McAllister H, et al. Sudden death in young athletes. Circulation 1980;62:218–229.

Thompson TR, Andrish JT, Bergfeld JA. A prospective study of preparticipation sports examinations of 2,670 young athletes: method and results. Cleve Clin Q 1982;49:225–233.

The Sports Medicine Committee, Colorado Medical Society. Guidelines for the management of concussion in sports. Denver: May, 1990.

Preparticipation Physical Evaluation

History

Date _____

Name _____ Sex _____ Age _____ Date of birth _____

Grade _____ Sport _____ _____ _____

Personal physician _____ _____ _____

Address   Physician's phone

Explain "Yes" answers below:

	Yes	No
1. Have you ever been hospitalized?	☐	☐
Have you ever had surgery?	☐	☐
2. Are you presently taking any medications or pills?	☐	☐
3. Do you have any allergies (medicine, bees or other stinging insects)?	☐	☐
4. Have you ever passed out during or after exercise?	☐	☐
Have you ever been dizzy during or after exercise?	☐	☐
Have you ever had chest pain during or after exercise?	☐	☐
Do you tire more quickly than your friends during exercise?	☐	☐
Have you ever had high blood pressure?	☐	☐
Have you ever been told that you have a heart murmur?	☐	☐
Have you ever had racing of your heart or skipped heartbeats?	☐	☐
Has anyone in your family died of heart problems or a sudden death before age 50?	☐	☐
5. Do you have any skin problems (itching, rashes, acne)?	☐	☐
6. Have you ever had a head injury?	☐	☐
Have you ever been knocked out or unconscious?	☐	☐
Have you ever had a seizure?	☐	☐
Have you ever had a stinger, burner or pinched nerve?	☐	☐
7. Have you ever had heat or muscle cramps?	☐	☐
Have you ever been dizzy or passed out in the heat?	☐	☐
8. Do you have trouble breathing or do you cough during or after activity?	☐	☐
9. Do you use any special equipment (pads, braces, neck rolls, mouth guard, eye guards, etc.)?	☐	☐
10. Have you had any problems with your eyes or vision?	☐	☐
Do you wear glasses or contacts or protective eye wear?	☐	☐
11. Have you ever sprained/strained, dislocated, fractured, broken or had repeated swelling or other injuries of any bones or joints?	☐	☐

☐ Head   ☐ Shoulder   ☐ Thigh   ☐ Neck   ☐ Elbow   ☐ Knee   ☐ Chest
☐ Forearm   ☐ Shin/calf   ☐ Back   ☐ Wrist   ☐ Ankle   ☐ Hip   ☐ Hand   ☐ Foot

	Yes	No
12. Have you had any other medical problems (infectious mononucleosis, diabetes, etc.)?	☐	☐
13. Have you had a medical problem or injury since your last evaluation?	☐	☐

14. When was your last tetanus shot? _____

When was your last measles immunization? _____

15. When was your first menstrual period? _____

When was your last menstrual period? _____

What was the longest time between your periods last year? _____

Explain "Yes" answers:

_____

_____

_____

_____

_____

_____

I hereby state that, to the best of my knowledge, my answers to the above questions are correct.

Date _____

Signature of athlete _____

Signature of parent/guardian _____

Preparticipation Physical Evaluation *continued*

Physical Examination

Date _____

Name _____ Age _____ Date of birth _____

Height _____ Weight _____ BP _____ / _____ Pulse _____

Vision R 20/____ L 20/ ____ Corrected: Y   N   Pupils _____

		Normal	Abnormal findings					Initials
COMPLETE	**LIMITED**	Cardiopulmonary						
		Pulses						
		Heart						
		Lungs						
		Tanner stage	1	2	3	4	5	
		Skin						
		Abdominal						
		Genitalia						
		Musculoskeletal						
		Neck						
		Shoulder						
		Elbow						
		Wrist						
		Hand						
		Back						
		Knee						
		Ankle						
		Foot						
		Other						

Clearance:

A.   Cleared

B.   Cleared after completing evaluation/rehabilitation for: _____

C.   Not cleared for: ☐ Collision

☐ Contact

☐ Noncontact   ____ Strenuous   ____ Moderately strenuous   ____ Nonstrenuous

Due to: _____

Recommendation: _____

_____

_____

Name of physician _____   Date _____

Address _____   Phone _____

Signature of physician _____

(Developed by the American Academy of Family Physicians, American Academy of Pediatrics, American Medical Society for Sports Medicine, American Orthopaedic Society for Sports Medicine and American Osteopathic Academy of Sports Medicine. Copyright © 1992.)

FORM CURRENTLY RECOMMENDED BY NCMS SPORTS MEDICINE COMMITTEE   (7/93)

SPORT PREPARTICIPATION HISTORY FORM

Patient's Name: _____   Age: _____

Athlete's Directions: Please review all questions with your parent or guardian and answer them to the best of your knowledge.

Physician's Directions: We recommend repeating the thirteen questions listed below and carefully reviewing details of any positive answers.

YES	NO	DON'T KNOW		
			1	Has anyone in the athlete's family (grandmother, grandfather, mother, father, brother, sister), died suddenly before age 50?
			2A	Has the athlete ever stopped exercising because of dizziness or passed out during exercise?
			2B	Have you ever been told you have a heart murmur or heart problems?
			3	Does the athlete have asthma (wheezing), hay fever, or coughing spells after exercise?
			4	Has the athlete ever had a bone broken, had to wear a cast, or had an injury to any joint?
			5	Does the athlete have a history of concussion (getting knocked out)?
			6	Has the athlete ever suffered a heat-related illness (heat stroke or heat exhaustion)?
			7	Does the athlete have anything he/she wants to talk to the doctor about?
			8	Does the athlete have a chronic illness or see a doctor regularly for any particular problem?
			9	Does the athlete take any medicine?
			10	Is the athlete allergic to any medications or bee stings?
			11	Does the athlete have only one of any paired organ? (eyes, ears, kidneys, testicles, ovaries, etc.)?
			12	Do you wear contacts or eye glasses?
			13	Date of last tetanus booster. DATE _____.

Elaborate on any positive answers:

I have answered and reviewed the questions above and give permission for my child to participate in sports.

Signature of Parent or Guardian _____

Date _____   Phone # _____

REQUIRED ELEMENTS ARE IN ASTERISK

EXAMINATION

PATIENT'S NAME: _____

* 1. BP _____ WT _____ HT _____ Vision (R) _____ (L) _____

* 2. Cardiovascular Exam ☐ Normal ☐ Abnormal Comments:

   Murmur ☐ Yes ☐ No Describe:

* 3. Musculoskeletal Exam Record laxity, weakness, instability, decreased ROM - if abnormal

Knee	☐ Normal	☐ Abnormal
Ankle	☐ Normal	☐ Abnormal
Shoulder	☐ Normal	☐ Abnormal
(Other Orthopedic	☐ Normal	☐ Abnormal
Problems, eg. neck, feet, scoliosis)		

4. Optional Exam - should be done if history is positive. Comments:

ENT	☐ Normal	☐ Abnormal
Chest	☐ Normal	☐ Abnormal
Abdomen	☐ Normal	☐ Abnormal
Genitalia	☐ Normal	☐ Abnormal
Skin	☐ Normal	☐ Abnormal

* ASSESSMENT: 5.A. ☐ No problems identified B. ☐ Other

* RECOMMENDATIONS: 6.A. ☐ Unlimited B. ☐ Limited to specific sports C. ☐ Deferred until: (e.g., rehab., recheck, consultation, lab, etc.)

* REEXAMINE: 7.A. ☐ Yearly and after any injury that limits participation for greater than one week. B. ☐ Other:

I certify that I have examined the above student and that such examination revealed (☐ conditions ☐ no conditions) that would prevent this student from participation in interscholastic sports.

Are you licensed to practice medicine in the United States? ☐ Yes ☐ No

Signature _____ Phone Number _____

Address _____ Date _____

If student not qualified, list reasons for disqualification: _____

(The following are considered disqualifying until medical and parental releases are obtained: acute infections, obvious growth retardation, diabetes, jaundice, severe visual or auditory impairment, pulmonary insufficiency, organic heart disease or hypertension, enlarged liver or spleen, hernia, musculoskeletal deformity associated with functional loss, history of convulsions or concussions, absence of one kidney, eye, testicle, or ovary, etc.)

APPENDIX E
RECOMMENDATIONS FOR PARTICIPATION IN COMPETITIVE SPORTS

	Contact/ Collision	Limited Contact/Impact	Noncontact		
			Strenuous	Moderately Strenuous	Nonstrenous
Atlantoaxial instability	No	No	Yes*	Yes	Yes
* Swimming: no butterfly, breast stroke, or diving starts					
Acute illnesses	*	*	*	*	*
* Needs individual assessment, e.g., contagiousness to others, risk of worsening illness					
Cardiovascular					
Carditis	No	No	No	No	No
Hypertension					
Mild	Yes	Yes	Yes	Yes	Yes
Moderate	*	*	*	*	*
Severe	*	*	*	*	*
Congenital heart disease	†	†	†	†	†
* Needs individual assessment.					
† Patients with mild forms can be allowed a full range of physical activities; patients with moderate or severe forms, or who are postoperative, should be evaluated by a cardiologist before athletic participation.					
Eyes					
Absence or loss of function of one eye	*	*	*	*	*
Detached retina	†	†	†	†	†
* Availability of American Society for Testing and Materials (ASTM)-approved eye guards may allow competitor to participate in most sports, but this must be judged on an individual basis.					
† Consult ophthalmologist					
Inguinal hernia	Yes	Yes	Yes	Yes	Yes
Kidney: Absence of one	No	Yes	Yes	Yes	Yes
Liver: Enlarged	No	No	Yes	Yes	Yes
Musculoskeletal disorders	*	*	*	*	*
* Needs individual assessment					
Neurologic					
History of serious head or spine trauma, repeated concussions, or craniotomy	*	*	Yes	Yes	Yes
Convulsive disorder					
Well controlled	Yes	Yes	Yes	Yes	Yes
Poorly controlled	No	No	Yes†	Yes	Yes‡
* Needs individual assessment					
† No swimming or weight lifting					
‡ No archery or riflery					
Ovary: Absence of one	Yes	Yes	Yes	Yes	Yes
Respiratory					
Pulmonary insufficiency	*	*	*	*	Yes
Asthma	Yes	Yes	Yes	Yes	Yes
* May be allowed to compete if oxygenation remains satisfactory during a graded stress test					
Sickle cell trait	Yes	Yes	Yes	Yes	Yes
Skin: Boils, herpes, impetigo, scabies	*	*	Yes	Yes	Yes
* No gymnastics with mats, martial arts, wrestling, or contact sports until not contagious					
Spleen: Enlarged	No	No	No	Yes	Yes
Testicle: Absence or undescended	Yes*	Yes*	Yes	Yes	Yes
* Certain sports may require protective cup.					
	Boxing	Baseball	Aerobic dancing	Badminton	Archery
	Field hockey	Basketball	Crew	Curling	Golf
	Football	Bicycling	Fencing	Table tennis	Riflery
	Ice hockey	Diving	Field		
	Lacrosse	Field	Discus		
	Martial arts	High jump	Javelin		
	Rodeo	Pole vault	Shot put		
	Soccer	Gymnastics	Running		
	Wrestling	Horseback riding	Swimming		
		Skating	Tennis		
		Ice	Track		
		Roller	Weight lifting		
		Skiing			
		Cross-country			
		Downhill			
		Water			
		Softball			
		Squash, handball			
		Volleyball			

HEAD INJURIES IN SPORTS

4

ABRAHAM MINTZ
ZEV DAVID NIJENSOHN

Pathophysiology of Brain Injury
General Management of Head Injury
General Evaluation and Triage Scoring
Neurologic Evaluation
Radiologic Evaluation
Pathology of Head Injury
Some Sports Statistics

The possibility of head injury exists in virtually all types of athletic activities. Although serious head injury occurs infrequently, it is often associated with contact sports such as football, rugby, ice hockey, and lacrosse; aquatic sports, gymnastics, and skiing also boast a comparable incidence of head injury. Although the severity of damage varies with each separate case, the types of injury have been divided into two categories: severe and minor. *Severe head injury* refers to intense structural damage to the brain, which could eventually lead to long-term disabling effects or possible death. *Minor head injury* or *concussion* occurs more frequently and can be defined as a traumatically induced alteration in mental status, not necessarily a loss of consciousness (LOC).

This chapter advises the physician on the athletic field with various guidelines to distinguish and manage the different types of head injury. The topic of management becomes compounded in the athletic arena, particularly when dealing with competitive sports because of the many outside factors that must play a role in decisions regarding the extent of the head injury suffered by the athlete and the amount of time advisable to wait before returning to practice or play. These factors include the results of your evaluation of the patient and the tendency of the athletes to minimize their symptoms out of fear or driven by the will to commence playing or practicing. As sport technology evolves, new equipment and laws have emerged with the hope of decreasing the chance of head injury (e.g., cyclists' helmet law). Because of the immense importance of head injury, the physician who sees the patient soon after the head injury must develop a practical knowledge of the initial care of this patient (1). Injuries to the head very often result in permanent damage to highly organized and integrated neural systems that generally cannot fully compensate through functional regeneration or neural reorganization. This permanent damage to the central nervous system (CNS) can occur immediately after an injury or sometime thereafter. Long-term deficits can ensue even from minor head injuries. Moreover, a single traumatic event that physically affects only one victim can have profound long-term financial, social, and emotional effects on the lives of many other persons. In terms of human suffering, social relationships, and economic burden, the effects of CNS trauma are incalculable. Ironically, most cases are also avoidable (2).

The care of the patient begins at the moment of injury and continues until the final outcome. Prehospital care is an important factor because it is the initial intervention in the entire sequence of care. Care during this time has a profound impact on the subsequent course of the patient (3).

PATHOPHYSIOLOGY OF BRAIN INJURY

The brain has minimal reserves to meet ongoing metabolic needs. If the constant and continuous flow of substrates is interrupted, the brain will rapidly lose the ability to maintain normal cellular function. The related principle is that neuronal damage occurs when metabolic needs are not met. Also, there may be areas of the brain that are in a "penumbra," that is, not able to function properly but able to maintain cellular integrity. The implication is that every effort should be made to ensure the availability of adequate substrate to meet cellular needs even under the stress of trauma to prevent a secondary brain injury.

The common pathway by which secondary events result in further damage is hypoxia or ischemia, which may be either global or focal. Some secondary effects are obvious—for example, a period of apnea, which may immediately follow a head injury (4). Other secondary events result from complex and occasionally even very delayed pathophysiologic events related to systemic and secondary intracranial mass lesions (5–7).

The brain needs an extremely high rate of energy production to maintain the neuronal integrity and ion exchange mechanism necessary for the generation and transmission of impulses. Actually, the brain's requirement for oxygen and glucose are out of proportion to that required by other organs. This fact, coupled with the paucity of energy and substrate reserves in neural tissue, makes neural tissue particularly vulnerable to impaired perfusion (2). Although the rate of cerebral metabolism varies enormously not only from area to area but also according to activity states, the brain consumes oxygen at an unusually constant rate, about 3 to 4 mL/100 g per minute (8).

The exact amount of time that must elapse from the primary brain injury to the onset of the secondary changes and then for these changes to become irreversible is difficult to know and obviously variable from individual to individual. For the same reason that this critical duration of time cannot be estimated, oxygen delivery must be assured as quickly as possible. This requires an adequate PaO_2, hemoglobin concentration, and cerebral blood flow.

The cerebral perfusion pressure (CPP) is the consequence of a dynamic relationship between the mean arterial pressure (MAP) and intracranial pressure (ICP) (2):

$$CPP = MAP - ICP$$

It is the critical determinant in delivery of oxygen and other substrates to the neural tissue.

GENERAL MANAGEMENT OF HEAD INJURY

It is generally accepted in dealing with trauma that if care is going to be useful, it must be administered in a timely fashion (9). In a study comparing the outcome of patients with severe head injuries, the difference in mortality between two centers—12.5% versus 4.8%—was felt to be due to the lack of prehospital emergency care and the delay between injury and treatment (10).

Of those conditions associated with severe head injury that can be readily prevented or treated in the prehospital phase, hypoxia and shock seem the most important. These complications are frequent and are clearly related to poor outcome. Personnel providing care for head-injured patients should be able to perform an accurate assessment of neurologic function, establish an adequate airway, institute a vascular access to treat shock, and prepare the patient for transport (e.g., log rolling; see Figure 5.7). It is important to recognize that the care of these patients is not a two-stage procedure but rather a smooth effort that begins on the field, with adequate stabilization of the patient, and continues in the emergency room with appropriate diagnosis and treatment of injuries followed by appropriate surgery, if indicated, and modern intensive care (3).

There is a significant incidence of hypoxia (PaO_2 less than 60 mmHg) in head-injured patients who are spontaneously breathing without any sign of respiratory distress. In one study, Frost and coworkers encountered it in 65% of patients (11). Also, there seems to be an association between hypoxia and the subsequent occurrence of elevated ICP (12). Thus, in terms of both hospital course and outcome, an adequate airway is crucial. This usually means that in patients with a Glasgow coma score of 8 or less (Table 4.1), control of the airway is indicated (3). This is accomplished by nasal or oral intubation. The nasal route does not require extension of the neck; it is an obvious benefit when spinal instability has to be ruled out. However, in a patient who is not able to localize painful stimuli or is in obvious respiratory distress, intubation by either route should not be delayed because of the possibility of an unstable neck (12). Intubation may require the use of paralytic drugs; lidocaine topically or intravenously should be used in an attempt to avoid sudden elevations of ICP. Once the airway is secured, moderate hyperventilation is carried out during the period of transportation until more definitive treatment can be given.

Ischemia is the other common insult that can further damage the injured brain.

Ischemia results primarily from blood loss from extracranial sources or intracranial hypertension, either separately or in combination (2,13). Adults with severe scalp or facial injuries may lose a considerable amount of blood, and these injuries may be the cause of shock. In infants and small children intracranial hemorrhage may be the cause of shock because of the disproportionately small blood volume in relation to intracranial volume. Shock may also occur from cardiac arrhythmias due to high levels of circulating catecholamines. Shock by itself is obviously detrimental, but when coupled with elevated ICP, inadequate levels of cerebral perfusion are quickly reached. It is imperative to maintain an adequate circulating blood volume with appropriate solutions (i.e., 0.9% normal saline solution); they should be administered at a rate necessary to keep an adequate blood pressure. There is little indication for fluid restriction (3).

Table 4.1. Glasgow coma scale

Eyes	Open	Spontaneous	4
		To speech	3
		To pain	2
		No response	1
Best motor response	To verbal command; to painful stimulus	Obeys	6
		Localizes pain	5
		Flexion/withdrawal	4
		Flexion/abnormal	3
		Extension/abnormal	2
		No response	1
Best verbal response		Oriented and converses	5
		Disoriented and converses	4
		Inappropriate words	3
		Incomprehensible sounds	2
		No response	1
		Total	3–15

GENERAL EVALUATION AND
TRIAGE SCORING

Several different triage scores have been introduced in an attempt to assess the extent and type of injury accurately and the degree of care required for the patient (14). A neurologic evaluation should answer three simple questions: 1) What is the baseline neurologic function of the patient? 2) Are there any focal signs? 3) Is the patient getting worse, better, or staying the same? The last question can only be answered with serial examinations. The most useful examination remains the Glasgow coma scale (GCS) (15). It provides a quick and accurate assessment, it can be performed by personnel with different levels of training, and it provides a quantitative measure of the patient's LOC (1,3,13).

The GCS is the sum of scores of three areas of assessment: eye opening, best motor response, and verbal response. Each is graded separately and the best response obtained is documented.

Scoring for eye opening is not valid if the eyes are swollen shut, of course. This fact must be recorded. The best response for any extremity is recorded even though worse responses may be present in other extremities. The worst motor response is also important but is not used for the GCS; the worst response should be noted separately. For patients not following verbal commands, a painful stimulus is applied to a fingernail or toenail. Scoring for the verbal portion is invalid if speech is impossible, such as the presence of an endotracheal tube (1).

The GCS itself can be used to categorize patients; a patient in a *coma* is defined as having no eye opening (E-1), no ability to follow commands (M-1 to M-5) and no word verbalization (V-1 or V-2). This means

that all patients with a GCS less than 8 and most of those with a GCS equal to 8 are in a coma. Patients with a GCS above 8 are not in a coma (1). Also, on the basis of the GCS, patients are classified as having:

* *Severe* head injury if GCS is 8 or less
* *Moderate* injury if GCS is 9 to 12
* *Minor* head injury if GCS is 13 to 15

The easiest method of treating intracranial hypertension and protecting the brain from ischemia is the establishment of a good airway, gentle hyperventilation, maintaining good CPP by maintaining good blood pressure, and rapid transportation to a facility that can treat the problem. Ideally, all patients should go to a level 1 or possibly a level 2 trauma center. This has been emphasized by the American College of Surgeons. In a patient without a severe head injury but in shock this may be lifesaving. However, in a patient with a mass lesion and elevated ICP, the result may be disastrous. It makes little sense to divert a patient with a severe head injury to a hospital that is 15 to 20 minutes closer to the scene but without neurosurgical support. With aggressive fluid resuscitation, adequate airway, and accurate assessment of the neurologic picture, the patient should be delivered to a facility that can treat all the injuries immediately. By doing this, the patient has the best chance for a favorable outcome (3).

NEUROLOGIC EVALUATION

The great majority of head injuries will be minor. Athletes will come to the sideline and a coach or fellow athlete will tell you that he or she is dazed or confused. Determine their level of confusion by assessing presence or absence of amnesia with questions like "Who are we playing?" "What's the score?" or "What quarter is it?" Have the trainer, coach, or another player help you with events the athlete should be able to remember. Sensory and motor examinations can be done by observing gait and movement and by assessing major muscle strength. The pupils should always be assessed to establish baselines for future evaluations. The great majority of athletes will have no neurologic defects and no amnesia. After an appropriate waiting period (20 minutes), they can return to the game. Be sure to observe that athlete during the rest of the game; any sign of confusion should lead to disqualification and further evaluation.

The more severe injuries, which include LOC even for a short period, require more extensive evaluation, probably in an emergency department setting. In the emergency department, initial evaluation should include information such as time, location, and mechanism of injury. Airway, breathing, and circulatory control must take priority (1). Care must be exercised in attributing changes in the patient's mental status to head injury if the systolic blood pressure is less than 60 mmHg or systemic hypoxemia exists. Similarly, a drug screen for alcohol and other CNS depressants may be required in certain circumstances. Altered consciousness is unlikely to be secondary to alcohol consumption when the alcohol blood level is less than 200 mg/ 100 mL (16).

The combination of progressive hypertension associated with bradycardia and diminished respiratory rate (Cushing's response) is a response to an acute and potentially lethal rise in ICP; in head-injured patients it is usually due to an expanding intracranial lesion demanding immediate operative intervention (1).

Direct blows to the head are more likely to cause epidural hematomas, whereas acceleration–deceleration injuries are more commonly associated with diffuse cerebral damage and subdural hematomas (17).

When neurologic and head examinations are performed, the patient's LOC should be noted using the GCS. It objectively quantifies the LOC and correlates with recovery from injury (15). The words stuporous, semicomatose, and obtunded should be avoided because they may have different connotations to different examiners. There are, though, some inadequacies in the GCS; the assessment of aphasic patients cannot be adequately done under its guidelines. Furthermore, because it assesses the best side, it fails to record unilateral deterioration.

The neurologic examination is adapted to the patient's LOC, but certain functions must be examined. Pupillary size, position, and response to light are observed. Preparticipation physical examinations should include pupillary size. Some individuals may have some difference in size normally. The trainer should have this information available during all athletic activity. *A difference of more than 1 mm in pupillary diameter is usually abnormal and, even though anisocoria is frequently due to blunt trauma to the eye, an intracranial injury must be excluded.* Light reactivity is evaluated by the briskness of the response; a sluggish response may indicate an intracranial injury. Spontaneous eye movements in lighter stages of coma are usually roving and may be conjugate or disconjugate. Horizontal eye movements indicate only that the midbrain and pontine tegmentum are intact. Oculovestibular response generally persists after oculocephalic response (doll's eyes maneuver) has. Conjugate gaze deviation to one side is abnormal and may indicate the presence of a mass lesion or a seizure. Pupillary light examination is important in the comatose patient. A brain injury severe enough to render a patient comatose with extensor posturing (decerebrate) is usually associated with unresponsive or poorly responsive pupils, whereas a patient in a coma from metabolic disease will generally have sparing of light reaction (18). Pinpoint pupils occur with pontine hemorrhages or narcotic intoxication.

A unilaterally dilated, unreactive pupil (fixed pupil) is usually indicative of a supratentorial expanding mass with midline shift, uncal herniation, and compression of the third cranial nerve (see below). Rarely, uncal herniation with paralysis of the third nerve may occur in an awake patient. The third nerve may be damaged by orbital trauma, and the optic nerve may also be injured. If the latter is the case, the pupil will not react directly to light but the consensual response will be preserved.

The purpose of the initial motor examination is to detect asymmetry. Spontaneous movements are observed; if they are minimal or absent, a painful stimulus is applied. A delay in onset of movement, less movement, or the need for a stronger stimulus on one side is significant. A clearly lateralizing weakness suggests an intracranial mass lesion.

The head should be palpated to identify lacerations, open fractures, compound fractures, cerebrospinal fluid (CSF) leaks, or exposed brain. The tympanic membranes should be visualized whenever possible.

Hemiplegia is usually contralateral to the lesion, and third nerve paresis is ipsilateral to the lesion. On occasion, the hemiplegia is ipsilateral to the lesion. For the most part, the third nerve is a more reliable indicator than the motor weakness in localizing the side of the mass lesion (13).

The initial neurologic examination is only the beginning, because the patient must be followed very closely. A change in the GCS of 2 points or more clearly means that the patient has deteriorated. A decrease of 3 points is catastrophic and requires immediate intervention (1).

RADIOLOGIC EVALUATION

Radiographs are reserved for the more severely injured athlete. Before any neuroradiologic procedure is performed, overall stability of the cervical spine must be determined by a lateral cervical spine x-ray. The entire cervical spine must be visualized, including C7.

The overall importance of skull x-rays in the early management of a patient with severe head injury has been the subject of considerable controversy. Skull x-rays are of little value in the early management of patients with obvious severe head injuries, except in cases of penetrating head injuries. They remain an acceptable tool for evaluation of depressed fractures or foreign bodies. For a patient with a minor head injury, skull x-rays may be recommended before considering the discharge of a patient from the emergency department (1) or to screen for skull fractures. Intracranial air or clouding of the sinuses may suggest a CSF leak.

Computed tomography (CT) has revolutionized diagnosis in patients with head injuries and is the diagnostic procedure of choice for patients who have or are suspected of having a serious head injury. This role was clearly demonstrated in the early use of CT (19). Except for patients with trivial injuries, all head-injured patients will require CT at some time. Intracranial hemorrhage as well as many skull fractures is evaluated by this modality. A major limitation is its inability to detect subtle nonhemorrhagic lesions in the white matter and brain stem (20).

Magnetic resonance imaging (MRI) has also changed almost every aspect of neuroradiology since its inception. This is true also for head injuries during the subacute and chronic phases. Also, it may be invaluable in the acute phase, in which the clinical picture is not explained by CT (20,21).

PATHOLOGY OF HEAD INJURY

Brain injury occurs in two stages. *Primary injury* is the damage occurring at the moment of injury. And *secondary injury* is the damage produced by complicating processes that are initiated at the moment of injury but are not present clinically for a period of time after the injury (22). The secondary injuries have been reviewed earlier in this chapter.

There are several different classifications of head injuries in the literature. The one in Table 4.2 is taken from the American College of Surgeons Committee on Trauma (1).

Skull Fractures

Skull fractures are not common athletic injuries. By themselves they do not cause neurologic disability. Many severe brain injuries occur without skull fractures, and searching for one should not delay patient management. On the other hand, it is important to diagnose a skull fracture because patients harboring them have a much higher incidence of intracranial hematoma (23). In one study of hospitalized patients with skull fractures, 67% had associated significant intracranial lesions (24).

Linear Skull Fractures

These fractures may be visualized by plain skull x-rays or by CT. They do not

Table 4.2. Classification of head injuries

A. Skull Fractures
    1. Linear, nondepressed fracture
    2. Depressed skull fracture
    3. Open skull fracture
    4. Basal skull fracture
B. Diffuse Brain Injuries
    1. Concussions
    2. Diffuse axonal injury
C. Focal Injuries
    1. Contusion
    2. Intracranial hemorrhages
        a. Meningeal hemorrhage
            I. Acute epidural hematoma
            II. Acute subdural hematoma
            III. Subarachnoid hemorrhage
        b. Brain hemorrhages and lacerations
            I. Intracerebral hematoma
            II. Impalement injuries
            III. Bullet wounds

require specific treatment other than observation if no other injuries are associated (Figure 4.1). Fractures over the temporal area and, more specifically, over the arterial groove of the middle meningeal artery should alert the physician to the possibility of an epidural hematoma. Patients with a skull fracture, with or without LOC, should undergo CT of the brain. If this is not feasible, then he or she should be admitted for observation. Jennet noted that in the small number of patients who were intact when first seen and then deteriorated, usually a skull fracture was present (25).

Depressed Skull Fractures

Depressed skull fractures develop when a significant kinetic energy is delivered to the skull in a relatively small area (Figure 4.2). They are frequently encountered after impact with a baseball bat, a golf ball, or a club. Their clinical significance usually de-

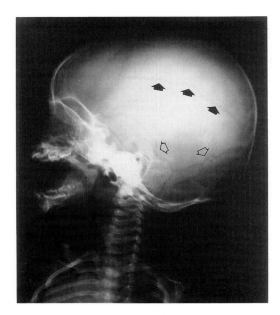

Figure 4.1. Linear skull fracture (*closed arrows*). Note that the fracture line is straighter than the meandering suture line (*open arrows*).

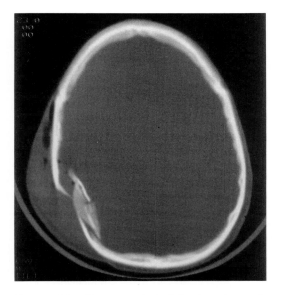

Figure 4.2. Depressed skull fracture is easily recognizable on CT scan.

pends on the underlying brain injury, if any. They can frequently be palpated although the physical examination may be entirely normal. These fractures are identified as a double density in the skull x-rays and are better delineated on the CT scan.

The management of these injuries has changed over the last two decades. Previously it was recommended that fractures that were depressed to a depth greater than the thickness of the skull should be surgically elevated. The rationale for this recommendation was that these fractures, if left untreated, produced a higher incidence of posttraumatic epilepsy. Braakman (26) and Jennet and colleagues (27) demonstrated no difference in the incidence of posttraumatic epilepsy regardless of the mode of treatment. Currently, many surgeons believe that the majority of these fractures need not be elevated surgically (28).

Open Skull Fractures

Open skull fractures may be linear or depressed (compound). Sometimes they can be diagnosed by inspection, that is, an obvious fracture under a large laceration. A subperiosteal hematoma to the inexperienced examiner may feel like a depressed fracture. In other unfortunate situations, CSF or brain matter can be seen extruding from a laceration. In any of these situations, or if there is clinical suspicion of a skull fracture, a CT scan and plain x-rays should be obtained. The information gained will help assess the extent of the injury and guide the treatment plan.

As in other types of skull fractures, a significant underlying hematoma or brain injury may or may not be present accompanying a fracture. Also, the associated injury may be in an area remote to the fracture. The fact that the fracture is open adds the possibility of infection to the injury.

Basal Skull Fractures

Usually diagnosed by clinical signs, basal skull fractures are often not apparent on skull films and sometimes even on CT (Figure 4.3). The patients may present with CSF leaking from the nose (rhinorrhea) or from the ear (otorrhea). A "ring sign" may be helpful to identify CSF mixed with blood; this is obtained by allowing a drop of fluid to drop on filter paper. The fluid will form a concentric ring around the blood remaining in the center (1). Raccoon eyes (periorbital ecchymosis) is usually due to a fracture in the cribriform plate, which can also cause rhinorrhea. Battle's sign is the ecchymosis seen over the mastoid that indicates, as does a hemotympanum, a basal skull fracture (Figure 4.4). Other signs due to dysfunction of any of the cranial nerves may occur, so the patient may develop anosmia, ocular palsies, facial paralysis, hearing loss, vestibular dysfunction, among others. These signs may also develop in any possible combination.

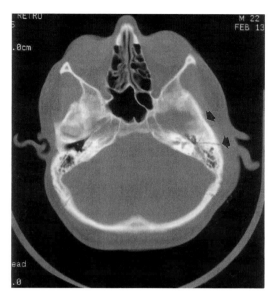

Figure 4.3. Basilar skull fracture indicated by arrows. These are typically straight or jagged.

Figure 4.4. Raccoon eyes (A) and Battle's sign (B) are indicative of basilar skull fractures.

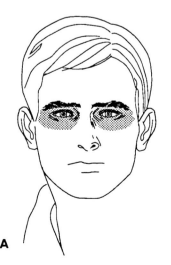

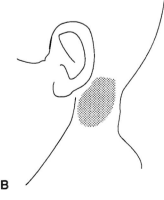

A   B

These signs may develop rather quickly, but it is not uncommon to discover them for the first time on follow-up examinations. *When a fracture of the floor of the frontal fossa is suspected, a nasogastric tube must not be passed because of the potential passage of the tube intracranially through the basal fracture* (29).

Basal fractures are of particular importance because the dura may be torn, creating a path between potentially contaminated chambers such as the paranasal sinuses and the CNS; also the creation of a CSF fistula is possible. Whether or not there is a CSF fistula, the dural tear in a basal skull fracture will predispose the patient to meningitis (30).

Diffuse Brain Injuries

Diffuse brain injuries are produced by rapid head motions, that is, the inertial or acceleration effects of the energy delivered to the head. They are the most common head injuries encountered in athletic competition. They can occur without an impact to the cranium and have little to do with the direct impact of an object against the skull, except if this impact produces acceleration or deceleration of the head. Their presence and severity are determined by the direction, magnitude, and speed in which the head moves or comes to rest during the injury sequence. The violent head motions are sufficient to produce stretching and even shearing of nerve fibers.

Diffuse brain injuries are associated with widespread or global disruption of neurologic function, which may be temporary, as in the case of a concussion, or permanent, as in severe diffuse axonal injury lesions (31). These injuries involve disturbances of consciousness. The mechanisms by which consciousness is maintained are rather complex; they involve a continuous interaction of the cerebral cortex, subcortical nuclei including the thalamus, and brain stem centers (reticular activating system). The functional isolation of one of these centers will produce alterations of consciousness. In general terms, unconsciousness can be produced by dysfunction of both cerebral hemispheres or dysfunction of the thalamic–brain stem axis (18).

Diffuse brain injuries span a continuum of progressively severe brain dysfunction due to increments in the acceleration force delivered to the head. At low levels of energy, function is disrupted, usually temporarily without pathologic changes in the brain (concussion). With higher forces delivered, function is interrupted first but anatomic changes also occur with diffuse axonal injury (DAI) (see below).

Diffuse brain injuries are the most common type of head injuries. Severe DAI is the greatest cause of severe disability and neurovegetative survivors (32). Also, severe DAI frequently accompanies injuries that are classified as focal. Patients who are rendered immediately unconscious with an epidural hematoma, and fail to improve despite immediate evacuation of the clot, have been found to have DAI (33).

Concussion

Concussion is a brain injury accompanied by transient loss of neurologic function, not necessarily LOC. Concussion has been divided into three grades (Table 4.3). In the mild forms, grade 1, it may only produce transient confusion and disorientation without amnesia (31). This syndrome—mild concussion—is completely reversible and not associated with any permanent sequelae. Slightly more severe injuries, grade 2 concussions, produce confusion with amnesia that develops after 5 to 10 minutes; the individual continues coordinated activities after the accident and is able

Table 4.3. Grading of concussion as developed by the Colorado Medical Society

Grade	Findings	Return to Play
1	Confusion without amnesia; no loss of consciousness	Remove from contest; examine every 5 min; may return 20 min after all symptoms resolve
2	Confusion with amnesia; no loss of consciousness	Remove from contest; no return; examine every 5 min; reevaluate next day; return 1 wk after symptoms resolve
3	Loss of consciousness	Transport from field by ambulance; C-spine immobilization if indicated; hospitalization may be necessary; return 2 wk after symptoms resolve

to recall it immediately, but if examined 5 to 10 minutes later, retrograde amnesia (forgetting events prior to the incident) will be present and he or she will not be able to recall the incident. The period of amnesia usually extends for several minutes before the event; it may shrink, but there will remain a period of permanent retrograde amnesia. The confusion often resolves within seconds. If the force delivered is even greater, confusion and amnesia will be present from the initial impact, although the subject can often continue performing the same task (boxing, playing football). Posttraumatic amnesia (forgetting the events after the impact) will be present along with retrograde amnesia. Although consciousness is preserved, it is obvious

that transient cerebral dysfunction occurs and the memory-acquiring mechanism (learning) is disrupted for a brief period of time. The force that produces these syndromes is not sufficient to functionally disconnect the brain cortex from the brain stem or to damage the brain stem, thus consciousness is not lost.

The most severe concussions, grade 3, are what have been termed the "classic cerebral concussion syndrome." These are defined by a transient posttraumatic period of unconsciousness that lasts for less than 6 hours (31). In these individuals, unconsciousness or coma is present from the initial injury and systemic changes such as pupillary dilatation, bradycardia, and even apnea may develop for a very brief period. It is always accompanied by retrograde and anterograde amnesia and full consciousness returns by 6 hours preceded by a period of confusion. Other lesions can be associated with any form of concussion. Following the concussion, the athlete may note difficulty concentrating and periodic headaches. School or job performance may be affected. This effect can remain for up to 3 months. The headache that remains is called "footballer's migraine."

Athletes and Concussions

As mentioned earlier, athletes are more frequently affected with minor head injuries or concussion. Football players and boxers face the highest risk. High school football players, for example, have a 19% chance of suffering a concussion each year (34). In the United States, approximately 1.5 million athletes participate in organized football each year (35). In addition to football other sports pose a risk for head injury. These include rugby, hockey, lacrosse, equestrian, and skiing among others.

The management of a minor head injury in the acute or initial stage is similar to the management of more serious injuries and is directed toward prevention of secondary brain injury due to intracranial mass lesion and elevated ICP. In patients with neurologic deficits or obvious penetrating wounds, a CT scan will be obtained once hemodynamic stability has been obtained. Also, particular attention to the cervical spine is needed because even though the patient may be awake, he or she may not report neck pain or other injuries. Following a concussion, the unavailability of a responsible adult to observe the injured athlete constitutes an indication for admission for observation. Also, any abnormality of the neurologic examination or persistence of confusion, nausea, and vomiting, even with a negative CT scan, should also indicate admission for observation and consideration for a follow-up CT scan in 24 hours to rule out the possibility of a delayed intracranial hemorrhage (36).

In athletics, the management of minor head injuries becomes confounded because of the many outside factors that play a role in decisions regarding the extent of the injury suffered by the athlete and the amount of time advisable to wait before return to play or practice. These decisions are complicated even further by the tendency of the athletes to minimize their symptoms out of fear of loosing their "edge" or by the will to play often at the behest of coaches and teammates.

The management of minor head injuries in the athletic competition field embodies three important aspects. First, recognize the injury. Second, identify the severity of the concussion to determine the need for additional medical treatment and testing. Third, determine how much time must the athlete wait before returning to a normal practice and competition (37).

Each injury embodies a separate and different event, making it very difficult to create a rigid set of guidelines for classification of the injury and advisability to return. More importantly, substantial evidence has been documented regarding the *second impact syndrome*, which identifies a minor head injury in an athlete still symptomatic from a previous injury as the cause of fatal brain swelling (38). Also, repetitive concussions can lead to brain atrophy and cumulative neuropsychological deficits (38).

The Colorado Medical Society developed a set of guidelines for the classification of degrees of minor head injuries and the advisable management for each level (see Table 4.3) (39). The Colorado model offers a working system for the observation and assessment of athletes sustaining head injuries and hopefully will be universally implemented to eliminate the incidence of further preventable injury.

The Colorado Medical Society divides head injuries in three categories: grade 1 concussions do not involve unconsciousness but do have confusion without amnesia. In accordance with these guidelines, athletes with grade 1 injury should be kept out of the game for a minimum of 20 minutes while being continually subjected to serial evaluation of neurologic function at 5-minute intervals. These should evaluate orientation and search for deficits in concentration, attention, and short-term memory. During the period of time out of the contest, the athlete should be consistently evaluated in search of continuing or new postconcussion symptoms. All signs and symptoms must clear before the athlete may return to competition.

Clinical Case #1

A high school linebacker makes a "great stick" in tackling the ball carrier during the first half of the homecoming game. He continues in the game for the rest of the series of downs, but reports some confusion to you on the sideline when he comes out of the game. He has full recall of the game and is intact neurologically.

Appropriate management requires 20 minutes out of the contest, with serial examinations at 5-minute intervals. As long as amnesia does not develop and he has complete resolution of all symptoms (such as headache, confusion, etc) he can return to play after 20 minutes. The persistence of confusion or headache precludes returning to competition.

The appearance of amnesia increases the level of injury to grade 2. The athlete should be removed from the contest *without the possibility* of return and subjected to frequent examinations in search of signs of evolving intracranial pathology. Following reexamination on the day after injury, the athlete can return to practice after 1 full week of rest only if no symptoms remain or appear (18).

Clinical Case #2

You are watching your daughter's high school soccer game from the stands. Two girls collide violently while going to head the ball. One girl is left motionless on the field and you rush to render aid. The girl is unconscious, face down, and bleeding from a scalp laceration.

As always, the first priority must be airway and pulse. Because the athlete is unconscious, you must treat her as if she has a neck injury. She must be turned supine, en bloc, with traction to stabilize her neck. (Log rolling is described earlier in this chapter, and is illustrated in Figure 5.7.)

An ambulance should be called immediately for transportation to the emergency room, even if she rapidly awakens and is neurologically intact.

Any loss of consciousness—even a momentary one—signifies a grade 3. The athlete should be transported from the field to the nearest hospital by ambulance with cer-vical spine immobilization if necessary. All athletes rendered unconscious should be closely observed, and neuroimaging of the brain should be considered. Focal neurologic deficits and persistent alterations in the mental status warrant hospitalization. If neurologic examination is normal, the athlete can be released to family with careful instructions for overnight evaluation. A low threshold for obtaining a CT scan should persist for any worsening of symptoms. If no symptoms persist, the athlete can return to practice only after 2 full weeks of rest (19).

Pressure from others as well as an athlete's competitive spirit can often lead the individual to reduce or deny symptoms such as severe headache or nausea, which could prevent a quick return to practice or competition. This must always be considered during evaluation and the determination of when an athlete can return safely to practice and competition. Teachers and trainers can often help you obtain information about the athlete's behavior.

Athletes use the term "dinged," which indicates that they have been dazed for a period of time. They do not like to tell anyone this has happened and at times they are not discovered unless one of the coaches or another player notices that they are acting "funny." The physician has a difficult job in helping these athletes because if he or she panics and keeps all grade 1 injuries from playing, the athletes will not want to impart any symptoms. A calm, deliberate assessment is crucial to your success as a team physician on the sidelines.

Careful observation during the remaining part of the athletic contest is mandatory for any athlete with a grade 1 injury whom you return to competition. If the athlete has any signs or symptoms no matter how subtle, remove the youngster from competition. Even with a grade 1 injury, reevaluate the athlete in 1 or 2 days to ensure that no changes have occurred. Athletes who are asymptomatic should be allowed to compete, but physicians should ensure that monitoring is ongoing.

One of the major complications and leading causes of morbidity and mortality after a head injury is brain swelling or cerebral hyperemia. It was first reported by Bruce and colleagues in 1981 (40). Brain swelling may occur with any type of head injury; the magnitude of the swelling does not correlate well with the severity of the injury. The second impact syndrome is felt to be caused by this mechanism; the first injury, even though it may be trivial, leaves the brain in a vulnerable position in which another trivial or modest injury can trigger brain swelling that has been known to be fatal (41). This is the reason for the strict requirements for delay in returning to athletics after grade 2 or grade 3 concussion.

Brain swelling may be triggered acutely by a severe head injury or may be delayed and not cause elevations in ICP for several days. The usual history is that of a patient suffering a mild head injury or concussion from which he or she recovers. Minutes to hours later the patient becomes sleepy and progresses to a coma. This is differentiated from a DAI because unconsciousness does not follow the head injury immediately, thus the axonal disruption is not present and the neurologic deficits are due to the loss of vasomotor autoregulation.

Diffuse Axonal Injury

This is the more severe global brain injury that is associated with structural injury to the brain. DAI is used to define the global injury with coma lasting more than 6 hours. In DAI axons and blood vessels are actually torn (42), as evidenced by small areas of hemorrhage that can be seen on a scan CT. DAI produces dysfunction of both cerebral hemispheres, which in turn produces un-

consciousness by breaking the interaction of the brain stem with the cerebral cortex. DAI represents significant neurologic injury that will require careful monitoring. Permanent neurologic loss or death may result from the injury.

Focal Injuries

Focal injuries occur in a localized area and the diagnostic tests in the early phase are directed to detect them because they frequently require emergency surgery to evacuate them. The reason for this is that they have the potential for causing rapid shifts of the intracranial contents with catastrophic consequences. The intracranial contents are divided in normal circumstances as shown in Table 4.4 (43). The relationship between ICP and intracranial volume is *not linear*, as shown in Figure 4.5. In the horizontal or initial part of the curve increases in volume are accompanied by minimal increments in ICP due to the compensatory mechanisms; then in the steep part of the curve, changes in volume of even 1 mL can change the ICP by 7 to 8 mmHg. When the compensatory mechanisms become exhausted, the curve shifts to the right and the patient deteriorates to a condition that becomes progressively irreversible.

Secondary intracranial developments following a head injury are associated with

Table 4.4. Normal intracranial contents

Tissue	Volume (mL)	Percentage
Glia	700–900	~45.5
Neurons	500–700	~35.5
Blood	100–150	~7.5
Cerebrospinal fluid	100–150	~7.5
Extracellular fluid	—	~3.5

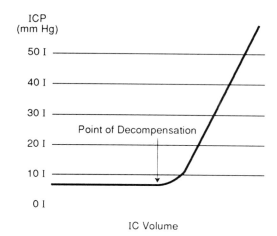

ICP
(mm Hg)

Point of Decompensation

IC Volume

Figure 4.5. Relationship between ICP and intracranial volume.

elevation of the ICP and are usually caused by a hematoma, hyperemia, edema, or any combination of them. Acute hydrocephalus may contribute by increasing the intracranial volume and not allowing the compensatory mechanism to work.

Cerebral Contusions

Cerebral contusions are focal areas of pulping, hemorrhage, infarction, and edema within the brain. They can develop at the site of an impact or at a distance from the impact (contracoup). The mechanism of formation of a contracoup contusion is the rapid acceleration of the skull followed by sudden arrest; the gelatinous brain still follows with the movement due to inertial forces resulting in compression at the site of contact between the brain and dura or bone (2–18). They most frequently occur in the basal surfaces of the frontal and temporal lobes.

The contusion may produce focal findings if it develops near sensitive areas; the deficit may be due to the contusion itself or to the edema that accompanies it. In the days after the injury, the contusion becomes homogeneous and by the end of the first week it begins to resolve.

Patients harboring contusions may have sustained a concussion and be intact at the time they are examined or a contusion may be part of a severe injury accompanying DAI or other kinds of intracranial hemorrhages. They are clearly seen on CT, and patients need hospital admission even if asymptomatic. There is a higher incidence of seizures with contusions and prophylaxis with dilantin is probably indicated for the first week (44). Treatment is usually conservative unless they are of significant size, in that case surgery for debridement may be indicated.

Intracranial Hemorrhages

Intracranial hemorrhages can be arbitrarily classified as meningeal or cerebral. Sometimes a subdural hematoma (meningeal) can actually be caused by rupture of an intracerebral hematoma into the subdural space or by a laceration of the surface of the brain. There are some "classic clinical pictures" of certain forms of hematoma but as in any kind of clinical practice, they do not always correspond to the presumed category of hemorrhage. CT has made the diagnosis of these hemorrhages quick and precise. Unless they are very small, they usually represent a neurosurgical emergency. An exception is the chronic subdural hematoma frequently seen in the geriatric population.

Acute Epidural Hemorrhage. This hemorrhage most frequently occurs from a fracture or acute deformity that strips the dura from the inner table of the skull and causes a laceration of the meningeal vessels, but it can be caused by tears of diploic veins or dural sinuses. Skull fractures are present in the majority of cases, but epidural hemorrhage (EDH) may develop without a

fracture (45). It represents 0.9% of coma-
producing head injuries and must always
be considered because it may be rapidly
fatal (1).

Patients usually present with signs and
symptoms of an intracranial mass and if
focal signs are present they will depend on
the location of the hematoma. The classic
history of a "lucid interval" after an initial
period of unconsciousness followed by deterioration is inconsistently present, and
probably represents a concussion from the
initial impact from which the patient recovers to deteriorate again, due to the expanding hematoma once the compensatory
mechanisms are exhausted. Usually, when
the "secondary deterioration occurs," the
patient will have an ipsilateral dilated pupil
with a contralateral hemiplegia.

The initial management will depend on
the patient's condition. If an intracranial
process is suspected and the patient
remains alert, the subject must be constantly monitored even while the emergency CT scan is being obtained (Figure
4.6). Neurologic deterioration requiring
intubation and support can occur without
any warning and in a matter of seconds.

This injury usually requires immediate
operative intervention. The underlying
brain injury if any, is frequently not serious
and if evacuated immediately the prognosis
is excellent. The outcome is related to the
condition in which the patient is before the
operation (1).

Some patients will have a very small
hematoma or no hematoma on admission.
In some series of EDH, delayed EDH has
accounted for up to 8% of the total number
(46). Thus, follow-up CT scan is recommended in any patient who has not
"cleared" after 24 hours or if any new
findings arise, no matter how subtle they
may be.

Posterior fossa EDH represents 3% to

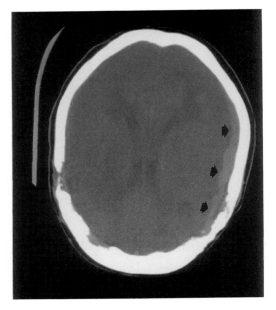

Figure 4.6. Acute epidural hemorrhage indicated by arrows. No fracture is evident.

13% of all EDH (47). It usually occurs after a
direct blow to the occipital area. Patients
usually complain about headache, nausea
and vomiting but can present also with
signs of obvious brain stem compression.
Treatment is surgical.

Acute Subdural Hematoma. This hematoma is
life-threatening. Seelig and colleagues (48)
found it in 22% of severe head-injured
patients and it accounted for 57% of the
intracranial lesions in their group of patients. The most common source is bleeding
from one of the bridging veins (from the
hemisphere to the superior sagittal sinus);
cortical vessels or cerebral contusions may
also become the source.

Subdural hematoma is frequently accompanied by an underlying brain injury that
varies in severity from a small contusion
to severe DAI or brain laceration. The
neurologic status of the patient on presentation varies and depends on both the

compressive effect of the hematoma and the underlying brain injury. Neurologic findings may help to localize the hematoma. CT will demonstrate a crescent-shaped high-density extra-axial collection with varying degrees of mass effect and accompanying lesions (Figure 4.7).

The initial treatment has been outlined earlier. The patient's hemodynamic status is optimized, and anticonvulsants should be considered. In general, steroids have not been found to be beneficial in brain traumatic injuries, but may have a place in the perioperative period. Emergency craniotomy is usually required; the goal is to decompress the brain by evacuating the hematoma and any other associated lesions. Mortality is higher than in epidural hematoma, ranging from 42% to 90% in different series (45). The outcome is many times determined by the underlying brain injury and not the hematoma.

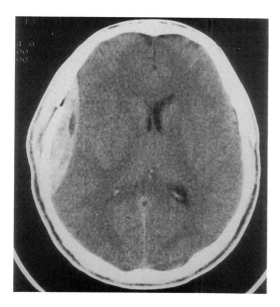

Figure 4.7. Acute subdural hematoma is obvious. The mass effect is evident.

Subarachnoid Hemorrhage. This hemorrhage is not unusual after head trauma. It results from trauma to a small superficial vessel. Headache, photophobia, and nuchal rigidity are the symptoms. The symptoms can be delayed 7 to 21 days.

Treatment is usually supportive. Steroids may help the meningitis caused by blood in the subarachnoid space. Acute or chronic hydrocephalus is a rare complication of this injury.

SOME SPORTS STATISTICS

Although head injuries are more common in contact sports, they have an incidence in almost every athletic activity. Skull fractures and intracranial injuries make up approximately 40% of the 500,000 yearly bicycle injuries. All of the deaths from head trauma are directly related to a persistent lack of helmet use both in the pediatric and adult populations. Helmet use reduces the risk of head injury by 85% (49). Lawmakers in Victoria, Australia reacted to these statistics by implementing mandatory helmet laws for all riders, resulting in a noticeable decrease in serious injury. Similar laws were passed in the United States, including Connecticut and Maryland, which now mandate the use of helmets in all children bicyclists under the age of 12. If similar legislation were enacted throughout the nation, it could possibly prevent 100 deaths and 56,000 emergency department-treated head injuries per year (50). Equestrian injuries and helmet use offer similar statistics. Football and boxing are associated with the highest incidence of head injury. The National Football Head and Neck Registry offers a good documentation of yearly deaths and concussions. On average, 5 to 10 people die yearly from football-related head injuries. Boxing injuries have been much more difficult to follow. Between 1945 and 1979, 335 were reported. Because the essence of boxing revolves around the attempt of each boxer to deliver a "knock-out punch," or concussion, boxing offers a "human laboratory" for the study of "chronic and acute brain injuries" (51). However, the cumulative effects of repeated blows to the head remain unknown. Neuropsychological testing of active and retired boxers may lead to further enlightenment regarding the results of these repeated injuries.

References

1. American College of Surgeons. Advanced trauma life support course for physicians. Chapter 6, 1989.

2. Dellen JR, Becker DP. Craniocerebral trauma, current concepts. Upjohn Company, 1988.

3. Ward J. In: Neurosurg Clin North Am 1991:2(2).

4. Becker DP, Miller JD, Ward JD, Greenberg RP, Young HF, Sakalas R. The outcome from severe head injury with early diagnosis and intensive management. J Neurosurg 1977;47:491–502.

5. Cooper PR. Delayed brain injury: secondary issues. In: Becker DP, Povlishock JT, eds. Central nervous system trauma status report. Washington, DC: National Institute of Neurological and Communicative Disorders and Stroke, National Intitutes of Health. 1985:217–228.

6. Miller JD, Becker DF. Secondary insults to the injured brain. J R Coll Surg Edinb 1982;Sept 2:292–298.

7. McCormick WF. Pathology of closed head injury. In: Wilkins, Rengachary SS, eds. Neurosurgery. New York: McGraw-Hill, 1985:1544–1570.

8. Mathern GW, Martin NA, Becker DP. Cerebral ischemia: clinical pathophysiology. In: Cerra FB, Shoemaker WC, eds. Critical care: state of the art. Fullerton, CA: The Society of Critical Care Medicine. 1987, vol 8, chap 2.

9. Cales RH, Trunkey DD. Preventable trauma deaths: a review of trauma systems development. JAMA 1985;254:1959–1963.

10. Colohan AR, Alves WM, Gross CR, et al. Head injury mortality in two centers with different emergency medical services and intensive care. J Neurosurg 1989;71:202–207.

11. Frost EAM, Arancibia CU, Shulman K. Pulmonary shunt as a prognostic indicator in head injury. J Neurosurg 1979;50:768–772.

12. Narayan RK, Kishore PPS, Becker DP, et al. Intracranial pressure monitor: to monitor or not to monitor. J Neurosurg 1982;56:650–659.

13. Eisenberg HM, Weiner RL, Tabaddor K. Emergency care and initial evaluation. In: Cooper PR, ed. Head injury, 2nd ed. Baltimore: Williams & Wilkins, 1987.

14. Baker SP, O'Neil B. The injury severity scale: an update. J Trauma 1976;16:882–886.

15. Teasdale G, Jennett B. Assessment of coma and impaired consciousness: a practical scale. Lancet 1974;2:81–84.

16. Galbraith S. Misdiagnosis and delayed diagnosis in traumatic intracranial haematoma. Br Med J 1976;1:1438–1439.

17. Bruce DA, Genarelli TA, Langfitt TW. Resuscitation from coma due to head injury. Crit Care Med 1978;6:254–269.

18. Plum F, Posner JB. The diagnosis of stupor and coma, 2nd ed. Philadelphia: FA Davis, 1972.

19. Lindenberg R. Pathology of craniovertebral injuries. In: Newton TH, Potts DG, eds. Radiology of the skull and brain. St. Louis: CV Mosby, 1977:3049–3089.

20. Crow W. Aspects of neuroradiology of head injury. In: Eisenberg H, Aldrich F, eds. Neurosurg Clin North Am 1991; 2:321–339.

21. Wilberger JE, Rothfus WE, Tabas J. Magnetic resonance imaging in cases of severe head injury. Neurosurgery 1987; 20:571–576.

22. Adams JH, Graham DI, Scott G, Parker LS, Doyle D. Brain damage in non-missile head injury. J Clin Pathol 1980;33:1132–1145.

23. Mendelow AD, Teasdale G, Jennet B, Bryden J, Hesset C. Risks of intracranial haematoma in head injured adults. Br Med J 1983;287:1173–1176.

24. Zimmerman RA, Bilaniuk LT, Gennarelli T, Bruce D. Cranial computed tomography in diagnosis and management of acute head

trauma. Am J Roentgenol 1978;131:27–34.

25. Jennet B. Some medicolegal aspects of the management of acute head injury. Br Med J 1976;1:1383–1385.

26. Braakman R. Depressed skull fracture: data, treatment and follow up in 225 consecutive cases. J Neurosurg Psych 1971;34:106–110.

27. Jennet B, Miller JD, Braakman R. Epilepsy after nonmissile depressed skull fracture. J Neurosurg 1974;41:208–216.

28. Van der Heever HJ, Van der Merwe JJ. Management of depressed skull fractures: selective conservative management of nonmissile injuries. J Neurosurg 1989;71:186–190.

29. Fremstad JD, Martin SH. Lethal complication from insertion of nasogastric tube after severe basilar skull fracture. J Trauma 1978; 18:820–824.

30. Cooper PR. Skull fracture and traumatic cerebrospinal fluid fistulas. In: Cooper PR, ed. Head injury, 2nd ed. Baltimore: Williams & Wilkins, 1987.

31. Gennarelli TA. Cerebral concussion and diffuse brain injury. In: Cooper PR, ed. Head injury, 2nd ed. Baltimore: Williams & Wilkins, 1987.

32. Graham DI, McLellan D, Adams JH. Neuropathology of the vegetative state and severe disability after non-missile head injury. Acta Neurochir 1983;(suppl)32:67–68.

33. Sahuquillo-Berris J, Lamarca-Ciurio J, et al. Epidural hematoma and diffuse axonal injury. Neurosurgery 1985;17:378–379.

34. Gerbich SG, Priest JD, Boen JR. Concussions, incidence and severity in secondary school varsity football players. Am J Public Health 1983;73:1370–1375.

35. Alves WM, Rimmel RW, et al. University of Virginia prospective study of football induced minor head injuries. Clin Sports Med 1987;6:211.

36. Gudeman SK, Kishore PRS, Miller JD, et al. The genesis and significance of delayed traumatic intracerebral hematoma. Neurosurgery 1979;5:309.

37. Wilberger J, Maroon J. Head injuries in athletes. Clin Sports Med 1989;8:5.

38. Kelly JP, Nichols JS, et al. Concussion in sports: guidelines for the prevention of catastrophic outcome. JAMA 1991;266:2867–2869.

39. Colorado Medical Society. Reports of the Sports Medicine Committee: guidelines for the management of concussion in sports (revised). Denver: Colorado Medical Society; 1991.

40. Bruce DA, Alavi A, Bilaniuk L, et al. Diffuse cerebral swelling following head injuries in children: the syndrome of "malignant brain edema." J Neurosurg 1981;54:170–178.

41. Saunders R, Harbaugh R. The second impact in catastrophic contact-sports head trauma. JAMA 1984;252:538–539.

42. Adams JH, Graham DI, et al. Diffuse axonal injury due to non-missile head injury in man. Ann Neurol 1982;12:557–563.

43. Langfitt TW. Increased intracranial pressure. Clin Neurosurg 1969;16:436–471.

44. Temkin NR, Dikmen SS, Winn HR. Post-traumatic seizures. In: Eisenberg H, Aldrich F, eds. Neurosurg Clin North Am 1991;2:425–436.

45. Obana WG, Pitts LH. Extracerebral lesions. In: Eisenberg H, Aldrich F, eds. Neurosurg Clin North Am 1991;2:351–372.

46. Borovich B, Braun J, Guilburd JN, et al. Delayed onset of traumatic extradural hematoma. J Neurosurg 1985;63:30–34.

47. Zuccarello M, Pardatscher K, Andrioli GC, et al. Epidural hematoma of the posterior cranial fossa. Neurosurgery 1981;8:434–437.

48. Seelig JM, Becker DP, Miller JD, et al. Traumatic acute subdural hematoma. Major morbidity reduction in comatose patients treated within four hours. N Engl J Med 1981;304:1511–1518.

49. Mandatory bicycle helmet use—Victoria, Australia. JAMA 1993;269:2967.

50. Cote TR, Sacks JJ, et al. Bicycle helmet use among Maryland children: effects of legislation and education. Pediatrics 1992;89:1216–1220.

51. Adelson PD, Thomas S, et al. Boxing fatalities and brain injury. Perspect Neurol Surg 1991;2:167–184.

Bibliography

Aldrich EF. Surgical management of traumatic intracerebral hematomas. In: Eisenberg H, Aldrich F, eds. Neurosurg Clin North Am 1991;2:373–385.

Black PM, Ojemann R. Hydrocephalus in adults. In: Youmans ed. Neurological Surgery,

3d ed. Philadelphia: WB Saunders, 1990:1277–1298.

Chestnut RM, Marshall L. Treatment of abnormal intracranial pressure. In: Eisenberg H, Aldrich F, eds. Neurosurg Clin North Am 1991;2:267–284.

Cooper PR. Post traumatic intracranial mass lesion. In: Cooper PR, ed. Head injury, 2nd ed. Baltimore: Williams & Wilkins, 1987.

Fackler ML. Wound ballistics: a review of common misconceptions. JAMA 1988;259:2730–2736.

Fleischer AS, Patton JM, Tindall GT. Cerebral aneurysms of traumatic origin. Surg Neurol 1975;4:233–239.

Gennarelli TA, Spielman G, Langfitt TW, et al. The influene of the type of intracranial lesion on outcome from severe head injury: a multicenter study using a new classification system. J Neurosurg 1982;56:26–32.

Jennet B, Miller JD. Infection after depressed fracture of skull. Implications for management in non missile injury. J Neurosurg 1972;36:333–339.

Kanter MJ, Narayan R. Intracranial pressure monitoring. In: Eisenberg H, Aldrich F, eds. Neurosurg Clin North Am 1991;2:257–266.

Mitchell DE, Adams JH. Primary focal impact damage to the brainstem in blunt head injury: does it really exist? Lancet 1973;2:215–218.

Quest D. Increased intracranial pressure, brain herniation and their control. In: Wilkins RH, Rengachary SS, eds. Neurosurgery. New York: McGraw-Hill, 1985:332–342.

Wilberger J, Chen D. Management of head trauma. The skull and meninges. In: Eisenberg H, Aldrich F, eds. Neurosurg Clin North Am 1991;2:341–350.

Zimmerman RA, Bilaniuk LT, Gennarelli TA. Computed tomography of shearing injuries of the cerebral white matter. Radiology 1978;127:393–396.

NECK INJURIES IN SPORTS

5

STUART C. BELKIN

Epidemiology of Sports-related Neck
    Injuries
Anatomy of the Cervical Spine
Diagnosis and Treatment of Cervical Spine
    Injuries: An Overview
Sprains, Strains, and Contusions
Fractures and Dislocations
Unstable Ligamentous Injuries
Neurologic Injury
Transient Quadriplegia
Return to Athletics After Neck Injury
Rehabilitation
Recommendations

Cervical spine injuries as a consequence of athletic activity range from the trivial and mundane to the catastrophic and tragic (1–10). The burgeoning athletic and exercise approach to health and well-being, though clearly beneficial to the public health, has produced substantial numbers of cervical spine injuries spanning the population, irrespective of age, sex, or athletic activity. Injuries can occur in organized sports or in pick-up games, team or individual, contact by design or maloccurrence. (3,5,8,11–16).

The acute treatment of cervical spine injuries is usually the responsibility of the primary care physician (11). Although the average primary care practitioner caring for athletes will probably never encounter a life-threatening or neurologically destructive cervical spine injury, the ability to critically assess and emergently care for such an injury is requisite for the sports physician.

The most commonly occurring cervical spine injury encountered by the primary care physician is a sprain or strain. A *sprain* is an injury to the ligamentous structures supporting the joints of the cervical spine; a *strain* is an injury to the muscle tendon units about the cervical spine. The vast majority of these injuries would be in continuity stretch injuries and functionally stable. Rarely, there might be more substantial ligamentous injury with pathologic lengthening of the ligamentous structure or even complete disruption producing instability and risk of injury to the neurologic structures.

Far more rarely, the primary care practitioner will be presented with a fracture, dislocation, or combination injury of the cervical spine. Although referral will be required, the initial critical care will frequently be the responsibility of the primary care practitioner.

Finally, a variety of sports-related neurologic injuries of the cervical spine may occur without a ligamentous or bony injury. The most common would be a brachial plexus injury, a "stinger" in football, which is usually a transient neurologic injury but can produce prolonged or even permanent sequelae depending on the degree of nerve injury (17–20). Another group of nerve root injuries can occur as a result of fractures, dislocations, or disk herniations involving the cervical spine. Finally, spinal cord injury complete or incomplete, transient, permanent, or fatal can result from spinal trauma in sports (1,3,5,6,9–11,14–16,21–24).

EPIDEMIOLOGY OF SPORTS-RELATED NECK INJURIES

Cervical spine injuries are reported in a multitude of sporting activities including football (3,6,10–13,21,25,26), hockey (16), track and field (27), rugby (28), boxing (10), wrestling (10,13), skateboarding (14), gymnastics (29), trampoline (5,13,15), skiing (29), diving (8,13,29,30), snowmobiling (29), volleyball (13), and baseball (13). These reports are placed in some perspective by Hodge (18), "Statistically, the risk of severe injury is greater driving the freeways of Los Angeles than participating in a high risk sport such as boxing, gymnastics, diving, ice hockey, wrestling or football." This is borne out by Dietrich and colleagues (13), whose 5-year retrospective review of pediatric cervical spinal fractures revealed a motor vehicle etiology in 54% and a sports etiology in 18%; Good and Nickels' (9) review of 1058 quadriplegic patients admitted to Rancho Los Amigos Hospital over 11 years with the majority of the injuries caused by motor vehicle accidents and 200 injuries caused by water sports as the second most common etiology; Kewalramani and Krauss' (10) review of 1305 spinal cord injury admissions over several years to institutions in Sacramento and Houston with the majority resulting from motor vehicle trauma and only 46 (3.5%) secondary to collision sports, such as football, boxing, and wrestling; and Mann and Dodds' (29) 8-year review of 57 pediatric cervical spine admissions to the University of Wisconsin Hospital with 46% of the injuries secondary to motor vehicle accidents and approximately 12% involving sports activities including gymnastics, diving, skiing, tobogganing, and snowmobiling.

It is of some importance to classify sports activities as contact or noncontact sports. The former include football, hockey, rugby, boxing, wrestling, and basketball; the latter baseball, gymnastics, water sports, skiing, skating, track and field, tennis, golf, and soccer. As Duffy Daugherty, the noted former Michigan State University football coach once stated, football is a collision sport, dancing is a contact sport. The distinction is, of course, germane to the epidemiology of cervical spine injuries because the violent forces placed on the cervical spine secondary to high-energy collisions produce the injuries in question.

Football, because of its great popularity in the United States and the collision forces intrinsic to the sport, has a primary place in the study and treatment of injuries to the cervical spine.

Schneider (31) reviewed football fatalities and serious injuries from 1959 to 1963 and found 60 deaths as a result of head trauma and 16 deaths secondary to cervical spine injuries. He concluded the football helmet was inadequate in protecting the player from direct trauma to the head and neck.

Mueller and Blyth (21) reviewed data from 1945 to 1984 from the Annual Survey of Football Injury Research collected by the American Football Coaches Association, receiving reports from public schools, colleges, and professional and youth programs. Over this interval there were 643 football fatalities, 433 (67.3%) from head injury and 111 (17.3%) from injury to the cervical spine. Further, they reported fatality totals of 42 neck injuries from 1965 to 1974 and 14 neck injuries from 1975 to 1984. This significant decrease was attributed to a 1976 rules change in high school and college football penalizing initial contact with the helmet or face mask in tackling or blocking, that is, "spearing." The authors firmly endorsed the need for coaches to teach "head up" blocking and tackling and recommended strengthening exercises for the cervical spine.

Albright and colleagues (25), reporting on nonfatal cervical spine football injuries in interscholastic football based on a 1973 questionnaire distributed to high school coaches, found a 1.2% incidence of neck injuries. These were most frequent in defensive backs and linebackers. There was a reinjury rate of 17.2% in the same season.

In a subsequent report on head and neck injuries in college football published in 1985, Albright and associates (12), reported on 342 college football players from 1978 to 1984. There was a 10.5% incidence of noncatastrophic neck injury with 42% of the players experiencing a second injury and 28% a third injury. If a player had an abnormality in history, physical examination, or x-ray with regard to the cervical spine in preseason evaluation, the cervical spine injury rate doubled from 7% to 13.5%.

Torg and coworkers (3) reported on cervical quadriplegia as excerpted from the National Football Head and Neck Injury Registry from 1971 through 1984. They noted that there were 34 permanent cervical quadriplegic patients secondary to football injuries in 1976 and 5 permanent cervical quadriplegic patients secondary to football in 1984. They also attributed this to the rule change banning "spearing" and the consistency in coaching and officiating in upholding the rule (Figure 5.1). Torg felt the axial load created by using the crown of the helmet in tackling or blocking produced the catastrophic cervical injuries in football and he further suggested the same mechanism would be responsible for catastrophic cervical spine injuries in diving, rugby, ice hockey, and gymnastics. Finally, Torg suggested changes in techniques and equipment in these sports might have the same beneficial result in limiting cervical spine injuries as the "spearing" rule had in football.

Torg and colleagues (23) expanded on the epidemiology of football-induced cervical spine trauma in 1990. They reported an incidence of fractures and dislocations of the cervical spine occurring in 1976 of 7.72 per

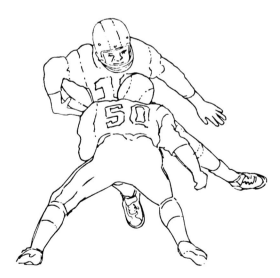

Figure 5.1. "Spearing," the use of the helmet in tackling or blocking, carries a risk of catastrophic neck injury and is now against the rules of American football.

100,000 in high school and 30.66 per 100,000 in college. These figures decreased in 1987 to 2.31 per 100,000 and 10.66 per 100,000, respectively. This represented a decrease of 70% in high school and 65% in college. Torg again emphasized the mechanism of axial compression producing fractures and dislocations of the cervical spine resulting in cervical spinal cord injuries. He pointed out that tackling or blocking with the head and neck flexed approximately 30° straightened the normal cervical lordosis, creating a segmented column that became compressed to failure when the helmet struck an immovable object while the body continued forward, crushing the cervical spine.

Tator analyzed ice hockey as a team contact sport responsible for substantial cervical spine injuries in Canada (16). A national survey in 1982 identified 42 ice hockey spinal injuries prior to that date. Thirty-nine of the 42 were injuries to the cervical spine. All injuries occurred secondary to axial compression as a result of a blow to the head. Twenty-five injuries occurred when the player's head struck the boards. Thirty-seven players were wearing helmets. Seventy percent of the injuries occurred at C5 or C6. Twenty-eight of the 42 players sustained spinal cord injuries. Twenty-two players were rendered wheelchair bound. Tator noted there were 4 cases of quadriplegia per year secondary to ice hockey injuries in Canada. On a per capita basis ice hockey in Canada produced three times the annual number of quadriplegics as football in the United States. Tator had several recommendations designed to decrease the incidence of cervical spine injury. He recommended enforcement of rules against boarding and cross checking and new rules against checking from behind, avoidance of head first checking, avoidance of smaller rinks, and greater emphasis on strengthening of the cervical spine musculature.

Water sports, particularly diving and body surfing, are responsible for substantial numbers of cervical spine injuries (8). Good and Nickel (32) reviewed 2104 spinal cord–injured patients admitted to Rancho Los Amigos Hospital from January 1965 to January 1976. Of these, 1046 were paraplegic and 1058 were quadriplegics. Water sports injuries produced 200 of the 1058 quadriplegics, second only to motor vehicle trauma as an etiology. Complete data were available on 152 of the 200 patients. Ninety-two percent were men, 65% between 16 and 25 years of age. Diving into an ocean caused 51% of the injuries and diving from a height produced 21%; another 21% occurred during body surfing and the last 7% were during surfboarding. Sixteen percent had been using drugs or alcohol prior to the injury. The injuries were devastating, with 54% complete cord syndromes and 41% incomplete with 5% neurologically normal.

Trampoline activities have produced a substantial number of cervical spine injuries. A recent limited review by Woodward and colleagues (15) reported on all trampoline injuries (114 patients) seen at Children's Hospital Medical Center in Salt Lake City, Utah from June 1989 to November 1990. The ratio of males to females was 1.2:1.0. The average age was 8 years. Thirty-seven percent of the patients sustained a head or neck injury including concussions, skull fractures, neck sprains, and a single cervical fracture. In an article from 1977 the American Academy of Pediatrics recommended a ban on all trampoline activities in public schools because of a rash of cervical spine injuries. This recommendation was revised in 1981, recommending school usage with seven precautions but no home use.

Torg and Das (5) reported results of a world literature review of catastrophic cervical spine injuries secondary to trampoline or minitramp accidents. The authors found 114 quadriplegic patients over 23 years. There were several reports of the patient "blacking out" prior to impact. The injured were frequently expert gymnasts. The injuries frequently occurred on thick mats and with spotters. The authors concluded there was "no place in recreational, educational or competitive gymnastics" for the trampoline or minitramp.

ANATOMY OF THE CERVICAL SPINE

The cervical spine is comprised of seven cervical vertebrae—C1 through C7. The first cervical vertebra, the atlas, articulates cranially with the occiput and caudally with the second cervical vertebra, the axis (Figure 5.2). The atlas is ring shaped and its relationship with the axis is stabilized by various ligaments. Fifty percent of rotation of the head and neck occurs between C1 and C2; 50% of the flexion occurs between the occiput and C1. The dens or odontoid process is the fingerlike cranial extension of the body of the axis, which is dorsal to the anterior arch of the atlas and ventral to the transverse atlantal ligament.

The remaining five vertebral bodies consist of solid cylinders of bone with posterior arches. Each pair of vertebral bodies from C2 to C7 articulates with an intervertebral disk and two facet joints (Figure 5.3). The joints are oriented in the coronal plane and thus allow for greater flexion and extension of the spine but are consequently less stable in flexion and rotation than the more sagittally oriented lumbar facet joints. The normal motion of the head and neck totals approximately 100° of flexion and extension, 80° rotation to the right and left, and

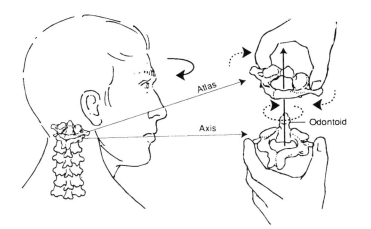

Figure 5.2. The ring shape of C1 (atlas) and the protruding odontoid process from C2 (axis) facilitate rotation of the neck.

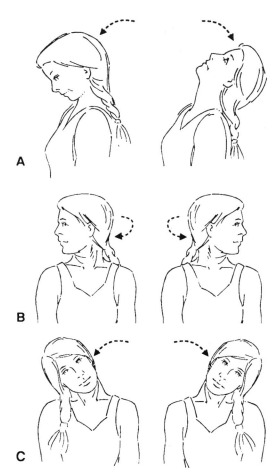

Figure 5.4. *A.* Normal range of neck flexion and extension (totals 100°). *B.* Normal range of neck rotation (80° in each direction). *C.* Normal range of neck lateral bending (40° in each direction).

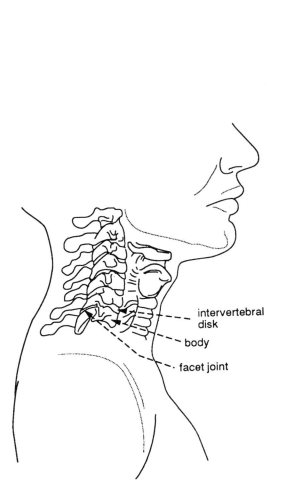

Figure 5.3. Anatomic relationships of the cervical vertebrae.

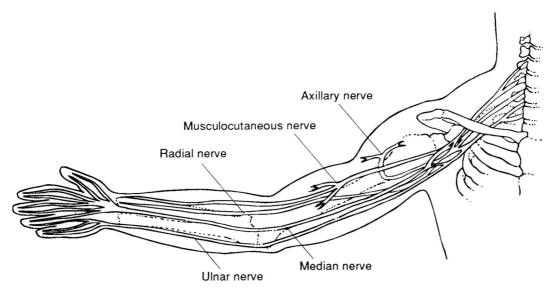

Axillary nerve

Musculocutaneous nerve

Radial nerve

Ulnar nerve

Median nerve

Figure 5.5. The brachial plexus and peripheral nerves.

40° lateral bending (Figure 5.4). These motions decrease with older age.

The spinal canal in the cervical region begins at the foramen magnum and is then bounded by the arch of C1 and the transverse atlantal ligament, then more caudally by each vertebral body and disk anteriorly and the vertebral arches laterally and posteriorly (see Figure 5.2). All of the vertebral structures are stabilized by the anterior longitudinal ligament, posterior longitudinal ligament, ligamentum flavum, capsules of the facet joints, and interspinous and supraspinous ligaments.

The cervical spinal cord traverses the spinal canal thus created by the column of vertebral bodies, disks, arches, and ligaments. Various patterns of spinal cord injury are produced depending on the forces across the cervical spine and the resultant deformities of bone, disk, and ligament producing spinal cord impingement.

The brachial plexus arises from the C5, C6, C7, C8, and T1 roots with occasional contributions from C4 or T2 (Figure 5.5). These roots innervate the musculature of the upper extremities. Injury to the neck via sports can commonly affect the brachial plexus, producing a variety of motor and sensory symptoms and signs of varying duration and severity.

DIAGNOSIS AND TREATMENT OF CERVICAL SPINE INJURIES: AN OVERVIEW

The evaluation of an injured athlete reflects the appropriate evaluation of any medical emergency. There must be immediate attention to potential life-threatening circumstances, then appropriate history, physical examination, and radiologic evaluation.

Patient History

Patient history is often helpful as to the exact mechanism of injury and an indication of the severity. The athlete must be asked to describe the exact sequence of events preceding the injury and as accurately as possible the forces applied to the head and neck and the direction and degree of resultant deformity. Ascertaining flexion, extension, axial compression, rotation, or lateral bending can give an initial hint as to the potential for neurologic injury and instability.

The nature, severity, and location of pain is next elicited. Radiating pain is more likely neurologic in nature. The burning of a "stinger" or "burner" down the arm is characteristic of a brachial plexus injury (Figure 5.6) (17–20). Severe neck pain may mandate spine board immobilization, whereas minor transient pain may allow immediate return to activities. Relentless excruciating pain after acute injury may indicate a fracture, dislocation, or disk herniation, but the degree of pain is not always proportional to the severity of the injury and some fractures or dislocations may be deceptively low key in presentation in a highly motivated stoic athlete.

Neurologic symptoms must next be elicited from the injured athlete. Subjective weakness may range from a vague generalized malaise to specific localized muscular dysfunction—for example, weakness in shoulder elevation with a C4–C5 disk herniation to quadriparesis. The symptom may be transient, lasting minutes to hours (e.g., brachial plexus neuropraxia or transient quadriplegia secondary to cervical spinal stenosis) or permanent (e.g., fracture dislocation with spinal cord injury). Sensory changes may vary in a similar fashion with hypesthesias, paresthesias, or

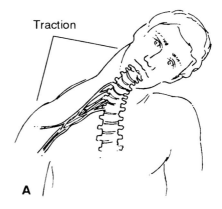

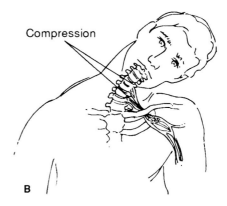

Figure 5.6. Lateral bending of the neck can lead either to traction on the brachial plexus (*A*) or compression of the plexus (*B*) causing a "stinger" or "burner."

anesthesia in dermatomal or quadriplegic distributions transiently or permanently.

Finally, the athlete unable to respond secondary to head injury and loss of consciousness must always be treated as having a cervical spine injury until proven otherwise. Even transient loss of consciousness or traumatically induced alteration in mental function mandates careful evaluation of the cervical spine.

Any athlete rendered unconscious by a head injury during athletic activity must be transported on a spine board with appropriate head and neck immobilization (Figure 5.7). In high-risk team sports, the responsible physician should anticipate significant head and neck trauma with the presence of a previously practiced plan of action, oral airway, spine board, sandbags,

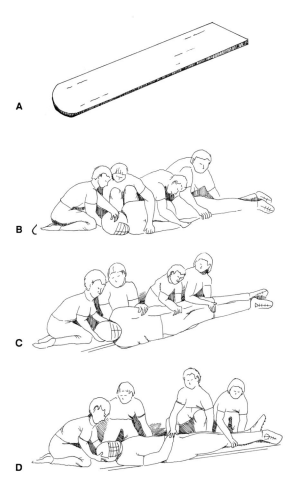

Figure 5.7. Technique for "log rolling." The team leader controls the athlete's head and gives commands while each of the other members rolls the athlete en bloc.

double action bolt cutters, and a fully equipped ambulance at the field or readily accessible.

Physical Examination

The physical examination follows the history in an effort to further elucidate the nature and severity of the injury. In a seriously injured athlete, the overriding principles of resuscitation must first be addressed. Particularly in the unconscious athlete, the airway must be assessed and maintained, the respiratory status must be ensured, and the circulation must be adequate (1,6,24,30,33). This must be done while protecting the cervical spine at all times and preventing iatrogenic injury.

Next, an assessment of the motor and sensory function, and reflexes can be easily performed on the field (Table 5.1). The C5 root (Figure 5.8) has a sensory innervation of the lateral arm. The motions are elbow flexion and power supination with the biceps and shoulder abduction with the deltoid. The biceps reflex is C5 innervated. The C6 root (Figure 5.9) has a sensory distribution to the thumb and index fingers. The motors are the radial wrist extensors. The C7 root (Figure 5.10) has a sensory distribution to the long finger. The motors are the radial wrist flexor, common finger extensors, and the triceps. The triceps reflex is also C7 innervated. The C8 root (Figure 5.11) gives sensory innervation to the little and ring fingers. The motor innervation is to the finger flexors, superficial and deep. The T1 root (Figure 5.12) gives sensory function to the medial arm and motor function to the interossei for abduction and adduction of the fingers.

In the event of obvious gross neurologic abnormality, the physician must next align and immobilize the cervical spine. This is done by placing the hands under the man-

Table 5.1. Neurologic levels of the upper extremity

Disk	Root	Reflex	Muscles	Sensation
C4–C5	C5	Biceps reflex	Deltoid, biceps	Lateral arm—axillary nerve
C5–C6	C6	Brachioradialis reflex (biceps reflex)	Wrist extension, biceps	Thumb and index finger—musculocutaneous nerve
C6–C7	C7	Triceps reflex	Wrist flexors, finger extension, triceps	Middle finger
C7–T1	C8	—	Finger flexion, hand intrinsics	Medial forearm—medial anterior brachialis, cutaneous nerve
T1–T2	T1	—	Hand intrinsics	Medial arm—medial brachialis, cutaneous nerve

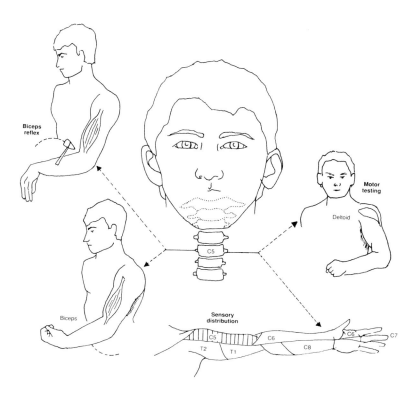

Figure 5.8. Motor, reflex, and sensory distribution of the C5 nerve root. (Modified from S Hoppenfeld. Physical Examination of the Spine Extremities. Norwalk, CT: Appleton & Lange, 1976: 120.)

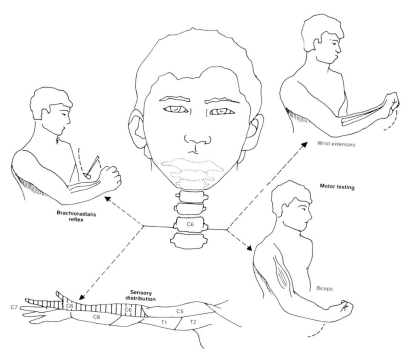

Figure 5.9. Motor, reflex, and sensory distribution of the C6 nerve root. (Modified from S Hoppenfeld. Physical Examination of the Spine Extremities. Norwalk, CT: Appleton & Lange, 1976: 121.)

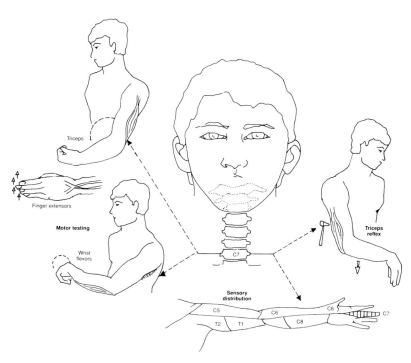

Figure 5.10. Motor, reflex, and sensory distribution of the C7 nerve root. (Modified from S Hoppenfeld. Physical Examination of the Spine Extremities. Norwalk, CT: Appleton & Lange, 1976: 122.)

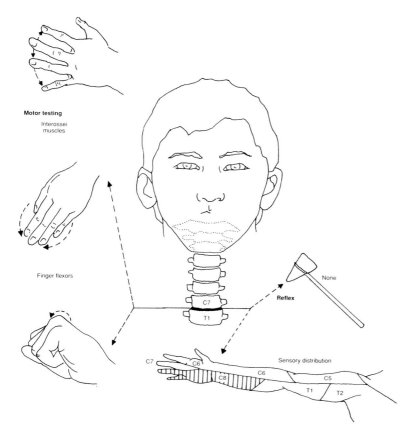

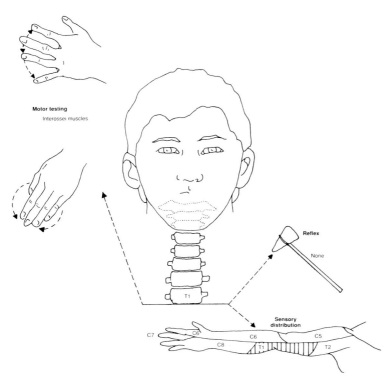

dible and occiput and holding gentle traction striving for a neutral alignment of head, neck, and trunk. The prone athlete must be log rolled supine with the help of two assistants on each side of the athlete controlling the trunk and extremities while the team physician controls the head and neck (see Figure 5.7). The athlete is then log rolled onto the spine board with the head and neck taped in neutral as to flexion, extension, and rotation or traction maintained by the physician. The helmet remains on and is taped to the board. Flexion must be avoided. The athlete is transported to the hospital on the spine board.

In the less severely injured athlete, who has not sustained loss of consciousness, a history and physical examination can be elicited more completely. Only the athlete with a normal neurologic examination and full painless range of motion of the cervical spine can be allowed to return to the competition. At any level of competition the physician's first responsibility is to protect the well-being of the athlete regardless of pressure to compete.

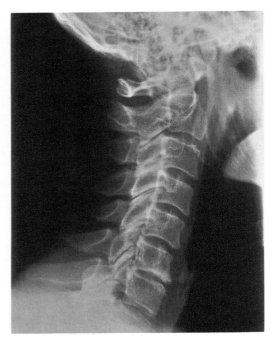

Figure 5.13. Lateral radiograph of the cervical spine must include the C7–T1 disk space to ensure normal relationships.

Radiologic Evaluation

Radiologic evaluation of the cervical spine, if indicated by the clinical suspicion of a significant injury, begins with a lateral x-ray from C1 to the C7–T1 disk space (Figure 5.13). In the athlete with muscular or obese shoulders the arms can be pulled down manually or with traction straps, or a "swimmer's view" can be obtained (Figure 5.14). Anteroposterior, open mouth, and oblique views are also obtained. If there is a question of instability in the face of otherwise normal x-rays, lateral flexion extension x-rays may be obtained.

There are several specific radiologic parameters of which to be aware. On the lateral x-ray the soft tissue shadow between the body of C3 and the trachea should be less than or equal to 5 mm in an adult. Children may have normally wider soft-tissue shadows when crying. There is usually a cervical lordosis, but Weir reported 20% of lateral cervical spine x-rays to show a straightened or kyphotic appearance, and if the chin is depressed 1 inch, 70% of cervical spines will be straightened (Figure 5.15). Consequently, assuming a straightened cervical lordosis is a result of spasm is not necessarily valid. The atlantodens interval (see Figure 5.20) should be less than or equal to 3 mm; an interval of 3 to 5 mm indicates rupture of the transverse ligament; an interval of greater than 5 mm indicates rupture of the accessory ligaments as

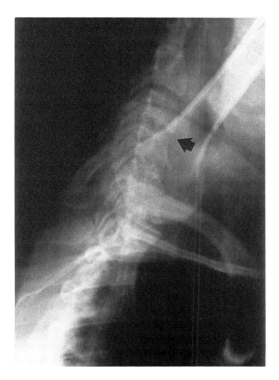

Figure 5.14. The "swimmers view" of the cervical spine clearly shows the C7–T1 disk space (*arrow*) and the accompanying vertebral bodies.

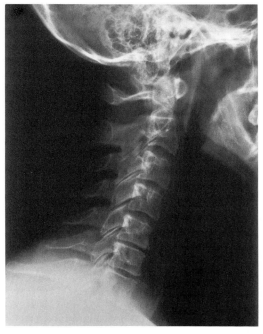

Figure 5.15. "Straightened" cervical spine, absence of the normal lordosis.

well. The vertebral bodies should form a smooth arc, viewing their anterior and posterior borders from the body of C2 to the body of C7. The facet joints should show a symmetrical appearance as well. Any step-off of the vertebral bodies or inequality of the facets may indicate a subluxation or dislocation.

The open mouth view should show an intact arch of C1 and symmetrical placement of the articular facets of C1 on C2. Asymmetry of the facets with the lateral masses of C1 subluxed on C2 can indicate a subluxation or fracture dislocation (see Figure 5.17). The open mouth view is also important in assessing the presence of an odontoid process fracture.

The anteroposterior view should reveal a smoothly undulating outline of the bodies and articular processes with the spinous processes in the midline. Displacement of a spinous process in the transverse plane may indicate a unilateral jumped facet, whereas displacement in the sagittal plane may indicate a bilateral jumped facet.

The oblique views reveal the patency of the neural foramina as well as the articular processes and facet joints, further revealing facet asymmetry in the presence of dislocation.

Depending on the athlete's history, physical examination, and plain films, further imaging may be required. The most likely studies would be computed tomography (CT) to elucidate bony injury and magnetic resonance imaging (MRI) to evaluate soft-tissue injury; myelography, tomography, and technetium scanning are less frequently useful.

SPRAINS, STRAINS, AND CONTUSIONS

Clinical Case #1

A high school soccer player was injured yesterday in a collision while trying to head the ball. She twisted her neck as she collided with her opponent. She had neck pain but was able to continue to play. She had no neurologic symptoms but has increased pain and stiffness of her neck now, 18 hours after the injury. Her examination shows painful but full motion of the neck. She is neurologically intact. She is tender in the trapezius muscle. Are radiographs indicated? When can she return to soccer?

The most innocuous cervical spine injuries will be sprains, strains, and contusions. A *sprain* is a ligamentous injury involving the facet joints. A *strain* entails injury to the muscles or tendons and a *contusion* involves a direct blow to these structures. These injuries may occur in contact sports such as football or wrestling or noncontact sports such as track and field or tennis. Each athlete is carefully evaluated as to the exact mechanism of injury; location, duration, and intensity of pain; neurologic symptoms; and whether play was continued. A complete physical examination of the cervical spine and upper extremities including neurologic evaluation is undertaken next. Radiologic evaluation is ordered only if the clinical situation so mandates (e.g., severe pain, decreased range of cervical motion, or neurologic abnormalities). The treatment regimen is ice for 48 hours followed by heat;

active range of motion to comfort; isometric to progressive resistive exercises to comfort; and medication including limited analgesics, muscle relaxants, and nonsteroidal anti-inflammatory drugs. The use of a soft collar is rarely indicated. The return to participation occurs when there is full painless range of motion of the cervical spine and a normal neurologic examination.

Our high school soccer player has had no sign of neurologic injury and has full range of motion of her cervical spine and no bony tenderness; therefore, films are not necessary. She should be kept out of soccer until her neck motion is pain free.

FRACTURES AND DISLOCATIONS

The more serious sports-related cervical spine injuries are fractures and dislocations. The initial evaluation may be critical to the ultimate well-being of the athlete. Any unconscious athlete must be assumed to be suffering from a cervical spine injury and must be immobilized and transported as previously noted. The conscious patient will be able to provide a history replete with mechanism of injury; quality, severity, and location of pain; and neurologic symptoms, which will alert the physician to the severity of the injury. Physical examination with observation, palpation, active motion, and neurologic examination will further elucidate the severity of the problem. After the cervical spine is appropriately aligned and immobilized with spine board transportation, appropriate radiologic or other imaging studies can be performed as indicated. The studies will always include lateral x-rays from C1 to the C7–T1 disk space, open mouth, anteroposterior, and oblique x-rays. Lateral flexion-extension x-rays, CT, CT myelography, or MRI may be obtained as indicated by the clinical picture.

Stable Fractures

Stable fractures of the cervical spine include avulsion fractures of the spinous processes or anterior wedge compression fractures. Spinous process avulsion fractures occur as a result of muscular traction forces on the spinous processes of the distal cervical vertebrae in weight lifters or football players tensing on contact. Anterior wedge compression fractures occur in contact or noncontact sports when the head is flexed and strikes an object with enough force to compress the anterior vertebral body but without enough force to disrupt the posterior ligaments or bony arch or create a burst fracture. Both types of stable fracture will produce immediate severe cervical pain and tenderness with the avulsion of the spinous process localizable posteriorly. Both will have limited cervical motion secondary to pain, but neither will produce any subjective weakness, numbness, or paresthesias and the injured athletes will be neurologically intact.

Radiographic evaluation will show localized soft-tissue swelling and the fractures themselves. In each case the injuries will be best demonstrated on lateral x-rays. When the acute pain has resolved, lateral flexion-extension x-rays are mandatory to rule out ligamentous instability, and they will be normal with these two types of injury.

The treatment of these injuries is similar, requiring ice, analgesics, and a soft collar for support. After 3 to 6 weeks, range of motion and isometric exercises are instituted as comfort allows (Figure 5.16). After full painless range of motion is regained with painless isometric exercises as well, progressive resistive exercises may be instituted. Return to contact sports should be withheld until the following season, that is, a minimum of 3 to 6 months.

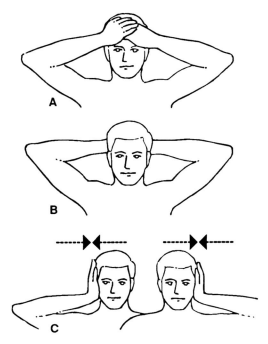

Figure 5.16. Isometric exercises for cervical spine. *A.* Resisted flexion: sit or stand upright with hands on forehead, push head against hands and hold for 7 seconds. Repeat 10 times. *B.* Resisted extension: sit or stand upright with hands behind head, push head back against hands and hold for 7 seconds. Repeat 10 times. *C.* Resisted side-bend: sit or stand upright with hand on right side of head, push toward it and hold for 7 seconds. Repeat 10 times. Then repeat exercise toward the left.

Unstable Fractures

The *Jefferson fracture* occurs as a result of axial compression to the top of the head with the cervical spine neutral. The ring of C1 is burst apart with fractures in two or more areas (Figure 5.17). The athlete will have immediate severe pain and decreased cervical motion. The neurologic examination is normal because the fracture frag-

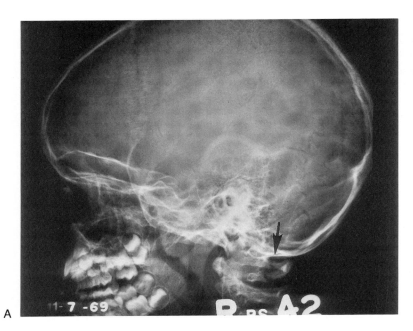

A

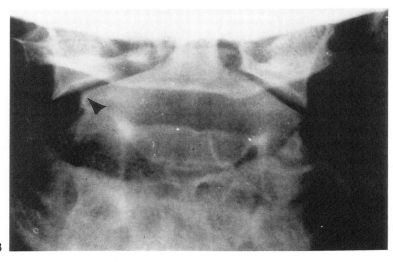

B

Figure 5.17. Jefferson fracture showing break in the ring of C1 (*A*) and displacement of the lateral mass of C1 at the arrowhead (*B*).

ments are displaced away from the spinal cord. The x-ray examination will be most revealing in the open mouth view where there will be an offset of the lateral masses of C1 from their normal articulation with those of C2. If the total lateral displacement of both lateral masses is greater than 7 mm the transverse ligament of the atlas is ruptured as well.

The *hangman's fracture*, a traumatic spondylolisthesis of C2 (Figure 5.18), is an extension distraction injury that can occur if the frontal area of the skull strikes an immovable object while the body is still accelerating. If the athlete is not immedi-

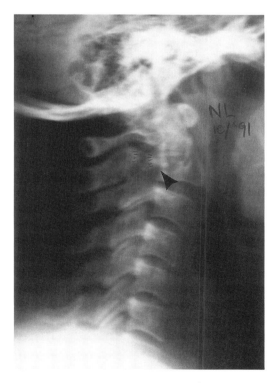

Figure 5.18. Hangman's fracture with the defect in the posterior elements highlighted.

ately killed by displacement and spinal cord injury there is severe pain and resistance to range of motion. The athlete is usually neurologically intact. Radiologic examination will reveal the fracture of the posterior elements of C2 seen on the lateral x-ray.

The *odontoid* may be fractured at its cephalad end, through the base of the odontoid or through the body of C2. The athlete will have immediate severe neck pain and loss of motion. There is usually no neurologic deficit. Radiologic examination is most revealing in the open mouth view and will reveal the fracture line.

The *burst fracture* may occur in any of the cervical vertebral bodies from C3 through C7 (Figure 5.19). This is an axial compression injury occurring with the head flexed approximately 30°, thereby straightening the cervical spine at impact and producing the burst of the vertebral body. There is a high incidence of spinal cord injury associated with this fracture pattern. The athlete will have severe neck pain and loss of cervical motion. He may also have pain, paresthesias, numbness, and paralysis of all four extremities. X-rays will show the fractured vertebral body with retropulsed bone, particularly on the lateral view. A cervical CT scan may be obtained to best evaluate the bony architecture and position of bone fragments in the spinal canal. A cervical MRI will best delineate the spinal cord and also best demonstrate possible retropulsed disk fragments impinging on the spinal cord.

Each of these unstable injuries will require protracted (up to 3 months) immobilization, with a complex device, such as a halo-vest. Surgery may be indicated to decompress the spinal cord. Following healing of the fracture, 3 months or more of rehabilitation is often necessary to regain

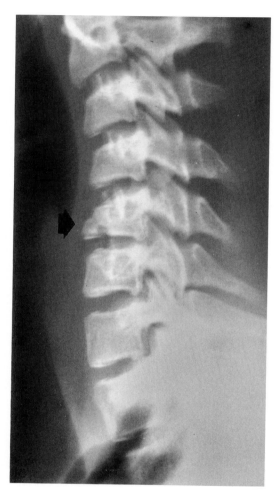

Figure 5.19. Burst fracture of C5 (*arrow*) with fragments displaced forward and posteriorly, toward the spinal cord.

flexibility and strength of the cervical musculature. Return to athletics should only be considered if there is complete healing of the fracture, the athlete is neurologically normal, and there has been no compromise of the spinal canal.

UNSTABLE LIGAMENTOUS INJURIES

Ligamentous injuries may result in cervical spinal instability without fractures. Instability at C1–C2 may occur with traumatic disruption of the transverse ligament (2,6). The athlete will complain of neck pain and decreased motion and will usually be neurologically normal. X-rays may be normal or may show an increase in the atlanto-dens interval (i.e., the space between the anterior arc of C1 and the dens on the lateral view) (Figure 5.20). This will increase in flexion and reduce in extension. The atlanto-dens interval should be less than or equal to 3 mm. If the interval is 3 to 5 mm, the transverse ligament is disrupted. An interval greater than 5 mm indicates disruption of accessory ligaments as well. Return to active sport mandates C1–C2 fusion, but cessation of sports in a neurologically intact and asymptomatic individual may obviate the necessity of surgery.

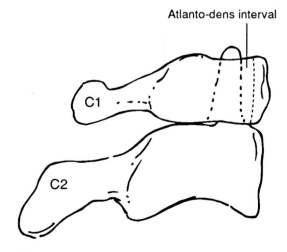

Figure 5.20. The atlanto-dens interval will be increased with ligamentous injury between C1 and C2. Flexion views may be needed to identify this.

Facet dislocation occurs as a result of a flexion rotation injury. The dislocation may be unilateral or bilateral. *The athlete will have severe pain and decreased range of cervical motion.* A unilateral "jumped facet" may produce no neurologic signs or symptoms or may compress a single root with consequent findings. Bilateral "jumped facets" will frequently produce signs and symptoms of spinal cord injury up to and including quadriplegia. X-rays will reveal a rotation of the spinous process toward the unilateral dislocated facet on the anteroposterior view and an anterior subluxation of the vertebral body less than or equal to 25% the width of the caudad vertebral body on the lateral view (Figure 5.21). The oblique view will show dislocation of the facet joint. The x-rays of the bilateral dislocated facets will show widening of the interspinous space on the anteroposterior view and a 50% subluxation of the vertebral body on the lateral view.

Each of these unstable ligamentous injuries will require reduction and surgical fusion. As with their bony counterparts, immobilization of up to 3 months and protracted rehabilitation periods are needed. Return to athletics can only be considered when the fusion is solid and the athlete is neurologically normal. Because fusion of two or more cervical spine levels increases the stress on the remaining cervical spine and the subsequent risk of serious injury,

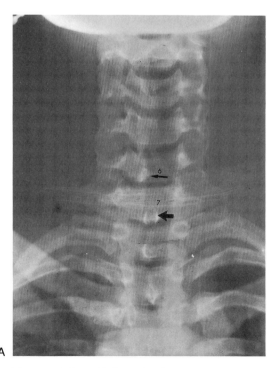

A

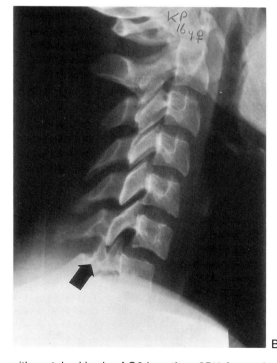

B

Figure 5.21. Unilateral "jumped facet." *A.* Anteroposterior view showing rotation of C6 spinous process in relation to C7. *B.* Lateral view with vertebral body of C6 less than 25% forward in relation to C7 and obvious displacement of facet joint (*arrow*).

collision-type contact sports (e.g., football, rugby, hockey) may be inappropriate.

NEUROLOGIC INJURY

Clinical Case #2

A high school football player comes to the sidelines with acute pain down his arm to his hand. He is shaking his arm to clear it. He had made the last tackle. He has never had a "stinger" before. He is neurologically intact to your examination on the sidelines. His pain and numbness resolve completely within 5 minutes. Can he safely return to the game?

The most common sports-related cervical spine neurologic injury involves the brachial plexus (1,6,18–20). The three degrees of injury in ascending order of severity are neurapraxia, axonotmesis, and neurotmesis. The mechanism of injury is a traction force on the brachial plexus produced by a force driving the shoulder caudad and the head into lateral flexion toward the opposite shoulder (see Figure 5.6). This is the common "stinger" or "burner" in football characterized by a burning paresthesia down the arm, usually involving the C5 and C6 nerve root distributions. If the athlete has symptoms in both arms, the injury is more central. A neurapraxia involves injury to the myelin sheath with an intact axon. The injury can produce paresthesias, weakness, and numbness in the arm and, particularly, tends to involve shoulder abduction, shoulder external rotation, and elbow flexion and supination through the deltoid, teres major, and biceps muscles. The symptoms usually resolve in minutes but may last 2 to 3 weeks with a neurapraxia before complete spontaneous resolution. An axonotmesis involves interruption of the axon with wallerian degeneration. The paresthesias, numbness, and weakness will persist from 3 weeks to several months but will usually spontaneously resolve. In the face of persistent signs or symptoms 3 weeks postinjury electromyography and nerve conduction velocity testing should be performed. These will show fibrillations and positive sharp waves in the affected muscles. Neurotmesis describes destruction of the nerve and the prognosis is nil for regeneration. In a high-velocity injury producing the signs and symptoms of severe acute brachial plexus injury myelography may show root avulsions. This may be amenable to microsurgical repair; also the athlete may be a candidate for future muscle transfer to improve function.

Most stingers are mild and the athlete will be able to return to play in the same game with no treatment. Return to play is not allowed until there is complete resolution of the neurologic signs and symptoms. For athletes recovering from brachial plexus neurapraxia and axonotmesis the initial treatment is ice, rest, and nonsteroidal anti-inflammatory drugs. As neurologic function returns the athlete works on resistive exercises to strengthen the affected extremity and range of motion. Return to sport is allowed when normal neurologic examination and full range of motion of the cervical spine and extremity are regained. The athlete should continue a long-term resistive exercise program to strengthen the cervical spine and shoulder girdles as a prophylaxis against future injury. In football the athlete should wear a collar to limit deviation of the head. In athletes with persistent signs or symptoms of neurologic dysfunction cervical spine films including lateral flexion-extension films, MRI, or CT myelogram may be indicated to further elucidate the problem.

Nerve root involvement may occur as a

result of sports injuries. The roots may be injured as a result of fractures, dislocations, subluxations, or disk herniations. The injury mechanism may occur as the result of purposeful (e.g., football) or incidental (e.g., diving) contact of the accelerating head and neck with an immovable object. The force usually produces some combination of flexion, compression, and rotation of the head and cervical spine.

The injured athlete will complain of immediate neck pain, loss of cervical spine motion, and numbness or weakness of the upper extremity. The anatomic specificity of the dermatomal sensory innervation and muscular innervation of the upper extremities makes the neurologic examination critical and frequently diagnostic as to the level of the injury.

Radiologic evaluation includes a cross-table lateral C spine for screening followed by anteroposterior, open mouth, and oblique x-rays. The need for flexion-extension lateral films to evaluate stability, CT scan for better bony detail, or MRI for better visualization of the spinal cord and roots is determined subsequent to the careful history, physical examination, and plain cervical spine films.

As previously noted, the treatment may vary from collar to halo to surgical procedures depending on the injury and its natural history.

The most catastrophic cervical sports injury is that resulting in injury to the spinal cord. The mechanism is virtually always an axial compression with some element of cervical flexion or rotation. More rarely, particularly in older patients with degenerative cervical spondylosis, an extension injury will produce spinal cord injury. The sports again are contact as in football or ice hockey, or noncontact as in diving or gymnastics. In each case the accelerating head and neck strike an immovable object with devastating consequence to the spinal cord.

The injured athlete will complain of neck pain and profound weakness or paralysis of the extremities. The head and neck must be carefully aligned and immobilized with collar, spine board, straps, and sandbags. The immediate care may be critical to recovery or may create an iatrogenically induced permanency.

The physical examination may show lacerations or abrasions about the head, indicating the area of impact and therefore the direction of the force. The neurologic examination, including motor power, sensory to touch, pin, temperature and vibration, deep tendon reflexes, bulbocavernosus and anal wink, and rectal examination, will indicate the level, pattern, and severity of spinal cord injury. If there is no neurologic function distal to the level of injury and no anal wink or bulbocavernosus reflex as well, the patient may be in spinal shock. This will resolve in 24 to 48 hours and be heralded by the return of the anal wink and bulbocavernosus reflex. At that time, absent motor and sensory function distal to the lesion will be permanent. Any slight sparing in perianal sensation or motor function in the extremities leaves the prognosis open ended for improvement.

Several patterns of spinal cord injury may occur. These are classified as *complete*, that is, with no neurologic function distal to the level of the injury, and *incomplete*, with some pattern of sparing. The incomplete lesions are further classified as anterior, posterior, and central cord syndromes and Brown-Séquard syndrome. The anterior cord syndrome is characterized by ischemic necrosis in the distribution of the anterior spinal artery with complete loss of motor function, pain and temperature sensation, and sphincter function distal to the level of the lesion. The central cord syndrome is characterized by more profound weakness in the upper extremities than the lower extremities. The upper extremities are flaccid, whereas the lower extremities are spastic. There is virtually always some degree of neurologic improvement and the majority of these patients regain sphincter function and ambulation. This syndrome is more common in the older athlete with cervical spondylosis who sustains a relatively low velocity hyperextension injury to the head and neck. Brown-Séquard syndrome is pathologically a hemisection of the spinal cord. There is ipsilateral loss of motor function on the side of the injury with contralateral loss of pain and temperature sensation. The great majority of these athletes will regain functional ambulation and sphincter function. Posterior cord syndrome is extremely rare and is characterized by a loss of proprioception, light touch, and vibration distal to the neurologic lesion with intact motor function, pain and temperature sensation, and normal sphincter control.

The complete cord syndrome, as the name implies, indicates absence of any motor, sensory, or sphincter function distal to the level of injury. Once spinal shock has resolved with return of the primitive reflexes the diagnosis of complete cord syndrome is made with a zero prognosis for neurologic improvement.

TRANSIENT QUADRIPLEGIA

Another rare but alarming and somewhat controversial spinal cord syndrome occurring as a result of sports trauma is transient quadriplegia (1,2). This is a syndrome characterized by routine cervical impact in football or other contact sports resulting in spinal cord neurapraxia with transient quadriplegia lasting 10 to 15 minutes, but occasionally requiring 24 to 36 hours to resolve. This occurs most commonly in the face of a congenital cervical spinal stenosis with occasional association of congenital cervical fusion, cervical instability, or cervical degenerative disk disease. Lateral x-rays of the cervical spine will show the ratio of cervical spinal canal diameter over the lateral diameter of the vertebral body (Torg ratio) to be less than or equal to 0.80 (Figure 5.22). This would be an absolute congenital cervical stenosis with a ratio of less than or equal to 1.0 being a relative stenosis. Another measure is the lateral diameter of the spinal canal, which should not be less than 15 mm.

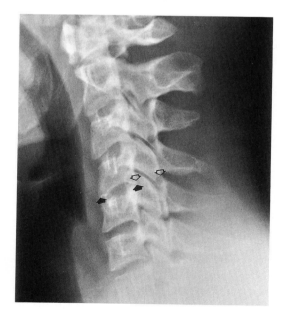

Figure 5.22. "Torg" ratio is the ratio of lateral spinal canal diameter (*open arrows*) over the lateral diameter of the vertebral body at the same level (*solid arrows*). The ratio of 0.8 or less is absolute spinal stenosis.

RETURN TO ATHLETICS AFTER NECK INJURY

Return to athletic activity subsequent to neurologic injury is controversial. The more conservative view was espoused by Bailes and Maroon (24) in 1989 who stated "... certainly no one would disagree that any athlete who suffers a neurologic injury to the spinal cord not be allowed to return." They further stated that any patient after cervical surgery, such as cervical disk excision with or without fusion, was unsuitable for contact sports. Specifically they stated patients with fractures or dislocations requiring a halo or surgery "best [be] considered not to have adequate strength to withstand subsequent contact sports."

Marks and colleagues (2) wrote that a decision on return to sport after cervical spine injury "is one of the most difficult decisions a physician has to make. Frequently, there is very little hard evidence on which to base such a decision, yet the consequences of making a wrong decision can be catastrophic."

In a 1993 article on the subject of return to collision sports after cervical spine injury, Torg (34) stated "... proposed criteria for return to contact activities in the presence of cervical spine abnormalities or after injury are intended only as guidelines. It is fully acknowledged that for the most part they are, at best, predicated on the anecdotal, and no responsibility can be assumed for their implementation."

Torg goes on to present a fairly comprehensive list of recommendations for congenital and acquired cervical spinal pathology as to collision sports. Interestingly Torg considers a solid C1–C2 fusion an absolute contraindication to the return to collision sport while Marks and colleagues (3) present an example of a football player with a C1–C2 instability who underwent C1–C2 fusion and returned to professional football as a "moderate" risk in their four-tier systems.

Torg (34) also feels athletes with two- or three-level stable, asymptomatic, posterior cervical fusions should rarely be returned to contact sports. Marks and coworkers place the two-level posterior fusion athlete whose fusion is solid and asymptomatic in the "moderate" risk group and would not be adverse to a return to contact sports by this athlete.

Certainly the decision as to whether an athlete may return to contact or potentially dangerous noncontact sports (e.g., skiing, skating, gymnastics) after a cervical spine injury is fraught with difficulty and potential catastrophic risk. Although the athletes and their parents must be given as much information as possible as to the pathology and natural history of the cervical spinal problem, the ultimate decision to "clear" the athlete lies with the physician. In view of the fact that hard data are unavailable in statistically significant numbers the dictum of *primum non nocere (first do no harm)* should rule. The role of the physician is always to protect the athlete as a patient first and as a competitor second. That is not to say that a physician treating athletes should not be cognizant of the importance of athletics. However, to err on the side of conservative care might produce emotional distress, whereas to err toward participation might produce quadriplegia. A careful, reasoned approach with a complete history, physical examination, x-rays, and scans; a knowledge of the sport; and an informed discussion with the athlete and family should lead to an appropriate decision as to the return to sports.

REHABILITATION

Rehabilitation of athletes with cervical spine injuries is critical to the return of the athlete to sport and the prevention of future injury (19,35). The goals of rehabilitation are to produce an athlete whose cervical spine has full painless range of motion and normal or increased strength, with a normal neurologic examination of the upper extremities.

In the acute painful postinjury phase the athlete may be treated with various modalities including ice, heat, ultrasound, phonophoresis, iontophoresis, or electrical stimulation. Massage and traction may be beneficial as well, assuming a stable injury. Subsequently as pain diminishes either after injury or after appropriate postoperative stability has been achieved, active and active assisted range of motion exercises are instituted as well as strengthening exercises.

The strengthening exercises are categorized as isometric or isotonic. Isometric exercises involve muscle contraction against an immovable object (see Figure 5.16). Isotonic exercises involve muscle contraction with motion of the adjacent joint (e.g., the use of free weights). Strength is increased by repetitive exercise over time with increasing resistance (i.e., progressive resistive exercises).

As range of motion and strength are restored, aerobic fitness must be addressed with appropriate exercises including jogging, swimming, bicycling, stair climbing, cross-country skiing, and rowing. These activities may be done on machines simulating the activities. Ultimately sports-specific training will be necessary prior to return to competition. Subsequently the athlete must maintain a program of cervical strengthening to best protect the cervical spine.

RECOMMENDATIONS

The health benefits, physiologic and psychological, of sports activity for men, women, and children of every age group are irrefutable. The role of the physician is to encourage the greatest participation in the safest manner. In view of the fact that athletes are becoming bigger, stronger, and faster the results of purposeful collisions in contact sports or accidental collisions in other sports produce a greater impact energy, which must be dissipated through the body of the participant. Particularly with regard to the cervical spine the risk of catastrophic injury is significant.

The effort to reduce injury must begin with the collection of epidemiologic data. Whether under the auspices of the National Football Head and Neck Injury Registry (3), professional organizations of coaches, or organizations of medical specialists in pediatrics, primary care, or sports medicine organizations, epidemiologic data are critical to assess the incidence and severity of cervical spine injuries and the attendant risk factors. The decrement in football-induced quadriplegia subsequent to rules outlawing "spearing" occurred as a direct result of the evaluation of epidemiologic data.

Once pertinent data are accumulated they must be disseminated to the athletes at large and the coaches and officials involved in the at-risk sports. This information can be used to educate as to proper techniques and equipment and in the case of organized sports to legislate rule changes to protect participants. Epidemiologic data will also allow the physician treating athletes to make more informed decisions as to the appropriate return to sports activity.

The challenge to motivate the patient-athlete to actively promote "wellness" by participating in sports can and should be addressed by the family practitioner. The primary caregiver should be a leader in educating and motivating the patient-athlete as to the benefit of sports activities.

References

1. Torg JS. Management guidelines for athletic injuries to the cervical spine. Clin Sports Med 1987;6.

2. Marks MR, Bell GR, Boumphrey FRS. Cervical spine fractures in athletes. Clin Sports Med 1990;9:13–29.

3. Torg JS, Vegso JJ, Sennett B, Das M. The National Football Head and Neck Injury Registry fourteen year report on cervical quadriplegia 1971–1984. JAMA 1985;254:3439–3443.

4. Cantu RC. Catastrophic injuries in high school and collegiate athletics. Surgical Rounds in Orthopedics 1988;2:62–66.

5. Torg JS, Das M. Trampoline related quadriplegia: review of the literature and reflections on the American Academy of Pediatrics position statement. Pediatrics 1984;74:804–812.

6. Marks MR, Bell GR, Boumphrey FRS. Cervical spine injuries and their neurologic implications. Clin Sports Med 1990;9:263–277.

7. Hodgson VR, Thomas LM. Mechanisms of cervical spine injury during impact to the protected head. In: The Twenty-Fourth Stapp Car Crash Conference, Society of Automotive Engineers, 1980:15–42.

8. Tator CH, Palm J. Spinal injuries in diving: incidents high and rising. Ontario Med Rev 1981;48:628–631.

9. Good RP, Nickel VC. Cervical spine injuries resulting from water sports. Spine 1980;5:502–506.

10. Kewalramani LS, Krauss JF. Cervical spine injuries resulting from collision sports. Paraplegia 1981;19:303–312.

11. Marzo JM, Simmons EH, Wheldon TJ. Neck injuries to high school football players in western New York State. NY State J Med 1991;91:46–49.

12. Albright JP, McAuley E, Martin RK, et al. Head and neck injuries in college football: an eight year analysis. Am J Sports Med 1985;13:147–152.

13. Dietrich AM, Grim-Pease ME, Bartkowski H, King DR. Pediatric cervical spine fractures: predominantly subtle presentation. J Pediatr Surg 1991;25:995–999.

14. Retsky J, Jaffe D, Christoffel K. Skateboarding injuries in children. Am J Dis Child 1991;145:188–192.

15. Woodward GA, Furuwal R, Schink J. Trampolines revisited: a review of 114 pediatric recreational trampoline injuries. Pediatrics 1992;89:849–854.

16. Tator CH. Neck injuries in ice hockey: a recent unsolved problem with many contributing factors. Clin Sports Med 1987;6:101–113.

17. Bailes JE, Maroon JC. Spinal cord injuries in athletes. NY State J Med 1991;91:44–48.

18. Hodge B. Common spinal injuries in athletes. Nurs Clin North Am 1991;26:211–221.

19. Vegso JJ, Torg E, Torg JS. Rehabilitation of cervical spine, brachial plexus and peripheral nerve injuries. Clin Sports Med 1987;6:135.

20. Hershman EB. Brachial plexus injuries. Clin Sports Med 1990;9:311–327.

21. Mueller FO, Blyth CS. Fatalities from head and cervical spine injuries occurring in tackle football: forty years experience. Clin Sports Med 1987;6:185–196.

22. Torg JS, Sennett B, Vegso JJ, Pavlov H. Axial loading injuries to the middle cervical spine segment: an analysis and classification of 25 cases. Am J Sports Med 1991;19:16–20.

23. Torg JS, Vegso JJ, O'Neil MJ, Sennett B. The epidemiologic, pathologic, biomechanical and cinematographic analysis of football induced cervical spine trauma. Am J Sports Med 1990;18:50–57.

24. Bailes JE, Maroon JC. Management of cervical spine injuries in athletes. Clin Sports Med 1989;8:43–57.

25. Albright JP, Moses JM, Feldrick HG, et al. Nonfatal cervical spine injuries in interscholastic football. JAMA 1976;236:1243–1245.

26. Andrish JT, Bergfeld JA, and Romo L. A method for the management of cervical injuries in football—a preliminary report. Am J Sports Med 1977;5:89–92.

27. Olerud C, et al. Cervical spine fracture caused by high jump. J Orthop Trauma 1990;4:179–182.

28. Williams P, et al. Unstable cervical spine injuries in rugby—a 20 year review. Injury 1987;18:329–332.

29. Mann DC, Dodds JA. Spinal injuries in 57 patients 17 years or younger. Orthopedics 1993;16:159–164.

30. Cantu RC. Transportation/immobilization. In: American Academy of Sports Medicine's Guideline for the Team Physician, Philadelphia, Lea and Febiger, 1991:151–152.

31. Schneider RC. Serious and fatal neurological football injuries. Clin Neurosurg 1965;12:226–235.

32. Marwick C. Administering methylprednisolone promptly appears to mitigate cord injury paralysis. JAMA 1990;263:2150–2153.

33. Vegso JJ, Lehman RC. Field evaluation and management of head and neck injuries. Clin Sports Med 1987;6:1–15.

34. Torg JS. Criteria for return to collision activities after cervical spine injury. Operative Techniques in Sports Medicine 1993;1:236–249.

35. Shaffer B, Welsh TR, and Wiesel S. Principles of rehabilitation techniques in the patient who has been injured or who has undergone surgery. Operative Techniques in Sports Medicine 1993;1:221–230.

ON-SITE ASSESSMENT OF EYE INJURIES: CAN THE ATHLETE RETURN TO PLAY?

6

MICHAEL EASTERBROOK

Anatomy
Instruments Required to Examine an
   Athlete on the Field, Court, or Rink
History
Specific Ocular Examinations

The purpose of this chapter is to enable a primary care physician to assess a player with an acute eye injury at the rink, on the field, or on the court to determine if the player can safely return to play, or whether the player should be referred for evaluation by an ophthalmologist.

ANATOMY

The eye is a relatively fragile structure, well protected by bone superiorly, inferiorly, and laterally, but not anteriorly or medially. The medial wall and floor of the orbit are paper thin over the ethmoids and roof of the maxillary sinus, but the eye is otherwise well protected by dense bone.

The eye itself (Figure 6.1) is enclosed by a coat of cornea blending into the white sclera, which is reinforced by the subconjunctival tendon insertion of the intraocular muscles. The structures within the eye, however, are extremely fragile. The vessels of the iris and the ciliary body rupture easily to produce a hyphema (blood in the anterior chamber). The lens of the eye, particularly if penetrated, may imbibe water to produce opacification (cataract). The retina is a particularly delicate structure subject to retinal tears and detachment, particularly in myopic patients. Patients who are myopic have larger eyes with a higher incidence of retinal holes and retinal thinning, which predispose to retinal detachment. The cornea itself is 1 mm thick and is difficult to penetrate unless a sharp object is used. However, the trend toward refractive surgery to remove glasses from patients so they may play sports is of particular concern to ophthalmologists. The older technique of radial keratotomy, where incisions are made al-

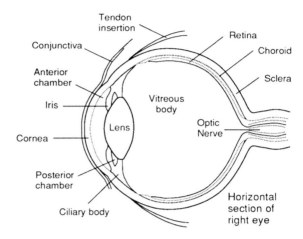

Figure 6.1. Normal eye.

most full thickness through the cornea, predispose the cornea to rupture of the eye, even with the slightest trauma. The incisions of radial keratotomy never completely heal and weaken the eye to injury. In 1994, at the International Congress of Ophthalmology in Toronto, Dr. Paul Vinger reported data on 26 patients previously undergoing radial keratotomy whose eye ruptured, often after minimal trauma. Most ophthalmologists recommend that patients who require refractive surgery and are athletic do not undergo radial keratotomy. The American military will not permit enlistment of any recruit who has undergone refractive surgery.

The newer technique of Excimer keratotomy, where the superficial 10% to 15% of the cornea is shaved, does not weaken the cornea to the same extent and is the treatment of choice should myopic or astigmatic athletes require refractive surgery.

With simple equipment, a proper history, and court or rinkside examination, it is possible to make a decision on the player's ability to return to play.

INSTRUMENTS REQUIRED TO EXAMINE AN ATHLETE ON THE FIELD, COURT, OR RINK

Visual Acuity Chart

Any examination of an athlete with an eye injury must include an assessment of visual acuity. If a visual acuity chart is not available, assessment of the athlete's vision with a flashlight, counting fingers, or reading a newspaper will at least provide, from a medicolegal viewpoint, some assessment of vision on the field.

A visual acuity chart should be on the wall in every dressing or training room (Figure 6.2). These visual acuity charts can be metric or nonmetric and can be designed for use at 10 or 20 feet viewing distance. If an athlete is unable to see the largest number on the visual acuity chart, then he or she should be asked to count fingers from 20 feet to 1 foot from his or her eye. If the athlete cannot count fingers, then a similar process with hand movements is carried out. If an athlete cannot see hand movements at 1 foot, then a penlight should be used. The athlete is instructed to look at the examiner's eye and point to the light as it is held above, below, and to each side. It is important to distinguish between light projection and light perception: with *light projection*, the patient recognizes light from different directions; with *light perception*, the patient recognizes light but cannot localize the source of the light. Light projection implies that the retina is functioning and is *not* detached. If the patient is very sensitive to light but the eye is not obviously ruptured, a drop of topical anesthetic may be administered to relieve the lid spasm, so that vision may be recorded.

Penlight

A penlight is not only useful for assessing anterior chamber depth and iris reaction, but it may also pick up small corneal abrasions, such as those caused by cinders at a track meet, or corneal foreign bodies. Modern halogen ophthalmoscopes contain a cobalt blue filter that can be used with fluorescein. If an ophthalmoscope is not available, a penlight such as the Cobalite

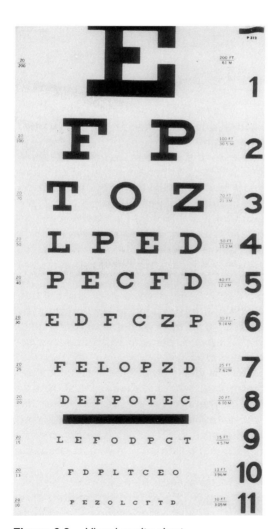

Figure 6.2. Visual acuity chart.

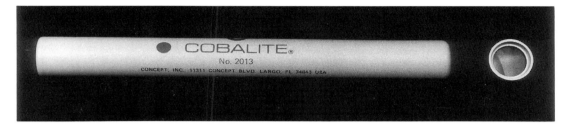

Figure 6.3. Cobalite penlight by Concept.

(by Concept) with a blue filter (Figure 6.3) is most useful for demonstrating even small corneal abrasions. These penlights cost less than $4 and are available in many stores. They are distributed in my practice to athletic trainers and trainers at hockey rinks and basketball and racquetball courts.

Cotton Applicators

The lid can be readily flipped with a cotton-tipped applicator; however, it is imperative to remind athletes *not* to squeeze the eye because tightening of the orbicularis oculi muscle will prevent such lid flipping. Patients are asked to look down, without closing the eye: a cotton-tipped applicator is then used as a fulcrum over which to flip the lid. The cotton applicator should be placed approximately 8 to 10 mm from the lid margin, while the eyelashes are pulled gently inferiorly prior to flipping the lid over the applicator. Often, small conjunctival corneal foreign bodies may be seen at this point.

Paper Clips

Paper clips are often recommended to provide a makeshift lid retractor (Figure 6.4). Patients complaining of a foreign-body sensation when the lid blinks may have either a corneal abrasion or a foreign body

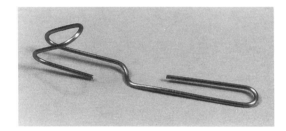

Figure 6.4. Paper clip bent to form a small retractor.

lodged under the upper lid, which is often seen when the eyelid is everted.

Fluorescein Strips

A corneal abrasion is best visualized with the blue light and the use of a fluorescein strip (Figure 6.5). The fluorescein strips should be moistened well with water and not inserted into the conjunctiva dry, which would cause patient discomfort. The paper strips are preferable because fluorescein solutions may be contaminated by *Pseudomonas* bacteria.

HISTORY

Almost all patients can be assessed at the courtside, on the rink, or on the field by history and examination with the tools

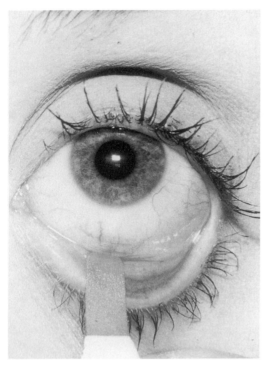

Figure 6.5. Fluorescein strips for corneal examination; *wet* before placing on the eye.

mentioned above. There are several questions that a practitioner should ask prior to examination of the patient.

Mechanism of Injury

Large objects such as soccer balls and basketballs and boxing gloves produce injury by transmission of force through the eye into the medial ethmoids and the floor of the orbit, producing a blow-out fracture. There may be associated eye injury, and all such patients with a dilated pupil should be examined at some point to rule out hyphema, dislocated lens, retinal hole, or retinal detachment. Very small objects such as a BB usually completely destroy an eye. A small projectile such as a pellet of war

games travels at 250 ft/sec and can produce enormous ocular injury. Larger objects such as a golf ball, because of its mass, may also completely explode an eye. Squash balls, badminton birds, and racquet balls often produce localized ocular injury without orbital fracture. A novice squash player strikes the ball at 80 mph. Tennis, squash, and racquetball "A" players have been clocked at 140 mph. In the last Olympics a professional badminton player was clocked at 180 mph with a direct smash. A hockey stick or a hockey puck can produce devastating ocular injury or slice the eye like a knife.

Was a Protector Worn?

It is apparent that so-called safety glass, streetwear plastic, and hardened prescription lenses may readily break into the eye (Figure 6.6), whereas polycarbonate will prevent almost all eye injuries in sport. Polycarbonate is a highly impact-resistant plastic used in police protective riot shields and jet canopies and is readily available in almost all prescriptions for our recreational and professional athletes.

There is no recorded incident of an eye lost in squash or racquetball with a lensed polycarbonate eye protector that meets the Canadian Standards Association (CSA) or the American National Standards Institute's impact standards (Figures 6.7 and 6.8). The open eye guard (Figure 6.9) still used in Europe by some players has been shown to be ineffective in preventing eye injuries in racquetball, where 90% of the injuries are caused by the ball. (In squash 60% of the injuries are caused by the ball.) The open eye guard may prevent some injuries by the racquet in squash but is ineffective in preventing injuries by the squash or racquet ball and probably by the badminton bird. These open eye guards should not

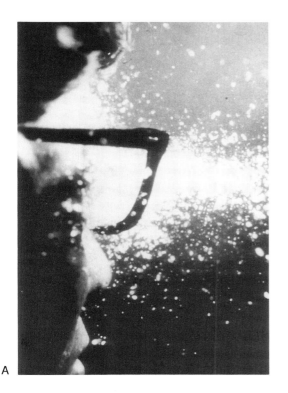

A

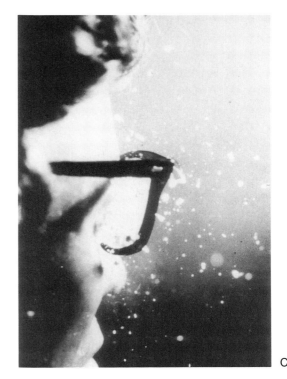

C

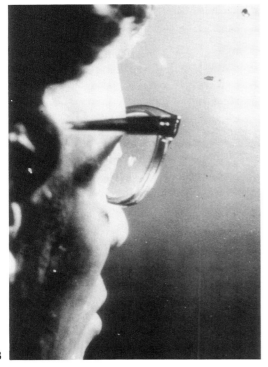

B

Figure 6.6. *A.* BB striking hardened safety glass. *B.* BB striking streetwear CR 39 plastic. *C.* BB striking polycarbonate lens.

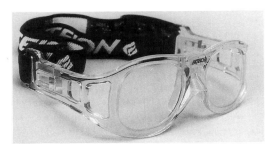

Figure 6.7. Lensed polycarbonate eye guard designed for racquetball players when a prescription is necessary.

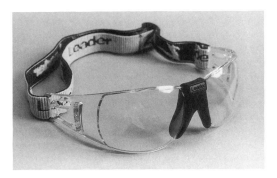

Figure 6.8. Lensed polycarbonate eye guard designed for racquetball players when no prescription is necessary.

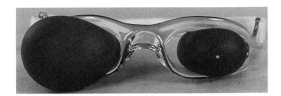

Figure 6.9. Open eye guard used in the 1970s and 1980s for squash and racquetball permitted penetration of the squash and racquet balls.

be permitted in the 1990s since good polycarbonate protection is available. Dr. Tom Pashby has reviewed data on 276 blind eyes in hockey players, none of whom was wearing a CSA- or Hockey Equipment Certified Council–certified full face protector.

The visor worn by older recreational and professional players should stop pucks and prevent most ocular injury: however, three players recently lost an eye when a hockey stick entered the space between their face and the visor.

Contact Lenses—Help or Hindrance?

A soft contact lens or a toric soft lens used for a patient with myopia or astigmatism will neither help nor hurt the athlete in terms of eye injury. The more rigid, gas permeable lens used for myopic patients with astigmatism may break and cut the eye and is a definite hazard to players, particularly in racquet sports. Any such player wearing contact lenses should also wear a polycarbonate protector while playing hockey and racquet sports. This includes doubles tennis and badminton.

Visual Loss—Transient or Permanent?

A player with transient or sustained visual loss should be evaluated microscopically by an ophthalmologist to rule out a hyphema, retinal holes, or retinal detachment.

Photophobia

Traumatic conjunctivitis does not cause photophobia. Photophobia implies traumatic iritis or a traumatic corneal abrasion and requires examination of the cornea with the penlight and the blue filter, or a slit lamp examination by an ophthalmologist if no changes are seen with the penlight and fluorescein strip.

Field Defects

If any player who has recently sustained an eye injury complains of floating spots or a field defect in one peripheral area, he or she should be referred immediately for evaluation by an ophthalmologist to rule out a retinal hole, retinal hemorrhage, or retinal detachment.

This is particularly common in patients who have been hit with a small object such as a squash ball, racquet ball, or badminton bird.

Double Vision

An athlete who is struck in the eye and complains of double vision often has a retinal hemorrhage, but on occasion may have a blow-out fracture of the orbit, either medially or inferiorly into the maxillary antrum. *Players who have been struck in the eye should be instructed not to blow their nose, because orbital emphysema may swell up the eyelids, preventing ocular assessment.* These patients may have infraorbital anesthesia from involvement of the inferorbital nerve, if the maxillary floor is involved. Diplopia may also occur if the inferior rectus or inferior oblique muscles are trapped in the blow-out fracture; however, most double vision is caused by orbital hemorrhage. Any player with diplopia should be referred to an ophthalmologist to rule out a blow-out fracture and should not be allowed to return to play until the diplopia subsides.

A patient who has been struck in the eye during a sport, who has no history of visual loss, no diplopia, no floaters, and no photophobia can return to play after being evaluated.

SPECIFIC OCULAR EXAMINATIONS

Lid Laceration

Lid lacerations must be examined carefully under bright illumination to rule out a laceration of the lid margin. If the laceration involves the lid margin, the athlete should be referred to the ophthalmologist for repair. A lid margin laceration that has not been adequately repaired may produce a lid notch with subsequent entropion or rubbing of the eyelashes on the cornea. A notch in the lid margin may be produced if exact apposition of the lacerated lid is not performed under the operating room microscope. The lid laceration involving the canaliculus is a much more serious event because persistent tearing may ensue if the canalicula laceration is not repaired promptly.

Cornea

Clinical Case #1

A 12-year-old Little League player comes to the office the day after a game. She got dust in her eye during the game and still feels there is something in there. Her mother looked for dirt in her eye but had not seen anything.

Foreign Body

At almost any athletic event we may encounter a corneal foreign body; classically this is the cinder at a track meet. A corneal foreign body can be removed with a 25- or 27-guage needle under topical anesthetic, *once vision has been assessed.* If a rust ring is present, instill antibiotic ointment, patch the eye, and refer the patient. Twenty-four hours later the surrounding epithelium will loosen and permit the removal of the rust ring under topical anesthetic with the slit lamp.

Corneal Abrasions

These are best seen with the use of fluorescein, with or without anesthetic. Small corneal abrasions may heal in a day or so with patching; however, larger abrasions involving more than 50% of the corneal surface may require 2 to 3 days to heal. Patients may return to play as soon as their foreign-body sensation and photophobia disappear.

Clinical Case #2

A 26-year-old recreational basketball player was struck in the eye by an opponent's finger. He had blurring of vision that has not resolved. Your examination reveals slight asymmetry in pupil size. You are unable to detect corneal abnormalities.

Corneal Lacerations

Any irregularity of the pupil or difference between the two pupils, in terms of size and reactivity to light, may implicate either a small corneal laceration or a hyphema. Small corneal lacerations may produce distortion of the pupil; larger lacerations are readily apparent. Almost all corneal lacerations, unless they are very tiny and located peripherally will produce blurring of vision. The athlete with a corneal laceration should be referred to an ophthalmologist.

Subconjunctival Hemorrhages

Subconjunctival hemorrhages are very common in sport; however, these patients have no change in their vision, no history of visual loss, no photophobia, no diplopia. They can return to play immediately. These patients will also have a normal pupil and normal iris details when examined by the penlight. Small subconjunctival hemorrhages will disappear in 2 to 3 days, but larger hemorrhages may persist for 1 to 2 weeks. No drops will speed up the process; these patients require no treatment and may return to the rink or court immediately.

Hyphema

Bleeding in the anterior chamber (hyphema) is common. The symptoms are mild pain and blurring of vision immediately after sustaining some type of trauma to the eye. Sometimes hyphema can be observed with a penlight, especially if the blood is layered out. After the athlete has moved, the layering will disappear and only slit-lamp examination will reveal the large number of red cells in the anterior chamber. A small hyphema may produce blurring of the iris details when examined by the penlight, often with normal vision. If there is a difference in pupil size after injury or blurring of iris details, the patient should be referred for slit-lamp examination by an ophthalmologist. Ophthalmologists are very concerned about the appearance of hyphemas because some 10% of hyphemas may rebleed between days 4 and 6. Patients with hyphemas have a lifelong tendency toward glaucoma and must be examined carefully to rule out associated lens and retinal damage. Patients who have a hyphema must not be allowed to return to play and must be either admitted to the hospital or be kept very quiet in the home for 6 or 7 days. The highest incidence of rebleeding occurs between days 4 and 6. Subsequent to resolution of the hyphema, these patients' eyes must be dilated to rule out traumatic cataract, retinal tear, or detachment. Upon clearing of the hyphema, the athlete may return to mild athletic activities within 2 weeks of the onset of the hyphema and may return to full physical contact 3 weeks from the onset of the hyphema.

Traumatic Cataract

An athlete who presents with traumatic cataract may often have an associated corneal laceration. These patients may have immediate loss of vision and an irregular pupil. They require immediate referral to an ophthalmologist.

Retinal Detachment

Clinical Case #3

After being struck in the eye by a ball, a 32-year-old recreational soccer player complains of floaters. Your examination reveals no pupil asymmetry or corneal lesions. His visual acuity is normal. He does appear to have a small lateral field defect. Should you be concerned?

An athlete with an eye injury from any sport, complaining of floaters, flashing of lights, or field defect must be examined with the pupil well dilated using the indirect ophthalmoscope to rule out a retinal tear or retinal detachment. One of the few ocular emergencies in ophthalmology is acute traumatic retinal detachment. The success rate for repairs of retinal detachment is over 90%. But if the detachment progresses to involve the macula, blindness can occur. A superior retinal detachment that is likely to progress to detachment of the macula must be repaired immediately before the macula comes off. An athlete who presents with poor vision, even 3 weeks after retinal detachment from a sports injury, is likely to have an excellent result when the retina is restored to its normal position. However, if the macula is off for more than 2 or 3 days, this may preclude useful vision and may produce a legally blind eye.

Blow-out Fracture of the Orbit

A blow-out fracture is often seen in patients who are struck by large objects, such as a basketball, a fist, or thumb. The force is transmitted through the eye into the weakest part of the orbit, the medial and inferior walls. If there is muscle entrapment, usually inferior rectus or inferior oblique, then the floor may require surgical repair. Many basketball or hockey players and boxers have returned to successful careers after repair of a blow-out fracture. Any patient with double vision should be referred for immediate assessment.

SUMMARY

A player struck in the eye can almost always be adequately assessed at rinkside, on the court, or on the field by the primary care physician if he or she asks the right questions and has a visual acuity chart and a flashlight. A player who has been hit in the eye, who has no history of visual loss, diplopia, photophobia, or floaters can almost always be safely returned to play if visual acuity is normal, extraocular movements are full, pupils are normal, and iris details and corneal examination are clear, when examined by flashlight. Any athlete with transient loss of vision, floaters, flashers, photophobia, change in vision, diplopia, or abnormal examination of cornea and iris by penlight, must be removed from play and immediately referred to an ophthalmologist.

References

1. Davis JK. Perspectives on impact resistance and polycarbonate lenses. In: Vinger P, ed. Prevention of ocular sports injuries, Int Ophthalmol Clin 1988:215–218.

2. Easterbrook M, Pashby T. Ocular injuries and war games. In: Vinger P, ed. Prevention of ocular sports injuries, Int Ophthalmol Clin 1988:222–224.

3. Vinger P. The eye in sports medicine. In: Duane T ed. Clinical ophthalmology, vol 5. Philadelphia: JB Lippincott, 1988:30.

4. Easterbrook M. Keeping an eye on sports-related injuries. Current Therapy. 1989;2:21, 33.

5. Easterbrook M. Eye protectors in racquet sports. In: Current Therapy in Sports Medicine, 2nd ed. Philadelphia: BC Decker, 1990:356–362.

6. Easterbrook M. Eye injuries in winter sports. In: Casey MJ, Foster C, Hixson DG, eds. Sports medicine. Philadelphia: FA Davis, 1990:195–210.

7. Easterbrook M. Standards for protective eye guards. In: Hermans GPH, Mostend WL, eds. Sports, medicine and health. Amsterdam: Excerpta Medica, 1990:1101–1106.

8. Easterbrook M. Prevention of eye injury in badminton. In: Hermans GPH Mostend WL, eds. Sports, medicine and health. Amsterdam: Excerpta Medica, 1990:1107–1110.

9. Easterbrook M. Eye protectors in racquet sports. In: Torg J, Welsh RP, Shepherd RJ. Current therapy in sports, 2d ed. Philadelphia: BC Decker, 1990:356–362.

10. Easterbrook M. Eye injuries. Modern Medicine of Canada 1991;46:14–18.

11. Pashby TJ. Eye injuries in racquet sports and recreational activities. Can J Ophthalmol 1992;27:226.

12. Easterbrook WM. Eye injuries in sports: prevention and cure. Can J Diag 1993:77–89.

THE CHEST AND THORAX

GREGORY TUTTLE

7

Rapid Injury Assessment
Soft-Tissue Trauma to the Neck
Tension Pneumothorax
Flail Chest
Cardiac Tamponade
Myocardial Contusion
Traumatic Aortic Rupture
Tracheobronchial Tree Injuries
Esophageal Disruption
Pneumomediastinum and
    Pneumopericardium
Pneumothorax and Hemothorax
Common Minor or Aggravating
    Conditions

Relatively few sports injuries involve the chest and thorax and most of these are minor and usually only a nuisance to the athlete. Because of their usual benign course and often subtle presentation, it is imperative that the physician who cares for athletes keeps a high index of suspicion for more serious pathology and rare life-threatening or potentially life-threatening conditions. This chapter provides a brief overview of these conditions, rapid on-the-field injury assessment, and the more common conditions the primary care physician will encounter.

RAPID INJURY ASSESSMENT

A rapid and systematic approach to injury assessment allows the physician to identify those injuries and conditions that may threaten an athlete's life (1). Here, the ABCDE mnemonic is especially useful. Using a 30-second primary survey (2) that incorporates the following areas of evaluation aids the physician in rapidly identifying and simultaneously managing a host of life-threatening conditions that may be encountered on the field, the sidelines, or in the locker room:

- Airway—assess patency, clear if necessary
- Breathing—assess and provide ventilatory support if necessary
- Circulation—assess, maintain adequate tissue perfusion, and control any hemorrhage
- Disability—assess neurologic status
- Exposure/environment—often need to undress; always be mindful of unfavorable climatic conditions

All of these areas of concern must be addressed and managed prior to the formal evaluation of the chest and thorax. The spe-

cifics of the primary and secondary surveys are well delineated in the current Advanced Trauma Life Support (ATLS) course core content (3). The physician may initially simply ask the injured athlete "What happened to you?" or "How did you hurt yourself?" and immediately gain significant information regarding the athlete's airway patency, ability to breath, circulatory sufficiency (adequate mean arterial pressure to perfuse the brain), and neurologic status. If the athlete answers these preliminary questions appropriately, then further evaluation can take place with reasonable dispatch and caution.

Some special concerns of athletes warrant brief mention. If the athlete is not breathing or is making sonorous or stridorous respirations, the airway may be obstructed. Causes may include inadvertently swallowed objects (e.g., chewing gum or tobacco, mouthguards, partial plates, or teeth), trauma to the neck and larynx, or a "swallowed tongue" or flaccid tongue and soft tissues caused by diminished levels of consciousness. As always, be cognizant of the possibility of alcohol use or other mind-altering substances. Usually a head tilt/chin lift or jaw thrust maneuver will reestablish the airway. If there is any suspicion of cervical spine injury, the jaw thrust maneuver with in-line traction of the head and neck is probably a better choice (4). If the entire lingual mass has been swallowed with severe trismus preventing opening of the mouth, an oral screw may be necessary to effectively open the jaw. A foreign body or debris may be removed with either the fingers sweeping the oral capacity, or a Magill forceps may be used with a good light source or laryngoscope if these are available.

It is a good idea for the team physician to always carry a mouth-to-mask device at athletic events. An oropharyngeal airway is also a simple and effective adjunct when airway patency is needed in an obtunded athlete. Athletes with presumed cervical injuries and lack of airway control with the previous techniques mentioned may best be managed with nasotracheal intubation. Again, it is imperative that the physician maintain immobilization of the head and neck until cervical spine injury can be ruled out. It is necessary to "log roll" any unconscious athlete to his or her back for transport (Figure 7.1).

There are some pitfalls in assessing hemodynamic status in athletes. The classic signs and symptoms of decreased organ–tissue perfusion (level of consciousness/mental status, pulse quality and rate, skin condition, thirst, orthostatic changes in blood pressure, etc) may not be manifested as clearly in athletes, especially in those who have undergone rigorous training routines (3). Well-conditioned athletes have changes in their cardiovascular dynamics, with blood volume increasing 15% to 20%, cardiac output increasing up to sixfold, and stroke volume increasing 50%. Resting pulse rate may be from 50 to 30. The elite athlete's ability to compensate for blood loss is remarkable. Significant blood loss may have occurred (either external or presumably internal) with a lack of the usual responses to hypovolemia until sudden cardiovascular collapse ensues. Thus, extra caution is warranted in evaluating these individuals for blood loss.

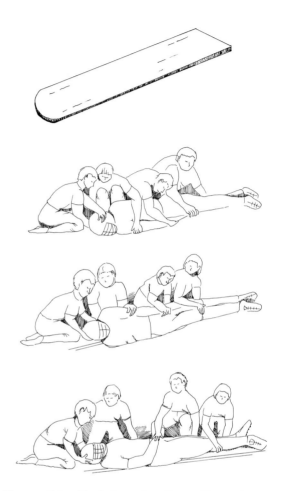

Figure 7.1. Technique for "log rolling." The team leader controls the athlete's head and gives commands while each of the other members rolls the athlete en bloc.

SOFT-TISSUE TRAUMA TO THE NECK

Thankfully, most injuries to the soft tissue of the neck in athletes are minor. Sudden flexion or extension movements cause compressive of shearing forces. Blunt trauma is more likely to cause soft-tissue damage and instability. Where the forces imposed are greater, such as in motor vehicle accidents or equestrian events, or from high-speed, contact sports, (e.g., football, soccer, rugby, lacrosse, ice hockey) the potential for more serious soft-tissue injury always exists. Laryngeal trauma resulting in structural damage and/or laryngospasm and edema with a compromised airway is a true emergency that team physicians must be able to evaluate and treat (5). Signs and symptoms indicating structural damage to the larynx include pain and tenderness, loss of normal laryngeal control, hoarseness or change in voice tone to aphonia, stridor, dyspnea, restlessness and agitation to extreme anxiety, subcutaneous emphysema, cough, hemoptysis, and cyanosis. If the patient is stable and time allows, lateral cervical spine x-rays with soft-tissue techniques may reveal retropharyngeal air (fracture of larynx and/or trachea) or elevation of the hydroid bone indicating laryngeal fracture. Any penetrating injury of the neck is potentially very serious and should be evaluated with the aid of a trusted surgeon. Laryngeal trauma may not be obvious in the athlete whose airway is not compromised (6). The initial signs and symptoms do not correlate well with the ultimate injury severity (7). Edema, usually maximal within 6 hours (8), may occur 24 to 48 hours after the injury (9). Late airway obstruction may result from the development of an expanding hematoma (10). Thus, laryngoscopy may not need to be performed on every athlete with more than trivial anterior neck trauma (10–12).

Treatment is centered on reassurance. Most laryngeal injuries respond well to straightening the airway and firmly moving the chin forward with pressure behind the angles of the jaw to relieve laryngospasm (5). This can be done if there are no obvious signs of cartilaginous fracture (flattening of laryngeal contour, especially the Adam's apple) (13), discontinuity of the airway (subcutaneous emphysema), or cervical vertebrae fracture. When airway obstruction is persistent, artificial airways may most easily be established by cricothyrotomy or needle-jet cricothyrotomy. Abelson (14) developed an emergency cricothyrotomy cannula that needs no other equipment. It can be in-

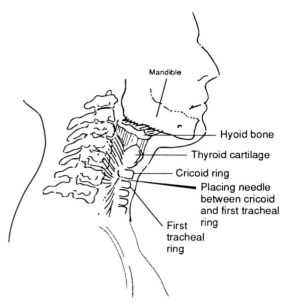

Figure 7.2. Needle cricothyrotomy.

serted through the cricothyroid ligament or membrane below the thyroid cartilage and above the cricoid cartilage. If a subglottic injury is suspected, a needle cricothyrotomy (using a large-bore, 14-gauge plastic cannula) can be performed with the insertion made between the cricoid cartilage and first tracheal ring (Figure 7.2). Once the athlete has an adequate airway in the field, he or she should be transported to the emergency room where further stabilization can take place. Revision to a more orderly and permanent tracheostomy can be achieved in a more favorable surgical environment.

TENSION PNEUMOTHORAX

Air leaks into the pleural space and a "one-way valve" air leak occurs either from the lung or through the chest wall. This air cannot escape and may completely collapse the affected lung. The mediastinum and trachea are displaced to the opposite side, decreasing venous return and hence cardiac output via compression of the vena cava. These may occur spontaneously with the rupture of an emphysematous or congenital bleb, with blunt trauma, and rupture of parenchymal lung tissue that fails to seal or via an open chest wound. The diagnosis is made clinically with the chief findings of anxiety, cyanosis, tachypnea and tachycardia, deviation of the trachea away from the affected lung, and possible distention of neck veins and hypotension. The involved hemithorax will reveal diminution or absence of breath sounds and hyperresonance to percussion. Treatment of this condition requires immediate decompression by inserting a needle (14-gauge angiocath is preferable for adults) into the second intercostal space in the midclavicular line of the affected hemithorax, converting the injury to a simple pneumothorax. Prepare for transfer to the nearest emergency room and reassess often.

FLAIL CHEST

The injury occurs when two or more ribs are fractured in at least two places, which allows a free-moving segment of the chest wall. These are usually lateral and can lead to paradoxical motion of the flail segment, which is the hallmark finding (injured segment goes in with inspiration and out with exhalation). There is usually considerable splinting of the chest wall because of pain; thus, it may be difficult to identify. Palpation of abnormal motion and palpable crepitus may aid in making the diagnosis. The major difficulty stems from the injury to the underlying lung, leading to hypoxia as well as restricted chest wall movement

because of pain. In the field, use gentle support and possibly sandbags to stabilize the segment.

CARDIAC TAMPONADE

This condition most commonly results from a penetrating injury but may occur due to blunt trauma such as a baseball striking the chest. The pathology is blood in the pericardial sac, and small amounts may restrict cardiac filling and activity. The clinical features in many ways resemble those described for tension pneumothorax, except that breath sounds are present, chest percussion is normal, and tracheal deviation does not occur. The heart sounds may be muffled or absent and distended neck veins may be present. Hussmaul's sign (a rise in venous pressure with inspiration when breathing spontaneously) is a true paradoxical venous pressure abnormality associated with tamponade. If cardiac tamponade is suspected, the initial administration of intravenous fluids will improve cardiac output transiently while transport to the nearest emergency room is being arranged. Pericardiocentesis via the subxyphoid route, by removing a small amount of nonclotting blood, may give the diagnosis and relieve symptoms temporarily while further definitive care (probably open thoracotomy) is being quickly arranged.

MYOCARDIAL CONTUSION

These are common and difficult to diagnose because there is no "gold standard" to rule these out. The athlete's complaints are often attributed to chest wall trauma. Look carefully for abnormalities on the electrocardiogram, especially multiple premature ventricular contractions, unexplained sinus tachycardia, atrial fibrillation, bundle branch block (usually right), frank ST-segment changes indicating myocardial infarction, or less specific ST-segment changes. Multigated angiography and two-dimensional echocardiography may be helpful (15).

In a myocardial concussion, the myocardium is "stunned" and there is no structural injury. However, the athlete may be transiently hypotensive. This may account for the small but significant number of sudden deaths seen in Little League players who are struck in the chest by a baseball. Coronary artery laceration from blunt trauma can result in myocardial infarction (16). Protective chest shields are now available for the younger athlete who is probably more vulnerable to this mechanism of injury due to the greater chest compliance. Although inconvenient to wear, they could prove to be lifesaving if used universally in this more vulnerable population.

TRAUMATIC AORTIC RUPTURE

These injuries require a major decelerating force usually associated with involvement in a motor vehicle collision or a fall from a great height. Sudden death is the usual outcome because of rapid exsanguination. If the adventitial layer of the aorta remains intact, salvage is frequently possible if the rupture is recognized and treated early. For survivors, specific signs and symptoms are often absent. A widened mediastinum is the most consistent finding on chest x-ray. Other adjunctive radiologic signs include fractures of the first and second ribs, obliteration of the aortic knob, deviation of the trachea to

the right, presence of a pleural cap, elevation and shift of the right mainstem bronchus, depression of the left mainstem bronchus, obliteration of space between the pulmonary artery and the aorta, and deviation of the esophagus (nasogastric tube) to the right. Transesophageal ultrasound may be useful, but angiography remains the "gold standard." Yates and Aldrete reported that a 25-year-old male rugby player suffered a ruptured aorta when a tackler's knee struck his chest (17). He had no immediate symptoms and continued to play, but 3 hours after the game, be developed dyspnea and chest pain. Other than motor sports accidents, reports of major vessel ruptures are rare in athletes. Certain congenital abnormalities of the aortic root (18) and collagen disorders, such as Marfan's syndrome (19), may predispose to this injury and should be uncovered where possible.

TRACHEOBRONCHIAL TREE INJURIES

Injuries to the larynx and trachea have already been discussed. Injury to a major bronchus is rare. Most result from blunt trauma and occur within 1 in. of the carina. Hemoptysis, subcutaneous emphysema, or a tension pneumothorax are frequent findings. Bronchoscopy will confirm the diagnosis. Suspicion of this injury warrants immediate surgical consultation.

ESOPHAGEAL DISRUPTION

Blunt injury is rare but may be lethal if unrecognized. A severe blow to the upper abdomen causes gastric contents to be forced into the lower esophagus producing a linear tear. Mediastinitis follows and ultimate rupture into the pleural space will result in empyema. This injury should be suspected in an athlete who has received a blow to the lower sternum or epigastrium and is in severe pain or shock. Chest x-ray may reveal mediastinal air or widening. Treatment is surgical.

PNEUMOMEDIASTINUM AND PNEUMOPERICARDIUM

These conditions are rare and usually self-limiting but have been described in athletes following forceful Valsalva maneuvers, especially weight lifting (20). Symptoms may be relatively mild to more severe, sharp or throbbing, substernal chest pain, dyspnea, dysplasia, and neck pain (21). Findings may include a pulsus paradoxus, hyperresonance over the precordium, decreased intensity of the heart sounds, Hammon's sign (a holo-systolic mediastinal crunch heard over most of the precordium—much like crackling cellophane), tachycardia, hypo-tension, and jugular venous distinction with rare tamponade, and subcutaneous emphysema. Chest x-ray usually reveals the radiolucent band outlining the heart or mediastinum, or both. Although these conditions are in and of themselves usually benign and self-limiting, when significant trauma has preceded their oc-currence, the physician must look closely for an injury to the larynx, trachea, major bronchi, pharynx, or esophagus. At minimum, an electrocardiogram and an echocardiogram to look for structural ab-normalities or a pericardial effusion should be obtained along with a complete blood count and erythrocyte sedimentation rate. Again, vigilance and careful consultations and follow-up are key (22).

PNEUMOTHORAX AND HEMOTHORAX

Clinical Case #1

A 22-year-old male varsity basketball player presented with persistent severe right an-terolateral chest pain and shortness of breath. During a game the night before, he was struck in the right lateral chest by an opposing player's knee while reaching for a loose ball. Examina-tion after the game revealed local chest wall ten-derness only and he was treated for a local chest wall contusion with ice and analgesics.

Examination the following day revealed a healthy young man with mild dyspnea and tachypnea and moderate splinting. His vital signs were stable. Examination of the lungs revealed decreased breath sounds and hyper-resonance to percussion on the right. The right anterolateral chest wall was diffusely tender, but there was no crepitus. Heart and abdominal examinations were normal. Chest x-ray revealed a right pneumothorax, moderately sized at 40% to 50%.

Blunt trauma to the thorax may produce varying degrees of air in the pleural space via rupture of alveoli or pulmonary blebs with or without associated chest wall in-jury. Similarly, lung laceration or laceration of an intercostal or internal mammary artery may result in hemorrhage in the pleural space. In the vast majority of cases, this bleeding is self-limiting. In athletic inju-ries, traumatic pneumothorax is not that uncommon. A simple pneumothorax may take a number of hours to develop. Thus, presentation may be delayed with the chief symptoms of shortness of breath, chest pain, decreased breath sounds, and hyper-resonance to percussion. If a standard pos-teroanterior inspiratory chest x-ray does not reveal a pneumothorax, repeat with the athlete in full expiration.

Treatment includes reassurance, supplemental oxygen, and observation if the pneumothorax is less than 10% to 15%. Chest tube placement in the fourth or fifth interspace just over the rib in the midaxillary line will probably be necessary for a moderate pneumothorax or when there is increasing dyspnea and hypoxia.

COMMON MINOR OR AGGRAVATING CONDITIONS

Chest Wall Contusions and Abrasions

Blows to the chest wall by a variety of foreign objects (e.g., field hockey and lacrosse sticks, parallel bars, helmets, baseballs) and various components of an athlete's anatomy (e.g., knee, elbow, foot) will produce an array of superficial skin damage and muscle and bone bruising, which although painful, do not usually interfere significantly with an athlete's play or performance. Occasionally the blow may be severe enough to "knock the breath" out of the athlete and he or she should be removed from competition and carefully evaluated before returning to play (Figure 7.3). Parameters allowing return would include full and equal bilateral chest motion, no dyspnea, and no suspicious findings on chest and abdominal examination (chest wall crepitus, rib step-off, any abdominal guarding, or any apparent chest wall splinting). If any suspicions remain, continue to monitor the athlete every several minutes if possible, until you are satisfied of full function and no significant injury.

Hematomas can be produced over the chest wall and supportive musculature, and they are treated in the usual fashion with ice and local compression, where possible, as are all general contusions. General first

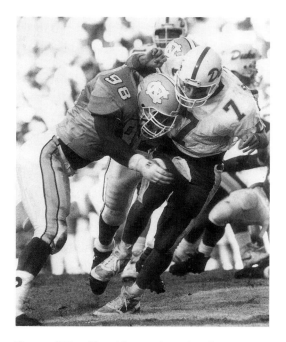

Figure 7.3. Shoulder pad to the thorax may "knock the wind out" of an athlete.

aid should also be given to abrasions, ensuring thorough cleansing and antisepsis and protective covering and antibiotic ointment to prevent or treat infection if warranted. These injuries are almost always self-limiting and mainly constitute a nuisance to the competitive athlete. Women have the potential for these same injuries to their breasts. Well-padded and fitted sports bras with good support and wide, firm elastic straps help to minimize extrinsic injury and injury secondary to rapid and forceful movement of the breast (Figure 7.4). The woman who has sustained a major insult to the breast must be followed closely for the possible development of a hematoma or duct blockage, which may culminate in mastitis. Warm compresses and oral antibiotics should be used for treatment.

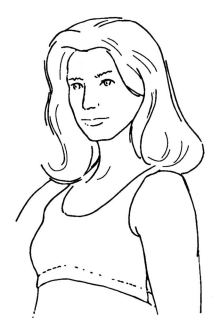

Figure 7.4. Sports bra, made of elastic and cotton, without stays.

In summary, chest wall contusion and abrasions are common and usually benign. Treat them conservatively and use ice and analgesics such as acetaminophen and nonsteroidal anti-inflammatory drugs (NSAIDs), along with good local care to ensure an athlete's prompt return to activity.

Chest Wall Strain and Costochondral Separation

These are also common sports injuries, especially in activities that entail rapid acceleration and deceleration and rapid and profound torque forces to the torso. They certainly are common in sports such as football and wrestling. The athlete is usually able to localize the area involved and should be asked to pinpoint the location

with a finger. Movement and occasionally breathing may increase the discomfort. Local tenderness is the norm. Muscle strains are treated in the usual fashion with ice, gentle stretching, and progressive motion as symptoms allow. Adjuncts such as NSAIDs and electrical stimulation are also helpful initially. After 3 or 4 days, the application of heat may be useful.

A forceful, violent motion or torso compression may produce a costochondral separation. These can be very painful and disabling and usually require several weeks to a month or two to resolve. Rib fracture and underlying visceral injury must be suspected and ruled out. The pain and point tenderness are usually localized and occasionally the rib and chondral separation can be palpated with both objective and subjective movement of the anterior free end of the rib appreciated. These often self-reduce or are easily reduced manually. Usually the separation is only partial. Pain is the main manifestation of this disabling and nagging injury. Rib fracture should be ruled out by x-ray if the pain is lateral. Local ice, analgesics, and compressive dressings are helpful. The return to athletics can be hastened by the use of a "flak-jacket" (Figure 7.5) to protect the painful area from repeated injury. If there is no fracture and full function, but persistent local tenderness, this area may be successfully injected with 3 to 6 mL of a long-acting local anesthetic such as bupivacaine to allow participation. Such a step should be reserved for the mature, adult athlete and only after all the potential risks have been carefully explained. If, several weeks after injury, the athlete's ability to move and perform are not returning, the physician may consider injecting a local anesthetic with a long-acting corticosteroid to reduce local pain and inflammation. Technique and experience are always invaluable, and the novice team physician

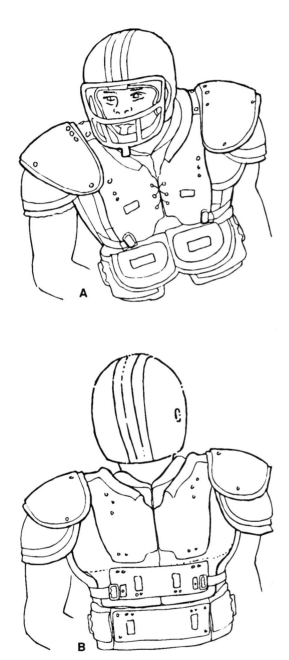

A

B

Figure 7.5. Current shoulder pad "flak jacket" combination will best protect the athlete for early return. It is routinely worn by most quarterbacks today.

should consider referring this athlete to a sports physician or orthopedic surgeon whom he or she trusts and make the experience both beneficial for the athlete and instructional for the primary care physician.

Fracture of the Thoracic Cage

Ribs are the more commonly injured bony element of the thorax, with ribs 4 to 9 most commonly fractured and these at the posterior angle and laterally. Local pain, splinting, and point tenderness with possible palpation and step-off of fracture fragment are the usual findings. Anteroposterior compression and lateral squeezing of the chest may help to clarify the picture where there is local tenderness and some swelling, but a definite fracture cannot be palpated (Figure 7.6). Pain away from the physician's pressing hands but localized to the area of tenderness raises the likelihood of fracture. Posteroanterior and lateral chest x-rays with rib detail films will usually settle the issue. (*Note:* costochondral separations or chondral fractures will not be visible and these may be just as or more disabling.) Be sure to look for injury to the liver or spleen if ribs 9 to 11 are fractured.

Treatment of rib fractures involves pain control, maintaining good pulmonary toilet, and possibly a properly fitted elastic rib belt with Velcro closure positioned below the level of the nipples. Return to activity will be slow and graded according to the athlete's symptoms. Healing generally requires 4 to 6 weeks. Return to any meaningful activity generally takes at least 2 to 3 weeks. There are many protective vests on the market that most athletic trainers are familiar with and can assist the team physician in obtaining and fitting properly when the physician determines return to activity

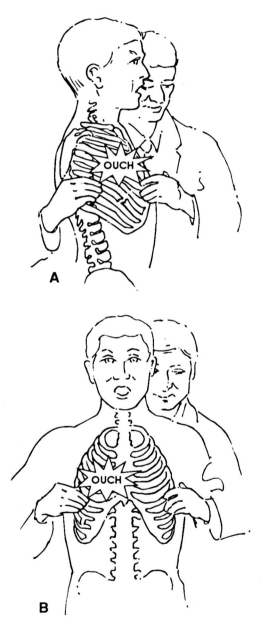

Figure 7.6. Front-to-back compression (*A*) and side-to-side compression (*B*) will lead to pain at the site of a fracture, but not a contusion.

is warranted (see Figure 7.5). If full contact is expected, the athlete should be symptom free and minimally tender over the fracture site.

Thoracic Vertebrae Fractures

Thoracic vertebrae fractures may occur in the athlete who has a sudden compressive force overload or acute flexion with a sudden stop or fall. Pain is usually immediate and quite severe (not developing over hours to days as in muscular insults). Point tenderness is the usual finding and x-rays often confirm the anterior wedging of the compressed vertebral body. Pain control with acetaminophen and narcotics may be warranted initially. Usually time is required for sufficient healing to occur and to allow the athlete to begin the rehabilitative process and ultimately return to full activity. Again, your orthopedic consultant can be helpful in managing these athletes, especially if the loss of vertebral height is greater than 1 to 2 mm or if there is any question of neurologic involvement or more complex spinal injuries. A simple compressive vertebral fracture will generally take 8 to 12 weeks to heal.

Runner's or Cyclist's Nipple

Frictional trauma from clothing and evaporative cooling from perspiration can work together or independently to cause chaffing and nipple irritation. Treatment is usually conservative and aimed at avoiding the irritant. This may involve a change in training routine, change in clothing, or special taping (using hypoallergic tape) or padding around the nipple (23). Petroleum jelly applied to the nipple before training may also reduce the irritation.

Precordial Catch Syndrome

These episodes of sharp, brief, occasionally stabbing anterior and lateral chest wall pains are commonly referred to as "stitches." The exact etiology is unknown (24), but it is seen more often in less well-conditioned athletes and probably involves some chest wall muscle or diaphragmatic spasm. Treatment involves rest, leaning into the side affected and grasping the area involved, along with short, shallow respiration. Ultimate treatment should focus more on prophylaxis, entailing better conditioning and training practices (e.g., not eating at least 3 hours prior to training).

Costochondritis

This fairly common condition describes pain and tenderness usually at multiple sites along the costochondral and costosternal articulations, usually from the second to the sixth costal cartilages. Swelling is not present and movement generally aggravates the symptoms. It may be precipitated by repetitive torso movement or direct trauma, but its exact etiology is unknown. It is differentiated from the rare Tietze's syndrome by involvement of multiple sites and a lack of swelling, whereas Tietze's syndrome usually affects only one site and is associated with some soft-tissue swelling. Treating is aimed at reducing inflammation and pain with ice, heat, and NSAIDs. Both conditions are generally self-limiting.

Slipping Rib Syndrome

This is a rare cause of lower anterior chest pain probably caused by some distant trauma and increased mobility of the costal margins of the lower, usually eighth to tenth, ribs. The inferior rib slips upward and rides over the superior ribs, producing pain and an audible and palpable click (21,25). The cartilage may be tender and moveable by palpation. Treatment is centered on recognition, reassurance, NSAIDs, and possibly an injection of corticosteroid, with surgical resection as a last resort (25).

Myofascial or "Trigger-Point" Pain Syndrome

These "injuries" are extremely common and usually more aggravating than truly debilitating. These areas of hyperirritable activity, once identified, can be treated with a host of physical therapy modalities and occasional fine-needle injections.

SUMMARY

Most injuries to the thorax in athletics are more aggravating than truly disabling or serious, but the purpose of this chapter has been to heighten awareness of the potential for more serious problems. Most conditions encountered are minor and self-limiting, but a number of simple interventions can safely expedite the return of function and performance while maintaining a degree of needed comfort for the athlete.

References

1. Hargarten KM. Rapid injury assessment: how to identify life-threatening emergencies. Phys Sports Med 1993;21:33–40.
2. Committee on Trauma, American College of Surgeons. ATLS program. Chicago: American College of Surgeons, 1989.
3. American College of Surgeons Committee on Trauma. Thoracic trauma. In: Advanced

trauma life support program for physicians. 1993 instructor manual, 5th ed. Chicago: First Impressions Publications, 1993:112–140.

4. Aprahamian C, Thompson BM, Finger WA, et al. Experimental cervical spine injury model: evaluation of airway management and splinting techniques. Ann Emerg Med 1984;13:584–587.

5. McCutcheon ML, Anderson JL. How I manage sports injuries to the larynx. Phys Sports Med 1985;13:100–112.

6. Leopold DA. Laryngeal trauma: a historical comparison of treatment methods. Arch Otolaryngol 1983;109:106–112.

7. Tarpy RF, Hick JN. Acute laryngeal trauma. J Med Assoc State Ala 1973;43:243–248.

8. Miles WK, Olson NR, Rodriquez A. Acute treatment of experimental laryngeal fractures. Ann Otol Rhinol Laryngol 1971;80:710–720.

9. Naham AM. Immediate care of acute blunt laryngeal trauma. J Trauma 1969;9:112–124.

10. Saletta JO, Folk FA, Freeark RJ. Trauma to the neck region. Surg Clin North Am 1973; 53:73–85.

11. Brandenberg JH. Management of acute blunt laryngeal injury. Otol Clin North Am 1979;12:41–51.

12. Maran AG, Murry JA, Stell PM, et al. Early management of laryngeal injuries. J R Soc Med 1981;74:656–660.

13. Birhazi H, Harcourt F. Management of fracture of the larynx. Ear Nose Throat Monthly 1974;53:23–28.

14. Abelson L. A cricothyrotomy device. Lett Emerg Med 1983;Oct:15–11.

15. Wisner DH, et al. Suspected myocardial contusion: triage and indications for monitoring. Ann Surg 1990;212:82.

16. Shears LL, et al. Myocardial performance after contusion with concurrent hypovolemia. Ann Thorac Surg 1993;55:834.

17. Yates MT, Aldrete V. Case report—blunt trauma causing aortic rupture. Phys Sports Med 1991;19:96–107.

18. Thiene G, Ho SY. Aortic root pathology and sudden death in youth: review of anatomical varieties. Appl Pathol 1986;4:237–245.

19. Maron BJ, Robert WC, McAllister HA, et al. Sudden death in young athletes. Circulation 1980;82:218–229.

20. Casamassima AC, Sternberg T, Weiss FH. Case report—spontaneous pneumopericardium: a link with weight lifting? Phys Sports Med 1991;19:107–110.

21. Stapczynski JJ. Life threatening signs and symptoms in adults. In: Tintinalli JE, Krome RK, Ruiz E, eds. Emergency medicine: a comprehensive study guide. American College of Emergency Physicians, 3rd ed. New York: McGraw-Hill, 1992.

22. Wilson RF. Thoracic trauma. In: Tintinalli JE, Krome RK, Ruiz E, eds. Emergency medicine: a comprehensive study guide. American College of Emergency Physicians, 3rd ed. New York: McGraw-Hill, 1992.

23. Hunter LY, Torgan C. The bra controversy: are sports bras a necessity? Phys Sports Med 1982;75:10.

24. Stamford B. A "stitch" in the side. Phys Sports Med 1985;13:187.

25. Reid DC. Sports injury assessment and rehabilitation. New York: Churchill Livingstone, 1992:678–681.

THE ABDOMEN

GREGORY TUTTLE

8

Overview and Anatomy
Initial Evaluation on the Field
Injuries to the Abdominal Wall Skin
Subcutaneous Tissue
Muscle
Blows to the Solar Plexus
"Hip Pointers"
Intra-abdominal Injuries: An Overview
Specific Organ Trauma
Other Injuries/Conditions
Protective Equipment and Other Measures

Injuries to the abdomen in athletics may be life-threatening and even fatal. Although these injuries are common, the vast majority are minor and self-limiting, and relatively few come to the attention of the physician caring for athletes. Most are superficial abdominal wall injuries and are recognized by the athlete as being trivial or a minor nuisance and are attended to by the athletic trainer. However, the potential for more serious internal or visceral injuries always exists, and the team physician should have a high index of suspicion for more serious injury. This chapter first gives an overview of sports-related trauma to the abdomen and the pertinent anatomy. Next is a discussion of the initial evaluation of the injured athlete and further diagnostic and therapeutic steps taken in the management of specific injuries to the abdomen and the genitourinary system. Several case histories that underline the more critical principles involved are also presented.

OVERVIEW AND ANATOMY

Sports-related trauma may cause up to 10% of all abdominal injuries (1). In contact sports, such as football, rugby, martial arts, and ice hockey, direct blows by opponent's bodies, equipment, or the ball or puck itself may injure the abdominal wall or its contents (Figure 8.1). Sports, such as wrestling, gymnastics, or cheerleading, that impose great torque forces to the torso may result in more significant abdominal wall injury. Alpine water skiing, speed skating, and horseback riding have the potential to impose great deceleration forces to the abdomen with resultant serious injury. Any sports that involve vehicles, from cycling to snowmobiles, may cause injuries that rival those encountered in motor vehicle accidents because of the energy that

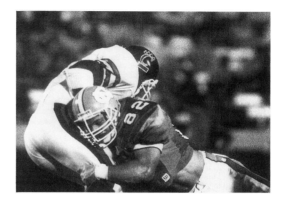

Figure 8.1. Shoulder pad to the abdomen may cause injury to the abdominal wall and contents.

must be dissipated in high-speed stops or collisions.

Abdominal injuries may be difficult to evaluate for a variety of reasons. The peritoneal cavity is a large potential reservoir for major occult blood loss (2), and the blood itself is not very irritating to the peritoneum. Initial signs and symptoms even in more serious visceral injuries may be absent or very subtle with a variety of presentations sometimes requiring hours or even days to manifest. Concomitant injuries may be more evident or painful. Altered or depressed mental sensorium from intracranial injury or chemical intoxicants may confuse the picture. A thorough evaluation is critical to avoid unnecessary morbidity and mortality. The most serious error is to delay surgical intervention when it is needed (3); thus, it is imperative to determine if an operation is required.

The abdomen is made up of three distinct anatomic compartments: the peritoneal cavity, the retroperitoneal space, and the pelvis. The peritoneal cavity is divided into the upper thoracic abdomen, which is located underneath the diaphragm and covered by the bony thorax (Figure 8.2). Contained within it are the liver, spleen,

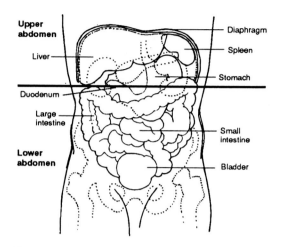

Figure 8.2. Peritoneal cavity.

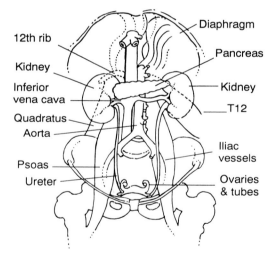

Figure 8.3. Retroperitoneal and pelvic organs.

stomach, gallbladder, and transverse colon. With full expiration, the diaphragm may rise to the level of the fourth intercostal space; thus, lower chest trauma may injure these viscera. The lower abdomen contains the small bowel and the remaining portion of the intra-abdominal colon (see Figure 8.2) (2). The retroperitoneal space contains

the inferior vena cava, aorta, kidneys, pancreas, and portions of the colon and duodenum (Figure 8.3). The pelvis contains the rectum, bladder, iliac vessels, and in women, the uterus, vagina, ovaries, and fallopian tubes.

In general, the muscular lower thoracic wall and ribs, the spine and its parallel supportive muscles and ligaments, the pelvis, and the abdominal musculature provide protection to the internal viscera. The strength of the abdominal wall resides in both the power of the muscles to contract and their ability to be flexible and absorb blows (4). The major muscle groups of the abdominal wall are the two rectus muscles running parallel from the costal margins to the pubis, the external and internal obliques, and the transversus muscles (Figure 8.4). Posteriorly, the sheaths of these muscles enclose the paravertebral muscles. Anterior to the lumbar vertebrae, the iliopsoas muscle traverses the retroperitoneal space bilaterally down the posterior pelvic wall with insertion into the lesser trochanters of the femur. The most vulnerable elements of the external genitalia in the male are the penis and the scrotum containing the testes, epididymis, and spermatic cord, and in the female, the vulva, primarily the labia majora.

INITIAL EVALUATION ON THE FIELD

Approach the injured athlete in a calm, confident manner and ask a very open-ended and general question such as "How did you get hurt?" or "Where are you hurt?" Because you must quickly assess for airway patency and adequate breathing and circulation, a quick and lucid response to this question establishes the athlete's initial presence. Always consider the possibility of spinal injury and protect the cervical

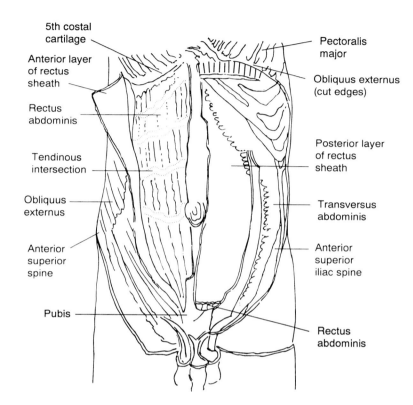

5th costal cartilage

Anterior layer of rectus sheath

Rectus abdominis

Tendinous intersection

Obliquus externus

Anterior superior spine

Pubis

Pectoralis major

Obliquus externus (cut edges)

Posterior layer of rectus sheath

Transversus abdominis

Anterior superior iliac spine

Rectus abdominis

Figure **8.4.** Abdominal wall, anterior layers on the right, deeper layers on the left.

spine accordingly. Next, evaluate the athlete's overall condition and vital signs. Most abdominal injuries seen in sports are due to blunt trauma, but penetrating injuries may be encountered, although extremely rare. A recent report (5) of three cases of penetrating javelin wounds involved one young man impaling himself with the lance entering through his upper midabdomen and exiting through his left flank. Any impaled object should be left in place. Its removal should not take place in the field, but in the operating room. The object should be secured to minimize any motion and the athlete should be rapidly transported to the emergency department via ambulance. With penetrating injuries, there is always the possibility of protrusion of fat, bowel, or muscle through the open wound. Cover

any such tissue with a moist, sterile dressing and gently secure in place.

If the athlete complains of severe, unremitting abdominal pain, coupled with marked abdominal tenderness, even abdominal rigidity, or signs of hypovolemic shock, transport the individual to the nearest emergency department.

The vast majority of blunt abdominal sports injuries will not unfold in such a dramatic fashion. If the athlete is lying supine, leave him or her in that position. If he or she is sitting up or standing, ask him or her to lie down on the ground or bench away from any area of play or competition. Expose the athlete's trunk and then ask for a description of what happened (kicked by opponent's foot in the epigastrium; landed with full weight on a football lying on the ground; received body check with lacrosse stick to the flank area, etc) and what symptoms are now present (local or diffuse pain, nausea, dizziness, shortness of breath, etc).

Pain and its location are usually the best indicators of local abdominal wall injury. If the athlete has rapid improvement in pain that is well localized, denies systemic symptoms, and has a normal examination, except for local superficial abdominal wall or flank tenderness, he or she may be allowed to sit up and then stand up while the physician carefully observes for any recurrence or increase in the original symptoms. The athlete should be instructed to begin a series of escalating activities off the field, and if both the athlete and physician have no further suspicions of significant injury, the athlete may be allowed to return to competition.

The physician should carefully observe the athlete's performance for any deterioration, guarding, or hesitancy that would mandate removal from competition and reevaluation. Indeed, serial examinations by the same physician are probably the most effective way to make a diagnosis. Knowing the athlete well, his or her personality, ability to tolerate pain or injury, underlying acute or chronic medical, psychological, and musculoskeletal problems over time allows the primary care physician to more accurately differentiate inconvenient or insignificant pain from more serious or debilitating injury. The vast majority of athletes with blunt trauma have little or no external signs of injury.

Knowledge of any recent viral syndromes, especially infectious mononucleosis, should greatly heighten suspicions of possible splenic rupture. Ask if there is any shoulder pain. Athletes who have irritation of the diaphragm from blood secondary to initial or delayed splenic rupture may have pain referred to the left shoulder

in up to 50% of cases of splenic bleeding (6). This finding is known as Kehr's sign and it may be elicited by placing the athlete in the Trendelenburg position or by palpation of the left upper quadrant (Figure 8.5) (7). Right shoulder pain secondary to right subdiaphragmatic irritation is not as common, but certainly possible in significant liver injury bleeding. Pain that is increased by coughing may signify early peritoneal or diaphragmatic irritation. If any of these symptoms are present, the physician must be suspicious of serious intra-abdominal injury.

The physical examination should begin by observing the athlete's trunk for any visible ecchymoses, abrasions, swelling, or lacerations. Ecchymosis around the umbilicus (Cullen's sign) or of the flank (Turner's sign) may indicate bleeding in the retroperitoneum. However, these visual signs usually take hours or days to develop (7). If a motor vehicle is involved and the athlete was wearing a seat or lap belt, look

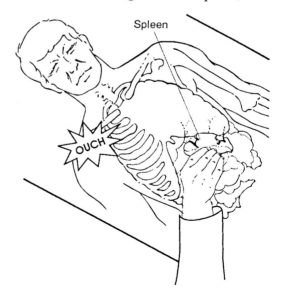

Figure 8.5. Palpation of a ruptured spleen may lead to pain referred to the shoulder.

carefully for a transverse area of ecchymoses and contusions across the lower abdomen (the seat belt sign) (8). This finding should raise the suspicion that the small intestines may be ruptured or that flexion fractures of the lumbar spine may be present.

Auscultation immediately after injury yields little clinically useful information. Background noise may make the enterprise difficult if not impossible, and the time spent listening carefully to all quadrants generally only delays more important diagnostic strategies. Bowel sounds may initially be normal despite hollow viscus perforation or intra-abdominal hemorrhage, and diminished or even absent bowel sounds do not always signal an intra-abdominal crisis. Dehydration, relative ischemia secondary to vigorous exercise, and major muscle blood pooling coupled with heightened sympathetic and decreased vagal tone may cause decreased bowel sounds (7).

Palpation is the next order of business and should begin in a gentle fashion away from the area that is most suspicious of injury or where there is an obvious contusion or abrasion. The lower chest should be palpated for any localized tenderness, swelling, or crepitus that might signal lower rib or costochondral fractures. The location of these injuries would heighten suspicion of an underlying organ injury. Grasp the iliac crests and gently rock the pelvis. If well tolerated by the patient, further compression and distraction of the crests along with compression of the symphysis pubis helps to rule out serious pelvis fracture. The thoracic and lumbar spine must also be palpated along with the flanks and costovertebral angles for tenderness that may signal an underlying fracture or kidney or retroperitoneal injury.

If pain, nausea, or referred pain to the shoulder is produced by the following maneuvers, then significant abdominal injury should be considered.

1. Ask the athlete to cough and bear down.
2. Strike the heel of the supine athlete with his or her leg extended and locked.
3. Shake the abdomen back and forth.

Most athletes with abdominal or genitourinary trauma that necessitates removal from competition and physician evaluation will have a "benign" initial examination and will request a return to action during the examination. If the sideline examination is normal and there are no systemic symptoms (nausea, dizziness, shortness of breath, etc) the athlete may be observed progressing through a series of physical tasks that place escalating demands on the cardiovascular and musculoskeletal system. If this activity produces no symptoms, then return to action may be considered. If the physician has any reservations, do not allow the athlete to return to competition. Proceed with further questions and serial examinations. For example, any hesitancy on the part of the athlete to return to competition should be taken seriously. Never allow an athlete to return to action if you are not absolutely convinced that the athlete is totally confident and willing to do so. If, after repeated serial examinations, there remains sufficient concern, then further work-up should proceed at a health care facility where needed diagnostic equipment is available.

INJURIES TO THE ABDOMINAL WALL SKIN

Because the abdomen is often exposed or only lightly covered in many athletic events, the skin is vulnerable to a variety of insults ranging from abrasions or friction ("cherry") burns to frank lacerations. Occasionally the skin may be chaffed by tight or ill-fitted equipment such as football shoulder pads that are too small or rib belts that are too large. Many protective dressing materials are available to cover the wound completely and reduce any further friction or chaffing. Fine-mesh gauzes impregnated with petrolatum are generally effective. Local antibacterial ointments or creams (avoiding those combination products containing neomycin) may be helpful in those wounds that appear more prone to infection (originally dirty and with some very early erythema and tenderness). Keep a close watch on those friction burns that appear deeper and more "angry." Superficial lacerations should be repaired in the usual fashion after thorough cleansing and debridement and irrigation if necessary. These lacerations are usually easy to cover and activity can resume promptly. Steri-Strips or butterfly-type closures are usually inadequate in the athlete who will be vigorously exercising and hence sweating profusely and where direct trauma or twisting forces will inevitably be encountered. If there is any question regarding the depth of the laceration or any penetrating wound (e.g., when muscle tissue is visible), then the athlete should have a more extensive evaluation.

SUBCUTANEOUS TISSUE

Direct blows may cause bleeding into the subcutaneous fat and connective tissue, which may present as a localized, tender mass. These hematomas may look impressive but are rarely serious. Standard ice and compressive dressings will usually contain the bleeding and any disability is usually minor. Custom protective padding may be engineered by the athletic trainer or physical therapist to minimize further local tissue injury and bleeding. If seemingly trivial trauma results in subcutaneous hematomas, investigate further for a bleeding diathesis. In the young and otherwise healthy athlete, consider leukemia or idiopathic thrombocytopenic purpura.

MUSCLE

Clinical Case #1

A 21-year-old male tennis player and team captain complained of a painful, tender area in his left anterior abdomen. He distinctly remembered a "muscle pull" in this area approximately 6 years earlier in high school. The symptoms have been intermittent and often nagging over the past 6 years, both during and after exercise, especially after hard overhead serves. He has noted some "lumps" in his anterior abdominal muscle, which will often disappear in hours to 3 to 4 days. The pain is occasionally severe enough to preclude further competition, even in the middle of a match. Over the years, these tender areas have been treated with varying degrees of success with various physical therapy modalities, including ultrasound, heat, ice, electrical stimulation and stretching. Nonsteroidal anti-inflammatory drugs (NSAIDs) had often been helpful episodically. Over the past year "stretching seemed to work the best."

During a time of considerable incapacitation, physical examination revealed a tall, thin, lanky man with a prominent left rectus abdominis muscle, obviously larger than the right muscle. It was felt to have more "tone" and it was diffusely tender to palpation with one area of point tenderness that he reported as causing a "deep ache" and a feeling of nausea. A poorly defined nodule approximately 1 × 1 cm located 4 cm superior and lateral to the umbilicus in the rectus abdominis muscle was palpated. Laboratory studies, including complete blood count, erythrocyte sedimentation rate, sequential multiple analysis, and creatine kinase, were all normal. Lateral soft-tissue abdominal x-rays were negative for any ectopic calcification. Ultrasound revealed an echogenic focus in the left rectus inferiorly, 5 cm below the umbilicus. It abutted the peritoneal line, but this demarcation was intact. Portions of this mass appeared "linear in contour."

Therapy ultimately involved an injection of 2 mL bupivacaine 0.5% with a long-acting corticosteroid directly into this probable area of scar tissue under ultrasound guidance. After this procedure, there was slight overall improvement, especially with normal activities of daily living, but then an attempt to return to full play resulted in a return of pain that limited any meaningful participation.

Repeat ultrasound 2 months later revealed a linear development extending inferiorly from the original mass and several other masses inferior to the initial mass. Magnetic resonance imaging (MRI) was reported to be totally negative—a finding difficult to explain given the abnormalities seen with the ultrasonogram. When he was last seen several weeks later, he reported feeling much improved and the previous treatment modalities were once again used, especially stretching and strengthening. Over the next 4 to 6 weeks, he was able to return to full activity without difficulty.

Muscle tears or strains may produce symptoms from trivial to considerable, and, sometimes, tumors must be sought after and excluded when suspicious clinical findings warrant, with MRI probably providing the greater clarity short of biopsy in this often pesky problem. Do not dismiss all such tender nodules as "trigger points." Careful follow-up is usually the key in making the correct diagnosis and not missing the rare soft-tissue tumor.

Because there are several large and major muscle groups investing the abdomen and trunk as delineated earlier, it is not surprising that strains to these muscles are common, especially in sports requiring great speed or force and marked torque or twisting movements. These movements are common in wrestling, gymnastics, tennis, cheerleading, and tumbling. Contusion and hematomas may be caused by direct blows and ultimate scar tissue may occur from acute or repetitive strains. The hematomas may calcify and can occasionally become irritated and inflamed. Treatment consists of rest, NSAIDs, local ice, electrical stimulation, and stretching and strengthening of the entire muscle group. These areas of fibrous scarring may be difficult to identify clinically, except for the area of localized tenderness (trigger point). Injection of a local anesthetic with or without a corticosteroid may help.

Strain or partial rupture of the rectus abdominis muscle is relatively common. If the epigastric artery or intramuscular vessels are damaged, a hematoma may form within the sheath itself. Eighty percent of rectus abdominis hematomas occur below the umbilicus (9). Occasionally, with violent stretching movements, the inferior epigastric artery ruptures and hemorrhages into the rectus abdominis sheath without accompanying muscle damage (4). Rarely, continued hemorrhage from the epigastric vessels has culminated in death (10). Usually these injuries are more of a nuisance with nagging pain and inability to perform at an optimal level. The hematoma itself is tender and usually palpable. It rarely crosses the midline.

Occasionally the location of the hematoma, coupled with the intense pain symptoms evolving over several days, may present a picture that closely mimics an acute intra-abdominal problem, and the white blood cell count is slightly elevated with genuine guarding and early rebound tenderness. Every effort should be made to make the diagnosis with the tender mass and, if still ill defined, the physician should perform a computed tomography (CT) scan prior to surgery to confirm the presence of the rectus sheath hematoma.

Clinical Case #2

An 18-year-old male cheerleader presented at the Student Health Service complaining of severe, intermittent, cramping right lower quadrant abdominal pain that had been steadily increasing over a 10-hour period. He was unable to sleep and felt nauseated with one episode of "dry heaves." He recalled performing a maneuver called a "back tuck" 8 days earlier when he felt he "pulled a stomach muscle" and, in fact, had seen his athletic trainer 2 days after this for evaluation and treatment of this "strain to the rectus abdominis." The pain was gradually subsiding with relative rest and physical therapy. His complete review of symptoms was essentially negative. Physical examination revealed an alert young man, in moderate distress, slightly diaphoretic with his legs drawn into his chest. Blood pressure was 146/80 and pulse ranged from 64 to 88; temperature was 98.5°F. Abdominal examination revealed tenderness in the right lower quadrant with marked guarding, positive peritoneal signs, positive rebound, and a positive psoas sign. He was intolerant of the attempted rectal examination. Laboratory studies revealed a white blood cell count of 13,400 with a slight left shift. Urinalysis, electrolytes, hemoglobin/hematocrit, platelets, prothrombin time, and partial thromboplastin time were normal. Intravenous fluids were started (Ringer's lactate); morphine sulfate and promethazine were given intravenously and immediate surgical consultation was obtained. The working diagnosis was "probable appendicitis/perforated."

The patient was admitted and prepared for surgery. Due to the above history and some observable asymmetry in his well-developed rectus abdominis muscles (the right side ap-

peared larger) a preoperative contrast-enhanced CT scan (intravenous and oral) was obtained (Figure 8.6). A small amount of free intraperitoneal fluid was noted in the right perirectal fossa, and there was a moderate enlargement of the right rectus abdominis muscle with a heterogeneous density consistent with a hematoma measuring approximately 3 ×5 cm. The patient was treated symptomatically, observed in the hospital for approximately 10 to 12 hours, and discharged for outpatient follow-up.

Recovery was slow but gradual over the next 8 to 10 weeks. However, he did develop a similar, but less severe, strain of his opposite left rectus abdominis muscle in the same distal one third region approximately 4 weeks after the right strain and hematoma. This, too, slowly improved until he experienced another similar strain and palpable hematoma in the proximal one third of his left rectus abdominis muscle 4 weeks after this second strain. Some 6 weeks later at follow-up he continued to experience some nagging left upper and lower rectus abdominis pain and was given maximal conservative physical and medical therapy.

In any clinical situation that involves abdominal wall pain and tenderness, it is

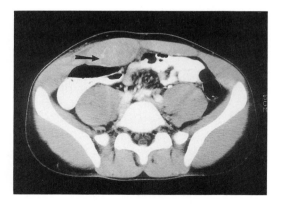

Figure 8.6. Hematoma of the recuts muscles (*arrow*).

imperative to try to distinguish between pain that is secondary to abdominal wall injury (contusion, hematoma, strain, etc) and pain that is secondary to deeper visceral trauma. Palpating the abdominal wall while the athlete contracts the rectus muscles by lifting the legs and head off the examining table or doing a partial (abdominal crunch) sit-up can help the examiner make this distinction. Increased pain with these maneuvers or with superficial palpation while the abdomen is tensed may indicate abdominal wall injury (11). With the tensed rectus muscles "guarding" the visceral organs, the athlete with visceral injury may have decreased pain with this maneuver. These maneuvers, at best, are only adjuncts to help clarify abdominal wall from deeper visceral injuries and are not definitive in themselves of locating or ruling out the exact location of the injury. In some situations, the athlete may have abdominal wall trauma combined with underlying visceral trauma.

BLOWS TO THE SOLAR PLEXUS

This injury is relatively common in athletes due to the open or unguarded anterior abdominal wall and the frequency with which blunt trauma is directed to this region, often when the abdominal muscles are relaxed in the unsuspecting athlete. This blow may result in having "the breath knocked out" of the athlete or the athlete "being winded." Both descriptions are used by the athlete who feels as if he or she is suffocating, unable to breathe, or even in danger of dying. The exact cause of the respiratory difficulty is uncertain, but diaphragmatic spasm and transient contusion to the sympathetic celiac plexus have been implicated by most authors (4). The pressure of the blow and the sudden con-

traction of the abdominal muscles force the diaphragm upward (12). At the same time, there is a violent reflex contraction of the intercostals and serrati muscles that pulls the rib cage down and stabilizes it. A forceful expiration results; at times, it is maintained for several seconds because of the muscle spasm. The athlete is acutely aware of the inability to take a breath and becomes anxious and agitated. Medical personnel who first arrive at the scene should quickly reassure the athlete while gathering associated clinical data such as pulse, color, patency of the airway, and so on. Be sure the airway is not compromised by the tongue or any foreign objects such as a mouthpiece or denture, and then loosen the belts or equipment around the abdomen. Rarely, the athlete may even convulse for a few seconds secondary to hypoxia before muscle relaxation occurs and allows for spontaneous recoil of the displaced structures and inspiration. The knees should be allowed to flex, and the athlete should be allowed to lean forward over the flexed knees while lying on his or her side. Sitting up and leaning forward is often helpful (4). Continued reassurance is in order. After several difficult breaths, normal respirations are usually rapidly restored.

This injury should not be regarded lightly because a force of considerable magnitude has been directed against an unprotected abdomen; hence, any number of more significant injuries are possible. After an initial evaluation, either on the playing field or at the scene where gentle, deep palpation of the abdomen has been completed, if the athlete reports minimal discomfort and no dyspnea, the athlete may be allowed to walk away from the playing area to an area conducive to a thorough evaluation of the abdomen. Full respiratory excursions with full inspiration and expiration should be observed for any guarding or asymmetry of motion. If the examination is normal and the athlete remains asymptomatic for 5 to 10 minutes, then sequential functional demands are made to ascertain normal running mechanics, normal trunk motion, especially flexion, extension, and twisting from side to side. If the evaluation continues to be negative, the athlete may be allowed to return to action under the physician's careful scrutiny. After the activity is completed, the athlete should once again be carefully evaluated. If all observations and repeat examination are negative, the athlete may be released with instructions to return for reevaluation in 24 to 48 hours, or sooner if any new or disturbing symptoms arise.

"HIP POINTERS"

The "hip pointer" is a contusion or hematoma along the upper or lower margin of the iliac crest where abdominal and lower extremity musculature attach (13). Usually, a fall onto the iliac crest or a blow by a firm object such as a football helmet causes this common injury. Hip pointers and bony pelvic injuries are covered in detail in Chapter 14.

INTRA-ABDOMINAL INJURIES: AN OVERVIEW

Clinical Case #3

A 22-year-old football linebacker was kicked in the epigastric area while he was flying through the air to make a tackle during an intercollegiate game. He complained of severe epigastric pain and nausea and was carried to the sidelines for further evaluation. He appeared pale and ashen and was slightly nauseated. His abdomen was firm with a great deal of muscular guarding and rigidity. His pain did not improve and he was taken to a local hospital emergency

room. His vital signs were stable. His abdomen was diffusely tender without bowel sounds. Notation was made by the examining surgeon that it was difficult to elicit peritoneal signs because of the extreme muscular habitus. The white cell count was 9900 with a left shift. Amylase was normal. Three-way abdominal x-rays were normal and contrast-enhanced CT showed "dependent fluid, probable hemorrhage within the pelvis." No visceral pathology was identified. He was admitted with a diagnosis of "abdominal injury of unknown etiology." Intravenous fluids were begun along with placement of a nasogastric tube and Foley catheter. The next morning his symptoms had slightly improved, but his abdomen remained rigid without bowel sounds. Repeat complete blood count revealed a leukocyte count of 18,000 with a further left shift. Exploratory celiotomy was scheduled that morning and hastened considerably when preoperative plain x-rays revealed a pneumoperitoneum. When the abdomen was opened, purulent fluid was obtained that ultimately grew two gram-positive cocci and a large growth of proteus. A transverse laceration at the proximal third of the jejunum was discovered at the antimesenteric border.

In assessing abdominal trauma, the accurate diagnosis of a specific type of injury is not of primary importance, but the determination that an intra-abdominal injury exists that requires further intervention and, in particular, operation is of critical importance. Athletes who present with recent abdominal trauma and pain coupled with signs of peritonitis such as absent bowel sounds, abdominal rigidity, referred abdominal pain and tenderness, and rebound tenderness do not need extensive diagnostic evaluations (14). They need a prompt exploratory and therapeutic abdominal operation. Because the vast majority of sports-related injuries are never this clear-cut regarding their management, the clinician must proceed methodically in the evaluation, relying heavily on the history and physical examination, especially serial examinations. Inspection and auscultation may be helpful, but palpation is the mainstay of the physical examination because signs of peritoneal irritation point strongly toward free blood in the abdomen (although, initially, blood is not very irritating to the peritoneum, and thus there may be several hours of delay in developing these signs) or a ruptured hollow viscus where the presence of bowel contents (hydrogen ions, digestive enzymes, bile, bacteria, digested or undigested food, etc) or bladder contents (urine) has occurred. If there is diffuse tenderness and pain to percussion, peritoneal irritation should be strongly suspected. A rectal examination is important for several reasons. If the prostate gland is "boggy" or "high riding," a urethral tear should be suspected. Gross blood may indicate acute bowel or rectal injury or pelvic fracture, whereas occult blood may indicate gastrointestinal luminal bleeding (especially with serial examinations over several days), stress ulcers, or even underlying or preexisting pathology. Loss of sphincter tone may indicate an associated spinal injury. Blood at the urethral meatus or in the scrotum may indicate a pelvic fracture or urethral tear.

The laboratory work-up should be tailored to the particular situation. Blood typing and cross-matching, along with a complete blood count, routine chemistries and coagulation studies, amylase, urinalysis, including dipstick and microscopic analysis, pregnancy testing for all females of childbearing age, and alcohol or other drug determinations are in order for the severely injured athlete. The white blood cell count is almost always elevated initially but usually drops within the first 12 hours.

If the rise continues, consider intra-abdominal viscus or retroperitoneal injury. Elevation of amylase and lipase suggests pancreatic injury, if there has been no injury to the salivary glands. Serial complete blood counts may aid in assessing ongoing bleeding, especially from the liver or spleen, and serial urinalysis can aid in the evaluation of injury to the kidney. All baseline tests can be important because subsequent changes may be indicative of occult injury (e.g., subphrenic, subdiaphragmatic, or intrahepatic abscess complicating a retroperitoneal hematoma) (15).

Radiographic assessment is also tailored to the clinical situation. Three-way abdominal x-rays may reveal extraluminal or intramural air or air under the diaphragm, which indicates hollow viscus, usually bowel, rupture or disruption. Chest x-rays may reveal rib or vertebral fractures or diaphragm injury if the diaphragm is not distinct. Abdominal contents within the chest cavity indicates diaphragmatic rupture. A single plain film of the abdomen may reveal signs of hemoperitoneum. These are the "flank-stripe sign" (collection of blood in the pericolic gutter), the "hepatic angle sign" (inferior lateral aspect of the liver blunted) and the "dog-ear-sign" (fluid density above and lateral to the bladder) (16). Lumbar spine fractures may be detected, and the loss of the psoas shadow may indicate retroperitoneal bleeding. Retroperitoneal air may be seen in injury to the duodenum, and hepatic parenchymal gas may be a manifestation of severe blunt trauma to the liver without infection (17). If the injury involves significant energy (fall from a horse, ejection from a bicycle or motor vehicle, etc), a film of the pelvis as a screening tool to exclude fracture is indicated. Further specialized contrast studies are often helpful.

An intravenous pyelogram (IVP) is indicated in significant flank, back, or abdominal trauma when urinalysis reveals more than 5 to 10 red blood cells per high-power field. High-dose intravenous bolus injection should provide evidence of relative kidney function in 5 to 10 minutes. Unilateral nonfunction implies massive parenchymal shattering or vascular pedicle disruption, but may be due to an absent kidney. Extravasation of dye indicates disruption of the collecting system. In the stable patient, CT is preferable to the IVP if there is suspicion of intra-abdominal or retroperitoneal injuries. Intravenous contrast studies should never be performed in the hypotensive, unstable patient. Finally, special upper and lower gastrointestinal contrast studies may help to identify isolated retroperitoneal gastrointestinal injuries.

Because up to 40% of athletes with significant abdominal injuries have unremarkable physical examinations, and the laboratory and radiographic studies are often not sensitive or specific enough, a diagnostic peritoneal lavage (DPL) or CT with both oral and intravenous contrast enhancement may be indicated. Both studies have special advantages and disadvantages in their applicability in given clinical situations and information obtained and are best regarded as complementary rather than competitive studies (18). DPL is considered 98% sensitive for intraperitoneal bleeding, but it cannot detect duodenal, pancreatic, or renal injuries. It can be performed rapidly and without delay in the emergency department where monitoring of the injured athlete's status may continue in an uninterrupted fashion. It is relatively inexpensive and does not require advanced equipment, but it is an invasive procedure and requires a physician skilled in its performance. The CT scan is noninvasive but more time consuming and thus should only be performed on stable patients. The CT scan provides information about specific organ injury and its extent and can assess retroperitoneal and pelvic organ injuries that may be missed with DPL. CT obviously requires special equipment and personnel and is expensive. CT with oral and intravenous contrast enhancement is probably the best imaging modality to evaluate the kidney, duodenum, and pancreas (2,19). CT may miss some gastrointestinal injuries (2). In the absence of liver or splenic injuries, the presence of free fluid in the abdominal cavity suggests an injury to the gastrointestinal tract or its mesentery and mandates early surgical intervention. Ultrasonography may be useful in demonstrating free intra-abdominal fluid or solid viscus injury but does not appear to be as sensitive or specific as contrast-enhanced CT (19). The role of laparoscopy is evolving (20). Where used it has a 10% to 15% incidence of missed enteric injury and tends to underestimate bleeding.

SPECIFIC ORGAN TRAUMA

Spleen

Clinical Case #4

A 21-year-old lacrosse player presented with continuing left upper quadrant abdominal pain, increased with deep inspirations and with associated nausea and anorexia. Three days earlier during a routine practice, he remembered having his own elbow thrust into his left upper abdomen with initial sharp pain and loss of breath. He continued to practice the following day, believing he had only "bruised some ribs." He did not bring this pain to anyone's attention until two days later when he saw an athletic trainer who performed a brief examination and quickly sent this young man to me. Examina-

tion revealed an enlarged, tender spleen, approximately 3 cm below the left costal margin with deep inspiration. His vital signs were stable. He also had some very mild left costovertebral angle tenderness. I immediately admitted this young man, began intravenous fluids, and consulted a trusted surgeon. Hemoglobin was stable and urinalysis revealed 20 to 40 red blood cells per high-power field. Mono spot was negative. This case occurred in 1983, so a liver-spleen radionuclide scan was obtained, revealing one large subcapsular and two intraparenchymal hematomas. The kidney-ureter-bladder x-ray revealed a soft-tissue density in the lower upper quadrant. The intravenous pyelogram was normal. Serial hemoglobin/hematocrits were stable; the urinalysis was normal 24 hours later, and he was discharged 3 days later with the diagnosis of traumatic splenomegaly and renal contusion.

Two days after discharge (8 days from the original insult) he had increasingly severe left shoulder pain. A CT scan revealed some subdiaphragmatic blood but the hematomas were stable. All laboratory values remained stable along with several repeat CT scans during this 5-day hospitalization for close observation. He was discharged feeling well after this disconcerting pain and malaise associated with liquefication of the splenic hematoma(s).

Three weeks later, he felt well and examination revealed a soft spleen tip, nontender, located 2 cm below the left costal margin. A repeat CT scan revealed the intrasplenic hematoma to have doubled in size. He was stable clinically but admitted for ultimate needle aspiration of approximately 750 mL of brown fluid from the liquefied hematoma under fluoroscopic needle guidance. Twenty-four hours later, he was again discharged for close daily follow-up.

Four weeks later (32 days since the initial insult), the tip of the spleen was palpable, but nontender. Ultrasound examination revealed a decrease in the size of the hematoma.

The organ most frequently injured by all blunt trauma to the abdomen is the spleen (21). Injuries to the spleen from sports-related trauma involve up to 8% of all adult and 20% of all pediatric spleen injuries (1,22). The spleen may be lacerated or contused with varying degrees of parenchymal injury leading to subcapsular or intrasplenic hematomas. Rarely, hilar vessels may be disrupted. The athlete usually relates a blow to the left upper abdominal quadrant or left lower chest wall anteriorly. Falls, body slams, elbows, lacrosse sticks, collisions, and kicks may all damage the spleen. The normal spleen is rarely injured even in sports that involve significant contact. After certain systemic disorders, especially viral infections such as infectious mononucleosis, the spleen can enlarge, making it more vulnerable to injury. Rib fractures of the lower posterior thorax make injury more likely. Initial symptoms may be vague with minimal pain. An initial sharp pain may be followed by a dull, left-sided flank or upper abdominal pain with malaise and anorexia. Pain upon deep inspiration or the development of left shoulder tip pain (Kehr's sign) may be present. Palpation of the abdomen should be deep but gentle. If the spleen is palpable, an injury must be ruled out. Avoid further palpation. If the athlete is hemodynamically stable, contrast-enhanced CT is the imaging modality of choice, although radionuclide scintigraphy may be indicated for pregnant patients and for those who are allergic to iodine (23). Ultrasound may detect free intraperitoneal fluid and posttraumatic cysts; however, both the spleen and liver can sustain severe injury that ultrasound cannot discern (24). Delayed rupture can follow injuries that cause subcapsular hematomas days to weeks after the traumatic event, thus signifying the need for close observation and monitoring of these individuals (25).

Most athletes with spleen injuries can be treated nonsurgically (26). Even significant trauma-induced bleeding rarely necessitates splenectomy. If surgery is necessary because of continued bleeding, partial splenectomy, salvaging as much splenic tissue as possible, is the procedure of choice (25). A pneumococcal vaccine should be administered to the athlete who has undergone total splenectomy.

In summary, beware of splenic injury, especially in the adolescent who may have undiagnosed infectious mononucleosis or other viral infection. The spleen is probably most vulnerable to injury 14 to 28 days after the onset of this systemic disorder (4), although delayed rupture has been reported, even at some months after the initial infection. Before the athlete is allowed to return to competitive activity, he or she should feel well and have regained normal strength, and the spleen should no longer be palpable (27). The length of time required for this recovery varies widely, but usually will require 3 to 6 weeks. If a return to athletics, especially contact sports, is strongly desired by the athlete, and if any doubt exists as to the size of the spleen, then ultrasound is the least invasive imaging tool to ascertain the size of the spleen.

Liver

The liver is the second most commonly injured organ in all blunt abdominal trauma (21), and it is the most commonly injured organ in all combined blunt and penetrating trauma (28). The liver is the third most commonly injured organ in sports-related abdominal trauma (8). A history of a direct blow to the right lower rib cage or right upper abdominal quadrant combined with right upper quadrant tenderness and guarding on gentle palpation should alert the clinician to a liver contusion or parenchymal injury. Rib fractures on the lower right (the tenth, eleventh, twelfth) are associated with liver injury. Children have poorly developed abdominal musculature and a smaller anteroposterior diameter, making them more vulnerable to compression-type injuries. Because the rib cage is more resilient in children, fractures occur less frequently, decreasing their value in predicting liver or spleen injuries. Massive blood loss may occur but is rare in nonvehicular sports activity. Subdiaphragmatic irritation from free blood may occur, giving rise to pain referred to the right shoulder, but this finding is uncommon. Placing the athlete in the Trendelenburg position for several minutes may elicit this finding. The use of liver function tests to screen for liver injury has been advocated by several authors (29,30), but this approach requires additional confirmation. Most injuries are minor contusions, and small subcapsular or intraparenchymal hematomas and will resolve spontaneously over 4 to 8 weeks. Contrast-enhanced CT is the diagnostic procedure of choice. Nonoperative management in stable patients consisting of bed rest and careful observation and repeat CT scans as indicated is the treatment of choice (31). Control of hemorrhage remains the dominant consideration in the treatment of major hepatic injuries (32) and thus early surgical consultation is essential in all such cases.

Pancreas

The pancreas is injured in 1% to 2% of all abdominal trauma (7) but is rare in sports-related activity. The history is usually significant for a very forceful "spear-like" direct blow to the epigastric region from a fist, hockey stick, or bicycle handlebar, which can crush the pancreas against the vertebral column. Karate training, which is now gaining popularity, may be responsible (33). Contusions, lacerations, hematomas, transections, or crush injuries may result, but the initial physical findings may be minimal with slow progression over 12 to 48 hours of systemic symptoms of nausea, vomiting, anorexia, and generalized malaise with increasing upper abdominal pain that may radiate to the back. Initial mild, local epigastric tenderness may increase along with diffuse abdominal tenderness and peritoneal signs. Ileus and abdominal distention will often develop. Serum amylase and lipase, if elevated, are helpful, but a normal serum amylase level does not exclude major pancreatic trauma (2). Even contrast-enhanced CT (intravenous and oral) may not identify significant trauma in the immediate postinjury period. Occasionally, endoscopic retrograde cholangiopancreatography may visualize ductal injury (7), and there may be an elevated amylase or lipase level in the fluid from peritoneal lavage, but early surgical consultation is mandatory when pancreatic injury is suspected, because abdominal exploration when delayed beyond 24 hours significantly increases morbidity and mortality (8). Complications are common and include persistent pancreatitis, fistulas, pseudocysts, and abscess formation (7).

Diaphragm

Most traumatic ruptures of the diaphragm are due to massive blunt abdominal injury and are rarely encountered in sports activity. The most common injury is 5 to 10 cm in length and involves the posterolateral left hemidiaphragm (2). Occasionally the traumatic defect is large enough to permit intrathoracic displacement of the abdominal viscera, which may lead to significant respiratory distress and collapse of the left lung. Chest and abdominal x-rays may be nonspecific, but usually a hemothorax will be identified, and the position of the nasogastric tube may identify an otherwise occult left-sided tear. The athlete's pain and abdominal tenderness are usually of significant magnitude to warrant early and aggressive emergency department work-up and surgical consultation when there has been herniation of abdominal contents into the hemithorax. Previous penetrating trauma (e.g., a stab wound) may predispose to future diaphragm injury and intrathoracic herniation of abdominal contents. Diaphragm injury can be missed when herniation does not occur. The physical examination and plain radiographs may be unremarkable. If the patient is stable enough to undergo MRI, this may be the best test for suspected diaphragmatic injury in the opinion of several authors (8).

Hollow Viscus

These injuries are rare in most sports but must be suspected when blunt trauma to the abdomen results in substantial persistent pain and progressive abdominal signs. Kicks and blows to the abdomen; pile-ons in football and rugby; spearing in hockey; falls from rodeo, equestrian, and skiing events; and landing awkwardly against the uneven parallel bar (8) as well as ejections and seat belt restraint forces in motor vehicle events can all deliver a powerful compressive force to an isolated and usually unprotected and relaxed area of the abdomen. When these injuries are followed by systemic signs of shock, there should be no delay in transporting the athlete to the nearest emergency room, preferably a level I or II trauma center. Sometimes symptoms may take hours or days to develop, mandating a high index of suspicion and careful evaluation and observation over time.

Stomach

It is very rare to rupture the stomach in sports. If this occurs, the low pH of the gastric contents causes early peritoneal irritation and accompanying physical signs. Blood is usually in the nasogastric aspirate and free air is usually seen on plain three-way abdominal x-rays. Treatment is a prompt laparotomy and repair of the injury. Stomach wall contusion usually produces local pain and tenderness, no peritoneal signs, and normal radiographs. Conservative therapy consisting of rest, avoidance of NSAIDs, and occasional use of an H_2 blocker will allow spontaneous resolution over 2 to 4 weeks.

Duodenum, Jejunum, and Ileum

The mechanism of injury is similar to that associated with pancreatic injury. The duodenum is usually injured at the second and third portions causing perforations or intramural hematomas (8). A bloody nasogastric aspirate or free intraperitoneal or retroperitoneal air should greatly raise suspicion of injury, especially in the patient with minimal early pain and physical findings. Indeed this injury can be overlooked because it is retroperitoneal with minimal initial intra-abdominal signs. Duodenal "C-loop" diatrizoate meglumine (Gastrografin) studies or double-contrast CT is indicated for the high-risk patient (2). The clinical picture of an intraperitoneal duodenal rupture may mimic that of a perforated duodenal ulcer (8), but an intramural hematoma may take days to develop signs and symptoms of proximal intestinal obstruction. Treatment of ruptures or perforations mandate prompt surgery and repair. Hematomas

may resolve spontaneously over days with nasogastric suction and intravenous fluids (8).

Athletes with small-bowel injury have little pain initially and will often have a normal examination (7). The pH content is almost neutral and the small intestine contains few bacteria; thus, peritoneal irritation is initially minimal. Injuries to the small bowel are particularly worrisome because symptoms may not appear for hours, days, or even weeks with a resultant increase in morbidity and mortality (34). Work-up should always include serial complete blood counts (watch for progressive rise in white blood cells or a left shift in the differential) and three-way abdomen and lateral decubiti radiographs to look for free air. Double-contrast CT is probably more sensitive for bowel injury (35), but some controversy remains in this area, with some authorities stating that peritoneal lavage is more accurate than CT in most cases of hollow viscus injury (36,37). Indeed, the false-negative rate of CT alone ranges from 5% to 12%. Although both studies have their advantages and disadvantages as discussed earlier, they are probably best used in a complementary fashion with both providing more information than either test alone (18). If duodenal rupture is missed, necrosis of the retroperitoneal tissues begins within 24 to 48 hours and up to half of these patients may develop an intra-abdominal abscess and septic shock and die (8).

Colon and Rectum

These very serious injuries occur most often in motor vehicle crashes and make up approximately 4% of all blunt abdominal trauma; they are rare in sports activity. Usual findings with rupture involve massive peritoneal contamination and an acute abdomen secondary to peritonitis. Occasionally, however, injuries may be asymptomatic initially, especially if retroperitoneal. The work-up should progress in much the same fashion as suspected small-bowel injury. The rectal examination may reveal gross blood. Treatment is usually surgical unless the athlete remains hemodynamically stable and frank rupture has not occurred.

OTHER INJURIES/CONDITIONS

Mesentery

The mesentery of the small bowel and colon may be torn by shearing forces in blunt trauma or contused with secondary hemorrhage, both leading to varying degrees of pain and physical findings (4,38). With major hemorrhage or vessel disruption, findings may mimic other serious intra-abdominal or retroperitoneal injuries with progressive peritoneal irritation and bowel ischemia. Under these circumstances aggressive work-up and early surgical consultation is warranted. Most mesenteric injuries are relatively minor and probably often go undiagnosed with spontaneous resolution in days to weeks. One thing to remember is that systemic infections such as infectious mononucleosis can lead to marked mesenteric adenopathy in some individuals. Such enlargement may lead to abdominal pain, nausea, and vomiting secondary to partial small-bowel obstruction. The other features of infectious mononucleosis are usually present and treatment is conservative.

Hernias

Even with the enormous forces imposed on the athlete's abdomen from direct trauma and through forceful contractions of the truncal musculature and diaphragm producing increased intra-abdominal pressure, the likelihood of developing any one of several different abdominal and inguinal and femoral hernias is probably no greater among athletes than would be found in nonathletes. Nearly all hernias develop on the basis of some congenital weakness in the arrangements of the abdominal muscles and fascia. Age, sex, and family history are thus more important determinants than any self-imposed or applied demands. A clear, concise discussion of the three most common hernias in adults (indirect and direct inguinal and femoral) and the common anterior wall hernias can be found elsewhere (62,63). An acute abdominal wall hernia caused by a large force directed on a small area is an unusual but serious injury (7). The so-called handlebar hernia occurs most commonly when a bicycle handlebar strikes the rider during a fall or crash (39). This hernia can be palpated as a tender defect within or just lateral to the rectus abdominis muscle. A loop of bowel may protrude through the defect.

Genitourinary System

Kidney

Clinical Case #5

A 19-year-old tall and relatively thin football quarterback was "sandwiched" between two opposing players while jumping into the air to throw a pass. He sustained a compression-type injury to his right lateral abdomen and flank area. He walked off the field, complaining of pain in the right upper quadrant and right lateral abdominal area and moderate nausea. He appeared ashen and described steadily increasing pain and "tightness" in the deep right flank area. The nausea subsided. He denied shoulder pain.

Examination revealed an alert man in no apparent distress, with return of his normal color. Blood pressure was 150/80 and pulse was 68. He had some slight tenderness over the right anterolateral rib cage. Abdominal examination revealed slight tenderness deep in the right upper quadrant with a tender liver edge. The liver was normal in size. The spleen was not palpable. There were some abrasions over the right lower flank and mild to moderate costovertebral angle tenderness. The first voided urine was grossly bloody with several clots noted. The complete blood count and amylase were normal. Three-way abdominal x-rays revealed a questionable decrease in the right psoas shadow but was otherwise within normal limits. Intravenous fluids were begun and a contrast-enhanced CT scan was obtained, which revealed a right perinephric hematoma and small right renal contusion. He remained hospitalized in the Student Health Service for approximately 19 hours, during which time he was given intravenous fluids and serial physical examinations. His hemoglobin and hematocrit remained stable and the gross hematuria resolved. He was discharged with urine dipstick 2+ for blood. He was followed as an outpatient with serial complete blood counts, urinalysis, and continuing normal blood pressures and creatinines. Sixteen days later, he was totally asymptomatic and his urinalysis was completely normal.

Injuries to the kidney are common, often frightening to the patient and physician when gross blood is urinated, and must be thoroughly evaluated. Most injuries will resolve spontaneously without surgical intervention. Remember to look for renal injury with any abdominal injury because the horseshoe configured, abdominal, or high pelvic kidney may be injured by direct blow to the anterior abdomen.

The location of the kidneys in the upper retroperitoneum partially under the rib cage, combined with their surrounding pericapsular fat and mucus, bulky posterior musculature and lumbar spine, and anterior abdominal organs and musculature, affords relatively good protection to these usually paired vital organs. Nonetheless, they are the abdominal organs most frequently injured in sports-related trauma (40,41). Children are particularly prone to renal damage due to the relatively large size of their kidneys and the increased resiliency and decreased strength of their rib cage (42). Approximately 30% of pediatric renal injuries are caused by sports activity (43). The most common injuries are contusions or minor lacerations caused by a direct blow (as in ice hockey, football, basketball, and rugby) or repeated blows (as in boxing). Pain in the flank is usually the chief complaint, but significant injury may be painless, particularly if the injury is confined to the substance of the kidney with bleeding into the renal collecting system rather than into the tissues around the kidney (14). Physical findings may vary tremendously from flank contusions or abrasions, local costovertebral angle tenderness, hematomas, or ecchymosis, to an expanding mass, peritoneal signs, or flank hypovolemic shock depending on the severity of the injury. The hallmark laboratory finding is hematuria, either microscopic or gross, although the degree of hematuria is not correlated to the degree of kidney injury.

There are five classes of renal injury (Figure 8.7) (4): 1) contusion, 2) cortical laceration, 3) caliceal laceration, 4) complete renal fracture, and 5) vascular pedicle injury. Chronically diseased kidneys, or large, malformed, or malpositioned (e.g., abdominal, pelvic or "horseshoe") kidneys are more likely to be injured. These athletes should be counseled to avoid those activities most prone to direct forceful contact.

A Contusion

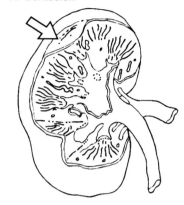

B Cortical laceration

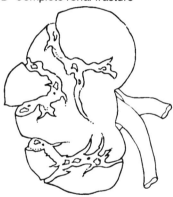

Figure 8.7. Five classes of renal injury. *A.* Contusion. *B.* Laceration. *C.* Caliceal laceration. *D.* Complete renal fracture. *E.* Vascular pedicle injury.

C Caliceal laceration

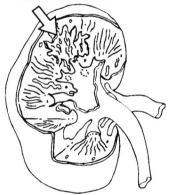

D Complete renal fracture

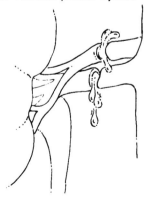

E Vascular pedicle injuries

Hematuria indicates renal injury (7), with the exception of renal pedicle avulsions, which often may not have blood in the urine. These avulsions are usually the result of severe deceleration accidents and are rarely seen in nonvehicular sports activity.

Any athlete with gross hematuria should receive further evaluation. The degree of renal trauma must be determined by IVP or CT evaluation. The greater the degree of renal injury, the more likely it is that the CT scan can determine the nature and extent of the injury better than IVP (42). In the athlete with blunt flank or back trauma, it is important to examine all urine in a serial fashion. Microscopic evaluation has not been proved superior to dipstick evaluation, with the latter associated with sensitivity higher than 97.5% and specificity for detection (42,44). The adult athlete who has gross hematuria and a benign physical examination should be followed clinically for 3 to 7 days. The hematuria should completely resolve within 2 to 3 days, during which time the patient should remain in bed, force fluids, and avoid exertion. Not all athletes with traumatic hematuria require imaging studies, but most authorities agree that IVP or CT is necessary when there is: 1) blunt trauma and gross hematuria, 2) blunt trauma with microscopic hematuria and systolic blood pressure less than 90 mm Hg, and 3) obviously penetrating abdominal flank trauma with hematuria (7,44). The initial magnitude of the blunt force, coupled with fractures of the posterior lower ribs or spinal transverse processes, and a large and possibly expanding flank hematoma, coupled with a falling hematocrit, are indications to proceed rapidly with IVP or CT evaluation. Where indications for IVP and CT are not straightforward, three-way abdominal x-rays may be helpful. The above fractures may be picked up along with loss of the usual sharp psoas shadow, implying peritoneal bleeding. The physician may note a "ground glass" appearance in the region of the renal bed, also suggesting renal injury (4).

If the kidney is not visualized on IVP, one must consider the following conditions: 1) total vascular pedicle avulsion, 2) arterial thrombosis, 3) vascular spasm, or 4) congenital absence of or previous surgical removal of the kidney (4). Should this occur, further aggressive work-up should proceed in consultation with the urologist because contrast-enhanced CT or renal arteriography, or both, and possibly surgery may be necessary. Contrast-enhanced CT has the advantage of also simultaneously examining other potentially injured abdominal and retroperitoneal structures.

Most athletic injuries to the kidneys are contusions or minor lacerations. The renal capsule remains intact and IVP, when obtained, is usually normal unless there is some underlying renal abnormality such as the presence of stones, horseshoe and pelvic kidneys, megaureter, renal malignancy, or ureteropelvic junction obstruction (44). Any subcapsular hematoma is usually limited in extent. Some authors believe that any degree of traumatic hematuria in a child should be investigated with some imaging study, usually IVP or CT, because up to 20% of these children will have a pre-existing renal abnormality (42).

Athletes with minor contusions and lacerations should be treated medically, with no strenuous activity allowed for 2 to 4 weeks. Follow blood pressure and urine closely during that time. Any athlete with a grade II injury or higher (cortical lacerations) should be considered for reevaluation by IVP at 3 to 6 months along with blood pressure checks to detect late complications such as renal vascular hypertension or hydronephrosis (4).

In more serious injuries where there is continuing hemodynamic instability, persistent retroperitoneal bleeding, urinary extravasation, nonviable renal tissue, or renal vascular pedicle injury, prompt surgical intervention is indicated to maximize kidney salvage and minimize patient morbidity and mortality.

Ureters and Bladder

Ureteral injuries are the rarest of all genitourinary injuries. They are usually seen in severe, blunt penetrating trauma where there are associated major pelvic or vertebral fractures or significant visceral injury. Injury may not be suspected until there are secondary major complications such as urinary extravasation.

The bladder is an intra-abdominal organ in a child, but in the adult it is situated in the pelvis, and when empty, it is rarely injured by blunt trauma. However, when distended, it may be injured, especially if there has been a fractured pelvis. The most common injury is contusion, which is usually evidenced by microscopic or gross hematuria along with suprapubic pain and tenderness. The cystogram shows an intact bladder outline. These athletes are treated with bed rest, good hydration, and observation. The second type of bladder injury is a frank rupture of the bladder contents. It is much more serious and is usually the result of a massive deceleration injury or direct kick or blow to the distended bladder. Findings will include severe lower abdominal pain and often guarding. Evaluation must include studies of the upper and lower tracts. The athlete may return to graded activity when symptom free and all hematuria has cleared. This injury can be prevented by instructing the athlete to empty his or her bladder prior to competition and at appropriate intervals during practice or competition. The athlete should not be instructed to "hold it."

In addition to direct blunt trauma, repetitive jarring of the bladder in runners and cyclists leading to varying degrees of hematuria has been well described in the literature as "biker's bladder" (42) and "runner's bladder" (4). Varying degrees of hematuria and proteinuria are also very common among athletes and even in the general population. Gardner coined the term "athletic pseudonephritis" in describing the hematuria and proteinuria appearing as smoke- or tea-colored urine after athletic activity in almost half of the football players studied (45). The vast majority of these exercise-related urinary findings will resolve completely in 24 to 48 hours and require no further evaluation, except for periodic repeat urinalysis. However, a small subset of such individuals, especially if over the age of 35, may have significant genitourinary tract pathology.

Male Genitalia

Even though the external male genitalia are potentially exposed to direct trauma, serious injuries are rare. Most injuries to the penis and scrotum in sports are a result of a direct blow that may impinge the testes against the symphysis pubis. A nauseating pain is experienced immediately, and the athlete will usually drop to the playing surface. The pain, although severe initially, usually clears rapidly and the athlete is able to return to competition in a short time. Scrotal supports (jock straps) usually help prevent serious damage. Athletes with a high risk of scrotal injury (e.g., hockey players, baseball catchers) should wear a rigid cup support to reduce the risk of injury. If the pain does not diminish, the athlete should be removed to a setting suitable to a more extensive examination. Carefully palpate the scrotum and testicle to be sure the capsule of the testicle is intact and similar in consistency to the uninjured testicle, except for perhaps mild swelling (46). If the epididymis can be readily distinguished and there is very little swelling in the tunica vaginalis sac (potential site for a hydrocele or hematocele) and if the testis is mobile and suspended loosely in its usual position within the scrotum, then a simple contusion is usually present. Conservative treatment using bed rest, scrotal support, ice packs, and analgesics will usually be sufficient. If the team physician is unable to differentiate the scrotal contents and cannot be certain of the integrity of the tunica albuginea because of severe pain and tenderness or severe and perhaps ongoing swelling, or if the diagnosis is not clear for any reason, the athlete should be promptly referred for definitive evaluation and therapy. The earlier the surgical intervention, the greater the extent of testicular salvage (47,48).

The nonerect penis is rarely injured. Urethral injuries are divided into those above (posterior) or below (anterior) the urogenital diaphragm. Posterior urethral injuries are usually associated with fractures of the pelvis (13), whereas anterior urethral injuries are more often the result of direct blows such as straddle-type falls, fall-astride injuries, or direct kicks. Most injuries involve contusions and are treated with ice and analgesics. If there is extensive perineal or meatal bleeding, then a digital rectal examination should be performed. A high-riding or detached prostate warrant urologic consultation for further evaluation and management.

An excellent discussion by York in *The Physician and Sports Medicine* (49) describes injuries to the male genitourinary system.

Female Genitalia

The female urethra is short and not fixed posteriorly. When blunt trauma occurs from gymnastic or cycling straddle-type injuries, the result is usually a contusion or laceration, rarely requiring surgical repair. The vulva is quite vascular, and direct blows to the perineal area may cause contusions of frank hematomas of the vulva. The usual treatment is the local application of ice and NSAIDs or acetaminophen.

A fall during water skiing may force water into the vagina under high pressure, resulting in contusions or lacerations of the vaginal wall (50). Additionally, air and water may be forced into the peritoneal cavity through the vagina, uterus, and fallopian tubes resulting in abdominal pain and tenderness and free intraperitoneal air on standard x-rays (51). Salpingitis may also result from this forced water douche (52). Abdominal pain is usually self-limiting, but the potential for intra-abdominal and genital infections exists, and the athlete with these distressing symptoms must be followed closely. Rapid infusion of water during a fall into the water can cause rectal bleeding in both men and women, but again, symptoms are usually self-limiting. Injuries such as these are easily preventable by wearing a nylon-reinforced suit, rubber pants, or wet suit.

PROTECTIVE EQUIPMENT AND OTHER MEASURES

Much could be said regarding the need for better protective equipment with regard to the abdomen and genital region, but most of the deficiencies involved in lack of optimal protection are a result of not using current prophylactic materials and devices to the extent possible. For example, protection for the spleen, liver, and kidneys may be best accomplished by use of padding stabilized from vertical slippage by being hung in the rear from the shoulders, independent of any shoulder pads (4). Standard athletic supporters and rigid metal scrotal cups offer excellent protection to the male external genitals. Future super lightweight flexible and breathable energy-absorbent material may offer greater hope than any currently known product to reduce torso impact forces safely, offering benefits both prophylactically in injury prevention and protectively when safe return to activity and contact is the goal.

Finally, not enough could be said for the protection afforded the abdomen and trunk in general by a balance of strong, flexible, supple, and resilient musculature coupled with a large cardiac reserve and high level of aerobic conditioning in the athlete whose proprioceptive and psychomotor skills are maximized through careful training and conditioning practices. Solid coaching techniques emphasizing adherence to injury-minimizing sports practices and rules of play can also aid in reducing certain injuries.

SUMMARY

Athletes in both contact (football, rugby, karate, etc) and noncontact (gymnastics, equestrian, and alpine skiing events) sports are constantly being bombarded by multiple body parts, balls, and apparatus over their torso and genitalia. The vast majority of these insults do not constitute reason to worry or panic, but the athlete is not totally immune from serious, even fatal consequences from such trauma. Rarely, the athlete may rupture solid viscera and proceed rapidly to shock and death if not attended to promptly. It is also possible for serious signs and symptoms to develop hours, or even several days, after the traumatic event. Vigilance by the team physician and the caring attitude transmitted to every mem-

ber of the team will lessen the likelihood for these potential catastrophes.

References

1. Bergquist D, Hedelin H, Karlsson G, et al. Abdominal trauma during thirty years: analysis of a large case series. Injury 1981;13:93–99.
2. American College of Surgeons Committee on Trauma. Abdominal trauma. In: Advanced trauma life support program for physicians. 1993 instructor manual, 5th ed. Chicago: First Impressions Publications, 1993:141–158.
3. Ney AL, Anderson RC. Abdominal Trauma. In: Tintinalli JE, Krome RL, Ruiz E, eds. Emergency medicine: a comprehensive study guide. American College of Emergency Physicians, 3rd ed. New York: McGraw-Hill, 1992:955–961.
4. Reid DC. Injuries to the thorax, abdominopelvic viscera and genitourinary system. Sports injury assessment and rehabilitation. New York: Churchill Livingstone, 1992:671–738.
5. Higgins GL. Case reports: penetrating trauma—managing and preventing javelin wounds. Phys Sports Med 1994;4:88–94.
6. Rutkow IM. Rupture of the spleen in infectious mononucleosis. Arch Surg 1978;113:718–720.
7. Colucciello SA, Plotka M. Abdominal trauma—occult injury may be life threatening. Phys Sports Med 1993;6:33–43.
8. Feliciano DV, Marx JA, Sclafani SJA. Abdominal trauma. Patient Care 1992;18:44–83.
9. Deshazo WF. Hematoma of the rectus abdominis in football. Phys Sports Med 1984; 12:73.
10. Ducatman BS, Ludwig J, Hurt RD. Fatal rectus sheath hematomas. JAMA 1983;249:924.
11. Halpern BD. Down man on the field. Prim Care 1991;18:833–849.
12. Whiteside JA. Field evaluation of common athletic injuries. In: Grana WA, Kalenak A, eds. Clinical sports medicine. Philadelphia: WB Saunders, 1991:130–151.
13. Common sports-related injuries and illnesses—thorax and abdomen. In: McKeag DB, Hough DO, Zemper ED, eds. Primary care

sports medicine. Dubuque, IA: Brown and Benchmark, 1993:343–397.

14. Diamond DL. Sports related abdominal trauma. Clin Sports Med 1989;1:91–99.

15. Fadel JN, Ambach JW, Fitzpatrick JD, Liebert CW. An intrahepatic abscess as a rare complication of a pelvic fracture from blunt trauma to the abdomen. Orthopedics 1985; 10:1254–1255.

16. Digowar and Digowar.

17. Panicek DM, Paquet DJ, Clark KG, Urretua EJ, Brinsko RE. Hepatic parenchymal gas after blunt trauma. Radiology 1986;159:343–344.

18. Kearney PA. Blunt trauma to the abdomen. Ann Emerg Med 1989;12:1322–1325.

19. Nagao S, Sugata S, Kondo T, et al. Role of CT and ultrasonography in acute blunt trauma of the abdomen. Nippon Igaku Hoshasen Gakkai Zasshi 1990;4:382–389.

20. Rossi P, et al. Role of laparoscopy in the evaluation of abdominal trauma. Am J Surg 1993;166–707.

21. Davis JJ, Cohn I, Nancy FC. Diagnosis and management of blunt abdominal trauma. Ann Surg 1976;183:672–677.

22. Muehricke DD, Kim SM, McCage CJ. Pediatric splenic trauma predicting the success of non-operative therapy. Am J Emerg Med 1987;5:109–112.

23. Berman BM, Nagle CE, Jafri SZH, Morden RS. Spleen injury in sports—Part I: what diagnostic imaging can reveal. Phys Sports Med 1992;3:168–179.

24. Chambers JA, Ratcliffe JF, Doig CM. Ultrasound in abdominal injury in children. Injury 1986;6:399–403.

25. Perkins RM, Sterling JC. Case conference: left lower chest pain in a collision athlete. Phys Sports Med 1991;3:78–84.

26. Morden RS, Berman BM, Nagle CE, Jafri SZH. Spleen injury in sports—Part II: avoiding splenectomy. Phys Sports Med 1992;4:126–139.

27. Eichner ER. Hematuria—a diagnostic challenge. Phys Sports Med 1990;18(11):52–62.

28. Feliciano DV, Jordan GL, Bitondo CG, Mattox KL, Burch JM, Cruse PA. Management of 1000 consecutive cases of hepatic trauma (1979–1984). Ann Surg 1986;10:438–445.

29. Hennes HM, Smith DS, Schneider K, et al. Elevated liver transaminase levels in children with blunt abdominal trauma and a predictor of liver injury. Pediatrics 1990;86:87–90.

30. Sahdev P, Garramon RR, Schwartz RJ. Evaluation of liver function tests in screening for intra-abdominal injuries. Ann Emerg Med 1991;20:838–841.

31. Durham RM, Buckley J, Keegan M, Fravell S, Shapiro MJ, Mazuski J. Management of blunt hepatic injuries. Am J Surg 1992;164:477–481.

32. Stain SC, Yellin AE, Donovan AJ. Hepatic trauma. Arch Surg 1988;123:1251–1255.

33. Nielsen TH, Jensen LS. Pancreatic transection during karate training. Br J Sports Med 1986;20:82–83.

34. Fossum RM, Descheneaux KA. Blunt trauma of the abdomen in children. J Forensic Science 1991;36:42–50.

35. Walters HL, Hupp J, McCabe CJ, Burke JF. Peritoneal lavage and the surgical resident. Surg Gen Obstet 1987;165:496–502.

36. Ceraldi CM, Waxman K. Computed tomography as an indicator of isolated mesenteric injury: a comparison with peritoneal lavage. Am Surg 1990;56:806–810.

37. Sherck JP, Oakes DD. Intestinal injuries missed by computed tomography. J Trauma 1990;30:1–5.

38. McCarthy P. Hernias in athletes: what you need to know. Phys Sports Med 1990;5:115–122.

39. Dreyfus DC, Flancbaum Z, Krasna IH, et al. Acute transrectus traumatic hernia. J Trauma 1986;26:1134–1136.

40. Bergquist D, Hedelin H, Karlsson G, et al. Abdominal injury from sporting activities. Br J Sports Med 1982;16:76–79.

41. Kenny P. Abdominal pain in athletes. Clin Sports Med 1986;6:885–905.

42. York JP. Sports and the male genitourinary system. Kidneys and bladder. Phys Sports Med 1990;9:116–129.

43. Mandour WA, Lai MK, Linke CA, et al. Blunt renal trauma in the pediatric patient. J Pediatr Surg 1989;16:669–676.

44. Mee SL, McAnich JW. Indications for radiographic assessment in suspected renal trauma. Urol Clin North Am 1989;16:187–192.

45. O'Brien K. Biker's bladder. N Engl J Med 1981;304:1367.

46. Blacklock NJ. Bladder trauma in the long-distance runner: "10,000 metres heamaturia." Br J Urol 1977;49:129–132.

47. Blacklock NJ. Bladder trauma from jogging. Am Heart J 1980;99:813–814.

48. Gardner KD Jr. Athletic pseudonephritis: alterations of sediment by athletic competition. JAMA 1956;161:1613–1617.

49. York JP. Sports and the male genitourinary system. Genital injuries and sexually transmitted diseases. Phys Sports Med 1990; 18:92–100.

50. Briner WW Jr, Howe WB, Jain RK. Scrotal injury in a high school football player: surgical exploration versus diagnostic testing. Phys Sports Med 1990;18:64–68.

51. Schuster G. Traumatic rupture of the testicle and a review of the literature. J Urol 1982;127:1194–1196.

52. Lee JY, Cass AS. Trauma to the genitourinary tract. In: Advanced trauma life support program for physicians. 1993 instructor manual, 5th ed. Chicago: First Impressions Publications 1993:141–158.

BACK INJURIES IN SPORTS

9

LARRY B. LIPSCOMB

Risk Factors for Back Injury
Anatomy
Sports-Specific Back Injuries
Patient History
Physical Examination
Differential Diagnosis
Basic Tenets for Radiologic Studies in
    Athletic Back Injury
Treatment

At any one time about a fifth of the adult population of the United States is affected by back pain. It is the fourth most common complaint in ambulatory medicine. It is also, after cancer and heart disease, the third most expensive disorder to treat when one considers such factors as the cost of diagnosis, cost of treatment, and lost productivity (1). It occurs at one time or another in 60% to 80% of the population between 25 and 69 years of age, the largest age group of physically active persons. It is second only to the common cold as a reason for sick leave, and low back pain causes workers to miss an estimated 93 million work days per year (2).

Although back pain is not the most common sports injury encountered (lumbar spine pain accounts for 5% to 8% of athletic injuries [3]), it is one of the most challenging to treat for the physician who cares for athletes. Thoracic, lumbar, and sacral injuries of the vertebral column and spinal cord segments have been described in a number of popular sports, including gymnastics, tobogganing, diving, skiing, and football (4,5); therefore it behooves the practitioner to become familiar with back injury care in his or her athletic patients.

To examine the frequency and types of back injuries sustained by athletes, the medical records of 4290 athletes, participating in 17 varsity sports over a 10-year period, were examined by Keene and colleagues (6). From this study, an average injury rate of 7 per 100 participants was shown (higher in football and gymnastics), and of 333 documented back injuries, 80% of the injuries occurred *in practice*, 14% of the injuries occurred *during preseason conditioning*, 6% of the injuries occurred *in competition*. Muscle strains with acute back injuries were more prevalent (59%) than extremity overuse injuries (12%) or injuries associated with preexisting conditions

(29%). *It is important, therefore, to note that 94% of the back injuries sustained in those athletes were injuries received in preparation of competition.*

RISK FACTORS FOR BACK INJURY

The primary care physician is often the first health care provider to see back pain secondary to exertional back injury, and does so in a variety of settings. He or she may care for the injured athlete 1) in the capacity of a school team physician, 2) in the employee health clinic, 3) on military installations, 4) in jail and prison clinics, or 5) in the private medical office. These patient populations, though somewhat dissimilar, have characteristic patterns of risk to the thoracic, lumbar, and sacral spine.

Certain factors that predispose the athlete to back injury and acute back pain are listed in Table 9.1. In children and adolescents, a growth spurt may lead to a muscle tendon imbalance (2) with tight hamstrings and lumbodorsal fascia posteriorly combined with weak abdominal muscles anteriorly. An abrupt increase in training intensity or frequency may result in muscle strains. Leg-length discrepancy may lead to acute facet joint sprains as well as muscle strains. Improper technique, particularly with weight lifting or other sports that concentrate high loads on the lumbar spine, may

Table 9.1. Factors that predispose the athlete to acute back injury

1. Growth spurt with muscle tendon imbalance
2. Abrupt increase in training intensity
3. Leg length discrepancy
4. Improper technique
5. Unsuitable sports equipment

Table 9.2. Factors that contribute to chronic
back injury

1. Poor strength of back extensor and
   abdominal musculature
2. Inflexibility of lumbar spine, hamstring, and
   hip flexors
3. Excessive lifting and twisting
4. Anatomic abnormalities

also cause muscle or ligament injury. The
use of unsuitable equipment of the wrong
size may lead to acute injury.

Factors that contribute to recurrent back
injury and chronic low back pain are listed
in Table 9.2. Poor strength of back extensor
and abdominal musculature leads to increased loads on the spinal column, predisposing to facet joint and disk injury.
Inflexibility of lumbar spine, hamstrings,
or hip flexors with resultant limitation of
mobility both concentrates stress and leads
to structural imbalance. Excessive lifting,
particularly with twisting, is the most common cause of sprains including injuries to
annulus. Anatomic abnormalities, such as
bony or neuromuscular disorders, may increase both the risk of injury and chronic
pain.

For example, vigorous exercise in sports
by poorly conditioned adults (usually overweight male "weekend warriors") creates
injuries that predispose them to disk disease. The combination of excessive weight
and poor abdominal muscle tone displaces
a person's center of gravity forward, resulting in increased lumbar lordosis and
thereby causing the patient to assume a
mechanically disadvantageous position (2).
Coupled with a deconditioned state, injuries to the back in these patients can become
serious. Even a history of sitting, which
places the most pressure on the intervertebral disk and is one of the most injuri-

ous activities for the painful back, is an important finding, especially in athletes who
primarily sit on or in something used in
their sport.

ANATOMY

Understanding injury to the back begins
with grasping important architectural and
functional aspects of its anatomy. The back
has two major components: the *vertebral column*, which provides the superstructure of
the back and the final layer of protection for
the nerves and vessels that traverse its
length, and the *muscular anatomy*, lending
motion, protection of bony and organ structures, mass, power, and stability to the
human frame.

Vertebral Column

The intervertebral disk consists of an
outer *annulus fibrosis* and an inner *nucleus
pulposus* situated in a slightly eccentric position posteriorly (Figure 9.1). The intervertebral disks, as a unit, are strengthened
by the anterior longitudinal ligament and
the weaker posterior longitudinal ligament
in the midline (7).

The annulus fibrosis is made of concentric fibrous lamellae, with adjacent lamellae
having fibers running in alternating directions, lending an increased resistance to
torsional strains. The nucleus pulposus is
soft and gelatinous, resisting compressive
forces. The mucoid content of the nucleus
pulposus is replaced from the second decade onward by fibrocartilage, reducing its
effectiveness and increasing the risk of
injury.

The spinal canal transmits the spinal cord
and nerve roots, with associated blood,
lymph, and specialized nervous ganglia.
The spinal canal is formed by the lamina

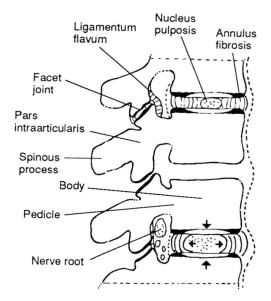

Figure 9.1. Anatomy of the lumbar spine, lateral view.

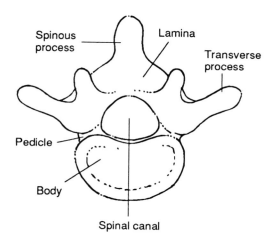

Figure 9.2. Bony spinal canal.

and ligamentum flavum posteriorly; the pars intra-articularis, pedicle, and intervertebral foramen laterally; and the vertebral body and annulus fibrosis anteriorly (see Figures 9.1 and 9.2). The spinal canal is roughly circular in the thoracic and upper lumbar regions and trefoil shaped in the lower lumbar region. The spinal cord ends as the conus medularis approximately at the L1–L2 disk space in the adult, with the cauda equina extending caudally. The nerve roots exit the spinal canal through the foramen just below the pedicle of the vertebra from which they are numbered (e.g., L4 nerve root exits just below L4 pedicle, and above the L4–L5 disk space [Figure 9.3]).

Musculature

The muscles of the back are divided into three functional groups: superficial, intermediate, and deep (8,9). The *trapezius, latissimus dorsi, levator scapulae,* and the

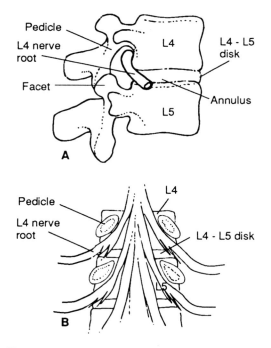

Figure 9.3. Relationship of nerve root to the vertebral bodies, disk space, and facet joint. *A.* Lateral view. *B.* Coronal view.

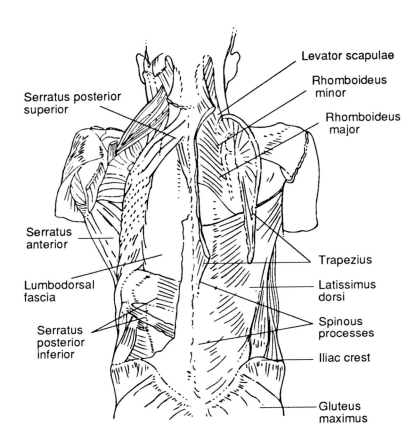

Figure 9.4. Muscles of the back—superficial on the right, intermediate on the left.

Levator scapulae

Rhomboideus minor

Rhomboideus major

Serratus posterior superior

Serratus anterior

Lumbodorsal fascia

Serratus posterior inferior

Trapezius

Latissimus dorsi

Spinous processes

Iliac crest

Gluteus maximus

rhomboideus minor and major comprise the *superficial* group; they originate along the vertebral column (with the exception of the levator scapulae) and insert on the shoulder girdle, and anchor the upper extremity to the axial skeleton, thereby allowing movement from the shoulder girdle (Figure 9.4).

The second functional group inhabit the intermediate layer of the muscular back and are comprised of the *serratus posterior, superior and inferior*, which originate from the spinous processes and insert into the rib cage. They act during inspiration to maximize the thorax by elevating the ribs while simultaneously drawing the lower ribs downward and backward to elongate the thorax. This action also fixes the lower ribs and thereby aids the downward movement of the diaphragm, which tends to pull the lower ribs upward and forward (see Figure 9.4).

The muscles of the deep functional group, the *erector spinae* and *transversospinal*, are considered the intrinsic or "native" muscles of the back. They originate and insert along the vertebral column and share nerve supply from the dorsal rami. The erector spinae muscle is a large complex muscle that fills the vertebral groove from the neck to the sacrum. It lies deep to the thoracolumbar fascia and has three columns: the medial *spinalis*, the intermediate *longissimus*, and the lateral *iliocostalis* (Figure 9.5). The erector spinae spans the whole length of the back but is formed by a series of fascicles that extend 6 to 10 spinal segments between bony attachments. The

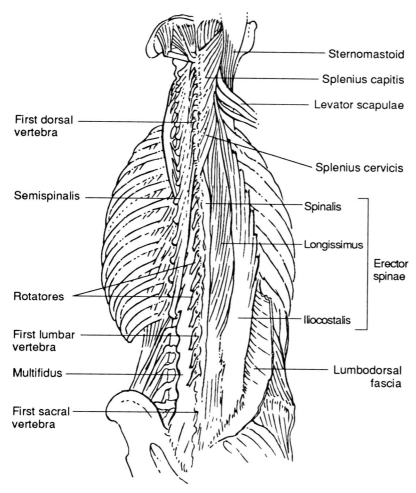

Figure 9.5. Deep muscles of the back.

Sternomastoid

Splenius capitis

Levator scapulae

First dorsal vertebra

Splenius cervicis

Semispinalis

Spinalis

Longissimus

Erector spinae

Rotatores

Iliocostalis

First lumbar vertebra

Lumbodorsal fascia

Multifidus

First sacral vertebra

erector spinae functions in synergy to extend and stabilize the spine and singly to bend the spine.

Deep to the erector spinae are the obliquely oriented *semispinalis, multifidus,* and *rotatores muscles* of the transversospinal group (see Figure 9.5). They arise from the transverse processes or sacrum and insert on the spinal segments above their origin. Acting in synergy they extend the spine and acting singly they rotate the vertebral column toward the opposite side.

Clinical Case #1

An active 67-year-old man, who has been an avid golfer most of his life, competed in a senior-level tournament over the weekend. After completing the first round of 18 holes, he began to notice a pain in his right side. Throughout the night, he had pain when he tried to lie on his side or tried to get out of bed. Concerned that this could keep him out of the competition, he consulted his physician. The physician discovered that his golf swing is characterized by a good right shoulder drop but, more often than not,

*little or no flexion of the right knee—causing
him to bend severely on his right side during
follow through. He admits that the pressure of
the tournament may have caused him to exaggerate his swing even more.*

This patient exhibits symptoms similar to
those encountered by baseball players and
fast-pitch cricket bowlers (10), where rapid
shoulder depression, trunk flexion, quadriceps drive, and poor technique combine to
produce inflammation and injury from
back muscle overuse. The muscle group involved in this case is the quadratus
lumborum (1), a flat muscle that lies just
lateral to the psoas major and transversospinal group of muscles. A lateral flexor
of the trunk, it extends from the lower
border of the twelfth rib and the tips of
the lumbar transverse processes to the
iliolumbar ligament. Pain secondary to
injury of this muscle manifests by painful
lateral bending. There is usually palpable
spasm along the quadratus lumborum
muscle and fairly marked tenderness at its
insertion at the iliac crest. Forward bending
does not elicit pain. Discomfort is usually
relieved by a local injection of bupivacaine
and betamethasone, which also help to
hasten recovery by anti-inflammatory action.

The musculoskeletal system of the back
provides the support required for the human frame to stand and locomote against
earth's gravity; protection for vital body
organs, the posterior costal bones as well as
their articulations with the bony spine and
associated spinal nerves, and the spinal column itself; greater range of motion; and
movement of the body through space,
thereby facilitating the unencumbered use
of the human hands. In the athlete, these
functions of the back are central to
performance.

SPORTS-SPECIFIC BACK INJURIES

Sports-related back injury crosses all
lines of age, gender, sport, and level of
participation. Some of the more popular
sports have documented patterns of injury
to the musculature and bony anatomy of
the back, usually directly related to the
types of stress that the sport places on the
participant.

Running

Back pain in runners, often due to a preexisting degenerative condition, usually occurs when the patient (often middle-aged)
increases mileage or hill running. Although
runners often complain of hip pain, in
many cases, they are actually referring to
symptoms or an injury in the buttocks,
pelvic area, or lumbar spine. Moreover,
running does not rupture vertebral disks
(11). With any sign of nerve root irritation
(weakness of toe extensors or reflex
changes), further evaluation is required
and running will need to stop temporarily,
possibly permanently.

Gymnastics

Over the last 15 to 20 years, gymnastics
has increased in popularity. The risk of
gymnastic injuries seems to be proportional
to 1) the level of the gymnastic activity, 2)
the more hours spent in practice, and 3) the
amount of exposure time to demanding
routines. Lumbar spine biomechanics research reveals that greater lumbar lordosis
increases the potential for both posterior
element failure at the pars interarticularis
and disk disorder. Gymnasts are especially
prone to these injuries because hyperlordotic mechanical low back pain is the
most common cause of all overuse of the

back in athletes (12). Spondylolysis and spondylolisthesis are discussed later in the chapter.

Back problems in gymnasts infrequently result from a single episode of macro-trauma, but more commonly from repeated microtrauma caused by specific impact loads during vaults and hyperextension. The combination of periods of rapid growth and intense training could provide for conditions where the gymnast is more injury prone (13). Nowhere is this more apparent than in elite female gymnasts, who train hard and early as their careers peak in the teenage years, and whose lumbar spines tend to assume increased lordosis as they grow.

Aerobic Dancing

Dancers, both aerobic and ballet style, frequently experience injuries at some time and about half have chronic injuries. The repetitive activities in aerobic dance lead to far more overuse injuries than traumatic injuries. Back injuries associated with dance activity include sprains, prolapsed or herniated intervertebral disks, and spondylolytic stress fractures (14,15).

Football

High-velocity impact from deceleration collisions and weight lifting lead to the majority of back problems in football players. These result in sprains, strains, disk injuries, and posterior element failure. In a study of discogenic injury of college football players, Day and colleagues followed 12 male players who required surgical repair for a suspected herniated lumbar disk (16). They found that:

- Weight lifting was associated with symptoms in 40% of cases.

- Symptoms consisted of low back or radicular pain.
- The most common player position affected was that of the down-lineman.
- Percutaneous diskectomy appears to be successful for disk herniations occurring at the L4–L5 space or higher.

Golf/Cricket

The golf swing and the pitch in cricket have similar actions, and both sports have surprisingly similar injury patterns. A prospective study conducted by Foster and coworkers found that in "fast bowlers," as they are called in the game of cricket, shoulder depression and horizontal flexion strength for the preferred limb and quadriceps power in the nonpreferred limb were significantly related to back injuries (10). Similarly, Batt reviewed the injury reports of some 461 amateur golfers, noting 57% of the reported injuries related to the wrist, the back, the elbow, and the knee were the most likely ailments to compromise a player's game. Overuse and poor technique appeared to be major etiologic factors (17). Both games require rapid shoulder depression, horizontal flexion strength, quadriceps power, and good mechanics to achieve reproducible results; expectedly, the brunt of the injuries of the amateur and the professional player result from these components of the game and their affect on the back.

The above examples illustrate different facets of back injury in the athlete. Low back pain is a leading cause of disability, with the most frequent causes being muscle and ligament strain, disk disease, and arthritis (18). Because the majority of back injuries in sports participants are caused initially by muscle strain and torsion, the physically active person has more opportunity to suffer such injury. The primary care provider must remain aware of the varied ways different sporting activities can result in back injury.

PATIENT HISTORY

The history that the patient provides continues to be the most secure foundation on which to eventually base the medical decision for treatment. Given ample opportunity, the patient is capable of relating what happened, providing the scenario of the injury. Next, how it happened should be elicited to define the mechanism of injury (fall? blow? lift injury? insidious? hyperextension/flexion injury?). Realize that the paravertebral extensor muscles of the spine are among the strongest muscles of the body, but when they are subjected to forceful stress, a muscle strain may ensue.

As the patient tells the story, the physician gains insight into the mechanism of injury and "finding the spot" is made easier. If early in the discussion the location of the pain is not stated, asking *where it hurts* may help localize the injury to either the vertebral column, muscular anatomy, or some other area of the body. Usually, the lumbar portions of the large muscles (i.e., erector spinae, iliocostalis, latissimus dorsi) are the areas athletes tend to experience pain, usually in the lower lumbar region. The corollary is that these areas are placed under the greatest mechanical stresses by the specific demands of the sport. However, much of what is thought to be back strain may actually be reversible damage to the intervertebral disk (2,19). Further, finding out if it hurts to move and which position feels best can help determine which disk or functional group of back muscles is affected and what compensatory mechanism has been put in place to prevent further injury. Finally, inquiry into how long has an injury

caused them back discomfort helps the physician decide to investigate occult spinal diseases, malignancies, or neurogenic sequelae of what the athlete felt was an innocuous event.

Injury to a lumbosacral nerve root will cause sciatica, pain radiating down the leg in the distribution of that nerve root. True radicular pain should go below the knee. Referred pain from other locations (e.g., facet joints or sacroiliac joints) will usually stop short of the knee.

Bladder and bowel functioning should be investigated because the patient will rarely volunteer this information. Any change in habits may indicate central pressure on the cauda equina.

PHYSICAL EXAMINATION

Medical observation, static and dynamic range-of-motion testing, palpation, and flexibility measurement are essential tools needed by the primary care physician who treats physically active patients. They provide the framework in which an accurate diagnosis can be reached and appropriate treatment can be instituted for the injured athlete.

With the patient standing, the back is symmetrical en face with an initial, gentle kyphotic curve that progresses to a lordosis that ends at the sacrum. The iliac crests are thus bisected by the spinal column and appear both even and level in the normal individual. This should be confirmed by palpation of the iliac crests. The iliac crests are at the L4–L5 disk level (Figure 9.6). A deviation of the spine to one side is called a *list*. This is easily observed in patients whose legs are of unequal length (one iliac crest will be lower). Diagnostically, leg-length discrepancy shows no predictive power for first occurrence of low back pain.

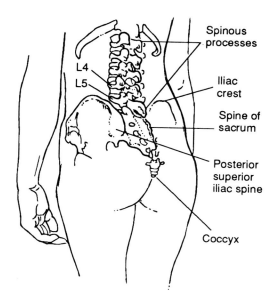

Figure 9.6. Anatomic relationships of the lumbar spine.

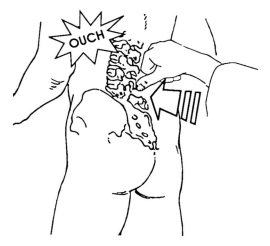

Figure 9.7. Spondylolisthesis.

However, a significant number of patients who have a history of low back pain also have had a leg-length discrepancy in contrast to patients without such history (20).

Lists may result from muscle spasms caused by herniation of an intervertebral disk or by acute strain of the paraspinal muscles. The trunk may list toward or away from the affected side in patients with sciatic pain. Occasionally the patient will list first to one side and then the other. Such lists disappear when the patient sits, or after the pain disappears. This is in contrast to the permanent list produced when scarring and fibrosis of the back muscles follow a fracture of a transverse vertebral process.

Palpation of the injured back establishes any changes of important landmarks. The spinous processes, the interspinous ligaments, and the paraspinal muscles should all be readily located by touch and position. Muscle spasm and pain on palpation of the muscles is often associated with fibrocytic nodules, a condition that may extend into the gluteal muscles. Pain over the spinous processes and interspinous ligaments is more indicative of disease of the spine. Percussion of the spine will produce pain in patients with osteoporosis, carcinomatosis, fractures, and infections of the bodies of the vertebrae. Tenderness to pressure in the midline at the lumbosacral junction is present in patients with herniated intervertebral disks and in patients with spondylolysis or spondylolisthesis. A palpable step, or shelf, may be present in patients with spondylolisthesis, in whom the body of a vertebra slips forward on the body of the vertebra below (Figure 9.7).

Another component of the back examination is the performance of a rectal examination, which is important to do in adult men because chronic prostatitis is a common cause of backache. Moreover, a digital rectal examination is the only way deformities and injuries of the coccyx can be evaluated. A pelvic examination should be performed in all cases of back complaints of adult women, which are not readily attributable to the musculoskeletal system.

Motion of the spine is best evaluated by observing the patient from behind as he or she bends forward, backward, from side to side, and rotates from side to side (Figure 9.8). Measurement of chest expansion is an indirect measurement of thoracic spine motion because rotation of the ribs occurs at the costovertebral joints, very near the facet joints. This is important, since a young adult male with ankylosing spondylitis may first present with back pain and the finding of chest expansion less than 2.5 cm is suggestive of this diagnosis. Because most injury to the back involves the lumbar portion, it is important to determine how flexible this part of the spine is. The importance of this is twofold: 1) to distinguish between intersegmental mobility and hip mobility and 2) help evaluate the patient's effort in performing measured movements (21).

Evaluating the possibility of disk herniation can prove to be the most important examination that is performed on the injured athlete. Careful neurologic examination of the lower extremities is indicated. The L4 nerve root provides sensory enervation to the anterior thigh, medial leg, and foot. It is the main motor enervation for the tibialis anterior muscle and the knee reflex is L4 innervated (Figure 9.9). The L5 nerve root has a sensory distribution from the lateral thigh and anterior leg to the dorsum of the foot. The most readily isolated muscle that is innervated by L5 is the extensor hallucis longus. The tibialis posterior reflex, although L5 specific, is so difficult to elicit as to not be reliable (Figure 9.10). The S1 nerve root has a sensory distribution from the posterior thigh, the lateral leg to the lateral border of the foot. The ankle jerk is the S1 specific reflex (Figure 9.11). Although a thorough, bilateral neurologic examination often helps locate the site of herniation,

many patients who have a herniated disk will have no hard neurologic findings. When that is the case, the distribution of pain alone is sufficient enough at *projecting* the site of herniation. The straight-leg-raising test (1) may help confirm disk herniation.

A classic straight-leg-raising test attempts to reproduce radicular pain while the patient is recumbent (Figure 9.12A). Passive elevation of a supine patient's straightened leg stretches the sciatic nerve. A positive test is one that reproduces radicular—not lower back—pain. The leg must be raised *passively* by the examiner rather than *actively* by the patient. It is helpful to try and get the patient to relax as best he or she can, and also carefully explain that the leg will be slowly elevated until the patient complains of pain. At whatever point radiating pain develops, that is the point at which the test is positive, regardless of the resulting amount of elevation.

The test is positive in 60% to 90% of patients with herniated disk, but it can be affected by examiner technique and experience as well as other causes of impingement (i.e., tumor, abcess, back trauma, or spinal stenosis). Therefore, to increase the specificity of the examination, a crossed straight-leg-raising test should follow. With this test, the examiner attempts to reproduce sciatic pain in the affected leg by raising the unaffected leg (Figure 9.12B). Over 90% of patients who have a positive crossed straight-leg-raising test have herniated disk (1).

Another test that offers similar benefits is the distraction test, which stretches the sciatic nerve while the patient is sitting. With the patient sitting, the physician casually straightens the leg in the course of apparently performing some other examination. If the patient leans backward to minimize

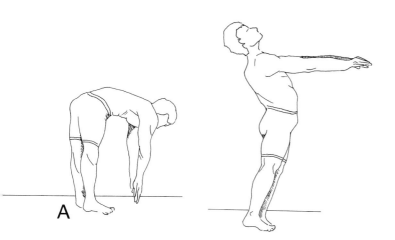

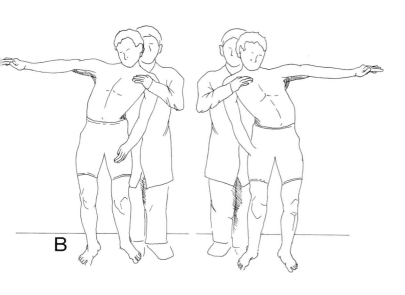

Figure 9.8. *A*. Flexion and extension of lumbar spine. *B*. Side-bending lumbar spine. *C*. Rotation of lumbar spine. *D*. Chest expansion. (Modified from S Hoppenfeld. Physical Examination of the Spine Extremities. Norwalk, CT: Appleton & Lange, 1976: 248–249.)

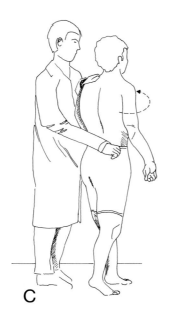

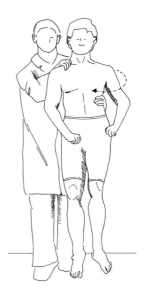

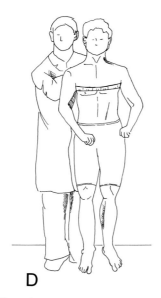

Figure 9.8. *Continued*

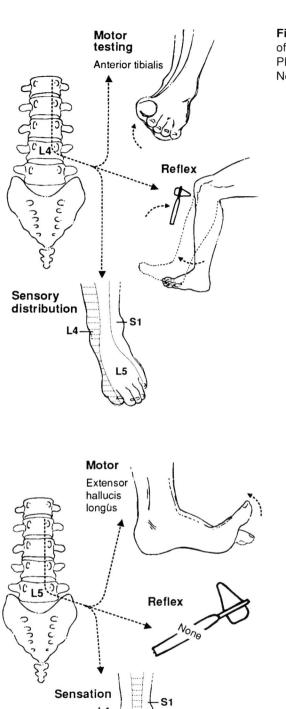

Figure 9.9. Motor, reflex, and sensory distribution of L4 nerve root. (Modified from S Hoppenfeld. Physical Examination of the Spine Extremities. Norwalk, CT: Appleton & Lange, 1976: 251.)

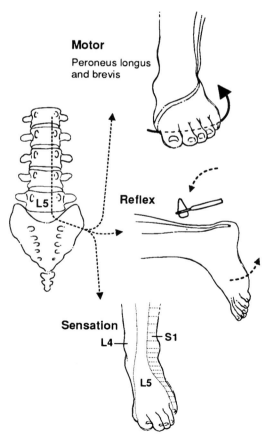

Figure 9.10. Motor, reflex, and sensory distribution of the L5 nerve root. (Modified from S Hoppenfeld. Physical Examination of the Spine Extremities. Norwalk, CT: Appleton & Lange, 1976: 252.)

Figure 9.11. Motor, reflex, and sensory distribution of the S1 nerve root. (Modified from S Hoppenfeld. Physical Examination of the Spine Extremities. Norwalk, CT: Appleton & Lange, 1976: 253.)

the stretch on the sciatic nerve, nerve root entrapment is confirmed. Failure to elicit a response suggests a functional component to the symptoms (Figure 9.12C).

Examination of the back also includes those maneuvers that evaluate the possibility of sacral injury (18). The sacroiliac joints are a hinge, extremely stable with very little motion, possessing a synovial membrane, and are joined by strong anterior and posterior ligaments—making them the strongest joints in the human body. When sacroiliac injury or inflammation is suspected, the patient often has pain on the affected side that increases when the patient lies on that side. Extension while standing is painful, whereas the same maneuver in a seated position improves the discomfort. It improves more when the patient sits on the affected buttock. Once a diagnosis of sacral injury is considered, a few maneuvers quickly and simply aid in confirming this problem.

Patrick's Test or FABER Test

Patrick's or FABER test (*f*lexion, *ab*duction and *e*xternal *r*otation) of the hip is performed by placing the patient in a supine position then resting either the right or the left foot on the thigh of the extended opposite leg. The pelvis is stabilized by one hand of the examiner on the opposite anterior superior iliac spine while the other hand gently applies downward pressure on the flexed, externally rotated, and abducted leg. The test is considered positive when pain at the sacroiliac joint is elicited with this maneuver (Figure 9.13).

Sacroiliac Compression Test

With the patient on his or her side and the bottom leg flexed, the examiner uses the sacroiliac compression test by simply pressing down on the lateral pelvis of the top leg. A positive test produces pain (Figure 9.14).

Iliac Compression Test

For the iliac compression test, the patient is supine with legs together. The examiner first attempts to push both iliac crests laterally, trying to spread them apart. Next, both crests are pressed medially. The test is positive when pain occurs in the affected joint (Figure 9.15).

Gaenslen's Extension Test

Gaenslen's extension test hyperextends the hip on the affected side against a stabilized pelvis, producing pain if the sacroiliac joints have been injured. The patient is supine and first pulls both knees to chest. The patient then hangs the leg on the affected side over the side of the examining table. The physician presses down on the thigh of the affected side while maintaining a knee-to-chest maneuver with the leg on the unaffected side (Figure 9.16).

Single-Leg Stand

In the single-leg stand, the patient stands on the leg of the symptomatic side and lifts the other leg off the floor. If the test is positive, pain will be elicited because stress is transmitted to the affected sacroiliac joint (Figure 9.17).

Of the maneuvers described, the more significant ones are those designed to compress or separate the iliac crests, and the more tests that are positive, the more accurate the diagnosis. This is important because other hip disorders and neuritides can cause these individual tests to be falsely positive.

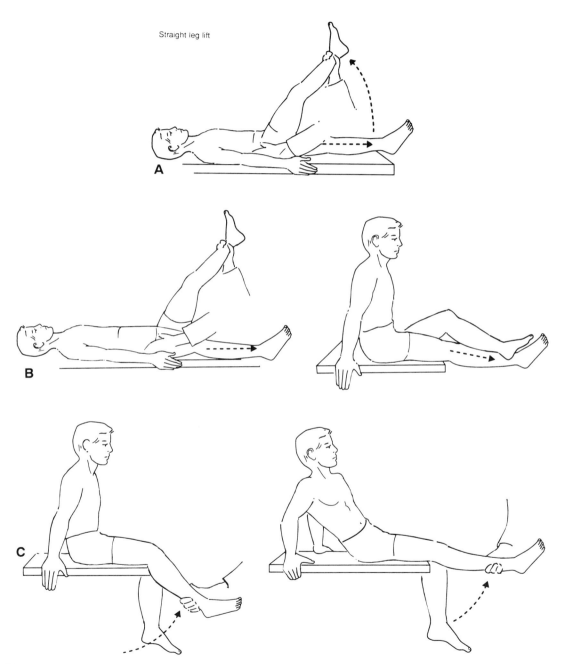

Straight leg lift

Figure 9.12. *A.* Straight leg lift causing ipsilateral pain radiation. *B.* Crossed straight leg lift causing contralateral pain radiation. *C.* Distraction straight leg lift. Lack of pain on the distraction test may indicate a functional component.

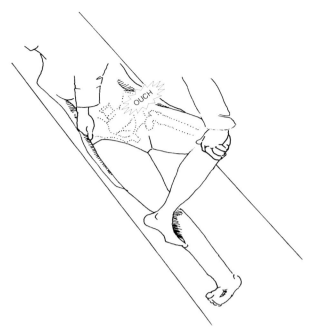

Figure 9.13. Patrick or FABER test. (Modified from S Hoppenfeld. Physical Examination of the Spine Extremities. Norwalk, CT: Appleton & Lange, 1976: 262.)

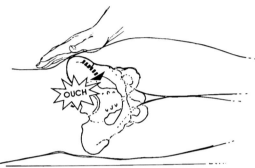

Figure 9.14. Sacroiliac compression test.

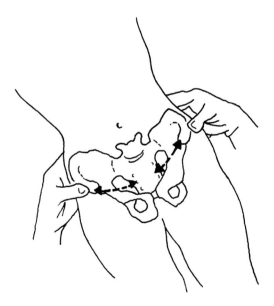

Figure 9.15. Iliac compression test. (Modified from S Hoppenfeld. Physical Examination of the Spine Extremities. Norwalk, CT: Appleton & Lange, 1976: 261.)

DIFFERENTIAL DIAGNOSIS

Pain along the vertebral column is such a frequent complaint that it is easy to overlook unusual or serious etiologies (22). The differential diagnosis of back pain in the athlete must encompass more than muscle strain and overuse syndromes. Among patients presenting with acute low back pain, herniated disks are found in less than 2%, vertebral cancer is present in about 0.6%, and osteomyelitis is diagnosed in only about 0.001% (23). In the athlete, some of the common causes of back pain are disk disease, facet joint syndromes, fractures and contusions, and spinal abnormalities.

Clinical Case #2

Concerned about his health, a 35-year-old man recently joined a health spa. Although he continues to have no active illnesses, his profes-

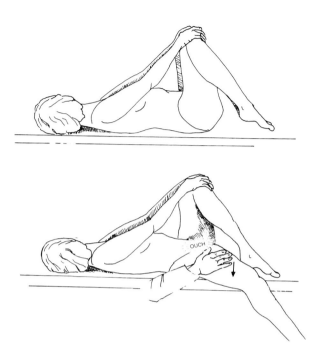

Figure 9.16. Gaensten's test. (Modified from S Hoppenfeld. Physical Examination of the Spine Extremities. Norwalk, CT: Appleton & Lange, 1976: 261.)

sional career has taken a toll on his level of fitness and he has gained approximately 60 lb over his ideal body weight. He wishes to regain some of his "lost youth" and is eager to start working out.

On his first day, he decided to start with an old weight training routine that he was taught in college. He did some cursory jumping jacks, but was so excited about "getting back to the gym" that he went right to work. He realized that he was too heavy to do pull-ups and push-ups right away, so he went to the squat rack. He felt so good that he put on about 225 lb to start with—he could do much more than this when he was in school. With some effort, he took it from its moorings and stepped back into position.

His right knee began to ache. As he proceeded to squat the weight, this ache became a sharp pain and he was unbalanced. The weight pulled him down and to the right, causing the weight to tip to the right while simultaneously extend-ing himself down to prevent the weight from falling on his neck. The weight continued to pull him down into a twisted, kneeling position before he was able to release it. He experienced immediate and excruciating pain on his right side and back and was unable to stand. He heard a "pop" in his back before he finally released the weight.

This case illustrates an all too common problem with adult athletes—ego. Often, the once elite athlete believes that the aging body will respond as before if only it is subjected to the same level of physical stress as received during his or her athletic prime. The individual will proceed with the assumption that if he or she exercises more, return to competition will be sooner. Although mentally conditioned to expect a certain amount of discomfort during the reconditioning period, the deconditioned athlete may try to compress this period by increasing the initial workloads—leading to muscle strain and sprain injuries.

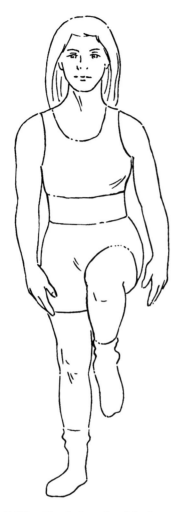

Figure 9.17. Single-leg stand test.

The individual in this case has obviously exceeded his body's ability to control and elevate the squat weight of 225 lb, causing his balance to falter and leaving his back musculature to compensate for the heavy weight. This generates tremendous pressures on the joint capsules and articular surfaces of the vertebral column, as well as the supporting muscular components of back motion, and invariably leads to muscular injury as the muscle columns instantaneously

seek to prevent further load or torsional damage to the bony spine. The high load and abrupt weight shift caused a severe, acute strain of his paravertebral muscles and possibly some deep muscular tears as a result. Activities associated with twisting while simultaneously lifting predispose to both muscular injury and disk injury, where the onset of pain may be acute or delayed for 6 to 12 hours after the injury (2).

Intervertebral Disk Disease

Risk factors associated with lumbar disk disease in common with the physically active patient include advanced age, history of back trauma, and cigarette smoking.

Miller and colleagues (24) correlated macroscopic disk degeneration grades with age, sex, and spine level in 600 lumbar intervertebral disks from over 200 cadavers (ages 0 to 96). The study concluded that lumbar disk degeneration first appears in the 11- to 19-year age range in boys, and one decade later in young women. By age 50 years, 97% of all lumbar disks exhibit degeneration, and when present, L3–L4 and L4–L5 are usually the most degenerated lumbar disks. Across most ages, male lumbar disks are significantly more degenerated than female disks. Calculations suggest greater compression loading and longer avascular nutritional pathways of the male intervertebral disk may contribute to its earlier and more severe degeneration.

Repeated microtrauma may lead to cumulative degeneration of the lumber disk; a history of back injury has been found to be a statistically significant factor in symmetrical degeneration of the disk. A history of back trauma also correlates with an increased incidence of annular rupture (25).

Several studies have suggested that smoking or coughing is a risk factor for prolapsed lumbar disk (26,27) and for back pain in general (28). The mechanisms for the association with smoking are not entirely clear; however, the most plausible mechanism is that smoking causes coughing, which in turn puts more pressure on the disk. The association of cigarette smoking is significant in that it is possible to completely eliminate this factor from the risk profile; therefore, smoking cessation can have a favorable effect beyond the cardiovascular, dermatologic, and respiratory systems.

Disk herniation is rare before skeletal maturity. When it occurs in the vigorous athlete, usually collegiate or older, it is posterior or posterolateral leading to acute sciatic symptoms. This is most common in football linemen or weight lifters. The athlete will often have little or no back pain but complain of significant leg pain. Neurologic examination should confirm nerve root involvement and straight leg-lifting will be positive.

Treatment of acute disk herniations is by a short course (2 to 3 days) of bed rest with nonsteroidal anti-inflammatory drugs (NSAIDs). This will usually get the athlete on the mend. Surgery is rarely necessary for the herniated lumbar disk in the athlete but may result in return to full participation (16).

Fractures and Contusions

Fractures of the thoracic and lumbar spine are uncommon in sports, but they must always be considered when there is bony tenderness and a history of axial loading, direct blow, or violent twisting. Fractures of the pelvic ring also require significant trauma. Avulsion fractures of either the pelvis or transverse process result from violent muscle contraction and should be considered when there is tenderness at a muscle origin.

Contusions to the back may involve more than the protective muscular canopy of the back and flank. Direct trauma to the posterior flank can cause muscle tearing, posterior rib disarticulation, gastrointestinal trauma, liver or spleen rupture, renal artery laceration, renal capsule hematoma, and renal laceration. Blows to the bony spinal column may create contusions or fractures that include compression fractures, comminuted fractures, fractures of the growth plate at the vertebral end plate, lumbar transverse process fracture, and fractures of the spinous process (6). It is important to remember that all of the major arteries and viscera of the body can be reached through the back; thus, injury to the back can be potentially lethal.

Spinal Abnormalities

Among the abnormalities that can lead to back pain in the athlete are alterations in mobility of the spine, bony abnormalities, and inflammatory conditions.

Hypermobility

Conditions that increase the range of motion of the vertebral spine are associated with cartilaginous changes. These conditions either alter the mechanical properties of joints or affect the osseous support of articular cartilage. For men, those with the greatest mobility in their lumbar spine and the shortest isometric endurance times have been shown to be the most liable to experience low back pain (29).

Conversely, studies by Howes and Isdale (30) suggest that hypermobility is important in the differential diagnosis of backache only in women. Until the data become more clear on this issue, it is well advised to consider hypermobility of the spine as a possible predictor of future low back pain in the athlete.

Bony Abnormalities

Spondylolysis is a defect in the pars interarticularis of the posterior elements of the spine between the superior and inferior facet joints (31). The cause is unknown, but there is some evidence that it has a genetic predisposition with an increased penetrance caused by inbreeding. Stewart described an incidence of 50% in Alaskan Eskimos, a finding which may result from inbreeding (32).

Repetitive jarring activities or hyperextension of the lumbar spine may also cause spondylolysis in the athlete. These include blocking in football, weight training, gymnastics, and diving. Jackson and colleagues (33) demonstrated an 11% incidence of spondylolysis in female gymnasts and indicated that the incidence may be 10% in several sports, twice that of the population at large. This suggests a stress reaction, similar to stress fractures in other areas, may also be a cause. The combination of intense training with repetitive hyperextension at a time of rapid growth seems to have a high association with symptomatic spondylolysis.

Spondylolysis usually presents as unilateral low back pain accentuated by hyperextension or rotation. Nerve root irritation or sciatica are rarely present. Often the athletes have marked flexibility and can place their palms on the floor.

Bilateral spondylolysis may result in the forward slipping of one vertebral body on the one below, creating a lesion called *spondylolisthesis* (Figure 9.18*A*). The most frequent site for this to happen is between L5 and the sacrum, but it may occur at L4–L5, or higher. A congenital variety of spondylolisthesis associated with an elongated pars interarticularis and defective facets allows forward slipping without a break in the pars.

Spondylolisthesis is usually associated with low back pain. The propensity to slip forward is exaggerated during the growth spurt, and the forward slip can be so severe that the vertebral body can fall off the one below. Irritation of the L5 and S1 roots is common and results in limitation in straight leg-raising with hamstring muscle spasm.

In children the condition is usually painless although the parents may notice an unduly prominent abdomen and buttock. In adolescents and adults, backache may be the presenting symptom. It is usually intermittent, coming on after exercise or strain, and in some cases there may be sciatica as a consequence of root pressure. There are two mechanisms for this root pressure: the first occurs with the displacement of the intervertebral foramina with root pressure; the second mechanism, producing first sacral root pressure, is the result of a protrusion of the disk or pressure by an irregular osteophytic margin about the defect in the neural arch. Probably the most commonly experienced pain is that which arises in the disk adjacent to the unstable vertebrae as a consequence of altered spine mechanics and increased forces on the disk.

Spondylolisthesis may be seen as a characteristic deformity that is the result of forward displacement of the involved vertebra and the vertebrae above. The spinous process above forms a "step-off" when palpated carefully (see Figure 9.7). The diagnosis of spondylolisthesis is best made from standing lateral roentgenograms of the lumbosacral spine. Diagnosis of spondylolysis requires oblique roentgenograms of the lumbosacral spine to show the defective pars interarticularis. Under normal circumstances the pars interarticularis and the superior articular facet form the outline of a "Scottish terrier" on the oblique radiograph. In the condition of spondylolysis

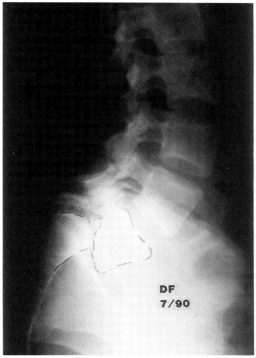

A

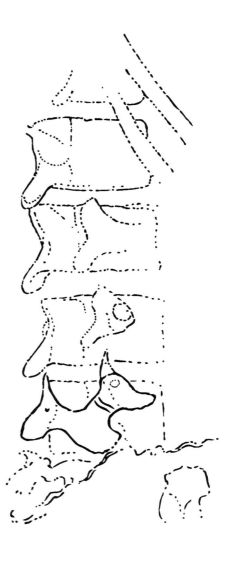

B

C

Figure 9.18. *A.* Spondylolisthesis with forward slip of L5 on the sacrum. *B.* Diagrammatic representation of spondylolysis. In the oblique view the "Scotty dog" wears a collar. *C.* In spondylolisthesis, the terrier is decapitated.

without slip, the terrier is seen to wear a collar of translucency as compared with the rest of the bone, whereas in spondylolisthesis, when there has been movement forward of the superior articular facet, the terrier is seen to be decapitated (Figure 9.18*B* and *C*). When roentgenograms are inconclusive, computed tomography (CT) scanning or radionuclide bone scan may be helpful.

Spondylolisthesis can be completely asymptomatic and may be found during examination for other complaints. It would be difficult otherwise to explain the discrepancy between the 5% incidence of the defect in adult skeletons in anatomic museums and the much smaller numbers of the general population who present for treatment. Many patients first appear for treatment in the middle or late decades of life but they have probably had the defect since early childhood.

Clinical Case #3

A 23-year-old woman went to her physician because of chronic back pain. She is recently married and plans to become pregnant within the year. This visit was prompted by concerns about how the pregnancy will affect her back. During the interview, the physician asked about recent or past injuries. She did not remember any recent injury to her back; she works as an administrative assistant and does no heavy lifting. But she did remember a fall from the balance beam when she was in competitive gymnastics as a 13-year-old girl. This fall was immediately preceded by a sharp pain in her back suffered while attempting a difficult back walk-over maneuver. At the time, it was treated like a bruise and she was told by her trainer to continue competing. But eventually the pain caused her to stop competing altogether. Periodically, she would try running or aerobics, but the pain in her back would eventually cause her to drop out. At that time, her doctor didn't think

it was anything more than a recurrent strain. Since, she has referred to her problem as a "delicate back condition."

Pediatric athletic injury assessment requires a high index of suspicion on the part of the examining physician. The pediatric patient can often only describe discomfort in general terms, especially when in a great deal of pain. Those injuries that initially appear to be of nominal consequence must be carefully evaluated and coupled with a high index of suspicion for more severe occult injury. In the above illustration, fracture of the pars interarticularis in the hypermobile spine of the adolescent has led to a cascade of problems for the adult, and a progression to the mind-set of being a "back cripple"— unable to participate in any physical exertion secondary to nonspecific back pain.

The hyperlordotic stresses of gymnastic exercise make the diagnosis of posterior element failure very important. As previously discussed, the combination of periods of rapid growth and intense training nurture conditions where the gymnast is more injury prone. Physical activity in later years may continue to aggravate the damaged pars interarticularis and supporting structures, keeping the athlete from exercising on a regular basis. Plane radiographs with oblique views would be indicated to assess for spondylolysis or spondylolisthesis.

Inflammatory Conditions

Symptoms of morning stiffness that ease through the day, worsening problems with the use of more than two pillows, and refractoriness to NSAIDs are typical of the seronegative spondyloarthropathies that share the HLA-B27 antigen. Epidemiologically, these diseases begin in the second or third decade at the height of athletic acuity, and the prevalence in men is three times that in women. They include ankylosing spondylitis, Reiter's syndrome, and psoriatic arthritis.

In the spine, the initial lesion consists of inflammatory granulation tissue at the junction of the annulus fibrosus of the disk cartilage and the margin of vertebral bone. The outer annular fibers are eroded and eventually replaced by bone, forming the beginning of a bony excrescence called a *syndesmophyte*, which then grows by continued enchondral ossification, ultimately bridging the adjacent vertebral bodies. The limitation of motion and increasing pain experienced by the patient in the above illustration reflects the degree of inflammation in the annulus fibrosus and at the facet joints. In ankylosing spondylitis, chest expansion is severely restricted. This may be the first clinical finding of this disease, which occurs primarily in young men. Involvement of the sacroiliac joints is common in all of the spondyloarthropathies and many of the tests of sacroiliac joint dysfunction will be helpful diagnostically.

Facet Syndrome

In most patients, the onset of back pain is acute and related to twisting motion with hyperextension or hyperflexion of the spine. Duplication of these motions particularly extrusion produces a "catching" sensation in the back (34). The facet joint is a true synovial joint formed by the superior articular process of one vertebra and the inferior articular process of the subjacent vertebra (Figure 9.19). It is encapsulated by a thin, fibrous layer. The anteromedial aspect of the joint capsule is formed by the ligamentum flavum, and the multifidus muscle covers the posterior aspect of the joint. Both structures maintain the integrity of the joint capsule.

The facet joint capsules are richly innervated by the dorsal ramus of the lumbar spinal nerve, but no nerve fibers have been found that penetrate the joint capsule. Each

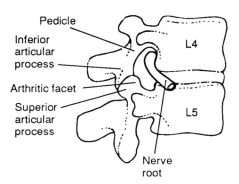

Figure 9.19. Facet joint, formed from the superior and inferior articular processes, in close proximity to the nerve root.

spinal nerve branches out to supply three facet joints; therefore, each facet joint has trisegmental innervation (35). An athlete performing certain movements in competition may entrap the facet joint capsule between the articular processes—particularly with hyperextension and rotation of the spine (36) (i.e., the "Fosbury flip" during a high jump). Also, like other joints, a nonspecific synovitis or degenerative joint disease may cause facet joint pain (37).

The typical athlete with facet syndrome will have back and leg pain, surprisingly sometimes demonstrating nerve root irritation and an altered neurologic examination. The pain is usually accentuated with hyperextension, relieved by ambulation, and reproduced by direct pressure on the facet joint. One half the patients respond to NSAIDs. Manipulative therapy can help dramatically, perhaps by liberating entrapped synovium. Facet joint injection with local anesthesia and a long-acting corticosteroid may also alleviate symptoms.

BASIC TENETS FOR RADIOLOGIC STUDIES IN ATHLETIC BACK INJURY

The majority of cases of low back pain are mechanical in nature (38), and 65% of patients with low back pain who are treated conservatively will recover within 2 weeks; 75% of patients will recover within 4 weeks (39). For these reasons, radiographs should generally be reserved for athletes with pain of more than 2 weeks' duration, significant acute trauma, focal neurologic signs, weight loss, or a history of previous non-dermatologic malignancy.

Computed tomography scanning is the diagnostic test of choice in cases of fracture, when plane films are inadequate to define the injury. It is also of practical benefit in cases of suspected malignancy. The technetium bone scan is an excellent screening tool for stress reaction or malignancy. The magnetic resonance imaging (MRI) scan, despite its cost, should be used in patients with suspected disk herniation (Figure 9.20) who have not responded to conservative therapy and are potential surgical candidates.

TREATMENT

Treating back injury in the athlete hinges on correcting the problems that interfere with the relationship of form and motion between the spinal column and the muscular canopy. Athletes tend to be more impatient with prolonged rehabilitation regimens and also tend to compete in the presence of an injury. These characteristics often have a positive effect on the rehabilitation program; however, athletes have to be protected from their own exuberance, because they will often proceed with the assumption that if they exercise more than instructed, they will return to competition sooner. This behavior can sometimes be detrimental to recovery. Table 9.3 provides a checklist example of acute and chronic treatment strategies for back injury in the athlete.

Treatment of the athlete with a back injury is somewhat different from the seden-

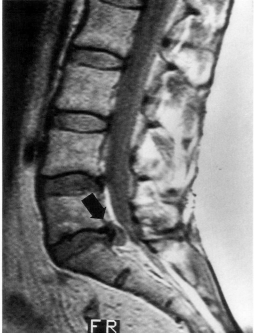

Figure 9.20. Magnetic resonance image of herniated L5–S1 disk (*arrow*).

Table 9.3. Treatment of acute and chronic back pain

Acute	Chronic

• Bed rest (up to 48 hr)
 • Cold therapy
 • Heat therapy
 • Nonsteroidal anti-inflammatory drugs
 • Sedative muscle relaxant
 • Manipulative therapy
 • Acupuncture
 • Exercise program
	• Exercise program
	 • Sports medicine approach:
	   • Work stimulation
	   • Passive and active stretching program
	   • Work hardening

tary population. The goals of treatment in the athlete must be directed not only at alleviating pain, but, wherever possible, at maintaining conditioning and promoting a rapid return to preinjury levels of performance.

The basic treatment for low back pain is rest. It has been shown that 2 days of bed rest are as effective as 7 days (40) and result in 45% less time lost from work. During the first 72 hours, application of ice prevents or reduces swelling (41,42), decreases nerve conduction velocity, and diminishes cellular and intracellular metabolism—thereby reducing pain and decreasing the effects of inflammation, respectively. When applied late in the healing process, heat increases circulation and cellular metabolism. Although heat and cold seem to provide symptomatic relief, no data indicate that ultrasonography or diathermy are effective. Moreover, no convincing data support benefits from lumbar corsets and braces; on the contrary, some studies show that braces cause unpredictable and often increased movements of the lumbar spine (43). The vast majority of patients with acute low back pain or injury will probably respond to short-term bed rest and NSAIDs.

High doses of NSAIDs should be given for the first 2 to 3 days because the anti-inflammatory dose is higher than the analgesic dose—usually about double. As the signs of inflammation subside, the dose of the NSAID should be reduced to an analgesic level for an additional 3 to 4 days. Pharmacotherapy should then be discontinued to test for the presence of exercise-stimulated pain and to determine if pain occurs on resting. If pain persists, an additional 3 to 7 days of NSAID therapy should be given. Thereafter, all medication should cease, the patient should be reevaluated, and the need for further therapy or referral should be assessed. Some patients may re-

quire more than 3 weeks of NSAID therapy (44).

Narcotics act at the opioid receptor level—the endorphin receptors—decreasing the perception of pain and inducing euphoria, as well as providing analgesia. They are effective in the treatment of moderate to severe pain, but because they have no anti-inflammatory effect and are potentially addictive and subject to abuse, they are not recommended for use in sports injuries.

Back injuries usually incur a significant amount of muscular spasm, so patient comfort and bed rest compliance can be enhanced with the addition of a sedative muscle relaxant, such as diazepam or cyclobenzaprine. The gold standard is 5 mg diazepam three times daily; however, cyclobenzaprine has proven to be as good as diazepam for relief of muscular spasm. It is more sedating than diazepam, which can be a benefit for a patient on modified bed rest. For both of these medications, only a very short course (3 to 5 days) is recommended.

Probably the most controversial form of treatment is manipulative therapy. Among the estimated 75 to 120 million annual visits to chiropractors in the United States, at least 50% are prompted because of low back symptoms (45). Historically, manipulative therapy has been performed by chiropractors and osteopathic physicians, but more clinicians in other disciplines are also now using this treatment. Manipulative therapy can be divided into manipulation, mobilization, soft-tissue massage, and point-pressure techniques. These various techniques have been evaluated by multiple critical trials that have compared manipulative therapy with other treatments, such as medication and sham therapy, and concluded that short-term manipulative therapy (no longer than 2 weeks' duration) may temporarily decrease pain and improve function, but that it has little or no lasting benefit. No studies have confirmed the effectiveness of long-term manipulative therapy, nor is there good evidence that it corrects spinal malalignment.

Acupuncture has been used increasingly by elite athletes to help speed healing and as an adjunct to any rehabilitation they may require. The limited amount of data on this form of therapy suggest that it is a useful modality for the relief of low back pain. How acupuncture works has yet to be elucidated, but it may be related to the release of endorphins or the stimulation of large myelinated nerve fibers.

Low back pain, either from injury or other etiologies, which persists through 2 to 4 months of passive and active conservative therapy, requires a more aggressive treatment approach. Conservative treatment should be tried before any invasive procedure is performed. For lumbar facet syndrome, prolonged pain relief may result from the intra-articular injection of a corticosteroid—which suggests an inflammatory etiology.

Exercises for chronic back pain are the foundation of any treatment for back pain. Following relief of severe pain an exercise program should begin. These exercises can be taught by the physician or an office nurse and can include the exercises noted in Figures 9.21 and 9.22.

Basic back exercises are divided into flexion and extension groups. With the exceptions of spondylolysis and spondylolisthesis, both types of exercises are indicated for most back conditions. The flexion group stresses abdominal strengthening, forward flexibility, and hamstring flexibility (see Figure 9.21), whereas the extension group concentrates on extension strength and flexibility (see Figure 9.22). If the pain is recurrent or your initial efforts are not working, then a more extensive exercise regimen is required. In spondylolysis or spondylolisthesis, exercises should be limited to the *flexion* program.

Evaluation and treatment by physical therapists is a valuable addition to your therapy and can be used initially or in recurrent or failed cases. Severity of the problem and ability to use resources will guide that decision.

For the more difficult patients an approach used by some physical therapists is called the sports medical approach to back rehabilitation. The sports medicine approach makes it possible to compare an individual's mobility, strength, lifting capacity, and range of motion in different planes with data bases developed from studies of people with healthy backs. These objective studies can be used to assess the patient's recovery at any point in the rehabilitation and to reassure him or her that despite pain and day-to-day frustration the rehabilitation effort is succeeding. The cornerstones of this approach are *work simulation* and *work hardening*.

Work simulation is designed to parallel the patient's premorbid activities as closely as possible. Motions and weight loads typical of the individual's job or sports activity are used in conjunction with nonpharmacologic pain control measures to restore function. Efforts to recondition the patient are also made by incorporating a program of isometric exercise and passive and active stretching. It is important to note that stretching is introduced to complement strength and conditioning exercises. By itself, stretching has little value and may cause injury (46).

Work hardening surpasses exercises and stretching of reconditioning programs in that it brings the entire body into activity. Work hardening should be highly individualized. For example, in work hardening, a

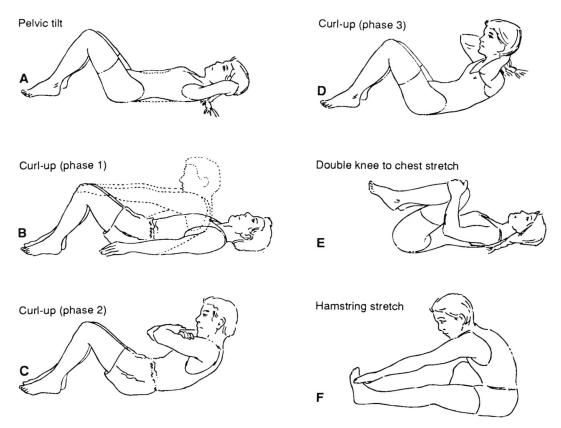

Pelvic tilt

A

Curl-up (phase 1)

B

Curl-up (phase 2)

C

Curl-up (phase 3)

D

Double knee to chest stretch

E

Hamstring stretch

F

Figure 9.21. *A.* Curl-up (level 1). Begin with arms at sides, knees bent. Tilt pelvis to flatten back. Raise shoulders and head from floor. *B.* Curl-up (level 2). Keeping arms folded across chest, raise head and shoulders. *C.* Curl-up (level 3). Hands behind neck, raise head and shoulders. *D.* Pelvic tilt. Knees bent, flatten back to floor by tightening buttocks and abdominal muscles. *E.* Both knees to chest. Pull both knees to chest until a gentle stretch is felt in the lower back. *F.* Hamstring stretch, one leg straight the other bent out. Reach toward the foot until a gentle stretch is felt in the back of the thighs.

therapist would actually supervise the patient lifting, carrying, and manipulating blocks or other heavy objects.

SUMMARY

Back pain ranks among the top ten disorders that prompt visits to the family physician's office. Musculoskeletal problems represent approximately 10 to 15% of all office visits to primary care physicians (22). The burden for both the physician and the athlete rests on how best to modify factors that cause or perpetuate injury to the back and coordinate caring, comprehensive, and accessible disease prevention, diagnosis, and treatment of acute injury, and responsible health management in the future.

Prone on elbows

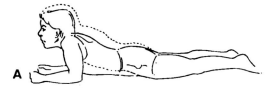

A

Upper body extension

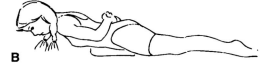

B

Hip extension on all-fours

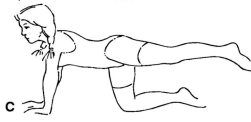

C

Angry cat stretch

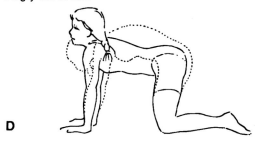

D

Figure 9.22. *A.* Prone press-up, raise up on elbows with hips on the floor. *B.* Thoracic extension, with abdomen on a thin pillow, clasp hands behind the back and lift chest from floor. *C.* Alternate hip extension. Kneeling on all fours lift one leg while keeping knee slightly bent and back flat. *D.* Angry cat stretch. Arch back by tightening abdomen and tucking chin.

References

1. Hockberger RS. Meeting the challenge of low back pain. Emerg Med 1990:99–127.

2. Shields CB, Williams PE Jr. Low back pain. Am Fam Physician 1986;33:173–182.

3. Harvey J, Tanner S. Low back pain in young athletes. A practical approach. Sports Med 1991;12:394–406.

4. Lehman LB. Neurologic injuries from winter sporting accidents. How they happen and how to minimize them. Postgrad Med 1986;80:88,93,96–98.

5. Lehman LB. Scuba and other sports diving. Nervous system complications. Postgrad Med 1986;80:68–70.

6. Keene JS, Albert MJ, Springer SL, et al. Back injuries in college athletes. J Spinal Disord 1989;2:190–195.

7. Vlok GJ, Hendrix MRG. The lumbar disc: evaluating the causes of pain. Orthopedics 1991;14:419–425.

8. Anderson JE. The back. Grant's atlas of anatomy, 7th ed. Baltimore: Williams & Wilkins, 1975.

9. Netter FH. Back. Muscles and fasciae. The CIBA collection of medical illustrations, vol 8. CIBA-GEIGY Corporation, 1987.

10. Foster D, Joan D, Elliot B, et al. Back injuries to fast bowlers in cricket: a prospective study. Br J Sports Med 1989;23:150–154.

11. Brody DM. Running injuries: prevention and management. In: Brass A, ed. Clinical symposia. Special orthopedics collection of clinical symposia. 1987;39:26–31.

12. Meeusen R, Borns J. Gymnastic injuries. Sports Med 1992;13:337–356.

13. O'Neill DB, Micheli LJ. Recognizing and preventing overuse injuries in young athletes. J Musc Med 1989;6:106–125.

14. Sohl P, Bowling A. Injuries to dancers. Prevalence, treatment and prevention. Sports Med 1990;9:317–322.

15. Belt CR. Injuries associated with aerobic dance. Am Fam Physician 1990;41:1769–1772.

16. Day AL, Friedman WA, Indelicato PA. Observations on the treatment of lumbar disk disease in college football players. Am J Sports Med 1987;15:72–75.

17. Batt ME. A survey of golf injuries in amateur golfers. Br J Sports Med 1992;26:63–65.

18. Leblanc KE. Sacroiliac sprain: an overlooked cause of back pain. Am Fam Physician 1992;46:459–463.

19. Macnab I. Disc degeneration and low back pain. Clin Orthop 1986;208:3–14.

20. Peltier LF. Examination of the back and extremities. In: Delp, Manning, eds. Major's physical diagnosis, 8th ed. Philadelphia: WB Saunders, 1975:637–656.

21. Deyo RA, Mayer TG, Pedinoff S, et al. The painful low back: keep it moving (E Richman, ed). Patient Care 1987;21:47–59.

22. Spoelhoef GD, Bristow M. Back pain pitfalls. Am Fam Physician 1989;40:133–138.

23. Frazier LM, Carey TS, Lyles MF, et al. Selective criteria may increase lumbosacral spine roentgenogram use in acute low back pain. Arch Intern Med 1989;149:47.

24. Miller JA, Schmatz C, Schultz AB. Lumbar disc degeneration: correlation with age, sex, and spine level in 600 autopsy specimens. Spine 1988;13:173–178.

25. Kelsey JL, Githens PB, White AA III, et al. Acute prolapsed lumbar intervertebral disc: an epidemiologic study with special reference to driving automobiles and cigarette smoking. Spine 1984;9:608–613.

26. Gyntelberg F. One year incidence of low back pain among male residents of Copenhagen aged 40–59. Dan Med Bull 1974;21:30.

27. Kamijo K, Tsujimara H, Obara H, Katsumata M. Evaluation of seating comfort. Society of Automotive Engineers technical paper series 820761, 1982:1–6.

28. Frymoyer JW, Pope MH, Costanaza MC, Rosen JC, Goggin JE, Wilder DG. Epidemiologic studies of low back pain. Spine 1980;5:419–423.

29. Biering-Sorenson F. Physical measurements as risk indicators for low back trouble over a one year period. Spine 1984;9:106–119.

30. Howes RG, Isdale IC. The loose back: an unrecognized syndrome. Rheum Phys Med 1971;11:72–77.

31. Taurog JD, Lipsky PE. Ankylosing spondylitis and reactive arthritis. In: Harrison's principles of internal medicine, 12th ed. New York: McGraw-Hill 1991:1451–1452.

32. Stewart TD. Age of incidence of neural arch defects in Alaskan natives, considered from the standpoint of etiology. J Bone Joint Surg [Am] 1953;35A:937.

33. Jackson DW, Wiltse LL, Cirincione RJ. Spondylolysis in the female gymnast. Clin Orthop 1976;117:68.

34. Destouet JM. Lumbar facet syndrome: diagnosis and treatment. Surgical Grand Rounds for Orthopaedics February 1988:22–27.

35. Selby DK, Paris SV. Anatomy of facet joints and its clinical correlation with low back pain. Contemp Orthop 1981;3:1097–1103.

36. Kraft GL, Levinthal DH. Facet synovial impingement: a new concept in the etiology of lumbar vertebral derangement. Surg Gynecol Obstet 1951;93:439–443.

37. Lewinnek GE, Warfield CA. Facet joint degeneration as a cause of low back pain. Clin Orthop 1986;213:216–222.

38. Liang M, Komaroff AL. Roentgenograms in primary care patients with acute low back pain: a cost-effectiveness analysis. Arch Intern Med 1982;142:1108–1112.

39. Troup JDG, Martin JW, Lloyd DCEF. Back pain in industry: a prospective survey. Spine 1981;6:61–69.

40. Deyo RA, Diehl AK, Rosenthal M. How many days of bed rest for acute low back pain? A randomized clinical trial. N Engl J Med 1986;315:1064.

41. Gieck JH, Saliba EN. Application of modalities in overuse syndromes. In: Hunter-Griffin LY, ed. Clinics in sports medicine. Philadelphia: WB Saunders, 1987;6:427.

42. Hunter SC, Poole RM. The chronically inflamed tendon. In: Hunter-Griffin LY, ed. Clinics in sports medicine. Philadelphia: WB Saunders, 1987;6:371.

43. Nachemson A, Schultz A, Andersson G. Mechanical effectiveness studies of lumbar spine orthoses. Scand J Rehabil Med 1983;9:139–149.

44. Amadio P Jr, Gates TN. NSAIDs in the treatment of overuse injuries. Fam Prac Recert 1991;13:18–45.

45. Frymoyer JW. Back pain and sciatica. N Engl J Med 1988;318:291–300.

46. Hubley-Kozey CL, Stanish WD. Can stretching prevent athletic injuries? J Musc Med 1990;7:21–31.

SHOULDER INJURIES IN SPORTS

TIMOTHY N. TAFT

10

Anatomy
Shoulder Motion and Biomechanics
Evaluation
Diagnostic Studies
The Clavicle
The Scapula
The Sternoclavicular Joint
The Acromioclavicular Joint
Shoulder Instability
The Rotator Cuff
Nerve Injuries
Muscle Injuries
Other Injuries
Shoulder Rehabilitation

Shoulder pain and instability are common problems in competitive and recreational athletes. Injuries and abuse of shoulder structures account for approximately 10% of all sports injuries. Athletes exerting maximum stress in the overhead position such as with throwing (baseball, football, javelin) or circumduction (swimming, tennis, volleyball) are particularly vulnerable to overuse and impingement-type syndromes. Violent sports such as football and wrestling are also hazardous for the shoulder.

Shoulder symptoms frequently begin insidiously without a clearly identifiable cause of the trauma. Repetitive movements that individually do not cause acute pathology frequently cause shoulder problems because of their cumulative nature. On the other hand, acute injuries caused by either direct or indirect forces are often followed by persistent symptoms that the clinician must sort out. With a careful history and physical examination, the physician can usually differentiate among the multiple causes of shoulder pain and prescribe a rational and effective treatment program.

ANATOMY

The shoulder is an extremely complex joint that defies brief description. The simple act of elevating the arm requires motion at four articulations and a sophisticated interplay of muscles including the deltoid, rotator cuff, and scapular stabilizers. A functional deficit in any part of the shoulder alters the biomechanics and places increased stress on other structures, leading to their eventual failure. It is important to recognize not only the functional deficit, but also the primary pathology. To do this requires a thorough understanding of basic shoulder anatomy and biomechanics.

The shoulder is comprised of three bones (clavicle, scapula, and proximal humerus), four articulations (sternoclavicular, acromioclavicular, glenohumeral, and scapulothoracic), and the muscles and tendons that bind them together into a functional unit. Normal shoulder function depends on the integrity of all of these units. Any single structure that is injured or dysfunctional will lead to a functional deficit of the shoulder as a whole.

Bones

The *clavicle* is an S-shaped strut between the sternum proximally and the acromion process distally (Figure 10.1). In addition to keeping the scapula on the posterior aspect of the thorax, it helps in preventing excessive anterior displacement of the glenoid. The clavicle is important in guiding the synchronous movement of the shoulder and it serves as the attachment for muscles, including the deltoid and trapezius. The clavicle overlies the brachial plexus and helps protect these nerves and associated vessels from anterior trauma.

The *scapula* is a broad, membranous bone

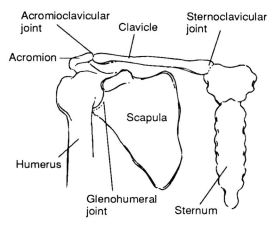

Figure 10.1. Bones of the shoulder girdle.

that serves as the origin or attachment for the muscles that power the shoulder. It has no bony connection to the thorax, and its concave undersurface glides over the muscles of the posterolateral chest wall. It also contains the glenoid articulation for the glenohumeral joint.

In addition to having one of the articular surfaces of the glenohumeral joint, the *proximal humerus* has the greater and lesser tuberosities, which serve as attachment sites for the rotator cuff.

Joints

The *sternoclavicular joint* is the only articular attachment between the upper limb and the axial skeleton. This diarthrodial joint is supported by a tough joint capsule, and the proximal clavicle is secured to the sternum by strong, circumferential, sternoclavicular ligaments. The anterior sternoclavicular ligament is the primary restraint to upward displacement, and the intra-articular disk is the primary restraint to medial displacement of the proximal end of the clavicle. The broad costoclavicular ligament between the proximal clavicle and the first rib also restricts vertical displacement.

Distally, the *acromioclavicular joint* (Figure 10.2*A*) is supported by two sets of ligaments. The horizontally disposed, circumferential, acromioclavicular ligaments support the superior and inferior aspects of this joint. Unlike the sternoclavicular joint, relatively little structural support comes from these ligaments. Their major function is to prevent horizontal displacement at the acromioclavicular joint. The conoid and trapezoid (coracoclavicular) ligaments extend from the coracoid to the undersurface of the clavicle and keep it from displacing superiorly. The conoid resists anterior and superior translation; the trapezoid helps re-

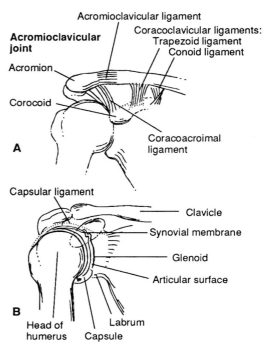

Figure 10.2. *A*. The acromioclavicular joint and supporting ligaments. *B*. The glenohumeral joint and supporting ligaments.

sist axial compression of the distal end of the clavicle. These ligaments also help prevent scapular tilt and thus limit rotation at the acromioclavicular joint. The entire upper limb is suspended from the clavicle by these two ligaments.

Although the *glenohumeral joint* is classified as a ball and socket joint, the anatomy is such that the large ball of the humeral head and the shallow socket of the glenoid provide relatively little inherent bony stability. Its configuration is said to resemble a golf ball sitting on a tee. Radiographs of the shoulder suggest that the glenoid surface is much flatter than that of the humeral head. This is a bit of a misperception because the articular cartilage is thicker at the margins and thus the joint surfaces are more congruent than it would seem on the radiographs.

The glenohumeral joint is the most mobile joint in the body and because of this it is also the most unstable. Stability has been sacrificed to gain mobility and this joint maintains a fine balance between functional mobility and adequate stability. Because of the bony configuration, this joint relies on the surrounding soft-tissue envelope (glenoid labrum, joint capsule, glenohumeral ligaments, and the rotator cuff) to provide stability through both dynamic and static restraints.

The static stabilizers are the joint surfaces, the glenoid labrum and the capsular complex of ligaments (Figure 10.2B). The glenoid labrum is a fibrocartilaginous wedge attached to the periphery of the glenoid and it roughly doubles the depth of the glenoid socket. It also serves as the glenoid attachment of the capsule and capsular ligaments.

The capsular ligaments are lax in all but the extremes of motion with different portions of the capsule being selectively tightened in different positions. At rest, with the arm in the dependent position, the superior portion of the capsule is taut, and the inferior region is lax. With elevation, this relationship is reversed. Similarly, the anterior portion tightens with external rotation, abduction and extension; whereas, the posterior capsule tightens with internal rotation and horizontal flexion. The anterior capsule is reinforced by three fairly substantial bands known as the superior, middle, and inferior glenohumeral ligaments. The superior glenohumeral ligament parallels the biceps tendon and helps support the dependent arm. The middle glenohumeral ligament, along with the inferior glenohumeral ligament and subscapularis tendon, resist external rotation

and provide anterior support to the shoulder. The most significant structure in preventing anterior displacement of the humeral head is the inferior glenohumeral ligament. This ligament is the primary restraint to external rotation and extension with the arm in abduction. Loss of integrity of the inferior glenohumeral ligament is thought to be a major cause of anterior glenohumeral instability. The dynamic stabilizers are the rotator cuff and scapular stabilizers.

The *scapulothoracic articulation* is not a true diarthrodial joint. Nonetheless, the scapula slides back and forth over the posterior thoracic wall as the shoulder moves through a full range of motion.

Shoulder motion can occur at either the scapulothoracic articulation or the glenohumeral joint. Normally, these two articulations work together synchronously to allow a smooth movement of the shoulder. Approximately two thirds (120°) of shoulder abduction takes place at the glenohumeral joint and approximately one third of the motion (60°) takes place between the scapula and thorax, as the scapula slides over the thoracic cage. Almost all shoulder pathology is associated with a disruption of the normally smooth, coordinated motion that occurs between these two joints as the shoulder is elevated.

Muscles

The shoulder is surrounded by large, powerful muscles. The *deltoid*, which is innervated by the axillary nerve, originates proximally from the spine of the scapula and the distal clavicle, and inserts laterally onto the proximal humerus. It elevates the arm after the glenohumeral joint fulcrum has been stabilized by the rotator cuff. The *pectoralis major*, along with the *latissimus dorsi* and the *subscapularis*, serve as the

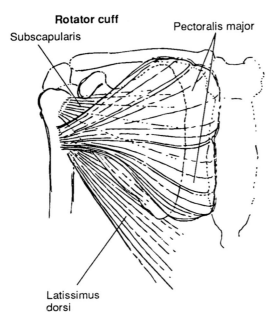

Rotator cuff

Subscapularis

Pectoralis major

Latissimus dorsi

Figure 10.3. Internal rotators of the shoulder.

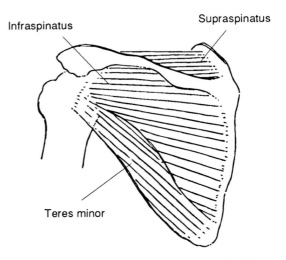

Infraspinatus

Supraspinatus

Teres minor

Figure 10.4. External rotators of the shoulder.

powerful internal rotators of the shoulder (Figure 10.3). These are balanced by the much weaker external rotators consisting of the *infraspinatus* and *teres minor*, which must be strengthened as part of any comprehensive rehabilitation program (Figure 10.4). The scapular stabilizers are the muscles that support the scapula. Of this group, the *serratus anterior* and the *rhomboids* seem to be the most important muscles to strengthen in a shoulder-conditioning and rehabilitation program. Weakness of the scapular stabilizers places additional stress on the rotator cuff and can lead to the development of shoulder pain and impingement.

The *rotator cuff* consists of the subscapularis anteriorly, the supraspinatus superiorly, and the infraspinatus and teres minor posteriorly (see Figure 10.4). These four muscles extend from the scapula to the proximal humerus and stabilize the hu-

meral head against the glenoid to provide a fulcrum through which the extrinsic muscles can work. The rotator cuff tendons envelope the humeral head anteriorly, superiorly, and posteriorly and provide dynamic stability for the shoulder joint.

The long head of the *biceps* tendon attaches to the superior aspect of the glenoid, passes through the shoulder joint, and exits through the bicipital groove between the greater and lesser tuberosities. It is held within this groove by a tough, transverse ligament. The location of the biceps tendon is such that circumduction of the shoulder makes it vulnerable to impingement between the humerus and the coracoacromial arch. The biceps also helps depress the humeral head.

Subacromial Space

The subacromial space is an extra-articular area bounded superiorly by the anterior coracoid process, the coracoacromial ligament, and the anterior acromion. This arch surrounds the rotator cuff, and along with

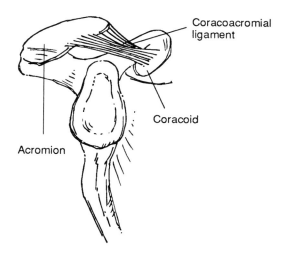

Coracoacromial
ligament

Coracoid

Acromion

Figure 10.5. The coracoacromial arch.

the acromioclavicular joint, defines the supraspinatus outlet. The subdeltoid bursa is just beneath the coracoacromial arch (Figure 10.5) and assists the gliding mechanism and cushioning of the shoulder. Beneath the subacromial bursa are the rotator cuff and shoulder joint capsule. The coracoacromial arch serves as a rigid roof, against which the bursa, rotator cuff, and biceps tendon may be impinged with elevation and circumduction of the shoulder. Any developmental, degenerative, or traumatic variation in the structure of this arch can have a role in the development of an impingement syndrome.

SHOULDER MOTION AND BIOMECHANICS

Shoulder elevation is customarily defined in three planes: sagittal (forward flexion and backward extension), scapular (neutral), and coronal (abduction). The scapular plane is parallel with the body of the scapula and approximately 30°

anterior to the coronal plane. Normal flexion and abduction (Figure 10.6) are approximately 170° while posterior elevation is approximately 60°. All of these motions occur because of combined movements at the glenohumeral and scapulothoracic articulations. This synchronized motion is referred to as *scapulohumeral rhythm*, and there is approximately 2° of glenohumeral motion to every 1° of scapulothoracic motion.

Forward flexion is restricted by capsular torsion and coronal abduction is restricted by impingement of the greater tuberosity on the acromion. Elevation in the scapular or neutral plane is recommended for both examination and rehabilitation of the shoulder.

Internal and external rotation occur primarily at the glenohumeral joint. The amount of rotation is partially determined by the amount of elevation. With the arm at the side, external rotation and internal rotation are approximately equal. At 90° of abduction, internal rotation exceeds external rotation, although this relationship may not hold true in overhead-throwing athletes. Loss of internal rotation because of shortening of the external rotators and posterior capsule can place additional stress on the rotator cuff and cause shoulder pain.

Shoulder Kinematics

Shoulder function during athletic activity has been analyzed using electromyography and digitized high-speed film analysis of motion. These data have supported the observation that athletes often experience a selective weakness of specific muscles rather than generalized muscle impairment. It is important to identify specific weaknesses in order to direct the appropriate rehabilitation.

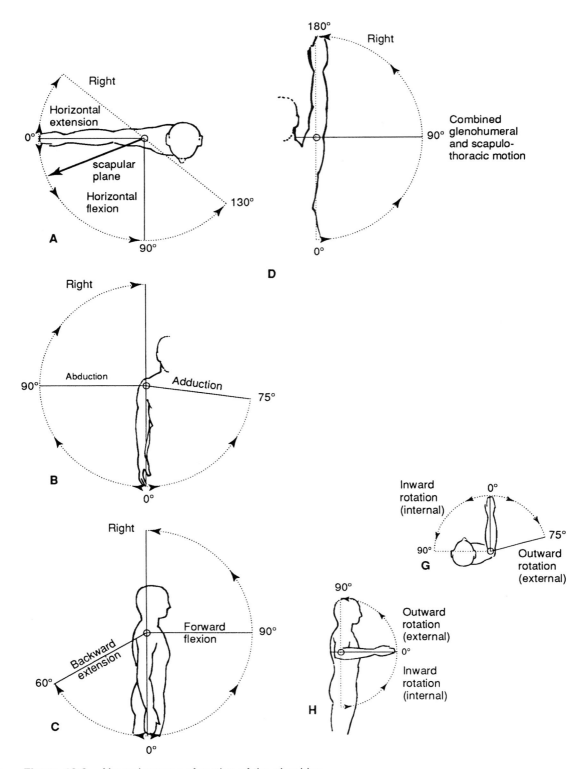

Figure 10.6. Normal ranges of motion of the shoulder.

Baseball Pitching

The baseball pitch (Figure 10.7) is divided into five phases. 1) The *windup* is the period of preparation and ends when the ball leaves the gloved hand. 2) *Early cocking* is the period of shoulder abduction and external rotation and ends with ground contact of the contralateral foot. 3) *Late cocking* is the period when the arm is maximally abducted and externally rotated and ends with the first forward movement of the arm. 4) *Acceleration* is the period of forward flexion and internal rotation of the humerus and ends with ball release. 5) *Follow-through* is the period between ball release and ends when motion stops (1).

All four of the rotator cuff muscles have peak electrical activity in late cocking when the shoulder is most vulnerable to anterior displacement (2). This indicates that these muscles are stabilizing the humeral head within the glenoid and providing stability to the fulcrum of motion. The infraspinatus and teres minor are also active in follow-through and thus help decelerate the ante-

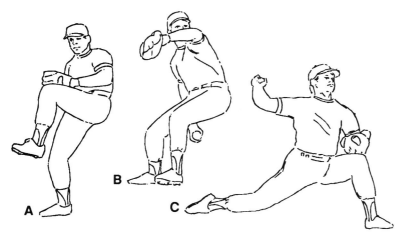

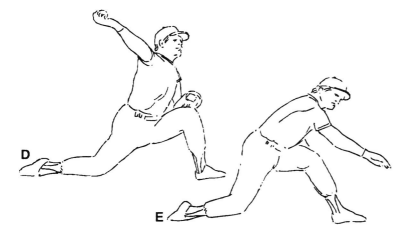

Figure 10.7. The throwing motion. *A.* Windup. *B.* Early cocking. *C.* Late cocking. *D.* Acceleration. *E.* Follow-through.

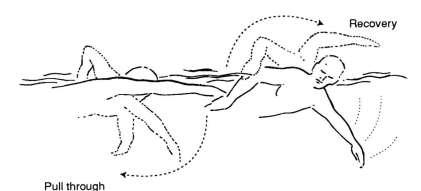

Figure 10.8. Freestyle
swimming stroke phase 1,
pull-through, and phase 2,
recovery (see text).

rior motion of the arm. The rotator cuff
muscles help the static anterior capsular
structures stabilize the shoulder during full
abduction and external rotation (3). As a
result of the action of the infraspinatus and
teres minor, the humeral head is actually
displaced posteriorly in the glenoid when
the arm is in the cocked position.

The serratus anterior, rhomboid, and
levator scapulae muscles all contract to
place the glenoid in the optimal position for
stability. If these muscles do not contract at
the proper time, shoulder subluxation or
impingement will occur.

Electromyographic (EMG) analysis reveals significantly different patterns of
muscle contraction in patients with instability or impingement when compared
with asymptomatic throwers (2). As a
general rule, the rotator cuff is less effective
in symptomatic patients than in nonsymptomatic patients. Imbalances between
the deltoid and the supraspinatus may
contribute to the impingement syndrome.

Increased activity of the biceps in patients with mild instability indicate its role
in helping to stabilize the shoulder (4).
This may help explain the frequency of
bicipital tendinitis in throwers with subtle
instabilities.

Swimming

The freestyle swimming stroke is divided
into two phases: 1) the *pull-through*, which is
further subdivided into a) hand entry, b)
mid–pull-through, and c) end pull-through;
and 2) *recovery*, which is further subdivided
into a) elbow lift, b) midrecovery, and c)
hand entry (Figure 10.8) (1).

Shoulder activity during swimming also
emphasizes the importance of a strong rotator cuff. The supraspinatus, infraspinatus,
and middle deltoid are the predominant
muscles in the recovery phase. EMG studies
reveal that the serratus anterior reaches
near maximal activity during every stroke
(5). Serratus contraction is necessary for the
acromion to rotate clear of the humerus and
to provide a stable glenoid for humeral
head rotation. Weakness or fatigue of
the serratus anterior has an adverse effect
on scapular rotation and leads to impingement.

Tennis

The tennis serve is divided into the same
five phases as the baseball pitch. The fore-
hand and backhand strokes are divided
into three phases: 1) *racquet preparation,*

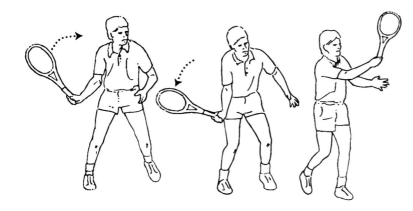

Figure 10.9. Three phases of the tennis stroke, racquet preparation, acceleration, and follow-through.

which begins with shoulder turn and ends with weight transfer to the front foot; 2) *acceleration*, which ends at ball impact; and 3) *follow-through*, which ends with completion of the stroke (1) (Figure 10.9).

As with throwing and swimming, EMG studies revealed that the rotator cuff muscles and serratus anterior were the muscles stressed the most during normal stroke (6,7).

Golf

The golf swing is divided into four phases: 1) *take away* begins with the initiation of motion and ends with the termination of the back swing; 2) *forward swing* starts at the termination of the back swing and continues until the club becomes horizontal with the ground; 3) *acceleration* is the period that ends with ball contact; and 4) *follow-through* continues until motion ceases (Figure 10.10).

Electromyographic studies in accomplished golfers reveal that the deltoid is electrically silent bilaterally through the entirety of the golf swing (8). As in other sports, however, the rotator cuff is extremely active with the subscapularis being more active than the other three. The

pectoralis major and latissimus dorsi are also very active.

Although each sport has its unique phasic pattern, all place heavy demands on the rotator cuff. The rotator cuff muscles do not always act synergistically with the deltoid, and although there are sports-specific differences, they all are active circumduction and throwing activities. Unskilled athletes consistently show greater rotator cuff activity than those of greater skill. This is particularly true if the serratus anterior is fatigued or weak. The importance of the serratus anterior and the other scapula stabilizers has been underemphasized in rehabilitation programs for patients with rotator cuff weakness or pain secondary to impingement or subluxation. Strengthening the scapula stabilizers should be part of any shoulder rehabilitation program (see Figures 10.42 through 10.45).

EVALUATION

Like all joints, the shoulder must have four basic mechanical characteristics to function normally. There must be a normal range of motion, normal stability, adequate

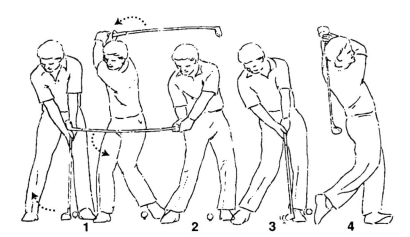

Figure   10.10. Four
phases of the golf swing,
(1) take away, (2) forward
swing, (3) acceleration,
and (4) follow-through
(see text).

strength, and smooth, congruent joint surfaces. Most clinically important shoulder disorders can be described as an abnormality of one of these necessary functions. The pathology can usually be established using only the history, physical examination, and plain radiographs. Shoulder pathology that can be defined in mechanical terms has a good chance of being treatable by nonoperative or operative means.

The physician has the responsibility of identifying and individualizing the best management approach for each patient. Every athlete who presents with a shoulder problem deserves a thorough clinical history and a comprehensive physical examination. A selected series of plain radiographs is usually appropriate. Special and invasive studies such as arthrography, computed tomography (CT), magnetic resonance imaging (MRI), examination under anesthesia, or arthroscopy are usually obtained only after a working diagnosis has been established and should serve as a tool for confirmation rather than discovery. There is the widespread misperception that accurate diagnosis of shoulder problems requires use of these special or invasive studies.

It is commonly taught that shoulder problems can be placed into one of three groups: 1) treatable, 2) diagnosable but untreatable, and 3) undiagnosable.

Treatable Problems

Most treatable disorders can be diagnosed from the basic evaluation that includes the clinical history, the physical examination, and sometimes plain radiographs. Special studies such as the MRI, arthrography, examination under anesthesia, or arthroscopy are seldom necessary to diagnose these conditions.

The need for treatment is based primarily on how much the condition adversely affects the patient's function. The diagnosis of instability, rotator cuff disease, frozen shoulder, or arthritis does not in and of itself mandate treatment unless these conditions adversely affect the patient's function or enjoyment of life. In addition, the success or failure of treatment is best measured in terms of the restoration of function. All treatment should be directed at improving patient function, and incremental improvement should result from treatment whether it is operative or nonoperative.

Diagnosable but Untreatable Problems

A variety of diagnosable shoulder conditions cannot be effectively treated. These include such conditions as remote midsubstance muscle tears, sternoclavicular instability, generalized ligamentous laxity, instability from movement disorders, habitual dislocations, brachial plexus neuritis, and massive rotator cuff tears in patients with paralysis. In these conditions, it is important to inform the patient of the limitations of existing treatment methods and then provide appropriate education, coping mechanisms, and vocational rehabilitation.

The Undiagnosable Shoulder

Unfortunately, some shoulder complaints elude diagnosis no matter how many tests are ordered. There is a risk in ordering endless tests when the basic evaluation suggests no shoulder pathology. The risk of this approach is that one of these tests may yield some "positive" finding that is unrelated to the patient's complaint. For example, labral fraying on arthroscopic examination or abnormal signals in the rotator cuff tendons on MRI or ill-defined laxity with examination under anesthesia do not help in the management of nonspecific shoulder complaints. It is important for the physician to identify those shoulders that will remain undiagnosable despite a plethora of medical tests. Whenever the basic evaluation, which includes a careful history, a good physical examination, and appropriate plain x-rays, does not suggest the existence of a definable problem, it is generally ill advised to proceed with advanced imaging, electrodiagnostic, arthroscopic, or examination under anesthesia evaluations because the yield is low in these circumstances. These special studies can be used to help confirm a diagnosis suspected by the basic examination but seldom yield helpful information if the diagnosis is not already suspected from the simpler tests.

As in all of medicine, special studies should not be obtained unless the results will somehow influence the recommended management. If a good history, a proper physical examination, and selected plain x-rays do not strongly suggest a specific diagnosis, it is unlikely that special studies will change the recommended treatment. Repeat clinical examination after several days or weeks often provides additional insight into the nature of the problem. It is quite acceptable to make a diagnosis of shoulder pain without identifiable pathology.

Using such labels as fibromyalgia, myofasciitis, painful trigger points, among others seldom helps provide meaningful treatment direction. These patients are generally best served with a program of vocational, social, and physical support.

Referred Pain

Before initiating the shoulder examination, it is important to remember that the shoulder is often the site of referred pain. Pulmonary pathology, cardiac abnormalities, diaphragmatic irritation, or intra-abdominal conditions can all cause shoulder pain. It has been reported that nearly 80% of patients with a Pancoast tumor of the lung had a chief complaint of shoulder pain and their initial physician contact was for shoulder pain. Problems external to the shoulder should be routinely evaluated and excluded. It is unlikely that any patient who has a full, painless range of motion and no tenderness of the shoulder has primary shoulder pathology.

Neurovascular problems of the cervical

spine commonly present with shoulder pain. Cervical spine pain is frequently characterized by a deep burning sensation in the posterior shoulder. The pain extends from the posterior shoulder down the arm and into the fingers and is characteristically associated with paresthesias. In contradistinction to pain of shoulder origin, the pain referred from the cervical spine is often improved with forward elevation of the shoulder. Interscapular pain (pain between the scapulae posteriorly) is a frequent complaint in athletes with cervical spine pathology. This is rarely a site of pain in athletes with primary shoulder pathology.

A careful examination of the cervical spine should be performed to exclude a cervical radiculopathy. Cervical radiculopathy can usually be confirmed with the Spurling test. This test involves lateral rotation and extension of the neck toward the painful shoulder followed by the application of axial compression. This maneuver reproduces the pain because of the encroachment of the cervical nerve roots as they exit the neural foramina. This test is better performed in a progressive fashion, beginning with axial loading in neutral, to extension without load, extension and lateral rotation without load, and finally extension and lateral rotation while loading. The test is positive if there is increasing pain or radiculopathy.

Neurovascular problems including thoracic outlet syndrome, axillary artery occlusion, and effort thrombosis of the axillary vein need to be similarly excluded.

DIAGNOSTIC STUDIES

The recent resurgence of interest in shoulder disorders has led to an increased understanding of shoulder pathology.

Despite this, the injured shoulder frequently presents a confusing picture. The most rewarding studies are an accurate history and a precise physical examination.

Medical History

The diagnosis of shoulder pain or injuries begins with the acquisition of a thorough medical history. Most athletes with shoulder pain will have symptoms with circumduction. The precise activity that causes symptoms, including the exact motion and position of the arm at the moment of pain, must be discovered and will give some clue as to the underlying pathology.

Pain is the most common complaint in athletes with shoulder problems (9). Characterization of the pain will assist greatly in making the proper diagnosis especially when its association with a specific athletic activity is carefully delineated. The pain of rotator cuff tears is often described as being dull and aching and present at rest. Night pain is characteristic of a rotator cuff tear. Red hot, burning pain is classically associated with acute calcific tendinitis or a brachial neuritis. Rotator cuff tendinitis is associated with progressive pain made worse by continued shoulder activity. Pain at the extremes of abduction, external rotation, and extension suggests instability, as does pain in the follow-through phase of throwing. Pain at the top of circumduction indicates impingement, and catching or locking symptoms suggest a labrum tear or loose body.

In the case of the throwing athlete with shoulder pain, it must be determined whether the pain occurs during windup, initiation of forward acceleration, ball release, or follow-through, and whether there is a difference in pain with different types of pitches and how the pain is influenced by the amount of shoulder elevation during throwing.

Pain at the time of ball release is characteristic of anterior capsulolabral pain or rotator cuff tendinitis caused by anterior instability. Pain during deceleration can be attributed to posterior rotator cuff pain, frequently isolated to the teres minor, and this too can herald subtle anterior instability. Patients with rotator cuff pathology often complain of pain near the deltoid insertion. Pain suddenly relieved at follow-through and localized to the inferior medial angle of the scapula is associated with scapulothoracic bursitis. Pain with forward flexion, horizontal adduction, and internal rotation is associated with and characteristic of posterior glenohumeral instability. Pathology of the acromioclavicular joint is characterized by pain on the top of the shoulder and is made worse with cross-chest adduction or the bench press.

Age is of critical importance in the athlete with shoulder problems. Athletes in the younger population (18 to 35 years) are typically overhand athletes with instability as a result of the repetitive stresses placed on their dominant shoulders. The cumulative microtrauma of these stresses leads to progressive instability, impingement, and finally a rotator cuff tear. Problems in older athletes (35+ years) can usually be attributed to degenerative changes. Proliferative changes in the coracoacromial arch compromises the subacromial space with resultant impingement, vascular insufficiency, and eventually a rotator cuff tear. In addition, the incidence of arthrosis of the glenohumeral and acromioclavicular joints increases with age.

The perception of instability should be specifically evaluated. The activity associated with subluxations and dislocations needs to be discussed in an effort to determine the direction of the instability. The perception of instability or pain with abduction, external rotation and extension characterizes anterior instability, whereas symptoms with adduction, internal rotation, and flexion suggest posterior laxity.

The mechanism of injury and the activity at the time of injury are both important. A fall onto the point of the shoulder often suggests a fracture of the clavicle or injury of the acromioclavicular joint. Falls onto the posterior aspect of the shoulder can cause scapula fractures.

Physical Examination

Physical examination of the shoulder begins with visual inspection followed by palpation, range of motion determinations, and muscle testing. Neurologic assessments and special stress tests for impingement or instability are necessary to complete the evaluation.

The examination room must be large enough for the patient to elevate and circumduct the arms simultaneously without bumping into furniture or the walls. The physician should have room to stand back and view the patient from a distance so as to gain a visual perspective of the symmetry of these motions. A sitting stool should be available for the patient so the examiner can view the shoulder from above and a firm, full length examination table is needed for the portions of the examination that are done supine or prone.

The patient must be disrobed so both shoulders can be examined and bilateral comparisons made. Female patients should wear a halter top. Disposable paper shorts can be modified into a simple but effective drape by cutting the crouch out of the pants and positioning the elastic waist band above the breasts. This allows free inspection and motion of both shoulders.

The physical examination includes the traditional techniques of inspection and palpation. Inspection includes appraisal of arm position and muscle atrophy. After this examination, the active and passive range of motion should be recorded. Motion of the shoulder occurs in the vertical, horizontal, and rotational planes. It should be determined whether these motions are associated with pain, weakness, or perceived instability. Limitation of passive motion suggests intrinsic joint pathology. Muscle strength should be rated according to the standard six-grade scale (Table 10.1). Often it is sufficient to measure the strength of a muscle group performing a specific function; however, occasionally the strength of individual muscles must be determined.

Inspection

Inspection begins with the first encounter with the patient and continues during the medical history. Observe the patient's use of the shoulder with arm gestures and while changing clothes. Observe for alterations in the normal smooth scapulohumeral rhythm and for muscle substitution patterns used to avoid pain or compensate for weakness. The shoulder should be inspected from the front, the back, and the side. Inspection should, of course, include a topical scan for deformities, blebs, discoloration, abrasions, scars, and other signs of present or previous pathology.

Observation should include evaluations of symmetry with particular attention to atrophy. Injuries such as clavicle fractures or dislocations of the acromioclavicular or glenohumeral joint are usually evident at a glance. Chronic problems, such as rotator cuff weakness or impingement, are frequently associated with atrophy of the supraspinatus or anterior deltoid muscles. A prominent scapular spine is the product of supraspinatus or infraspinatus wasting and is often an indication of rotator cuff pathology or entrapment of the suprascapular nerve, especially in overhand athletes. In throwing athletes, the dominant shoulder is normally hypertrophic with respect to the nondominant side, and the shoulder is held slightly lower than the nondominant side. Many shoulder pain problems are associated with shrugging, and the patient will elevate the symptomatic shoulder. The position of the scapula should be evaluated and excessive rotation or winging noted. Thoracic scoliosis can also cause shoulder asymmetry.

Dynamic inspection is directed at evaluating asynchrony of scapulohumeral rhythm. Elevation or movement of the scapula before movement of the humerus is a subtle and early sign of rotator cuff dysfunction and can be detected by close observation.

Table 10.1. Muscle grading chart

Muscle Gradations	Description
5–Normal	Complete range of motion against gravity with full resistance
4–Good	Complete range of motion against gravity with some resistance
3–Fair	Complete range of motion against gravity
2–Poor	Complete range of motion with gravity eliminated
1–Trace	Evidence of slight contractility. No joint motion
0–Zero	No evidence of contractility

Palpation

One of the fundamental principles of physical examination is that there is point tenderness directly over the injured structure. A knowledge of anatomy combined with precise localization of tenderness will usually lead to a correct diagnosis. This concept is sometimes difficult to apply to the shoulder in muscled or overweight athletes who have injuries to the deep structures.

The shoulder should be carefully and completely palpated to localize the point of maximum tenderness. Sometimes this is easier to do if the patient is seated and the examiner is able to stand above the shoulder and move from front to back. Crepitation, deformity, and temperature are also assessed.

Palpation should specifically include the entire clavicle with the sternoclavicular and acromioclavicular joints. Careful palpation should differentiate problems of the clavicle from those of its joints. The scapula including its medial border, spine, acromion, and coracoid should also be palpated. The greater tuberosity and bicipital groove should be examined. The bicipital groove is anterior and medial to the greater tuberosity. It is best palpated if the arm is externally rotated so as to expose the groove anteriorly (Figure 10.11). Excessive digital pressure will cause pain in all patients. This must not be overinterpreted as representing pathology.

Palpation should include the soft tissues as well as the skeletal structures. Tenderness along the anterior margin of the acromion or the coracoacromial ligament suggests impingement of the supraspinatus against the coracoacromial arch. The greater tuberosity should be palpated for evidence of supraspinatus tendinitis. This is facilitated by placing the arm in slight

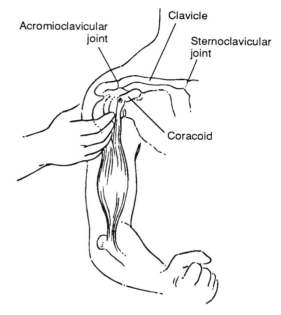

Figure 10.11. Palpation of the biceps tendon in its groove.

extension and internal rotation such as placing the hand on the ipsilateral iliac crest. Tenderness near the cuff insertion onto the greater tuberosity suggests a rotator cuff tear. Of the rotator cuff muscles the supraspinatus is most commonly ruptured.

In addition to locating points of tenderness, palpation should include evaluation of the muscles for integrity. In particular, ruptures of the pectoralis major can be diagnosed by the palpable defect in this muscle as it forms the anterior wall of the axilla. This is sometimes not evident by inspection alone. Similarly ruptures of the biceps can be detected by palpation.

Range of Motion

Both active and passive range of motion should be evaluated. In active testing, the patient uses his or her own muscles to complete the range of motion, whereas in passive testing, the examiner moves the patient's relaxed limbs through the range of motion. Passive testing should be carried out whenever a patient has difficulty performing the active tests. As a general rule, if the patient is able to perform a complete active range of motion without pain or discomfort, there is little need to proceed with passive tests. The emphasis here is on "complete" because more detailed passive range of motion testing is indicated if active range of motion is either limited or excessive.

Many different authors have suggested specific values for the normal range of shoulder motion. When evaluating a given patient, it is best to compare the range of motion on the affected side with the range of motion on the unaffected side. In this way, one can determine individual deviations from normal. Skilled overhead throwers often develop an adaptive shift in the arc of motion toward external rotation in excess of 15° to 30°, and this should not be considered abnormal (1).

Humerothoracic position is determined by measuring the angle between the long axis of the humerus and the longitudinal axis of the thorax. The angle between these lines is the angle of humerothoracic elevation. Humerothoracic motion and rhythm depend on normal function in both the glenohumeral and the scapulothoracic articulations. Alterations in either of these will cause limitations of humerothoracic positioning and abnormal shoulder function.

Shoulder motion is quite complex (see Figure 10.6), and the terminology used to describe all shoulder movement is frequently confusing and misunderstood. *Elevation* is the movement of the arm away from the body, whereas *adduction* is the movement of the arm toward the body or the midline. *Abduction* is elevation in the

coronal plane (to the side). *Flexion* is forward elevation in the sagittal plane, whereas *extension* is backward elevation in the sagittal plane. With the arm held at any given degree of elevation (e.g., at 90°) flexion and extension also refer to the forward or backward movement of the shoulder, respectively. Neutral or scapular elevation (called scaption by some) is elevation in the plane of the scapula. The glenoid is not oriented perpendicular to the coronal plane but is offset anteriorly approximately 30°. Thus, elevation in the coronal plane (true abduction) places the shoulder in approximately 30° of extension relative to the plane of the glenoid. Evaluation of neutral elevation is the most useful and significant for the overhead athlete. Internal and external rotation occur primarily at the glenohumeral joint and can be measured in any degree of elevation.

The patient must be relaxed during these evaluations. The patient can be examined standing, sitting, or supine but the examiner must be positioned comfortably and be able to move easily around the patient. Some authors recommend that this portion of the examination be done with the patient sitting or supine. This minimizes the subtle and possible misleading compensatory action of the spine or pelvis.

Six quick tests will determine full active range of motion of the shoulder. First, have the patient abduct the arms in the coronal plane to 90° while keeping the elbows straight. The palms should then be turned up and elevation continued until the hands touch each other in the overhead position such as signaling a safety in football (Figure 10.12*A*). This tests abduction and allows bilateral comparison. Next the hands are placed behind the neck and the elbows pushed posteriorly as far as possible to further test abduction and external rotation. Bilateral adduction and internal rotation

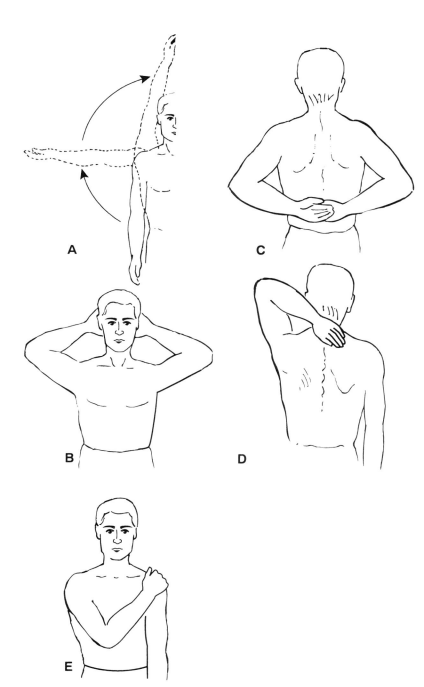

Figure 10.12. Quick range of motion tests for the shoulder. *A.* Bilateral abduction. *B.* Bilateral abduction external rotation. *C.* Bilateral adduction internal rotation. *D.* Unilateral abduction external rotation arc. *E.* Unilateral adduction.

A

B

C

D

E

can be simultaneously evaluated by having the patient reach up the back as high as possible (Figure 10.12*B*) with both hands. Unilateral movements can be quickly tested by having the patient touch the superior medial angle of the opposite scapula, by reaching both behind the head (abduction and external rotation) and also in front of the face (adduction). Elevating the arms to the full overhead position in the sagittal plane will test flexion. The patient should repeatedly abduct and adduct the shoulders to assess for smooth scapulohumeral rhythm.

If the patient is unable to fully perform any of these motions or if there is any asymmetry, a more detailed evaluation of passive range of motion must be undertaken. Limited active motion may reflect weakness, joint laxity, capsular tightness, or bone deformity. If the joint moves through a full passive range of motion, but there is limited active range of motion, the examiner can conclude that muscle weakness is the cause of restriction. Bone pathology or soft-tissue laxity or contracture will lead to asymmetry of passive range of motion.

Differences between active and passive range of motion should be noted. Passive range of motion should be divided into the glenohumeral and scapulothoracic components with the combination being the sum of these two (Figure 10.13). To evaluate glenohumeral motion, the scapula must be stabilized. This can easily be done by placing the hand over the top of the shoulder and stabilizing the clavicle anteriorly and the spine of the scapula posteriorly. The arm is then elevated. Glenohumeral motion has ended when the scapula begins mov-

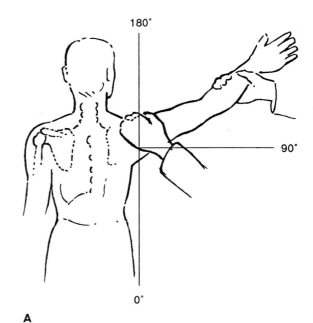

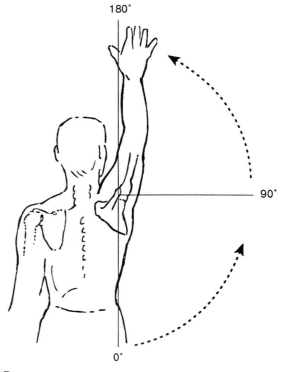

Figure 10.13. Shoulder motion is a combination of glenohumeral motion (*A*) and scapulothoracic motion (*B*).

ing. Another way to evaluate this is to hold the inferior angle of the scapula to determine when movement occurs as the arm is being elevated and rotated.

Internal and external rotation should both be measured in neutral (arm at the side) and in 90° neutral elevation. These motions should be compared to the contralateral normal side for both restricted motion and excessive movement (see Figure 10.6).

While moving the shoulder through a range of motion, the examiner must determine the difference between pain and apprehension. The former is usually an indicator of some type of impingement, while the latter is generally an indication of instability.

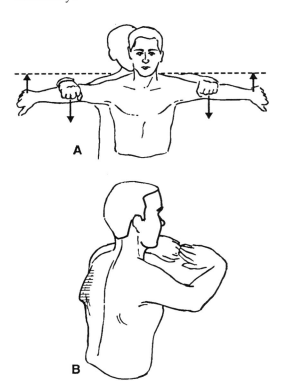

A

B

Figure 10.14. *A.* Test for supraspinatus strength. *B.* Winging of the scapula.

Manual Muscle Testing

Dysfunction of individual muscles or muscle groups can be a cause of shoulder pain. Weakness alters normal mechanics and thus places additional stress on the adjacent structures. This results in pain and additional dysfunction. Weakness is also the by-product of most shoulder injuries and abnormalities. Muscle strength testing evaluates the integrity of the musculotendinous unit while also assessing neurologic function.

Documentation should include strength measurements in forward flexion, abduction, and external and internal rotation. Classically abduction and external rotation strength are diminished in the presence of rotator cuff disease.

Specific testing of the supraspinatus is done in the scapular plane by abducting the arm to 90°, forward flexing to 30°, and maximally internally rotating the shoulder (Figure 10.14*A*). The arm is then pushed down against the upward pressure of the patient. Subtle comparative weakness without pain during this test indicates early rotator cuff disease. While doing this test, it is best to evaluate both shoulders simultaneously so that the patient does not rotate out of the testing position.

Of particular importance in throwing athletes is the strength of the scapular stabilizers and rotators. Serratus anterior weakness is associated with scapular winging during such provocative maneuvers as doing a wall push-up (Figure 10.14*B*).

Subscapularis weakness is documented by the so-called lift-off test. The athlete internally rotates the shoulder so as to place the back of the hand over the ipsilateral back pocket. The athlete then attempts to lift the hand off the back. Asymmetry or failure to do this maneuver indicates weakness of the subscapularis.

As a general rule athletes with weakness will be in the "good" or grade 4 range. It is important to consider the athlete's size and expected strength before assigning a strength rating. Seemingly normal strength may be weakness for a well-conditioned competitive athlete. They may be as strong as most nonathletes but this still represents weakness for their activities.

Because the manual muscle examination of the shoulder is detailed and complex, it requires skill and practice. Careful manual muscle examination of the shoulder by a physical therapist trained in this technique is often helpful in identifying subtle weakness.

If there is no evidence of muscle contraction the patient needs a comprehensive neurologic examination to rule out a nerve injury. If the muscle is seemingly weak, it is incumbent on the examiner to determine whether the weakness is real or the result of guarding because of pain. Sometimes it is impossible to determine whether the weakness is due to real weakness or secondary to pain.

Motor strength of these motions should then be assessed looking for asymmetry to the opposite shoulder. As a general rule the nondominant side is approximately 10% weaker than the dominant side.

Provocative Tests

Provocative tests can help discover shoulder pathology. These tests stress the shoulder and are designed to uncover a specific pathology such as impingement or instability.

The drop arm test detects full thickness rotator cuff tears (Figure 10.15). It is also useful, but less reliable, for partial-thickness cuff tears. The patient is instructed to slowly lower the abducted arm. At approximately 90° the arm will drop to the side. A patient with a rotator cuff tear is unable to lower the arm smoothly and slowly from the abducted position. If the patient can hold the arm horizontal, a gentle tap on the forearm will cause the arm to fall to the side. The drop arm test is rarely positive in the young athletic population.

Bicipital tendinitis is diagnosed by direct palpation of the biceps tendon and by the provocative tests of Speed or Yergason. The bicipital groove is brought into anterior prominence by externally rotating the humerus 15°. The groove can then be palpated

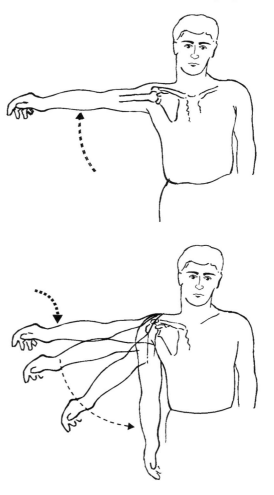

Figure 10.15. Drop arm test.

in even the most muscular patient. Speed's test is positive if the patient has pain with resisted shoulder flexion with the elbow fully extended and the wrist supinated. The starting position for Yergason's test (Figure 10.16) is with the elbow fully flexed and pronated. The examiner forcefully extends the elbow and supinates the forearm against the patient's resistance. The presence of pain indicates bicipital tendinitis or instability of the tendon in the bicipital groove.

Chronic anterior instability can be discovered with the apprehension test (Figure 10.17A). The shoulder is placed into 90° of abduction and 90° external rotation and then extended. If the shoulder is ready to subluxate or dislocate the patient will have a look of apprehension and will flinch so as to resist further motion (10–12). This test is more reliable than any examination under anesthesia. Similarly posterior laxity is evaluated by observing for apprehension when the shoulder is placed into flexion, adduction, and internal rotation.

Similarly, posterior apprehension is evaluated with the shoulder in 90° of forward flexion and then adducted and internally rotated (Figure 10.17B). A posteriorly directed force on the elbow adds further provocation of apprehension and may lead to subluxation. With either of the apprehension tests, further confirmation is given when the athlete notes that these reproduce the symptoms.

Inferior laxity of the glenohumeral joint is usually a component of multidirectional instability, and rarely, if ever, identified by itself. Inferior laxity is most easily identified by the sulcus sign (Figure 10.17C), where inferior traction with the arm relaxed at the side leads to inferior subluxation of the humeral head and a sulcus beneath the acromion.

Further diagnostic help can be obtained by diagnostic injections of lidocaine into the structures around the shoulder. One can anesthetize a known area, and by evaluating the patient's response, gain information as to the contribution this area makes to the overall pain syndrome. Injections into the acromioclavicular joint, the subdeltoid bursa, the shoulder joint, and along the coracoacromial ligament will help localize the area of pain and irritation. Once the area of pain is identified, treatment can be more specifically directed.

Imaging

It is uncommon for specialized imaging techniques to discover unsuspected pathology. For the most part, the specialized studies should be used to confirm a specific diagnosis rather than requested in hopes that something might be uncovered. Such fishing expeditions are seldom rewarding and are quite expensive. The imaging

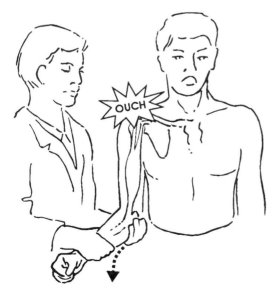

Figure 10.16. Yergason's test for biceps tendonitis or instability.

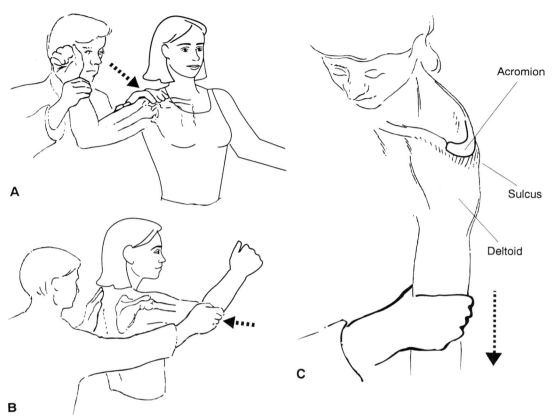

A

B

C

Acromion

Sulcus

Deltoid

Figure 10.17. *A.* Apprehension test for anterior shoulder instability. *B.* Apprehension test for posterior shoulder instability. *C.* Sulcus sign for inferior laxity.

techniques used for evaluating the shoulder are rather specific and vary widely in their ability to detect a particular defect. Some are more effective for one pathology, whereas others are better in evaluating different problems. An inappropriate study might fail to reveal the symptomatic lesion. Because these specialized studies are often invasive, painful, and expensive, they should be selected with great care and tailored to the clinical problem so as not to waste the patient's time and money. Nonetheless arthrography, CT, computed arthrotomography, subacromial bursography,

ultrasound, and MRI studies can help clarify pathology in the shoulder region.

Plain Radiography

Plain radiography, in addition to the history and physical examination, is usually sufficient to correctly diagnose most shoulder pathology. The acquisition of a so-called shoulder series is often of little value because the views requested lack specificity and may not adequately evaluate the area in question. Different techniques and positioning are used to study the sternoclavicular, acromioclavicular, and glenohumeral joints. Similarly radiographs of the clavicle, scapula, and proximal humerus are taken with much different techniques and must be individualized. Even

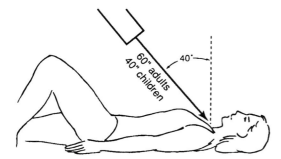

Figure 10.18. Hobbs or Heinig view to visualize sternoclavicular joint.

with significant pathology, "routine radiographs" may not reveal a structural disorder and thus they can provide a false sense of security. Specific radiographs of the shoulder should be ordered selectively and specifically to investigate the area of suspected pathology.

Evaluation of the sternoclavicular joint is done with special positioning or the use of the Hobbs or Heinig view (Figure 10.18). Even so, the sternoclavicular joint is often difficult to evaluate because of other overlying structures. CT scans are often necessary to thoroughly evaluate the sternoclavicular joint and proximal clavicle.

Routine radiographs of the shoulder will usually overpenetrate the distal clavicle and acromion, making evaluation of the acromioclavicular joint difficult. If pathology of the acromioclavicular joint is suspected, the physician should order "acromioclavicular joint" films. These radiographs are taken with the beam aimed approximately 15° to 20° cephalad and the power reduced by approximately one third. This allows evaluation of the acromioclavicular joint and distal clavicle. Acromioclavicular joint separations are most accurately assessed by weight-bearing stress views (Figure 10.19).

Routine radiographs of the glenohumeral

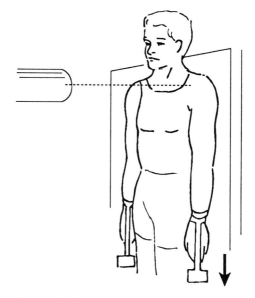

Figure 10.19. Stress (weight-bearing) views to assess acromioclavicular joint separations.

joint should include biplane views of the proximal humerus as well as the glenoid itself. A "true anteroposterior" (Figure 10.20*A* and *B*) (Grashey view) of the shoulder is taken so that the x-ray beam parallels the face of the glenoid. This eliminates overlap of the humeral head on the glenoid rim. Many so-called anteroposterior radiographs of the shoulder are, in fact, taken with the beam in the sagittal plane and thus perpendicular to the coronal plane of the body. This oblique view of the shoulder joint causes the humeral head to be superimposed on the glenoid, making interpretation of glenohumeral pathology more difficult. These anteroposterior views, taken with the humerus in internal and external rotation, give biplane views of the humerus (Figure 10.20*C* and *D*).

The axillary (Figure 10.21) and outlet (Figure 10.22) views complete the routine radiographic series of the glenohumeral joint. These complete the biplane imaging

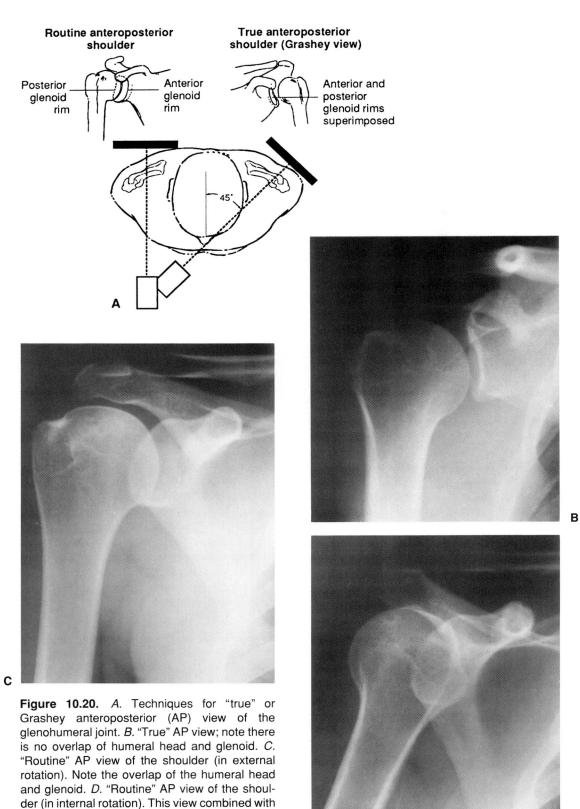

Figure 10.20. *A.* Techniques for "true" or Grashey anteroposterior (AP) view of the glenohumeral joint. *B.* "True" AP view; note there is no overlap of humeral head and glenoid. *C.* "Routine" AP view of the shoulder (in external rotation). Note the overlap of the humeral head and glenoid. *D.* "Routine" AP view of the shoulder (in internal rotation). This view combined with C gives biplane views of the proximal humerus.

Within the figure:

Routine anteroposterior shoulder

Posterior glenoid rim — Anterior glenoid rim

True anteroposterior shoulder (Grashey view)

Anterior and posterior glenoid rims superimposed

45°

A

B

C

D

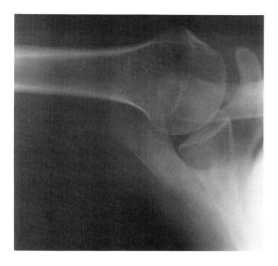

Figure 10.21. Axillary lateral view of shoulder.

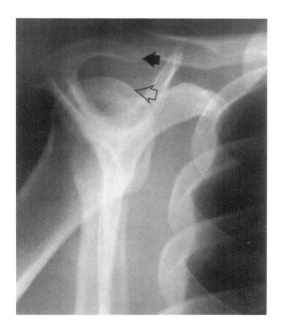

Figure 10.22. Outlet view of the shoulder shows the subacromial space between the acromion (*solid arrow*) and humeral head (*open arrow*).

of the glenoid and scapula, allowing assessment of the subacromial space.

Changes noted on routine views may provide clues to soft-tissue pathology such as rotator cuff tears, impingement syndrome, and other articular abnormalities. The presence of bony eburnation or osteophytes inferior to the acromioclavicular joint should raise the question of impingement or acromioclavicular arthritis. Sclerosis or erosion of the greater tuberosity has been noted in 95% of patients with rotator cuff tears and these changes are often present in patients with impingement. A decrease in the humeroacromial distance (normally 0.8 to 1.0 cm on the external rotation anteroposterior view) is also common in patients with rotator cuff tears. Sclerosis of the inferior surface of the acromion can be seen in patients with impingement or rotator cuff tears. The shoulder impingement syndrome may be suggested by flattening or sclerosis of the greater tuberosity or by bony excrescences arising from the anterior inferior aspect of the acromion.

Arthrography

Shoulder arthrography remains a useful tool in diagnosing full-thickness rotator cuff tears. Double-contrast techniques (radiopaque contrast material and air) provide the most information. The addition of CT to the double-contrast arthrogram (arthro-CT) provides the best technique for assessing the glenoid labrum.

Extravasation of contrast material into the subacromial space on arthrography is diagnostic of a full-thickness rotator cuff tear. Unfortunately, the size of the tear cannot be accurately estimated by arthrography.

Not only can adhesive capsulitis be diagnosed by arthrography (markedly reduced capsular volume), but the procedure may have therapeutic value. The distention of the capsule by contrast material and air, accompanied by the manipulation of the examination, may substantially improve shoulder mobility.

Computed Arthrotomography

Combining double-contrast arthrography with CT will provide valuable additional information. Rotator cuff tears, the size and shape of the labrum, labrum tears, loose bodies, defects in the articular cartilage, adhesive capsulitis and superior labrum anterior and posterior (13) lesions can all be detected. Biceps tendon abnormalities can be difficult to define, but dislocation and rupture of the tendon as well as tenosynovitis may be noted. These defects are better assessed with this technique than with arthrography alone.

Double-contrast arthrotomography is useful in evaluating patients with shoulder instability. Both the Hill-Sachs and Bankart lesions can be seen. Capsular enlargement, loss of demarcation between the subscapular and axillary recesses and defects in the middle and inferior glenohumeral ligaments are all characteristic of anterior shoulder instability and can be detected with this imaging technique.

Certain subtle lesions of the bony and soft-tissue structures will be more easily defined with this method than by any other presently available diagnostic procedure.

Subacromial Bursography

Single- or double-contrast subacromial bursography may help identify partial-thickness tears of the superior surface of the rotator cuff. The size of the bursa is said to be decreased in the presence of an impingement syndrome, and some authors have suggested that a normal bursogram excludes chronic impingement associated with fibrosis. Prior to the description of the outlet view, this technique was used to evaluate the shape of the anterior lip of the acromion. In current practice subacromial bursography is of limited clinical usefulness.

Ultrasonography

Ultrasonographic evaluation of the rotator cuff can reveal full- and partial-thickness rotator cuff tears. The technique is noninvasive, but requires great skill on the part of the ultrasonographer to be of value. The echogenic pattern of tissue changes within a nontorn tendon can mimic those of a small or medium-sized tear. Large full thickness can usually be identified with this technique. Except in the most skilled hands, ultrasonography is inferior to both arthrography and the MRI in evaluating the rotator cuff.

Magnetic Resonance Imaging

There is considerable disagreement in the orthopedic and radiologic literature regarding the effectiveness of MRI in evaluating the rotator cuff. The radiographic literature suggests that this technique is equal or possibly superior to computed arthrography in assessing the shoulder joint. Numerous reports in the orthopedic literature disagree, pointing out that the MRI falls short of computed arthrography in assessing the rotator cuff, the labrum, and the articular surfaces. The major advantage of the MRI is that it is noninvasive and it may be helpful in identifying inflammatory changes within the rotator cuff. The disadvantages are that it requires a cooperative patient, is costly, and has been disappointing in revealing a partial- or full-thickness rotator cuff tear. This technique is also less effective than double-contrast arthrotomography in evaluating the shoulder for articular cartilage lesions, loose bodies, and labrum detachments.

At the present time, there is some confusion about the significance of an abnormal signal coming from the substance of the supraspinatus tendon. Double-contrast computed arthrography, bursography, arthroscopy, bursoscopy, and surgical exploration with biopsy have often failed to discover pathology suggested by the MRI. A complete understanding of the significance of these signals remains a mystery. The MRI seldom reveals pathology that was not suspected or demonstrated by the history, physical examination, and plain radiographs.

Arthroscopy

The history and physical examination are at the core of accurate diagnosis of shoulder injuries. Arthroscopy is a powerful tool in confirming diagnosis and is most exciting as techniques of minimally invasive surgery evolve. Because shoulder arthroscopy is both expensive and invasive, it should be used as a diagnostic technique only when all less invasive means of reaching a diagnosis have been exhausted.

Arthroscopic surgical techniques of subacromial decompression, distal clavicle excision, rotator cuff repair, and shoulder stabilization all continue to evolve. Although technically demanding for the arthroscopist, these procedures facilitate recovery of the patient. The use of arthroscopy for these procedures will steadily decrease the amount of open surgery necessary for athletically related shoulder injuries.

THE CLAVICLE

Fractures

Fractures of the clavicle occur commonly in sports. Because of the characteristic history, the localized tenderness, and the customary deformity, the diagnosis is usually evident on the sideline. In most instances closed treatment is effective, and most clavicle fractures will unite regardless of the treatment used (14,15).

Anatomy

The clavicle is an S-shaped strut that maintains the width of the shoulders. It is anchored medially to the sternum and laterally to the scapula by both capsular and extrascapular ligaments.

There is no generally accepted classification for clavicle fractures, but it should be recognized that the deforming muscle forces are different, depending on whether the fracture is in the proximal, middle, or distal portion of the bone. If the fracture occurs in the medial clavicle, the proximal portion remains affixed to the sternum while the sternocleidomastoid displaces the distal fragment superiorly. When the fracture occurs in the middle third, the sternocleidomastoid pulls the proximal fragment superiorly, while the weight of the arm pulls the distal fragment inferiorly. The displacement of distal fractures depends on whether the fracture is proximal or distal to the coracoclavicular ligaments. If the fracture is proximal to the coracoclavicular ligaments, the distal fragment is displaced inferiorly while the proximal fragment is pulled superiorly by the neck muscles. If the fracture is distal to the coracoclavicular ligaments, the fragments are not significantly displaced unless the ligaments have been disrupted. In this case there may be wide separation at the fracture.

Clinical Case #1

A 17-year-old wide receiver was tackled while attempting to catch a pass. The defender drove his right shoulder into the turf. The other athlete experienced immediate severe pain in the shoulder region. He walked off the field with assistance holding his right arm to his side with the

*left hand. After cautious removal of the shoulder
pads, a deformity and tenderness were obvious
on the midshaft of his clavicle.*

Medical History

Approximately 90% of clavicle fractures
occur following a fall onto the point of
the shoulder with the remainder being divided between a fall onto the outstretched
hand and a direct blow. The mechanism
of injury is the same for fractures of the
proximal, middle, and distal thirds. The
patient presents with a characteristic
mechanism of injury and has often perceived the fracture occurring. There is pain
at the fracture site.

Physical Examination

The athlete with a fractured clavicle
characteristically holds the arm against
the body by supporting the elbow. This
minimizes painful motion at the fracture
site. The visible fracture deformity can be
confirmed by palpation. It is important
to remain alert so as not to miss a
posterior sternoclavicular dislocation or a
minimally displaced fracture of the lateral
clavicle.

The brachial plexus lies immediately
beneath the clavicle. It seems surprising
that more neurovascular injuries do not occur with this common fracture. Nonetheless, a complete neurovascular examination
is necessary to rule out injuries of the
brachial plexus and adjacent vessels. A
pneumothorax is uncommonly associated
with clavicle fractures.

Radiographic Evaluation

Fractures of the shaft of the clavicle
are best evaluated by an anteroposterior
view with a 45° cephalic tilt. This moves
the projection of the clavicle away from the
rib cage and allows better assessment of

the fracture. A chest x-ray may be helpful
in screening for associated rib fractures or
the uncommon pneumothorax. Fractures
of the distal third of the clavicle can be
evaluated using the acromioclavicular
technique. Axillary views are needed to
assess the horizontal displacement of the
fragments.

Fractures of the medial clavicle may be
difficult to detect on plain x-rays although
the 45° cephalic tilt view can be helpful. If
this fracture is suspected clinically, but cannot be identified on routine radiographs, a
CT scan is indicated.

Treatment

Closed treatment is usually successful in
the treatment of clavicle fractures (14,15).
Comfort and pain relief during healing are
the goals because obtaining and maintaining anatomic alignment by closed means
is difficult if not impossible. Fortunately,
anatomic reduction is not necessary for an
excellent end result with normal pain-free
function. It is generally reasonable to accept
the bump that results from a clavicle fracture. In most instances, a simple sling or a
figure-of-eight dressing is sufficient. The
functional and cosmetic results are comparable between these two treatment methods, and both yield excellent union rates.
Many patients find a simple arm sling is
more comfortable and this avoids the skin
and axillary irritation of a figure-of-eight
harness. Pendulum exercises are begun as
soon as tolerated, with active elevation
above 60° avoided as long as there is pain
or motion at the fracture site. External support is used for 3 to 6 weeks as symptoms
dictate.

There are few indications for open reduction and internal fixation, and surgical
treatment of clavicle fractures is associated
with a high complication rate. It is not uncommon for the scar to be unattractive and

painful. Thus, one must be very cautious about advising surgery for the stated goal of eliminating the bump. The indications for surgical fixation are uncommon, but these include 1) open fractures, 2) polytrauma patients, 3) neurovascular injury that requires early exploration, 4) severe displacement with tenting of the skin, 5) posteriorly displaced fractures of the medial clavicle, and 6) displaced distal clavicle fractures. Fractures of the distal clavicle combined with tears of the coracoclavicular ligaments are associated with a high rate of nonunion and painful dysfunction. It is generally agreed that this fracture should be treated surgically so as to eliminate these problems.

Fortunately, nonunion of clavicle fractures is uncommon, but when it does occur it most often follows refracture, severe trauma, or soft-tissue interposition. Open reduction with internal fixation of nonunions is difficult and has a high complication rate.

Criteria for Return to Sports

The duration of treatment depends primarily on the amount of displacement and the location of the fracture. As is usually the case, the athlete should not return to sports and athletics until the fracture is radiographically healed and nontender, and the athlete has a full, painless range of motion and normal strength. For noncontact sports, this usually requires at least 6 weeks. The contact in collision sports places the clavicle at risk for refracture and should be avoided until the union is solid, which often takes 2 to 4 months. Following union, no special bracing is necessary.

Osteolysis of the Distal Clavicle

Osteolysis of the distal clavicle is characterized by pain, resorption of bone, and de-struction of the clavicular surface of the acromioclavicular joint. The acromial side of the joint is generally preserved. This osteolysis seems to be an atypical response to trivial or significant acromioclavicular trauma or repetitive overuse. It may be precipitated by a single, seemingly minor, or unremembered injury or by more violent trauma with disruption of the acromioclavicular joint.

The sports traditionally associated with osteolysis of the distal clavicle are judo (thought secondary to repetitive falling), softball pitching (thought secondary to the windmill type action), and weight training with repetitive overhead lifting. Although reported in female athletes, this condition occurs predominantly in men.

There is controversy about the exact pathology of this osteolysis. Aseptic necrosis of the distal clavicle is the most widely supported causative theory. Evidence against the avascular necrosis theory is the observation that there is increased isotopic uptake with a bone scan. It has thus been suggested that the underlying etiology is a subchondral stress fracture. It may be that both stress fractures and avascular necrosis are part of the pathology, but it is difficult to know which preceded the other because each can lead to the other. A third suggested etiology is that acromioclavicular synovitis is the primary underlying cause. Biopsies have revealed vascular proliferation and vilus hypertrophy of the synovium in many cases, but in others there are no synovial changes.

Although the etiology of this condition remains obscure, its identification and treatment are reasonably straightforward.

Medical History

With careful questioning, the examiner can usually elicit some form of shoulder trauma as the inciting incident. This is most commonly a direct blow to the point of the shoulder, which caused moderate to severe initial pain, but cleared spontaneously. The fact that most competitive athletes can recall some type of mild shoulder injury during training and competition makes the significance of this historical finding uncertain. The onset may be insidious with the pain being aggravated after bench pressing, dips, push-ups, or doing the military press. Most athletes with this condition participate in weight training at least three times a week and present with pain over the distal clavicle and restricted motion of the shoulder.

Physical Examination

There is usually no obvious deformity, and the color and temperature of the skin is normal. Point tenderness over the distal clavicle and acromioclavicular joint are characteristic. Cross-chest adduction and other maneuvers that stress the acromioclavicular joint generally cause pain (see Figure 10.26). There is often crepitus of the acromioclavicular joint and ballottement of the acromioclavicular joint usually causes pain. Selective injection of 1 to 2 mL of local anesthetic into the acromioclavicular joint will usually alleviate these symptoms.

Radiographic Evaluation

The mainstay of diagnosis of this condition is the plain anteroposterior x-ray. Demineralization of the distal clavicle, with loss of the subarticular cortex, is characteristic. Cystic erosions on the clavicular side of the acromioclavicular joint are often present. As the osteolysis of the distal clavicle progresses, there is an apparent widening of the acromioclavicular joint space. Frequently, the symptoms of osteolysis may precede the radiologic changes, and repeat radiographs should be taken if symptoms persist.

Acromioclavicular views of the shoulder are necessary for adequate visualization of the distal clavicle. A misdiagnosis can be made because the distal clavicle and acromion are washed out with routine shoulder views.

Treatment

The treatment options are basically two. The first is nonoperative and consists of avoiding the aggravating activity. The second is surgical excision of the distal clavicle.

The natural history of untreated osteolysis of the distal clavicle is poorly described in the literature. Some articles have suggested a self-limiting course of 1 to 2 years, whereas others suggest persistent symptoms if this condition is treated nonoperatively. Most athletes are unwilling to pursue a lengthy nonoperative course with no assurance that this will lead to resolution of the problem. Nonetheless, a nonoperative program should be used for as long as the patient will comply. A short period of sling immobilization may be used, and nonsteroidal anti-inflammatory drugs (NSAIDs) are prescribed. The response to this program is variable and it seldom produces the desired result in competitive athletes. Seasonal relief can usually be obtained by alternating between the training program and rest periods. Elimination of weight training is often necessary. Intra-articular corticosteroid injections usually fail to provide long-term benefit, and some have suggested that the catabolic effect of the corticosteroids may accelerate the osteolytic process.

The patient will eventually indicate when this program is unacceptable, at which time surgical excision of the distal clavicle is undertaken. Most competitive athletes prefer the surgical alternative because it offers a faster and more certain resolution to their symptoms. The surgery may be performed arthroscopically or via open techniques.

Postoperatively, a weight-training program is continued for the other three extremities, and light weight training on the involved shoulder is begun at 3 weeks. More aggressive training is resumed at 6 weeks, and preinjury strength has usually recovered by 8 weeks. Sports participation should be curtailed until the patient has regained full motion and normal strength, and the pain has subsided.

THE SCAPULA

Fractures

Fractures of the scapula are uncommon. Although these fractures are usually the result of severe high-speed trauma, they can occur in sports following a fall. For the most part, the critical determinant of treatment is whether or not the fracture extends into the glenoid. As a general rule, fractures that are extra-articular are treated nonoperatively, and those involving the glenoid are treated surgically (16,17).

Anatomy

The broad, flat scapula is enveloped by multiple layers of muscles that provide a protective cushion for the scapula. This helps explain the low incidence of fracture. The rich vascular supply of this muscular envelope provides excellent circulation for fracture healing.

The scapula arises from several separate ossification centers that coalesce during embryologic development and early childhood. The acromion is a coalescence of two or three ossification centers that appear in early adolescence, but often do not fuse

until mid twenties. In approximately 5% of patients, the anterior acromion ossification center fails to fuse to the scapular spine, giving rise to an os acrominale. This apophyseal growth plate is evident on the axillary radiograph and should not be mistaken for a fracture of the acromion (Figure 10.23). Interestingly enough, there is an increased incidence of rotator cuff tears in patients who have an os acrominale.

Medical History

Direct blows, such as falling on the scapula, can be forceful enough to fracture the scapula. Glenoid fractures can occur during a violent glenohumeral dislocation. Patients who have fractures of the acromion will complain of localized pain. The pain from fractures of the coracoid, glenoid, spine, neck, or body of the scapula is less precise. The athlete is often unable to localize the vague, deep-seated pain and may even report anterior chest wall discomfort.

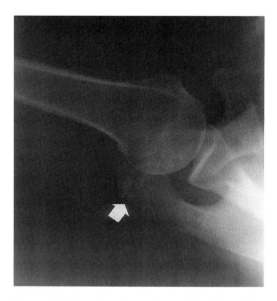

Figure 10.23. Apophyseal growth plate of the acromion, not to be mistaken for a fracture.

Physical Examination

Because abduction is usually painful, the athlete will hold the arm adducted against the side and protect the shoulder against all movement. There is seldom deformity, ecchymosis, or skin temperature change. Marked local tenderness is present if the fracture involves a subcutaneous portion of the scapula. The tenderness is not well localized if the fracture involves the glenoid, neck, or body of the scapula. Pain with deep inspiration is due to the pull of the serratus and pectoralis minor muscles. Resisted function of the rotator cuff or other muscles that attach to the scapula causes pain.

Radiographic Evaluation

A true anteroposterior view of the scapula (Grashey) (see Figure 10.20A and B) combined with an axillary (see Figure 10.21) and a true lateral (see Figure 10.22) of the scapula will adequately demonstrate most scapula fractures. In young adults, it may be helpful to obtain films of the contralateral shoulder if there is difficulty distinguishing between a fracture and an unfused apophysis.

When evaluating the athlete with a glenoid rim fracture, it is important to determine whether or not there is instability of the glenohumeral joint. The athlete does not always relate a history of instability, and careful questioning by the physician is necessary.

Treatment

Unless excessively displaced, extra-articular fractures of the scapula are generally treated nonoperatively. Intra-articular fractures, especially those associated with glenohumeral instability, are usually managed operatively.

Extra-articular Fractures

Because of the rich vascular supply provided by the surrounding muscular envelope, scapula fractures generally heal rapidly and completely. This envelope also provides some support to the scapula, and it is uncommon for the fracture to displace more than the displacement evident at the time of the original injury. The most common type of scapula fracture is that of the body. These fractures heal and apparent malunion is rarely associated with clinical symptoms. Scapula body fractures are treated symptomatically and nonoperatively with range of motion exercises instituted as soon as symptoms permit.

Fractures of the acromion are uncommon, and the physician must distinguish a minimally displaced or nondisplaced fracture from an os acrominale. The shoulder outlet view can be helpful in evaluating the subacromial interval. Solid osseous union is the rule for acromion fractures, and nonoperative treatment of the symptoms is preferred.

Treatment of coracoid fractures depends on the integrity of the acromioclavicular joint. If the acromioclavicular joint is intact, the coracoid fracture is stable. Symptomatic treatment with an arm sling is sufficient. Range of motion exercises are encouraged as soon as symptoms permit. Strengthening exercises of the muscles that attach to the coracoid are deferred for 4 to 6 weeks following the injury. Coracoid fractures associated with acromioclavicular dislocations are unstable and usually displaced. Open reduction with internal fixation is indicated.

Intra-articular Fractures

Most authors base their treatment recommendations of glenoid fractures on the presence or absence of shoulder instability.

Good functional results are reported with significantly displaced intra-articular glenoid fractures that were not associated with instability. Shoulder instability in combination with a glenoid fracture is an indication for open reduction and internal fixation.

Criteria for Return to Sports

The athlete with a scapula fracture that has been treated nonoperatively may return to sports following return of a full, painless range of motion and normal strength. This is usually 6 to 10 weeks. Following open reduction and internal fixation, the athlete should wait for fracture healing, full and painless range of motion, and restoration of normal strength. This normally requires 8 to 12 weeks.

"Snapping" Scapula

"Snapping" scapula refers to a variety of periscapular, bursal, ligamentous, muscular, and bony abnormalities that cause a snapping sensation in the scapulothoracic articulation. This may or may not be painful. In the absence of skeletal abnormalities, such as an osteochondroma or an exostosis, this can be a perplexing problem. The diagnosis may be difficult to discover, and at best the treatment is imprecise.

In the case of a specific skeletal abnormality, such as a scapular exostosis that bumps over the ribs, the problem is easily diagnosed and the treatment noncontroversial. Surgical excision is recommended.

Most cases of snapping scapula are due to abnormalities of the soft tissues interposed between the scapula and the rib cage. A variety of fibrous bands and flaps have been described although surgical exploration has often failed to discover these abnormalities.

Enlargement of a bursa, particularly at the inferior angle of the scapula, has been proposed as a cause of scapular snapping, as well as scapulothoracic pain with throwing. O'Donoghue suggested that inflammation of the bursa between the serratus anterior and the chest wall was the source of pain and crepitus.

Medical History

Symptomatic snapping of the scapula most commonly occurs in the dominant shoulder of young adults involved in throwing sports. The snapping may or may not be painful, and if present, usually occurs during the early and late cocking phases of throwing. The pain, if present, is alleviated at follow-through.

Physical Examination

Careful palpation during the maneuver that causes the snapping will usually distinguish bony incongruities from a soft-tissue etiology. Long thoracic nerve function must be assessed. Scapulothoracic bursitis is most common at the inferior medial angle of the scapula although it may occur at the superior medial angle as well.

Radiographic Evaluation

Routine scapular radiographs are usually normal. A true lateral x-ray of the scapula is crucial to identify a subscapular exostosis. Comparison views of the contralateral shoulder are often helpful, and CT scans are sometimes necessary to identify skeletal irregularities on the scapula or the ribs.

Treatment

Scapular or costal exostoses can be excised with good results. The treatment is more difficult if no skeletal abnormality is identified. Reassurance is appropriate if the snapping is painless. Periscapular strengthening exercises will sometimes decrease the snapping and pain.

Corticosteroid injection into a palpable bursa at the angle of the scapula can affect symptomatic relief. Rest, ice, physical therapy modalities, as well as stretching, strengthening, and anti-inflammatory medications have met with variable success. Corticosteroid injection seems to be slightly more effective than phonophoresis or ionophoresis in treating bursitis. In the extreme circumstance, the offending portion of the scapula can be excised, but this is a large procedure and is often met with disappointing results. Arthroscopic excision of the subscapular bursa has recently been described and, in the future, may offer a less invasive surgical technique for recalcitrant cases.

THE STERNOCLAVICULAR JOINT

The sternoclavicular joint is one of the least commonly injured joints in the body with acute dislocations accounting for only 3% of all dislocations around the shoulder. These injuries are important, however, because posterior dislocations of the sternoclavicular joint are potentially life-threatening (18,19).

Subluxations and Dislocations

Sternoclavicular joint subluxations and dislocations are classified according to the anatomic location of the dislocated medial clavicle with respect to the sternum. Anterior subluxations and dislocations occur 10 to 20 times more commonly than posterior dislocations although the later are potentially more severe and can be life-threatening. If the clavicle is displaced posteriorly, pressure may be placed on the trachea and other adjacent structures. Sometimes these patients have an airway obstruction and are unable to talk. If the athlete is wearing shoulder pads, the deformity is not immediately evident, but this diagnosis should be considered whenever an acute airway obstruction occurs during contact athletics.

Anatomy

The sternoclavicular joint is a true diarthrodial joint and the only actual articulation between the upper limb and the axial skeleton. Interestingly, the opposing joint surfaces are relatively incongruent, and this joint has the smallest bone-to-bone contact of any of the major joints in the body. It relies on a dense set of ligaments for most of its stability. In addition to the sternoclavicular ligaments, the joint is supported by a short, strong costoclavicular ligament between the proximal clavicle and the first rib. Because of these strong ligaments traumatic dislocations of the sternoclavicular joint occur only after significant direct or indirect forces have been applied to the shoulder.

The medial epiphysis of the clavicle is the last of the long bone epiphyses to appear and to close. The medial clavicular epiphysis ossifies in the late teens and does not close until the mid to late twenties. Some of the so-called sternoclavicular dislocations in this age group are in fact fractures through the unfused physeal plate. These injuries should always be suspected in the case of injuries to the proximal clavicle and sternoclavicular joint in young adults.

Medical History

A fall onto the point of the shoulder or a direct blow to the chest can cause a dislocation of the sternoclavicular joint. Most sternoclavicular dislocations follow the indirect mechanism, such as when a force is applied to the lateral aspect of the shoulder. As the shoulder is compressed centrally, the proximal clavicle dislocates anteriorly. This injury can occur when the player falls to the ground landing on the shoulder or when the player is crushed side to side in a pileup. Posterior dislocations are likely to occur when a blow is applied to the posterior aspect of the flexed shoulder and the proximal end of the clavicle is driven posteriorly. Similarly, an anterior dislocation may occur when the anterior aspect of the shoulder is struck with the shoulder in extension, causing the medial clavicle to lever anteriorly.

The direct injury occurs when force is applied to the anteromedial aspect of the clavicle. This pushes the medial clavicle posteriorly behind the sternum and into the mediastinum. These dislocations can occur when the athlete is kicked or struck by another player, or after a fall onto a stationary object.

The patient complains of localized anterior chest pain with both anterior and posterior dislocations. If the posteriorly dislocated clavicle compresses the trachea, the patient may have difficulty talking and display other signs of airway obstruction.

In older athletes, particularly those participating in racquet sports, it is not uncommon for atraumatic anterior subluxation of the sternoclavicular joint to develop, possibly related to repetitive stresses on an aging ligament complex. In these athletes, pain and swelling over the sternoclavicular joint develop atraumatically as the clavicle subluxes anteriorly.

Physical Examination

In a mild to moderate sprain, the only physical findings will be local swelling and tenderness directly over the sternoclavicular joint. No deformity is present. All movements of the arm will cause localized pain.

The deformity of a sternoclavicular dislo-

cation is usually apparent by inspection and palpation. All shoulder movement causes pain, and axial compression of the shoulders is particularly painful. The head is usually tilted toward the side of the dislocated joint, and the discomfort is often exaggerated when the patient lies supine. In the case of an anterior dislocation, the medial clavicle is prominent anterior to the manubrium (Figure 10.24).

Posterior dislocations of the sternoclavicular joint can be more difficult to diagnose. There is a palpable defect immediately lateral to the manubrium in the area vacated by the medial clavicle and the articular corner of the sternum is more easily palpated than on the normal side. This is sometimes difficult to detect in the muscular athlete. The symptoms associated with posterior dislocation can be more severe. The posteriorly displaced clavicle can put pressure on the superior mediastinal vessels, causing venous congestion or arterial compression of the vessels to the arm and head. Of greater immediate consequence is that the clavicle can compress the trachea, causing airway obstruction.

Radiographic Evaluation

Although the distinction between an anterior and posterior sternoclavicular dislocation is usually evident by physical examination, the amount and direction of displacement can be confirmed by radiography. Radiographs of this region can be difficult to obtain and interpret. A variety of special projections may help determine the exact relationship between the medial clavicle and the sternum. The most popular view is the one described by Hobbs (see Figure 10.18).

The CT scan is the best technique for evaluating suspected injuries to the sternoclavicular joint. The patient is placed supine in the CT gantry, and the scan in-

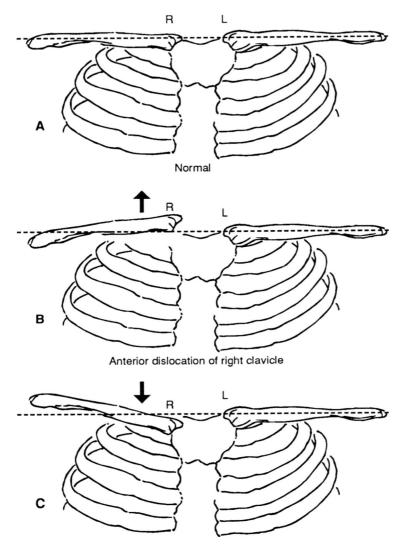

R   L

A

Normal

B

Anterior dislocation of right clavicle

C

Posterior dislocation of right clavicle

Figure 10.24. Schematic representation of the sterno-clavicular joint. *A.* Normal. *B.* Anteriorly dislocated clavicle. *C.* Posteriorly dislocated clavicle.

cludes both sternoclavicular joints so that a direct comparison between the normal and abnormal sides can be made. This scan is especially helpful in diagnosing fractures of the physeal plate.

Treatment

The mild to moderate sprains are treated symptomatically with rest, ice, and analgesics. Patients will usually obtain relief with the use of an arm sling or a figure-of-eight bandage combined with an arm sling.

Anterior dislocations of the sterno-clavicular joint are usually easy to reduce. The patient is placed supine, and a 5- to 6-in pad is placed between the shoulder blades. Pressure is applied directly over the anteriorly displaced medial clavicle. Although reduction is easy, it is often difficult to maintain. If the reduction is stable, the patient can be immobilized for 6 weeks in a figure-of-eight dressing. If the reduction remains unstable, a sling is prescribed for 2 weeks and the patient encouraged to begin range of motion exercises as soon as comfort permits. The patient should be informed that a permanent bump will be present on the front of the chest. The alternative is surgical reconstruction, which is hazardous and often associated with a poor result.

A posterior sternoclavicular dislocation can be a life-threatening injury. Immediate reduction is often necessary to relieve airway obstruction. This can be done by placing a firm object such as a football, a helmet, or the physician's knee between the scapulae and pulling backward on both shoulders simultaneously. This will cause the proximal end of the clavicle to displace anteriorly, thus relieving pressure on the vital mediastinal structures. If this maneuver is unsuccessful, the anterior clavicle may be pulled forward with a towel clip. Once reduced, the joint is usually stable, and reduction can be maintained by a figure-of-eight dressing. If closed reduction cannot be obtained and maintained, operative intervention may be indicated. Many adult patients do not tolerate significant posterior displacement of the medial clavicle and surgery must be considered even though it is associated with a high complication rate.

If airway obstruction does not exist, the posterior dislocation should not be reduced until the mediastinal structures have been evaluated. If the clinical and radiographic evaluations suggest vascular injury or mediastinal bleeding, it is wise to obtain an arteriogram before reduction. Cases have been reported in which the clavicle impaled one of the major vessels, and because the clavicle remained within the vessel, the bleeding was reduced. Had the injury not been suspected, a closed reduction would

have opened the dike to exsanguination.

The treatment of physeal injuries to the medial clavicle is similar to that described for anterior and posterior dislocations. Residual deformity is usually less with physeal injuries because of the capacity for remodeling.

Criteria for Return to Sports

Following a mild to moderate sprain the athlete may return to sports and athletics after regaining a full, painless range of motion and normal strength. This normally occurs within 1 to 2 weeks. If the joint has been subluxated or dislocated anteriorly, contact sports should be avoided for approximately 6 to 8 weeks until the supporting structures have consolidated. Noncontact sports may be resumed as symptoms permit, which is usually approximately 4 weeks.

After a posterior dislocation, return to contact sports should be delayed for 10 to 12 weeks to allow adequate soft-tissue healing. The complications associated with chronic or recurrent posterior dislocations are so severe that complete ligament healing must be ensured before return to risky activities.

Following a physeal fracture noncontact sports can be begun at 6 weeks or when the athlete has regained full, painless range of motion and the fracture site is no longer tender. Contact sports should be avoided for an additional 4 to 6 weeks to allow remodeling and strengthening of the medial clavicle.

THE ACROMIOCLAVICULAR JOINT

Acute Injuries

Injuries of the acromioclavicular region are common in sports. In fact, one of the earliest reported cases of acromioclavicular dislocation was that of Galen who diagnosed his own acromioclavicular dislocation, which he sustained while wrestling in the Palaestra.

There is considerable controversy regarding the treatment of acromioclavicular dislocations. Urist likened the use of surgery in this injury to shooting a dove with an elephant gun. This admonition not withstanding, dozens of surgical procedures have been described (20–23).

Traditional teaching holds that a grade I acromioclavicular injury is a partial tearing of the acromioclavicular ligament with no displacement of the acromioclavicular joint. A grade II sprain is said to occur when the acromioclavicular ligaments are completely torn, the coracoclavicular ligaments are incompletely damaged, and the acromioclavicular joint is subluxated on stress radiographs. A grade III sprain or acromioclavicular dislocation is associated with complete disruption of both the acromioclavicular and the coracoclavicular ligaments. Many physicians further subdivided the grade III injuries in their own minds, but this classification was not formalized until Rockwood's classification was introduced in 1984. In the grade IV injury, the clavicle is displaced posteriorly into or through the trapezius. A grade V is an exaggeration of the grade III with severe vertical displacement of the clavicle with respect to the scapula. In the grade VI injury, the clavicle is dislocated inferiorly into either the subacromial or subcoracoid position (Figure 10.25).

Anatomy

The acromioclavicular joint is a true diarthrodial joint between the distal clavicle and the medial edge of the acromion. The horizontally directed fibers of the acromioclavicular ligaments, in combination with the attached muscles, control the horizontal stability of the joint. Anterior, posterior, or rotational displacement may occur if these ligaments are divided. Unlike the sternoclavicular joint, the capsule surrounding the acromioclavicular joint provides relatively little support against superior displacement of the distal clavicle.

Vertical stability is controlled by the two vertically directed coracoclavicular ligaments, the conoid and the trapezoid. The entire upper limb is suspended from the clavicle by these two ligaments.

Acromioclavicular dislocations, such as seen in the grade III to VI injuries, occur following disruption of both the acromioclavicular and coracoclavicular ligaments. The severe displacement observed in the grade V injuries results when significant muscle stripping of the deltoid and trapezius from the distal clavicle is added to the ligament disruptions.

Clinical Case #2

A high school wrestler comes to your office complaining of pain in his left shoulder. Yesterday he was thrown to the mat by another wrestler and his shoulder was the point of contact. He was unable to continue competing. Your exam reveals tenderness over his left acromioclavicular joint and pain when attempting to cross over his left hand to his right shoulder.

Medical History

The acromioclavicular joint is most commonly injured when a person falls onto the point of the shoulder. The direct pressure onto the acromion drives the scapula downward. The clavicle moves with the scapula until it strikes the first rib at which time the clavicle stops moving. If the forces continue, the acromioclavicular and subsequently the coracoclavicular ligaments

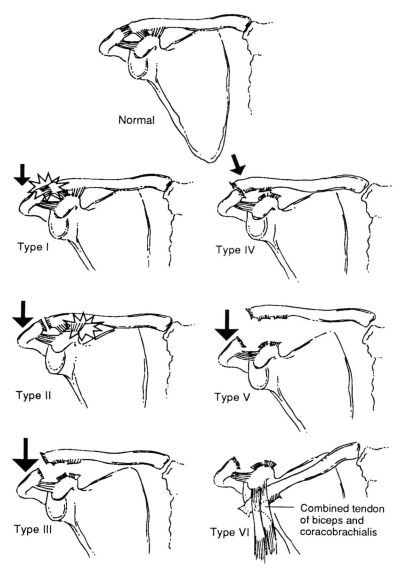

Figure 10.25. Schematic representation of ligamentous injuries of the acromioclavicular joint (see text).

Normal

Type I

Type II

Type III

Type IV

Type V

Type VI — Combined tendon of biceps and coracobrachialis

may be ruptured, leading to a subluxation or dislocation of the acromioclavicular joint. Less commonly, the acromioclavicular joint can be injured as a result of a fall onto the outstretched hand, in which case the force is transmitted up the arm, causing shear stress on the acromiocla-

vicular ligaments. This mechanism can produce a grade I or grade II acromioclavicular injury because the coracoclavicular ligaments are rarely injured with this mechanism.

The athlete with this injury complains of local pain that is aggravated by all movements of the shoulder. Frequently the grade II injuries are more painful than those of higher grades.

Physical Examination

As in other extremity injuries, the patient will have point tenderness directly over the injured structures. A meticulous examination of the shoulder should give considerable insight as to the exact pathology. The acromion, distal clavicle, acromioclavicular joint, and coracoclavicular interval should be carefully palpated for tenderness.

The patient should be examined in the standing or sitting position with the arm hanging free. Gentle downward stress on the arm will exaggerate the deformity. Although the injury is classified by the appearance of the stress radiographs, the degree of elevation of the distal clavicle gives some indication as to the amount of muscle injury and stripping. All shoulder motion will produce localized pain. Pain with the "crossover" test is typical in acromioclavicular separations (Figure 10.26).

Manual manipulation of the distal clavicle will reveal excessive motion in both the

horizontal and vertical planes. In the grade I and grade II injuries, the deformity may not be evident, especially in the muscular athlete. The diagnosis is made by the location of tenderness and the amount of displacement discovered on the stress radiographs.

The patient with a grade III injury characteristically supports the elbow so as to elevate the arm and reduce the acromioclavicular displacement. The distal clavicle is prominent, and there is tenderness at both the acromioclavicular joint and coracoclavicular interval. The distal clavicle is unstable, both horizontally and vertically. In the grade IV injury, the distal clavicle is palpated posteriorly. Pain with movement is often severe. The vertical displacement is often less noticeable than in the grade III injuries because the distal clavicle is held down by the trapezius muscle through which it has buttonholed. The skin may be tented posteriorly.

The grade V injury is easy to diagnose because of the exaggerated elevation of the distal clavicle. One gets the feeling that the major restraining tissue for this injury is the skin. The exaggerated upper displacement is the result of elevation of the distal clavicle and the downward displacement of the scapula because of the weight of the arm. This displacement occurs because of the extensive muscle stripping from the distal clavicle.

The grade VI injury is extremely uncommon and is suspected when the medial side of the acromion is excessively prominent.

Except for the grade I injuries in which there is no displacement, inspection reveals elevation of the distal clavicle. This can be accentuated by pulling the arm downward. The degree of elevation of the distal clavicle gives an indication of the amount of associated muscle injury and stripping. As a general rule, the greater degree of elevation, the

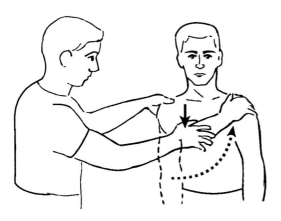

Figure 10.26. "Crossover" test.

greater amount of tissue injury. Palpation confirms tenderness directly over the injured structures and gives an indication of the degree of involvement of the acromioclavicular and coracoclavicular ligaments. The crossover test helps evaluate the acromioclavicular joint (see Figure 10.26).

Radiographic Evaluation

Radiographs of the acromioclavicular joint, which use routine shoulder techniques, will overpenetrate this joint, making it difficult, if not impossible, to discover small fractures and subtle displacements. Specific x-rays of the acromioclavicular joint should be requested so that the radiographer can use the appropriate technique.

Three views should be routinely obtained. These are an anteroposterior view with the patient standing or sitting, a lateral, and an anteroposterior stress view (see Figure 10.19). Comparative views of the contralateral shoulder may need to be taken to allow direct comparison of the acromioclavicular joint anatomy and comparative measurements of the coracoclavicular interspace.

Lateral x-rays are necessary. The importance of biplane imaging in evaluating radiographs is an established concept. The axillary view should be taken of both the injured and the contralateral side. This will reveal the anterior or posterior displacement of the clavicle with respect to the acromion. On some occasions, this is only an abnormal view of the grade IV injuries.

The importance of stress positioning cannot be overemphasized. Subluxations and dislocations may be reduced if the patient lies supine, and a dislocation may appear to be a subluxation unless weights are suspended from the wrists. A 10-lb weight should be strapped to both wrists rather than held by the patient because the in-

creased muscular effort required to hold the weight may mask the degree of displacement. Stress films are necessary to accurately evaluate and categorize the degree of displacement.

The radiographic findings in the grade I injury are essentially normal. The findings in the grade II injury reveal widening or subluxation of the acromioclavicular joint. The coracoclavicular interval measures the same bilaterally.

In the grade III injuries, the acromioclavicular joint is dislocated and the coracoclavicular interval is widened. The normal interval between the superior surface of the coracoid and the inferior surface of the clavicle is 1.1 to 1.3 cm. This interval should be compared to the contralateral normal side. If the interval is increased by 25% to 100%, a grade III injury is diagnosed. The most striking feature of the grade IV injuries is posterior displacement of the distal clavicle as seen on the axillary x-ray. The characteristic finding in a grade V injury is extreme elevation of the distal clavicle with the coracoclavicular interval being two to three times the normal width. The grade VI injury is diagnosed because the distal clavicle is inferior to the acromion.

Treatment

Management of acromioclavicular joint injuries depends on the degree of ligament injury. A grade I (no displacement) or grade II (subluxation) injury of the acromioclavicular joint is best treated with analgesics and an arm sling until the symptoms subside. Range of motion exercises are begun as soon as the patient tolerates them and similarly strengthening exercises are begun promptly. Resumption of activity is usually permissible within 1 to 3 weeks.

Several recent reports have suggested that untreated or undertreated grade I and grade II injuries may lead to chronic acromioclavicular pain and posttraumatic arthritis (22). The medical literature describes more than 35 forms of nonoperative treatment with the duration of treatment varying from 2 to 3 days to 2 to 3 months. Symptomatic treatment with early mobilization is generally recommended for most grade I and grade II injuries. If symptomatic posttraumatic arthritis or symptomatic osteolysis of the distal clavicle occur, the patient can be effectively treated by excision of the distal clavicle (23).

The greatest controversy concerns the treatment of grade III injuries. Both operative and nonoperative intervention have strong and vocal advocates. A whole host of splints, straps, and surgical procedures have been designed, and the recommended length of treatment varies from several days to several months. Comparative studies have shown little difference in the long-term functional results in patients treated operatively as compared to those treated nonoperatively.

Numerous methods of nonoperative treatment have been described. The two most popular methods are closed reduction with application of a sling or harness to maintain reduction for 10 to 12 weeks versus "skillful neglect." Such devices as the Kenny Howard splint will elevate the elbow and pull down on the distal clavicle so as to obtain and maintain reduction. These harnesses have been associated with skin breakdown because of the pressure and time needed to maintain reduction. Immobilization is necessary until ligament strength is sufficient to hold this position. The second method is short-term sling immobilization followed by early range of motion exercises and resumption of activities as motion, strength, and pain permit. This program of "skillful neglect" is increasingly popular. The convenience,

shorter rehabilitation time, and general dissatisfaction with surgical reconstruction have led more and more physicians to treat grade III injuries with this method. Athletes treated in this manner can often be back to competition within several weeks, and there are few reported cases of injury aggravation.

Surgical alternatives include open reduction with internal stabilization during the time of ligament healing. The acromioclavicular complex can be stabilized by transarticular acromioclavicular pins, by fixing the coracoid to the clavicle with a screw or loop, by excising the distal clavicle, or by dynamic muscle transfers. Of these methods, the coracoclavicular stabilization is more popular and predictable.

Excision of the distal clavicle so as to avoid the complication of posttraumatic arthritis is advocated by some. This procedure is not done in isolation, but in combination with one of the stabilization procedures.

The high-performance throwing athlete falls into a special category. Although normal motion and strength are reported following the nonoperative treatment of acromioclavicular dislocations, the issue of muscle fatigability has not been addressed in the literature. It seems logical that surgical reconstruction of the coracoclavicular ligaments and restoration of the acromioclavicular complex would be beneficial in the restoration of synchronous scapulothoracic motion. Operative reduction with coracoclavicular ligament repair and reconstruction should be considered for high-caliber throwing athletes who have a grade III acromioclavicular dislocation.

Grades IV, V, and VI injuries are generally treated surgically. Without surgery the grade V injuries are often associated with persistent deformity, weakness, and discomfort, and it is beneficial to restore normal scapuloclavicular relationships. Although not supported by scientific documentation, the trend in clinical practice is to operate on acromioclavicular disruptions that involve extensive soft-tissue avulsions.

Criteria for Return to Athletics

The athlete must have regained full motion, be relatively pain free, and have normal strength. This usually takes 1 to 2 weeks in grade I injury, 2 to 3 weeks in grade II injury, and 3 to 4 weeks in grade III injury. The absence of pain on the crossover test (see Figure 10.26) as well as normal deltoid strength in this position are good criteria for return to sport.

Acromioclavicular Arthritis

The intra-articular meniscus and articular surfaces can be damaged by a fall onto the point of the shoulder that causes minimal injury to the supporting structures. This type of injury may subsequently lead to posttraumatic degenerative arthritis of the acromioclavicular joint or osteolysis of the distal clavicle.

A common sequela of grade I or II acromioclavicular injuries is the development of posttraumatic arthritis in the acromioclavicular joint. This condition develops when there is residual incongruous contact between the distal clavicle and the acromion and is not seen if the joint remains dislocated, such as in a grade III or grade V injury. Posttraumatic degenerative changes are also seen in osteolysis of the distal clavicle, and it may be impossible to determine whether the arthritic changes preceded the osteolytic changes or vice versa. This debate is of academic importance only since the presentation and effective treatment of these two conditions is the same.

Medical History

Although most patients can recall a specific injury, many cannot. The pain over the top of the shoulder is well localized and aggravated by overhead activity. Powerful movements in front of the body, especially with the bench press, characteristically increase the pain.

Physical Examination

The examination is characterized by point tenderness over the acromioclavicular joint and increased pain with horizontal adduction of the shoulder across the front of the body. Ballottement of the distal clavicle also produces pain.

A diagnostic injection of a local anesthetic directly into the acromioclavicular joint helps clinch the diagnosis. Following the injection, the patient is instructed to perform the exercises that usually cause the pain. Those patients whose pain is confined to the acromioclavicular joint will have relief of symptoms following the diagnostic injection.

Radiographic Evaluation

Although the radiographs are occasionally normal, they usually reveal degenerative changes in the acromioclavicular joint. The joint is often narrowed and sclerotic, with cystic formation on one or both surfaces. Periarticular osteophytes are occasionally present and there may be osteolysis of the distal clavicle.

Treatment

Ice, rest, and anti-inflammatory medications may provide temporary relief, but seldom offer a permanent solution to the problem. Similarly, a corticosteroid injection may provide temporary symptomatic relief. Multiple corticosteroid injections should be avoided. The definitive treatment for this problem is excisional arthroplasty.

SHOULDER INSTABILITY

The glenohumeral joint is noted for its wide range of motion. Bony constraints are minimal, and the surrounding soft-tissue envelope confers stability to the shoulder joint. The capsule, which is reinforced by the glenohumeral ligaments, provides static restraints. The capsule is reinforced by the dynamic forces of the musculotendinous rotator cuff. Should any of these structures be weakened or damaged the shoulder becomes vulnerable to symptomatic instability. During the routine activities of daily living, most shoulder motion occurs in the midrange positions and the supporting structures are not stressed. In sports and athletics power is needed at the extremes of position. The high forces generated by throwing, swimming, weight training, and circumduction can stress the stabilizers to their physiologic limits and thus lead to instability and pain (4,9).

Classification

To be clinically useful, a classification system should give information that helps determine treatment plan and prognosis. Shoulder instability may be classified on the basis of frequency, etiology, direction, and degree of instability.

Shoulder instabilities may be described as initial or recurrent. If the capsule or labrum are damaged with the first dislocation, the patient may subsequently present with recurrent episodes. Chronic dislocations—those that have been dislocated for several days or weeks—are not seen in the sporting population.

Shoulder instability may follow trauma or be secondary to generalized ligamentous laxity. Traumatic instability may be traced to a single event or be the result of the repetitive microtrauma of overuse or abuse. Because some patients are unable to relate the onset of their symptoms to a single traumatic event or to repetitive overuse, they are said to have the atraumatic variety of instability. If the patient has generalized ligamentous laxity, the supporting capsular structures may be inadequate to assist the rotator cuff in maintaining proper glenohumeral alignment.

The instability may be anterior, posterior, or inferior, in which case it is probably multidirectional. Although anterior laxity is the most common type of instability, posterior and multidirectional instabilities are increasingly recognized as a cause of shoulder symptoms. The signs and symptoms of these instabilities are often more subtle than those seen in patients with unidirectional anterior instability. As a general rule, anterior dislocations follow a single traumatic event. This is not to say that all patients with anterior laxity have had such an injury. The cumulative microtrauma associated with repetitive stress can also stretch the capsule and lead to anterior instability, especially in swimmers and throwers. Posterior or multidirectional instability is more commonly associated with multiple submaximal injuries or with patients who have generalized ligamentous laxity.

The articular surfaces may be completely (dislocation) displaced or incompletely (subluxation) separated. During a subluxation the humeral head translates so that it is perched on the rim of the glenoid but it slips back into the glenoid rather than dislocating over the edge. Reduction following an initial dislocation usually requires assistance from medical personnel, whereas most subluxations will reduce spontaneously or with minimal assistance. This provides a clue to the diagnosis. When the athlete reports that the shoulder has "jumped out" but that it "popped back in," the diagnosis is usually a subluxation. This history is uncommon with a first time dislocation. Patients with generalized ligamentous laxity may never actually dislocate the shoulder, but rather present with repeated episodes of subluxations.

The traditional teaching has been that patients who can voluntarily dislocate the shoulders need psychiatric rather than orthopedic treatment. There is increasing recent evidence to show that some patients without underlying psychiatric abnormality can voluntarily demonstrate their instability.

General Medical History

A careful history and physical examination remain the cornerstone of diagnosis in shoulder instability. Patients with the initial traumatic dislocation will usually present to an emergency room for reduction. In contrast, patients with a subluxation or recurrent dislocations often seek help from friends, therapists, or their primary care physician. The patient should describe the position that reproduces the symptoms of instability. Anterior instability becomes symptomatic when the shoulder is abducted, externally rotated, and extended. This position is reproduced when attempting to throw or to reach powerfully overhead, such as with rebounding a basketball.

Posterior instability will often be noted when the shoulder is in 90° of forward flexion and longitudinal pressure is placed along the axis of the arm. This occurs in such activities as the bench press or pass blocking in football (24).

Multidirectional instability may be more subtle with complaints of diffuse aching and laxity especially during or after overhead activities. These patients state the shoulder feels loose and "moves around" with certain activities, especially with ab-

duction, external rotation, and extension, which coincidentally is the position of risk for anterior instability.

General Physical Examination

Instability is a dynamic problem and therefore is best diagnosed by a comprehensive physical examination. Inspection, palpation, range of motion determination, manual muscle test, and assessment of neurologic function are all routine. Specific tests that assess stability are then performed. The shoulder should be stressed in all directions, attempting to elicit apprehension or to reproduce the patient's symptoms. It is this reproduction of symptoms that is most diagnostically accurate in determining the direction or severity of the instability. During stress testing the patient must be relaxed because guarding can interfere with the interpretation of these findings (11,25).

The anterior and posterior drawer tests evaluate the translation of the humeral head on the glenoid (Figure 10.27). In neutral rotation, translation is normally equal in both directions. These tests are best performed with the patient supine and the arm in 60° of abduction and neutral rotation. The examiner supports the elbow in one hand and grasps the proximal humerus in the other. As the shoulder is extended, the humeral head is pulled forward, and similarly as the shoulder is flexed, the humeral head is pushed posteriorly. The amount of translation is identified and the presence of apprehension noted. Translational laxity observed on examination is a normal finding and is of no significance unless it causes pain or apprehension (26).

The sulcus sign test evaluates the superior glenohumeral ligament and the inferior glenohumeral ligament complex (see Fig-

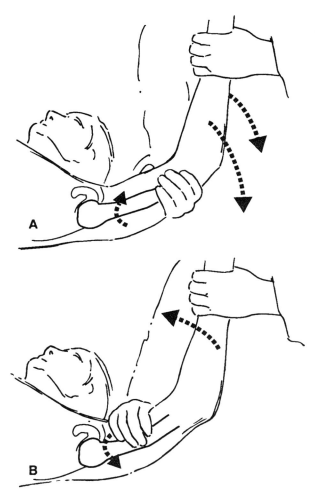

Figure 10.27. Anterior (*A*) and posterior (*B*) drawer tests to evaluate translation of the humeral head.

ure 10.17*C*). Both arms of the standing patient are simultaneously pulled downward and the examiner looks for a sulcus at the inferior margin of the lateral acromion. If positive this test indicates inferior instability and is said to be pathognomic of multidirectional instability. Stress radiographs to demonstrate the sulcus sign can sometimes be helpful.

Both anterior and posterior instability are best assessed clinically by apprehension tests, which are designed to induce anxiety in the patient as the joint is brought into the position associated with instability (see Figure 10.17*A* and *B*). The anterior apprehension test is performed with the arm abducted, externally rotated. The shoulder is gradually extended as the examiner's thumb pushes the humeral head forward. This movement levers the humeral head forward on the glenoid. The posterior stress test is performed with the arm adducted, internally rotated and forward flexed 90°. Pressure is placed along the longitudinal axis of the humerus so as to push the humeral head posteriorly. These tests are positive if the patient becomes apprehensive and resists as the shoulder approaches the position of impending subluxation or dislocation.

The relocation test is also helpful in evaluating for anterior instability (Figure 10.28). The examiner places the hand over the anterior aspect of the shoulder of the supine patient. The humeral head is pushed posteriorly so as to prevent anterior translation of the head. The shoulder is then abducted, externally rotated, and extended into the position associated with apprehension. This test is said to be positive if apprehension is eliminated by holding the humeral head posteriorly. In essence, the

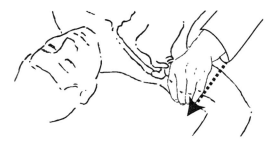

Figure 10.28. The relocation test for anterior instability.

examiner is blocking the anterior translation of the humeral head and resultant subluxation.

Variable results are reported following examination under anesthesia. In some patients without apprehension or instability symptoms, the shoulders are remarkably lax when examined under anesthesia. Similarly, some patients with extreme subluxation symptoms and marked apprehension have seemingly snug shoulders. Evaluations under anesthesia can be misleading and must be interpreted very cautiously.

Anterior laxity is best evaluated by the apprehension, relocation and anterior drawer tests. Posterior instability is often difficult to assess. The posterior drawer test can be negative but should be done because it occasionally provides helpful information. A regular or wall push-up with the position held at maximum push away is sometimes helpful in reproducing the symptoms of posterior instability. The key to multidirectional instability is the presence of inferior laxity which is confirmed by the sulcus sign.

General Radiographic Evaluation

Following an initial dislocation, as with any trauma to the shoulder, a trauma series of radiographs should be obtained. This should be done prior to reduction to document the direction of dislocation and rule out an associated fracture. Prereduction radiographs are not always needed for a recurrent dislocation. The standard series in evaluating shoulder instability should include a true anteroposterior radiograph of the shoulder (Grashey), and a lateral view, which is either an axillary or a transcapular lateral (Y view). The axillary view is the most effective method of determining the position of the humeral head relative to the glenoid fossa and is preferred; but, the lateral scapular view may be used in the patient who does not tolerate the amount of abduction necessary to obtain the axillary view. Postreduction radiographs for both initial and recurrent dislocations are necessary to confirm concentric reduction and rule out a fracture.

For recurrent instability true anteroposterior views with the shoulder in internal and external rotation, as well as an axillary lateral (West Point view) are indicated. These help define the presence and size of a posterolateral humeral head impression fracture (Hill-Sachs lesion).

Arthrography is helpful in evaluating patients over 45 years old, especially if they seem slow to recover after a dislocation. These patients are more likely to have a rotator cuff tear in addition to the dislocation and the arthrogram will help evaluate the torn rotator cuff. CT arthrography can add significant information in confusing cases. Specifically, labral and capsular abnormalities can be identified with this technique. The role of magnetic resonance imaging in such cases has not yet been defined.

General Treatment

Numerous studies have recently confirmed that no single lesion is uniformly responsible for glenohumeral instability. The pathology varies from patient to patient and is different for different degrees and types of instability. Treatment should be directed at the specific pathology for a specific patient. Nonoperative treatment consists of changing the form during athletic activity and performing strengthening exercises. Physical therapy should be directed at improving the strength and tone of the rotator cuff, deltoid, and scapular stabilizers. Surgical intervention may be considered if the nonoperative regimen fails. The rationale for the strengthening program is that the shoulder is at least partially dependent on the muscles for stability. Even if the supporting capsule and ligaments are attenuated the surrounding muscles, if strengthened, can often control the symptoms, especially if they occur only with athletic activity.

As a general rule, patients who have recurrent shoulder subluxations will respond adequately to the appropriate rehabilitation program. The appropriate rehabilitation program for shoulder instability includes balanced strengthening of the rotator cuff and the scapular stabilizers. Adequate internal and external rotation strength is required to provide anterior and posterior stability (4,12).

Traumatic instability in patients under the age of 30 is less often responsive to physical therapy and may require surgery to control the instability. Nonetheless a regular rehabilitation program is more effective than generally reported in the literature. Nontraumatic instability is the most difficult to treat surgically, but fortunately is more responsive to a nonoperative rehabilitation program.

Anterior Glenohumeral Instability

Anterior instability of the glenohumeral joint is the most common of the shoulder instabilities. Approximately 95% of shoulder instabilities are due to anterior displacement of the humeral head either in isolation or in conjunction with another type of laxity.

Dislocation follows complete failure of the restraining structures. Some variation of the Bankart lesion is a prominent feature in up to 65% of patients who have anterior shoulder instability. This most commonly includes avulsion of the capsule and cartilaginous labrum from the anterior portion of the glenoid rim. Less commonly, the capsule and labrum avulse a small piece of bone from the anterior, inferior glenoid rim.

Anterior instability can present in one of four ways: 1) acute anterior dislocation, 2) recurrent anterior dislocation, 3) acute anterior subluxation, and 4) recurrent anterior subluxation.

Acute Anterior Dislocation

Indirect forces are the most common cause of anterior dislocations. The shoulder is placed into an extreme of abduction, external rotation, and extension. Most of the literature fails to emphasize the importance of extension in the production of this injury. Extension is the mechanism that levers the humeral head over the anterior rim of the glenoid.

The diagnosis of anterior dislocation is usually evident on visual inspection and by palpation. The arm is supported by the other hand and held slightly abducted. All movement is painful especially adduction or internal rotation. The humeral head may be visible or palpable anteriorly, and the distal acromion is more prominent yielding a squaring off of the lateral shoulder. The neurovascular examination should be performed both before and after the reduction. The axillary nerve is the most frequently damaged neurologic structure after an anterior dislocation.

Biplane radiographs should be taken to confirm the direction of dislocation and rule out fractures. Radiographs should always be taken after reduction to confirm reduction and evaluate the glenoid and proximal humerus for the possibility of fracture.

A variety of successful reduction maneuvers have been described. Most involve the concept of traction and countertraction originally advocated by Hippocrates (Figure 10.29). Gradual traction is placed on the arm with counter-traction placed against the chest wall. It is important that the countertraction not be placed into the axilla so as not to damage the brachial plexus. The arm is slowly pulled into abduction, forward flexion, and internal rotation. Even with sedation and muscle relaxation it can sometimes be difficult to reduce a shoulder dislocation in a muscular athlete.

If you are present on the field at the time an athlete suffers an anterior shoulder dislocation, it is appropriate to relocate the shoulder prior to transportation of the athlete to the emergency room or clinic. At this time, before the onset of muscle spasm and increasing pain, one gentle attempt at reduction using a traction-countertraction technique is appropriate. This should only

be attempted if you are sure of the diagnosis and comfortable with the technique. The pain spared the athlete will be most appreciated.

With Stimson's method (Figure 10.30), the patient lies prone with the arm hanging off the edge of the table. A 10-lb weight is strapped to the wrist. With gradual sedation and relaxation, the humeral head spontaneously reduces. Some refer to this as the 10-10-10 method because 10 lb of weight are used for 10 minutes after administering 10 mg morphine.

The double-sheet method is performed with the patient supine (Figure 10.31). One sheet is tied around the patient's chest and then secured on the contralateral side to an assistant or the table. A second sheet is wrapped around the physician's waist as he

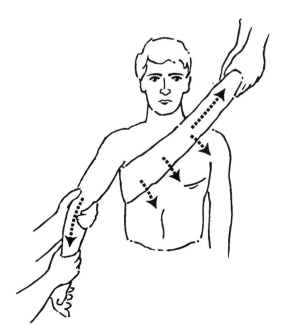

Figure 10.29. Traction-countertraction technique for reduction of an anterior dislocation of glenohumeral joint.

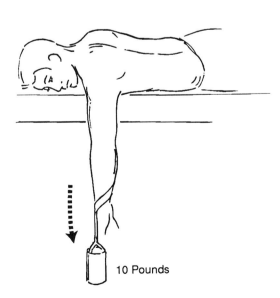

10 Pounds

Figure 10.30. Stimson technique for reduction of an anterior dislocation of the glenohumeral joint.

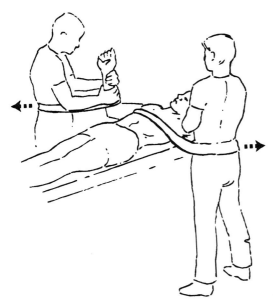

Figure 10.31. Double-sheet technique for reduction of an anterior dislocation of the glenohumeral joint.

or she stands in the axillary region. The elbow is flexed to 90° and placed beneath the sheet around the physician's waist. Traction is applied to the upper limb by the physician leaning backward, and the arm is gently rotated back and forth until the shoulder reduces.

The effect of immobilization and rehabilitation on recurrence rates is controversial. Most authors immobilize young patients who suffered a traumatic anterior dislocation for 3 weeks. This is followed by a rehabilitation program that emphasizes rotator cuff and scapular stabilizer strengthening. Positions of extreme abduction and external rotation are avoided for approximately 3 months, and return to athletics is permitted after this time provided full range of motion and normal strength have returned. A protective harness may be used in sports

that place the athlete at risk of abduction, external rotation, and extension, but is often not well tolerated by the athlete.

In patients over 40 years, the immobilization is discontinued as soon as symptoms subside. The rehabilitation program is begun as soon as possible. If the progress with therapy seems slow, an arthrogram should be obtained to rule out a rotator cuff tear.

Open reduction is necessary for shoulders that cannot be reduced with closed methods. More recently, some authors have suggested early surgery to repair the damaged structures. The role of operative repair following acute dislocation remains controversial. Young, male athletes are at high risk for recurrence. Although the standard of care in most circumstances does not use immediate capsular repair, surgical treatment may be appropriate for selected individuals. In young athletes engaged in throwing or contact sports, early restoration of the disrupted anatomy may provide the best opportunity for continuing the sport without losing more than one season.

The incidence of recurrence following the initial dislocation varies widely, depending on the literature cited (12,27). A large study in the Swedish literature suggests that patients under 22 years of age have a recurrence rate of 50%, whereas the recurrence rate is 25% in patients over the age of 22. The type and duration of immobilization had no effect on the incidence of recurrence. In most cases, the recurrence occurred within 2 years of the original injury.

In a Minnesota study, approximately 66% of patients under the age of 20 had recurrence, whereas none of the patients over the age of 40 had a recurrence. There was a higher incidence of recurrence in athletes, and restricting athletic activity for 6 weeks following the initial episode seemed to be beneficial in reducing the rate of recurrence.

An important prospective study of 254 patients confirmed that age at the time of initial dislocation was the most important factor with regard to prognosis. During the 5-year follow-up, two or more recurrences occurred in 55% of patients 12 to 22 years old, in 37% of those 23 to 29 years old, and in 12% of those 30 to 40 years old. Immobilization did not reduce the recurrence rate. Although longer follow-up may increase the recurrence rate, these statistics represent reasonable estimates of anticipated outcome after an initial anterior dislocation (28).

Of note is that the incidence of recurrence in these studies is high, but lower than that reported in the past. An even more optimistic outlook is presented by a study done at the Naval Academy where 15 of 20 midshipmen had successful treatment without recurrence when internal rotation strengthening exercises were prescribed and activities limited until the goals of rehabilitation were achieved. These highly motivated, young, athletic men had a high compliance rate with the prescribed program.

Several factors seem to influence the rate of recurrence following an anterior dislocation. Age at the time of the original dislocation seems to have the major effect. The younger the patient at the time of the first dislocation the more likely the chance of recurrence. The rate of dislocation is higher in patients who have the atraumatic variety. Recent data suggest that the type and duration of immobilization after reduction has little effect on the likelihood of recurrence. Early initiation of strengthening exercises seems to be beneficial. Patients who were able to reduce the shoulders themselves are also at increased risk. Men have a higher rate of recurrence than women. Athletes have a higher recurrence rate than non-athletes. Patients with greater tuberosity fractures have a lower rate of recurrence.

Recurrent Anterior Dislocations

The diagnosis of recurrent anterior dislocations is generally simple and is made primarily on the basis of the patient's history of repeated dislocations. Patients with recurrent anterior dislocations usually refuse to use the arm in the unstable or overhead position.

Physical examination is essential in establishing the diagnosis of recurrent anterior instability. A positive apprehension test is elicited when the arm is placed into abduction, external rotation, and extension (see Figure 10.17). The patient's complaints are exaggerated when the humeral head is pushed forward by the examiner's thumb. The anterior drawer and relocation tests are also positive (see Figures 10.27 and 10.28). Multidirectional instability is ruled out when the sulcus sign is absent (see Figure 10.17).

Radiographic confirmation of recurrent anterior instability may be difficult because the radiographs are often normal. The two areas that must be evaluated are the posterolateral aspect of the humeral head and the anteroinferior aspect of the glenoid. The Hill-Sachs lesion on the humeral head is best demonstrated by an anteroposterior view of the humerus in internal rotation. The glenoid rim is best evaluated by the West Point axillary. Superimposition of bony structures, obesity, large patient size, and difficulty in positioning can obscure the injury and make these views difficult to interpret.

A recurrent dislocation is treated with immobilization in an arm sling for several days until the discomfort subsides. Anti-inflammatory medications are often helpful. There is no evidence to show that prolonged immobilization provides any therapeutic benefit.

The rehabilitation program is begun as

soon as possible and emphasizes rotator cuff and periscapular strengthening. Decreased strength of the serratus anterior adds to the stress on the anterior restraints and the need to include this muscle in the rehabilitation program cannot be overemphasized. Selective strengthening of weakened muscles is performed. Muscle endurance as well as strengthening needs to be achieved. Shoulder strengthening can be accomplished with free weights, rubber tubing, isokinetic machines, or body exercises such as push-ups and chin-ups. It is essential to have the shoulder properly positioned when the exercises are being performed so that the weak muscles can be specifically isolated and selectively strengthened. It is easy for the patient to cheat on these exercises and thus specific muscles or muscle groups can get ignored or avoided.

Recently Townsend has described four specific exercises to strengthen the glenohumeral muscles. These are 1) elevation of the arm in the scapular plane with the arm internally rotated and the thumb down, 2) elevation of the arm in the sagittal plane, 3) horizontal adduction from the prone position with the arms externally rotated, and 4) the press-up exercise in which case the patient lifts himself straight upward from a chair while in the seated position. The first of these may aggravate rotator cuff symptomatology and should be avoided if rotator cuff pathology is suspected.

Throwing is not permitted until strength and range of motion have returned to normal. Pitching mechanics should be evaluated by a skilled coach. Correction of form abnormalities may also help resolve this problem.

In sports that do not require circumduction activity, an adduction harness may be worn to prevent elevation of the arm above 90°. Straps or laces extend between a chest corset and an arm cuff. These prevent extreme position of the arm and thus protect the shoulder. In football players, straps can also be used to prevent abduction by holding the arm to the shoulder pads.

Surgical reconstruction of the anterior structures is recommended for those who fail a nonoperative program. Relative contraindications to surgery are older patients or patients with voluntary anterior instability. Patients who are reluctant to participate in a preoperative rehabilitation program are often reluctant to do the necessary exercises postoperatively.

Arthroscopic management of anterior shoulder instability is in its infancy. Short-term follow-up data report a 20% redislocation rate. The standard by which these newer surgical techniques must be judged is the Bankart repair, which has a success rate of approximately 95% without significant limitation of motion or subsequent arthritis.

It is important to rule out voluntary dislocations as a cause of this pathology. These patients may need psychiatric evaluation and therapy as part of their treatment program.

Anterior Subluxations

The diagnosis of recurrent anterior subluxation is often more difficult than that of recurrent dislocation (26). This diagnosis can be easy if the patient reports repeated episodes of "popping out." In some patients, however, the chief complaint may be subtle, such as a sensation of abnormal movement, pain, or clicking with certain activities. Frequently the pain is posterior due to stretching of the posterior capsule as the humeral head displaces anteriorly. The so-called dead arm syndrome is also an indication of anterior subluxation. In this condition, the patient experiences a sharp pain followed by loss of control of the extremity and the sensation that the arm has gone dead. The pain usually occurs in the provocative position of abduction, external rotation, and extension. The acute severe pain subsides almost immediately, but the shoulder remains sore and weak for several hours to several days. With recurrent anterior subluxations the arm may also be described as "going dead" when throwing hard or doing forceful circumduction activity. On occasion, the athlete may drop an object or a ball because of dysesthesias in the hand.

It is not necessary that an athlete have had an acute traumatic subluxation or dislocation to have problems with recurrent subluxations. This problem may arise from the repetitive forceful use of the arm in the overhead position.

Physical examination findings are also subtle. Characteristically, these athletes have tenderness over the anterior shoulder capsule, but it is not uncommon to have tenderness over the posterior capsule as well. Many will have a 10° to 15° loss of internal rotation, indicating an external rotation contracture. The anterior apprehension test position of abduction, external rotation and extension usually causes more pain than apprehension (see Figure 10.17), but the pain is usually relieved with the relocation test. The patient is often unilaterally weaker when trying to hold abduction at 90°.

Rotator cuff impingement symptoms often accompany anterior subluxations and instability. Differentiating pure impingement, pure instability, and mixed pathology can be difficult (4). Patients with pure impingement usually do not experience pain relief with the relocation test. Patients with pure instability should have a negative impingement sign (see Figure 10.33). The impingement test (injection of local anesthetic into the subacromial space) localizes the process to the subacromial space and should provide temporary relief of symptoms in patients who have pure impingement. Patients with pure instability will continue to have pain after this injection.

Radiographs are almost always negative for osseous pathology. Tomographic arthrography may demonstrate a patulous capsule or defect in the inferior glenohumeral ligament. MRI has been unreliable in demonstrating subtle labral-capsular and osseous lesions. Arthroscopy is occasionally helpful in this evaluation. Arthroscopy and bursoscopy allow visual inspection of both the acromial (superior) surface and articular (inferior) surfaces of the rotator cuff. The glenoid labrum and capsular ligaments can be seen and palpated, not only for tears but for the attenuation that often occurs in nontraumatic subluxation.

The initial treatment is a nonoperative program that allows most athletes to avoid reconstructive surgery. The recent trend is toward early motion and strengthening with resumption of activity when symptoms permit. The rehabilitation consists of a four-phase program that begins with rest, to allow an inflamed and stretched capsule to recover. This can be complemented by anti-inflammatory medications. A strengthening program is then initiated for the rotator cuff and parascapular muscles, with emphasis on the internal rotators and serratus anterior. The exercises should be done in the scapular plane, avoiding extension. An endurance program is then begun. Finally, a throwing program is initiated with slow progression to competitive distance, speed, duration, and frequency.

Those for whom a rehabilitation program fails may require surgery. Many procedures have been developed to correct subtle glenohumeral instability. The overall success of surgical stabilization in allowing the throwing athlete to return to a competitive level has generally been disappointing.

Posterior Glenohumeral Instability

Posterior instability is difficult to diagnose and treat. Although recognized more frequently, it is neither as common nor as well understood as anterior instability (24). The literature would suggest that posterior dislocations constitute somewhat less than 5% of all shoulder dislocations, but recent evidence suggests that this may be understated. Recurrent posterior subluxations and dislocations are frequently associated with multidirectional instability. This diagnosis is often missed by the physician who first sees the patient.

A careful history is often the most revealing component of the evaluation. Although a direct blow to the anterior shoulder can produce a posterior dislocation, it is the indirect forces such as adduction, flexion, and internal rotation that place the shoulder at greatest risk. A fall onto the outstretched hand can cause an acute posterior dislocation. Pain or the sensation of laxity while doing the bench press, pass blocking in football, or with the arm in the adducted position suggest posterior instability. Shoulder posturing during seizures can also produce a posterior dislocation.

The patient who has an acute posterior dislocation holds the arm in internal rotation and guards against abduction and external rotation. The anterior prominence of the coracoid may be noted in thin patients, but the deformity is not as evident as in those who have an anterior dislocation. Frequently these patients will have a limitation of forearm supination with the elbow fully extended. The apprehension test for recurrent posterior instability is performed by applying internal rotation and adduction forces to the shoulder, which is flexed beyond 90°. Apprehension or pain is interpreted as a positive test. The posterior drawer test usually demonstrates increased posterior translation. Forward elevation will also test for posteroinferior laxity.

Radiographs of the patient with a posterior dislocation of the shoulder have often been misinterpreted as being normal. Distortion of the elliptical overlap between the humeral head and glenoid may be the only abnormality on the routine anteroposterior view. Thus the anteroposterior projection may suggest but, by itself, is not diagnostic of a posterior dislocation. The inability to see the clear space between the humeral head and the glenoid on the true anteroposterior radiograph of the shoulder should be a tip off to a posterior dislocation. The definitive view is the axillary in which the posterior location of the humeral head is easily seen. A lateral or axillary view was never obtained in a large series of missed posterior dislocations. This again emphasizes the importance of biplane radiographs in the initial evaluation. The transcapular lateral can be difficult to interpret because of the overlapping bone densities. The complete series of radiographs is also necessary to rule out fractures that are common in posterior dislocations. Routine radiographs are usually normal in patients with recurrent posterior laxity.

Closed reduction is sometimes difficult, and sedation is usually warranted. Occasionally general anesthesia is necessary to achieve reduction. The patient is positioned supine and posterior pressure is applied to the humeral head while longitudinal traction is placed on the adducted arm. This unlocks the humeral head from the glenoid.

The head is lifted back into the glenoid as the arm is rotated. Open reduction is indicated if closed reduction maneuvers fail.

Recurrent instability after a posterior dislocation is less common than following anterior dislocation. If the reduction is stable, the shoulder should be immobilized for 3 to 5 weeks prior to initiation of an aggressive strengthening program that emphasizes the external rotators and the posterior deltoid. Older patients are immobilized for a shorter period of time to avoid significant problems with stiffness. Provocative activities should be avoided for 8 to 12 weeks.

Multidirectional Glenohumeral Instability

The term multidirectional instability implies a shoulder that has a component of symptomatic inferior instability in addition to anterior or posterior instability (12,25). The medical history is somewhat different from those with anterior subluxations. Patients with involuntary multidirectional instability complain of discomfort or fatigue when carrying heavy objects that apply a downward force on the shoulder. The inability to throw, swim, or work in the overhead position is characteristic of this condition. Although many patients with multidirectional instability have evidence of generalized ligamentous laxity, most can recall a discrete episode that initiated the instability, although many cannot and the history of a specific injury is variable. Many of these patients are athletically active and it can be difficult to differentiate this condition from unidirectional instability. The sulcus sign is positive. Radiographs are customarily normal.

The first step in the treatment of recurrent multidirectional instability is a rigorous physical therapy program to strengthen the internal and external rotators. This, in conjunction with educating patients about the condition, may eliminate symptoms. Enlisting the help of a knowledgeable coach to suggest form or style changes so as to avoid or modify the provocative movements is often helpful. Only when a program such as this fails should surgery be considered. Surgery in such cases has generally been less successful than surgery in unidirectional anterior instability, perhaps because of stretched and deficient capsular tissues, a mild connective tissue disorder, or an unrecognized emotional disturbance manifested as voluntary instability.

Inferior Glenohumeral Instability

Traumatic inferior dislocation of the shoulder (luxatio erecta) (Figure 10.32) is rare especially in sports. Forceful hyperabduction causes this injury, and the patient usually presents with the arm held in the overhead position. All movement causes pain. The anteroposterior radiographs confirm the inferior position of the humeral head. General anesthesia with muscle relaxation is often necessary before reduction can be achieved. The method of reduction is upward traction on the extended arm with countertraction on the top of the shoulder. The arm is then slowly moved to the side of the body. There is a high incidence of brachial plexus injuries with this dislocation, and frequently pain and weakness persist for months or years. Treatment of acute inferior instability is the same as for that of anterior instability.

Inferior subluxations occur when lifting a heavy weight at the side or when the arm is stressed in the full overhead position. Anterior capsular tenderness with pain and apprehension with abduction, external rotation, and extension are common. Thus, both the history and examination are

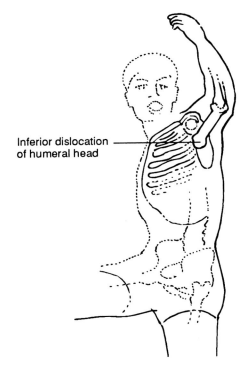

Inferior dislocation
of humeral head

Figure 10.32. Inferior dislocation of the shoulder (luxatio erecta).

similar to that for anterior instability. The inferior component of this instability is differentiated from anterior instability by the presence of a positive sulcus sign.

Internal Derangements of the Glenohumeral Joint

Included in this group are miscellaneous conditions which affect the intra-articular structures of the glenohumeral joint, unrelated to instability. The most notable are loose bodies and glenoid labral tears. Although these conditions are often associated with instability, they may occur primarily.

Medical History

The athlete usually has vague complaints of pain associated with catching or clicking.

If the injury involves the superior labrum these are called SLAP lesions (superior *l*abrum *a*nterior and *p*osterior to the biceps anchor). The cause of these and other labral tears may be from a single traumatic event, or the recurrent overstressing of overhead sports.

Physical Examination

Anterior or posterior instability testing may elicit the click or catch of a labral tear and reproduce the athlete's pain. In SLAP lesions, superior pressure on the humerus, likewise, may be provocative of the athlete's symptoms. Instability should be ruled out as a cause of labral pathology.

Radiographic Evaluation

Routine radiographs should be obtained and will identify an intra-articular calcified loose body if present. Arthro-CT is the imaging technique most likely to identify labral pathology. MRI scanning has been less helpful in clearly delineating pathology of the labrum or loose bodies.

Treatment

Because these conditions represent mechanical derangements within the joint, surgical treatment is usually necessary. Rest and NSAIDs may quiet the symptoms temporarily but will rarely give any long-term relief. Arthroscopic removal of the loose body or cartiliguous labrum usually resolves the symptoms.

THE ROTATOR CUFF

Most athletes with shoulder pain have some type of disorder of the rotator cuff. The challenge for the physician is to determine whether the rotator cuff pain is the primary problem or if it is secondary to some other pathology.

Impingement Syndrome

When the anatomy of the shoulder is reviewed, the mechanism of impingement becomes obvious. The subacromial space increases and decreases in size as the arm is moved. With abduction or internal rotation, the prominent greater tuberosity sweeps under the anterior acromion and the coracoacromial ligament, thus narrowing this interval. With this circumduction the tendons of the rotator cuff and the long head of the biceps get pinched between the greater tuberosity below and the unyielding coracoacromial arch above. In the case of repetitive overhead motions such as throwing or swimming, this repeated abuse takes its toll. The region of maximum impingement occurs near the hypovascular area of the supraspinatus tendon. This area is just proximal to the cuff's insertion into the greater tuberosity. As in any hypovascular area, the healing capacity of this region is limited. The subacromial bursa is interposed between the rotator cuff and the coracoacromial arch, but does not provide sufficient protection for the repetitive wear and tear of repeated overhead activity (29).

If scapular rotation is not synchronous with the movements of the proximal humerus, the impingement of the rotator cuff between the greater tuberosity and the coracoacromial arch is increased. With repeated overhead activity, the patient develops an inflammatory tendinitis. The hypertrophy associated with inflammation further diminishes the space available and thus aggravates the impingement compression. The pain from tendinitis leads to disuse atrophy of the supraspinatus muscle, which decreases its depressor function. The humeral head rides higher, resulting in a cycle of increasing impingement.

In the simple overuse group, there is inflammation of the subacromial bursa, the tendons of the rotator cuff, the biceps, the capsule, or any combination of these structures. Athletes particularly prone to develop cuff tendinitis are those involved in sports requiring frequent overhead use of the arms such as swimmers, tennis players, pitchers, and quarterbacks.

Subacromial disease and rotator cuff injuries in particular present a continuum of progressive disease severity. These injuries may be partial thickness (on only the inferior or superior surface), incomplete (involving only a portion, e.g., the supraspinatus), or complete. Although more frequent in patients over 40 years of age, impingement symptoms do occur in young adults, especially those with subtle instability. The cause may be acute trauma or degeneration of tendon tissue. Clinical manifestations vary from minimal discomfort to severe pain, weakness, and loss of shoulder function. There is some correlation between the severity of the symptoms and the amount of damage but it is often impossible, on the basis of history and physical examination alone, to separate the athlete with tendinitis from one with a partial-thickness tear. Full-thickness tears are rare in the youthful athlete.

Medical History

Pain with circumduction activity is the customary complaint of athletes with rotator cuff pathology. Other complaints such as fatigue, functional catching, stiffness, the perception of instability, grinding, and general deterioration in function are other common complaints. Except for the bilateral sports, such as swimming and gymnastics, the symptoms are characteristically in the dominant shoulder.

Athletes with rotator cuff pathology tend to fall into two major categories: 1) symptoms following an acute injury, or 2) symptoms following overuse or abuse. In the acute presentation, it is important to identify as clearly as possible the exact mechanism of injury. In the case of overuse, it is necessary to analyze the pattern of repetitive training so as to identify the inciting activity. It is often helpful to get historical information from observers beside the patient. Frequently the parents, the coach, or even other athletes can provide helpful information as to the duration of symptoms and the precipitating activity.

The pain is often poorly localized and it commonly radiates into the upper arm, particularly the region of the deltoid insertion. Anterior pain radiating along the course of the biceps muscle usually indicates involvement of the biceps tendon.

Blazina's classification is used to grade the severity of symptoms. The modified classification is as follows:

Grade I—pain (not disabling) during activity
Grade II—pain during and after activity (not disabling)
Grade III—pain (disabling) during and after activity
Grade IV—pain with activities of daily living

Rotator cuff pain can be particularly difficult to evaluate because impingement may be the primary pathology or it may be secondary to another primary condition. Abnormalities, such as subtle instabilities or weaknesses, can alter the stresses placed on the shoulder joint and cause secondary rotator cuff symptoms. The main concern in evaluating the athlete with shoulder pain is to rule out glenohumeral instability of one type or another. In younger athletes most impingement symptoms are due to some type of subtle instability which, combined with rotator cuff or biceps tendinitis, causes progressive shoulder dysfunction and pain.

Physical Examination

An organized and comprehensive approach to the physical examination is necessary. Inspection pays particular attention to remote acromioclavicular injuries and muscle wasting of the supraspinatus or infraspinatus.

Tenderness in the bicipital groove is a reliable sign of bicipital tendinitis. Tenderness over the supraspinatus insertion just distal to the anterolateral border of the acromion is an indication of impingement. Anterior or posterior joint line tenderness may suggest capsular stretching due to instability.

Discrepancies between the active and passive range of motion suggests a rotator cuff tear. In throwing athletes there is normally increased strength and range of motion on the dominant side. Particular attention is paid to passive internal rotation in abduction. Loss of internal rotation suggests a posterior capsular contracture and is indicative of anterior laxity.

The assessment of shoulder stability is very important in evaluating the patient with suspected rotator cuff pathology. The rotator cuff symptoms are often a secondary manifestation of an underlying instability. This can be confirmed by the apprehension and relocation tests and the sulcus sign.

A number of special tests will help confirm the diagnosis of impingement. These include a painful arc between 70° and 120° of elevation in the scapular plane. Increased pain in the "impingement position" of 90° abduction, 30° flexion, and maximum internal rotation with forced elevation is indicative of rotator cuff impingement (Figure 10.33). Biceps tendon involvement can be demonstrated by Speed's or Yergason's test (see Figure 10.16).

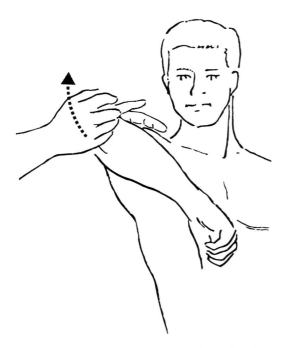

Figure 10.33. Impingement test, forced abduction with the shoulder in 30° forward flexion and maximum internal rotation.

The main differential is between instability and primary rotator cuff pathology. Often these conditions overlap and the physician is confronted with answering the difficult chicken and egg question about tendinitis versus instability.

The impingement test is performed by injecting a local anesthetic into the subacromial bursa and evaluating the patient for pain relief. This diagnostic injection should be part of the physical examination when evaluating the athlete with a painful shoulder. It is important to remember that the subacromial space lies under only the anterior third of the acromion. Sometime it is actually easier to inject the bursa by inserting a 3-in. needle posteriorly and passing it under the acromion while aiming at the anterior margin of the acromion. Subjective relief of the impingement signs after injecting a local anesthetic into the subacromial bursa suggests supraspinatus tendon impingement is a part of the pathology. It must be emphasized that this test is nonspecific. In some cases, the acromioclavicular joint communicates with the subdeltoid bursa, and in the case of a rotator cuff tear, the glenohumeral joint and biceps tendon sheath may similarly be anesthetized.

Radiographic Evaluation

Plain radiographs of the athlete with shoulder pain are customarily normal. The routine views are taken to rule out conditions such as arthritis, calcific tendinitis, fractures, and tumors, which might be a cause of discomfort. The supraspinatus outlet view is helpful to determine the shape of the acromion and determine if a hook or osteophytes on the anterior margin are contributing to impingement (see Figure 10.22) (30).

Double-contrast arthrography is helpful in ruling out rotator cuff tears. In combination with CT, a double-contrast arthrogram will also evaluate the labrum, articular surfaces, biceps tendon, and help discover loose bodies. MRI is occasionally helpful in identifying edema of the rotator cuff. MRI will delineate massive cuff tears, but it has been notably inaccurate in evaluating the rotator cuff for smaller tears.

Chronic rotator cuff impingement cannot be differentiated from a partial-thickness cuff tear without specialized studies. Double-contrast arthrography may reveal a partial-thickness tear on the articular side of the cuff. Bursography has been disappointing in showing tears of the superior surface. MRI similarly has been disappointing in its ability to reveal partial-thickness tears. This study will confirm cuff edema but has failed to reliably demonstrate partial-thickness cuff tears.

Treatment

As a general rule, the treatment of rotator cuff tendinitis is nonoperative. The factors that help determine treatment are the etiology of the problem, the sport and time of the season, and the severity of symptoms.

In the athlete the initial treatment should include diminution of the inflammation with rest, ice packs, anti-inflammatory medications, and physical therapy modalities such as ultrasound. After the inflammatory phase has subsided, shoulder strengthening exercises (including both rotator cuff and scapular stabilizing muscles) should be initiated to improve function and diminish impingement. In the overhead athlete, anterior subluxation is a common cause of secondary impingement. Strengthening the rotator cuff and serratus anterior will often help control shoulder stability and thus diminish impingement symptoms.

Local steroid injections do diminish pain and inflammation but also impair tissue metabolism. Injecting the subacromial-subdeltoid bursa in impingement lesions is more frequently successful than injection of trigger (or tender) points.

First and foremost, the best treatment is prevention. It is important that the athlete realize that the rotator cuff and scapular stabilizer muscles must be in good condition prior to circumduction activities. An off-season and preseason stretching and strengthening program is mandatory. It is also important not to change activity levels dramatically and thus overuse and abuse the tissues.

In patients in whom nonoperative treatment has failed, excision of the coracoacromial ligament and anterior acromioplasty may be indicated. In those athletes with impingement alone (and no instability) the surgical treatment of subacromial decompression is effective. When the tendinitis is secondary to subtle instabilities, subacromial decompression does not address the primary pathology and is not of benefit. Accurate diagnosis of any instability is key to successful treatment. Hopefully, some of the uncertainties as to which athletes will benefit and how frequently performance will be improved by surgical treatment will be resolved in the next several years.

Impingement and Associated Instability

Many athletes with chronic impingement have an underlying concomitant instability (4). Because the capsule is lax, the rotator cuff muscles and the scapular stabilizers must work overtime to provide stability to the shoulder. Selective fatigue and impairment of these muscles has been demonstrated in athletes with glenohumeral instability. The dysfunction resulting from muscle fatigue causes impingement of the humeral head on the coracoacromial arch.

Most athletes with impingement associated with instability are 16 to 35 years old and participate in overhead activities such as throwing, tennis, volleyball, or water polo. It is well recognized that the impingement symptoms will persist if the underlying instability is not treated. Often, patients with subluxation describe pain during the late cocking and acceleration phases of throwing. This differs from the nonspecific pain that progresses with repeated throwing in the athlete who has rotator cuff tendinitis alone. Pain associated with subluxation is usually along the posterior glenohumeral joint, and can be confused with infraspinatus tendinitis.

The signs of subluxation are often subtle. The impingement signs of secondary rotator cuff tendinitis are more obvious and dramatic and may obscure the diagnosis of instability. A positive anterior apprehension sign and evidence of instability on palpation confirm the diagnosis of instability. Unfortunately these tests are often equivocal. The anterior apprehension sign may produce pain only at the posterior glenohumeral joint and there may be no sense of impending subluxation. The "relocation test" has been helpful in confirming findings of instability in subtle cases by relieving pain (see Figure 17.28). Athletes with rotator cuff disease have a positive impingement sign and pain with supraspinatus strength testing.

Radiographs do not help differentiate the patients with isolated instability from those with isolated impingement or from those with a combination of the two. In some patients, an examination under general anesthesia and an arthroscopic evaluation are useful to confirm the diagnosis.

Proper management is also difficult in patients who have impingement combined with instability. The rehabilitation appropriate for the instability will usually reduce the symptoms of both the instability and the impingement. Undetected instability should be ruled out in any athlete with impingement findings. If instability is diagnosed, it should be addressed primarily.

NERVE INJURIES

It is important not to overlook nerve injuries as a cause of shoulder pain or dysfunction. Isolated injuries of the axillary, suprascapular, spinal accessory, and long thoracic nerves as well as the brachial plexus have been reported in athletes, and proper functioning of these structures must be routinely evaluated.

Thoracic Outlet Syndrome

Compression of the neurovascular bundle at the thoracic outlet may produce shoulder pain, dysesthesias, weakness, or muscle atrophy. At least seven different types of fibromuscular bands in and around the scalene muscles have been described. In athletes these abnormal constriction bands can be the result of healing of torn muscle fibers. Characteristically the neck, shoulder and arm are involved with paresthesias extending into the ulnar three digits. Symptoms are aggravated by circumduction and overhead postures of the arm. Special maneuvers, such as Adson's or Wright's test, should be performed with the understanding that their absence does not absolutely preclude the presence of thoracic outlet syndrome. Similarly obliteration of the radial pulse and the presence of a subclavian bruit may be present in normal individuals. As a general rule, neurologic symptoms are predominant over vascular symptoms. Even so, EMG abnormalities are rare.

In Wright's test, the neck is extended while the shoulder is hyperabducted and externally rotated. In Adson's test, the patient's neck is extended and turned toward the affected side while the patient is asked to inspire deeply. In each test, a thoracic outlet syndrome is suspected if the radial pulse is diminished or the neurologic symptoms reproduced. A careful history and physical examination are the best tools in establishing this diagnosis. Relief of symptoms following infiltration of local anesthetic into the anterior or middle scalene muscles may be the best confirmatory test.

Nonoperative treatments include pos-

tural and muscle strengthening exercises.
If the symptoms do not respond, surgical
decompression is advised.

Brachial Plexus Injuries

The brachial plexus may be injured by
traction or a direct blow. The traction injuries occur when the shoulder is pushed
downward as the head is being forced to
the contralateral side. This same mechanism may cause the brachial plexus to be
pinched between the clavicle and first rib.
The resulting "stinger" may present as
shoulder and arm pain, and the symptoms
can mimic those of shoulder subluxation
(see Chapter 5 on the cervical spine). When
confronted with a patient who has a "dead
arm" (Figure 10.34), the physician must distinguish between a brachial plexus injury
and a shoulder subluxation or dislocation
that has spontaneously reduced. Brachial
plexus injuries more commonly have
dysesthesias and persistent weakness after
the event. Shoulder instability is usually
associated with a positive apprehension
sign.

Axillary Nerve

Axillary nerve palsies are characterized
by absent deltoid function and decreased
sensation over the "shoulder patch" area.
Many athletes with complete deltoid paralysis following an axillary nerve injury
are able to strongly abduct the shoulder
through a complex substitution pattern.
In the chronic case deltoid atrophy will be
obvious because of the flattened shoulder
and the lateral acromion will be prominent.

The axillary nerve is located on the inferior aspect of the shoulder and vulnerable
to injury during an anterior dislocation,
especially if the dislocation follows a traction injury or a violent fall. The reported

incidence of an axillary nerve palsy after an
anterior shoulder dislocation ranges from
8% to 18%. Recovery is generally complete
unless the neuropraxia follows blunt
trauma, in which case the potential for recovery is diminished. Approximately half
of these patients have permanent partial or
complete axillary nerve palsies.

Not all patients who are unable to abduct
the arm after the reduction of a shoulder
dislocation have an axillary nerve palsy.
This finding may also be secondary to pain

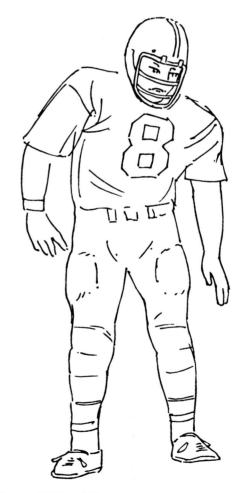

Figure 10.34. Athlete with a "dead arm."

inhibition or a rotator cuff tear, especially if the patient is over 40 years old. Shoulder patch sensation helps evaluate the axillary nerve. If the nerve is intact, an arthrogram to look for rotator cuff tear should be obtained. If a tear is present, rotator cuff repair is the recommended treatment.

Violent or repeated blows to the top of the shoulder can contribute to the entrapment of the axillary nerve in the quadrilateral space. Permanent paralysis is the rule following this injury, but surgical decompression is occasionally helpful.

Suprascapular Nerve

Suprascapular nerve palsy may cause paralysis of the supraspinatus and infraspinatus muscles or the infraspinatus muscle alone, depending on the location of injury. The nerve may be injured as it passes through the scapula notch, in which case both muscles will be affected. If the nerve is injured as it passes the spine of the scapula, then only the infraspinatus muscle is involved. The mechanism of injury is usually forceful scapular protraction or a direct blow.

The diagnosis is often difficult. The athlete complains of a vague, deep, diffuse pain at the posterior and lateral aspect of the shoulder. There may or may not be radiation into the neck and the arm. Weakness of external rotation due to denervation of the infraspinatus may be difficult to detect in the muscular athlete. It may be difficult to determine if the apparent weakness is due to pain or infraspinatus dysfunction. The patient with chronic suprascapular nerve dysfunction will present with infraspinatus atrophy and weakness. Adduction of the arm across the body may aggravate the symptoms, and deep palpation over the suprascapular notch frequently causes pain. Supra-

spinatus atrophy may be difficult to see, and its weakness is not as easily determined as that of the infraspinatus. Infraspinatus atrophy is usually visible and palpable. The diagnosis is confirmed with an EMG of the supraspinatus and infraspinatus.

The patient with a closed acute suprascapular nerve injury is followed expectantly. Rest during the acute episode with return to activity as symptoms permit is usually recommended. Because only 30% to 40% of the maximum strength of the infraspinatus is used during throwing, patients with a partial nerve injury are often able to return to high-performance athletics. Surgical exploration of a well-localized lesion may be considered if atrophy develops or nonoperative management of 3 to 6 months fails to alleviate symptoms.

Spinal Accessory Nerve

The spinal accessory nerve (cranial nerve XI) is a pure motor nerve that innervates the trapezius and sternocleidomastoid muscles. Trapezius paralysis causes drooping of the shoulder, asymmetry of the neck line, winging of the scapula, weakness of forward elevation, and pain. This nerve is relatively superficial and thus vulnerable to blunt trauma as it crosses the floor of the posterior triangle of the neck. Traction such as from wrestling or football can also cause injury. Thorough neurologic and EMG examinations are necessary for an acute diagnosis.

Closed injuries should be followed for 6 months and exploration of the nerve considered if no recovery has occurred. If the diagnosis is made within 1 year of injury, surgical exploration with neurolysis or repair is usually recommended.

Scapular winging (see Figure 10.14) is less obvious and often less disabling with trapezius palsy than with serratus anterior palsy. Shoulder function with an accessory nerve palsy may or may not be adequate for return to competition.

Long Thoracic Nerve

Palsy of the long thoracic nerve causes paralysis of the serratus anterior muscle with resultant winging of the scapula. The loss of this important scapular stabilizer places additional stress on the rotator cuff and leads to altered shoulder mechanics and pain.

This disabling condition is often associated with brachial plexus neuritis. This clinical syndrome of unknown etiology is usually unilateral and the pain generally precedes loss of function. Recovery, while good, may take several years. Backpacking, shoveling, and improper use of crutches can also cause long thoracic nerve palsies. The outcome following acute traction injuries is usually good.

The diagnosis is suspected when examination reveals scapular winging. Winging of the scapula can be demonstrated by having the patient remain in the up position after doing a push-up. Less stress with similar scapular prominence can be demonstrated with a wall push-up (see Figure 10.14). The diagnosis can be confirmed with EMG studies.

Treatment consists of discontinuing the inciting activity and watchful waiting. This is often a career-ending condition if nerve recovery does not occur.

MUSCLE INJURIES

Although injuries to the musculotendinous unit are common in sports, it is uncommon to have a complete avulsion, or disruption, of the major muscles around the shoulder. When these injuries occur, however, they cause substantial functional disability. Shortening with contracture of the muscle will lead to permanent dysfunction and significant alteration of joint mechanics unless appropriate anatomic repair is carried out within the first several days of the injury.

The injury may vary in severity from a mild strain with some inflammation, to a complete avulsion or disruption of the musculotendinous unit. The tendon may be avulsed from the bone or it may pull a fragment of bone with it as it pulls loose.

Muscle ruptures occur when an actively contracting muscle group is overloaded. This overload can occur acutely with a single large force. Or, it can follow a smaller force which is applied to a structure that has been weakened by repetitive overuse and abuse. A minuscule amount of damage occurs to the musculotendinous unit during each exercise session. If the unit is repeatedly stressed before this damage is repaired, there is a gradual weakening of the structure and failure may occur with a submaximal stress.

In the normal state, the tendon is stronger than both the muscle belly and the tendon attachment to bone. Repetitive overuse as well as scar and granulation tissue within the substance of the tendon alters this normal situation. The tendon is weakened and likely to rupture with overloading. The use of anabolic steroids further weakens the musculotendinous unit, and increases the risk of injury. Similarly injections of corticosteroids into the substance of the tendon weakens it, predisposing the tendon to rupture.

Muscle strains are characterized by pain and tenderness at the site of injury. Resisted activity of the injured muscle accentuates the complaints of pain. Similarly, passive stretch of the injured muscle causes increased pain. The muscle should be palpated for continuity because complete disruptions are usually associated with a palpable defect or visible deformity.

Incomplete tears are treated nonoperatively with ice, rest, and antiinflammatory medications until the acute symptoms subside. A structured therapy program is used to restore motion and strength.

Complete disruptions are treated with early surgical repair or reconstruction. Surgical repair can be difficult because of the problems with the direct suturing of muscle. Nonetheless, repair in the acute phase is recommended whenever possible. Early surgery is indicated because it is often difficult, if not impossible, to restore the muscle length if the repair is delayed more than 7 to 10 days. Careful protected exercise programs are used to optimize the result following surgery.

Rupture of the Pectoralis Major

Ruptures of the pectoralis major are relatively rare. Weight lifting, especially the bench press, is the most common mechanism of injury. The majority of pectoralis major strains are incomplete and occur within the muscle belly or at the musculotendinous junction. Complete disruptions usually occur as avulsions from the humerus with only 25% of these cases being disruptions of the musculotendinous junction or the muscle belly.

Patients with an acute complete rupture of the pectoralis major note a sharp, tearing sensation at the site of rupture. An audible pop and burning are often reported.

The physical findings depend on the site of rupture. Early swelling and ecchymosis occur in the chest and upper arm. The muscle belly retracts toward the axillary fold causing a prominent bulge on the anterior chest wall. Tendon avulsion produces asymmetry of the anterior axillary fold as the muscle retracts medially. A palpable defect at the site of injury is usually present, but this may be obscured by swelling. The examiner needs to be careful not to mistake the intact fibers of the fascial layer overlying the tendon for an intact tendon. Attempts to adduct the arm against resistance will increase the bulge of the muscle on the anterior chest wall and the absence of tendon bulk in the anterior axillary wall becomes more apparent. In chronic cases, the balled up retracted muscle belly is very prominent and side-to-side asymmetry is noticeable. The defect in the anterior axillary fold gives a webbed appearance to the axilla.

Plain x-rays of the shoulder, chest, and scapula are normal, and in one series, the diagnosis of tendon avulsion was not detected by MRI in two of three cases.

There is uniform agreement that partial ruptures of the tendon and incomplete tears of the muscle belly itself should be treated nonoperatively. Ice and rest, followed by a program of progressive range of motion and strengthening exercises, will lead to recovery in 6 to 8 weeks. Nonoperative treatment of complete disruptions is similar to that described for incomplete injuries, although strength deficits and cosmetic deformities usually result. If the tear is an avulsion or near the musculotendinous junction, early surgical repair leads to better results. It is difficult, but possible, to restore the muscle length if the repair is delayed for more than 3 weeks.

Rupture of the Subscapularis

The subscapularis may be partially or completely torn during an anterior dislocation of the glenohumeral joint. If the subscapularis has been ruptured, the likelihood of recurrent anterior dislocations is increased.

This diagnosis is difficult to make. It is especially difficult in the acutely injured shoulder. Incompetence of the subscapularis is demonstrated by a positive lift-off test. During this test, the patient places the dorsum of the hand on the sacrum. The inability to internally rotate the arm sufficiently to lift the hand off the back demonstrates weakness or incompetence of the subscapularis. In the acute situation, pain may give a false positive test. The MRI may be useful in confirming this diagnosis, but this study often fails to conclusively demonstrate defects in the muscle or tendon.

Acute ruptures of the subscapularis are treated surgically with simultaneous reconstruction of the shoulder capsule. Reconstruction of both the tendon and capsule are indicated in the case of chronic deficiency.

Rupture of the Biceps

Acute ruptures of the biceps occur because of forceful contraction of the muscle against resistance. Usually there is an avulsion of the tendon of the long head from its attachment at the superior glenoid, although the muscle may be torn within its substance, at the musculotendinous junction, or it may be pulled free from its distal attachment on the coronoid process.

Complete ruptures of the long head of the biceps occurs most commonly in patients over 40 years. Although causing a cosmetic deformity, this injury seldom causes functional deficits in this population. In the youthful athlete, however, a biceps rupture is associated with detectable weakness of shoulder flexion as well as elbow flexion and supination. In addition the athlete may develop impingement symptoms due to the loss of this humeral head depressor.

A tearing or popping sensation in the anterior shoulder is followed by pain, swelling, and loss of strength. Ecchymosis extends into the arm and with attempts at contraction the characteristic arm bulge of the balled up biceps is evident. Examination reveals tenderness at the site of tearing and the wad of muscle is palpable in the arm. Radiographs are usually normal although sometimes a small piece of bone is pulled loose with the tendon avulsion. This fragment serves as a marker to identify the location of the tendon end.

As a general rule, acute ruptures in young, active athletes should be considered for surgery providing the surgery can be completed within several days of the injury. No attempt should be made to restore the attachment to the glenoid. In the case of a proximal avulsion, the long head of the biceps should be attached to the proximal humerus in such a way that early rehabilitation can be initiated. Attempts at reconstruction several weeks or months after this injury produce unsatisfying results.

Patients over the age of 35 are treated nonoperatively with hematoma aspirations and immobilization until the acute reaction subsides. Physical therapy is then initiated to restore motion and strength and one can expect normal motion and functional strength in this population.

Subluxation of the Biceps Tendon

Most sports medicine texts discuss subluxation of the biceps tendon and imply that this is a common condition. Although biceps tendinitis (often associated with impingement) is relatively common, actual displacement of the biceps tendon out of the bicipital groove is infrequent. The literature descriptions of this condition make it indistinguishable from tenosynovitis, which is a more common and a more likely explanation for anterior/superior shoulder pain and snapping.

Contusion

Contusions occur because of direct blows. In many sports, the shoulder is well protected by shoulder pads; thus, contusions are infrequently seen.

The treatment of a contusion is similar to that anywhere else in the body. Cold, compression, anti-inflammatory medications, and rest with gradual resumption of activity through a structured rehabilitation program are prescribed. The criteria for return to sporting activity is recovery of full range of motion and normal strength.

OTHER INJURIES

Axillary Artery Occlusion

Occlusion of the axillary artery characteristically involves the pectoralis minor muscle in throwing and other circumduction activities. The diagnosis may be difficult with the athlete complaining only of fatigue, muscle ache, or decreased endurance. Severe cases including loss of pulse, cyanosis or claudication are easier to diagnose and are frequently associated with a bruit. This diagnosis is confirmed by an arteriogram.

Effort Thrombosis

Repetitive, strenuous overhead activity can injure the axillary vein leading to intramural damage, thrombophlebitis and thrombosis. Under normal conditions the collateral circulation around the shoulder is sufficient to drain the arm and the patient is asymptomatic. With activity, however, the athlete develops pain and swelling because of the inadequate venous drainage. Venous distention is often present. The diagnosis is confirmed with a venogram.

SHOULDER REHABILITATION

As had been noted in earlier sections of this chapter, many conditions caused by athletic injury are treated conservatively with a program that includes improving flexibility and strength. For these exercises to be effective they must be done properly.

Stretching the Capsule and Rotator Cuff

Improving flexibility is the initial key to treating most of the inflammatory conditions about the shoulder. Stretching contracted structures is important and should precede the strengthening exercises. Stretching the anterior cuff and capsule is best done lying supine on a table (Figure 10.35). Stretching the posterior and inferior cuff and capsule can be performed either sitting or standing (Figure 10.36).

Strengthening Specific Muscles

The rotator cuff muscles are relatively small and are easily overwhelmed by the larger shoulder girdle muscles (deltoid, pectoralis major, latissimus) unless these exercises are carefully done to isolate specific muscle groups.

Rotator Cuff

Strengthening the three positions of the cuff (anterior, posterior, and superior) should be done with light weights, 1 to 5 lb, in a slowly progressive fashion. The *supraspinatus* is strengthened with the arm in the plane of the scapula (30° forward of

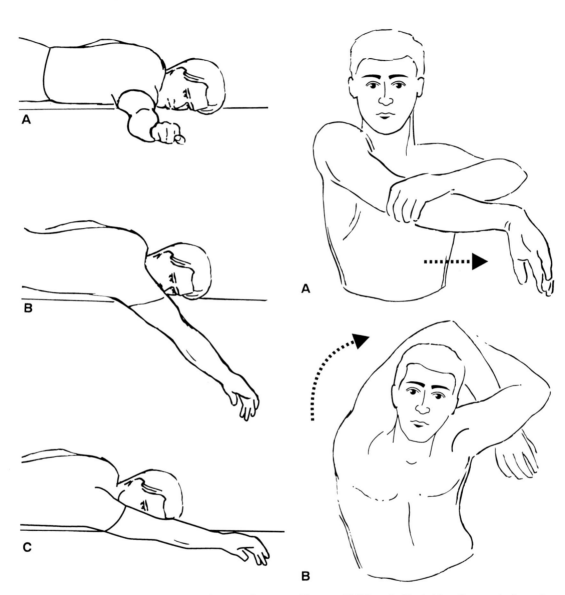

Figure 10.35. Stretching the anterior rotation cuff in various positions. *A.* 90°. *B.* 135°. *C.* 180°.

Figure 10.36. *A.* Stretching the posterior rotator cuff. *B.* Stretching the inferior rotator cuff.

the coronal plane) with the elbow extended and the thumb down (Figure 10.37). The athlete lifts the weight 60°, holds for 5 seconds then lowers slowly. The *subscapularis* is strengthened with the athlete supine, the arm at the side and the elbow flexed 90° (Figure 10.38*A*). The athlete lifts the weight (1 to 5 lb), holds for 5 seconds, and lowers slowly. The *infraspinatus* and *teres minor* muscles are strengthened with the athlete lying with the affected side up, arm at the side and elbow flexed 90° (Figure 10.38*B*). The athlete lifts the weight (1 to 5 lb), holds for 5 seconds, and lowers slowly. Each of these exercises can also be done against the resistance of latex tubing or Theraband (The Hygienic Corporation, Akron, OH) (Figure 10.39).

Shoulder Girdle Large Muscles

These muscles include not only the muscles which move the glenohumeral joint (e.g., deltoid, pectoralis major, and latissimus dorsi), but also the scapular stabilizers (e.g., serratus anterior, rhomboids, and levator scapulae). The *deltoid* muscle has three separate functional parts (middle, anterior, and posterior) and each needs to be strengthened independently. Each exercise can be done with weights or elastic mate-

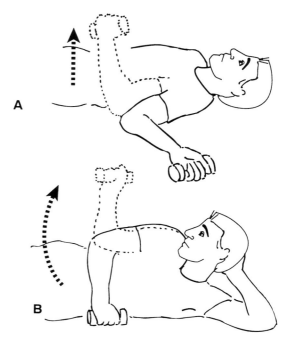

Figure 10.38. Light weight (1 to 5 lb) strengthening of the subscapularis muscle (*A*) and infraspinatus and teres minor muscles (*B*).

rial. The middle deltoid is strengthened with abduction in external rotation, having the thumb up (Figure 10.40*A*). The anterior and posterior deltoid are strengthened with forward flexion and extension respectively (Figure 10.40*B* and *C*). The *pectoralis major* can be strengthened well with either of two exercises: the bench press or fly (Figure 10.41). Both exercises are done supine. The sitting press-up (Figure 10.42) works the *latissimus dorsi* and also works all of the scapula stabilizers.

There are three basic exercises for strengthening the *scapula stabilizers*. The corner push-up (Figure 10.43) works the serratus anterior. The prone extension (Figure 10.44) works the rhomboids. The shoulder shrug done with weights in the hands (Figure 10.45) works the levator scapula.

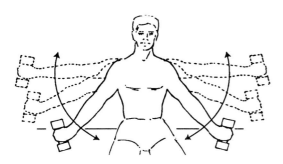

Figure 10.37. Supraspinatus muscle strengthening with a light weight (1 to 5 lb).

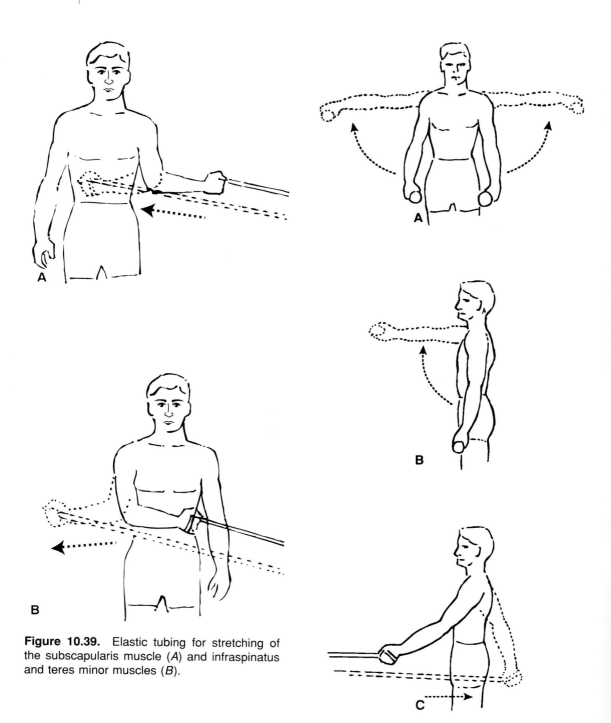

Figure 10.39. Elastic tubing for stretching of
the subscapularis muscle (*A*) and infraspinatus
and teres minor muscles (*B*).

Figure 10.40. Strengthening the three functional parts of the deltoid muscle (*A*) middle, (*B*)
anterior, and (*C*) posterior.

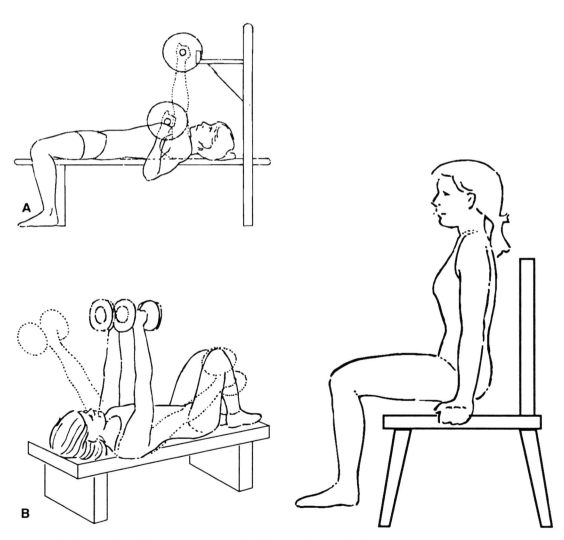

Figure 10.41. Strengthening the pectorali major with the bench press (*A*) and the fly (*B*).

Figure 10.42. Strengthening the latissimus dorsi with the sitting press-up.

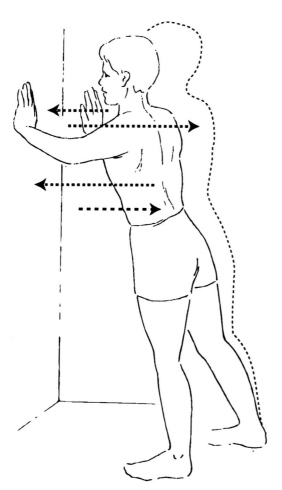

Figure 10.43. Strengthening the serratus anterior with the corner push-up.

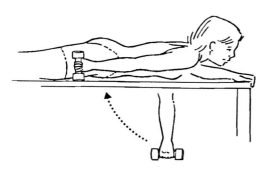

Figure 10.44. Strengthening the rhomboids with prone extension.

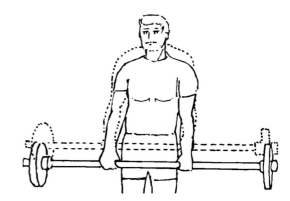

Figure 10.45. Strengthening the levator scapulae with the shoulder shrug.

References

1. Perry J. Anatomy and biomechanics of the shoulder in throwing, swimming, gymnastics, and tennis. Clin Sports Med 1983;2:247–270.

2. Glousman R, Jobe F, Tibone J, Moynes D, Antonelli D, Perry J. Dynamic electromyographic analysis of the throwing shoulder with glenohumeral instability. J Bone Joint Surg 1988;70A:220–226.

3. Jobe FW, Bradley JP. Rotator cuff injuries in baseball: prevention and rehabilitation. Sports Med 1988;6:377–386.

4. Jobe FW, Kvitne RS. Shoulder pain in the overhead or throwing athlete: the relationship of anterior instability and rotator cuff impingement. Orthop Rev 1989;18:963–975.

5. Pink M, Perry J, Browne A, et al. The normal shoulder during freestyle swimming: an electromyographic and cinematographic analysis of twelve muscles. Am J Sports Med 1991; 19:569–576.

6. Morris M, Jobe FW, Perry J, et al. Electromyographic analysis of elbow function in tennis players. Am J Sports Med 1989;17:241–247.

7. Ryu RK, Jobe FW, et al. An electromyographic analysis of shoulder function in tennis players. Am J Sports Med 1988;16:481–485.

8. Jobe FW. Electromyographic shoulder activity in men and women professional golfers. Am J Sports Med 1989;17:782–787.

9. Jobe FW, Jobe CM. Painful athletic injuries of the shoulder. Clin Orthop 1983;173:117–124.

10. Garth WP, Allman FL, Armstrong WS. Occult anterior subluxations of the shoulder in noncontact sports. Am J Sports Med 1987;15:579–585.

11. Hawkins RJ, Mohtadi NG. Clinical evaluation of shoulder instability. Clin J Sports Med 1991;1:59–64.

12. Hawkins RJ, Mohtadi NGH. Controversy in anterior shoulder instability. Clin Orthop 1991;272:152–161.

13. Snyder SJ, Karzel RP, Del Pizzo W, et al. SLAP lesions of the shoulder. J Arthroscopy Rel Surg 1990;6:274–279.

14. Post M. Current concepts in the treatment of fractures of the clavicle. Clin Orthop 1989;245:89–101.

15. Stanley D, Norris S. Recovery following fractures of the clavicle treated conservatively. Injury 1988;19:162–164.

16. Ada JR, Miller ME. Scapular fractures: analysis of 113 cases. Clin Orthop 1991;269:174–180.

17. Wilbur MC, Evans EB. Fractures of the scapula—an analysis of forty cases and review of literature. J Bone Joint Surg 1977;59A:358–362.

18. Nettles JL, Linscheid R. Sternoclavicular dislocations. J Trauma 1968;8:158–164.

19. Salvatore JE. Sternoclavicular joint dislocation. Clin Orthop 1968;58:51–54.

20. Bearden JM, Hughston JC, Whatley GS. Acromioclavicular dislocation: method of treatment. Am J Sports Med 1973;1:5–17.

21. Behling F. Treatment of acromioclavicular separations. Orthop Clin North Am 1973;4:747–757.

22. Cox JS. The fate of the acromioclavicular joint in athletic injuries. Am J Sports Med 1981;9:50–53.

23. Rockwood CA Jr. Injuries to the acromioclavicular joint. In: Rockwood CA Jr, Green DP. Fractures in Adults, vol. 1. Philadelphia: JB Lippincott, 1984:860–910.

24. Hindenach JCR. Recurrent posterior dislocation of the shoulder. J Bone Joint Surg 1947;29B:582–586.

25. Harryman DT, Sidles JA, Clark JM, McQuade KJ. Translation of the humeral head on the glenoid with passive glenohumeral motion. J Bone Joint Surg 1990;72A:1334.

26. Rowe CR, Zarins B. Recurrent transient subluxation of the shoulder. J Bone Joint Surg 1981;63A:863–872.

27. Rowe CR. Prognosis in dislocations of the shoulder. J Bone Joint Surg 1956;38A:957–977.

28. Carr CR. Prognosis in dislocations of the shoulder (discussion). J Bone Joint Surg 1956;38A:977.

29. Jobe FW. Impingement problems in athletics. Instr Course Lect 1989;38:205–209.

30. Bigliani LU, Morrison DS, April EW. The morphology of the acromion in its relationship to rotator cuff tears. Orthop Trans 1986;10:228.

ELBOW INJURIES IN SPORTS

11

LOUIS C. ALMEKINDERS

Anatomy
History
Physical Examination
Acute Conditions and Treatment
Chronic Conditions and Treatment
Elbow Exercises

Traumatic injuries to the elbow in sports tend to be less common than injuries to knee, ankle, or even the shoulder. However, in certain sports that require vigorous motions of the upper extremity, elbow injuries are definitely not a rarity. In particular, contact sports, racquet sports, and sports requiring repeated throwing motions have a relatively high incidence of elbow injuries. In a survey of tennis players, nearly 50% of avid tennis players indicated they had experienced elbow problems (1). Studies of Little League pitchers have revealed an incidence of elbow pain of approximately 20% (2). Other sports with a relatively high incidence of elbow injuries include gymnastics (3), roller skating, and skate boarding.

The injuries in the racquet and throwing sports generally fall in the category of repetitive motion or overuse injuries. The cumulative effect of the repetitive motion eventually can cause a chronic injury to the tendons, ligaments, or joint surfaces. Examples of such injuries are tendinitis, ligamentous laxity, and osteochondritis dissecans. In other sports the elbow injury is often due to a single traumatic event in a previously normal elbow. These injuries generally result in acute fractures, dislocations, and ligament tears. In growing children these acute injuries usually do not result in ligament injuries but cause fractures around the elbow. The cartilaginous growth plates are often involved with these fractures because they are weaker than the ossified part of the bones and the ligaments surrounding the joint. In young adults ligament injuries become more common as the growth plates are closed following cessation of longitudinal growth. In older adults fractures will again become more common because of the gradual weakening of the bone as a result of senile osteoporosis. This chapter discusses the examination, diag-

nosis, and treatment of both acute injuries as well as chronic overuse injuries in and around the elbow joint.

ANATOMY

The elbow joint is a unique joint consisting of multiple articulations within one common joint space (4). The articulation between the distal humerus and proximal ulna (Figure 11.1) has the characteristics of a classic, uniaxial hinge joint. The proximal ulna or olecranon has a semicircular sigmoid notch that fits into the trochlea of the distal humerus. Posteriorly in the distal humerus the olecranon fossa accommodates the olecranon of the ulna when the elbow comes to full extension. Anteriorly the coronoid process of the ulna adds to the stability of the joint and can prevent posterior dislocation. This ulnohumeral articulation generally allows motion from 0° to approximately 150° of flexion. Occasionally 5° to 10° of hyperextension is possible in normal individuals.

Elbow flexion can be achieved by asking the patient to bend the elbow and touch the front of the shoulder with the hand. Normal is 135° to 150° (Figure 11.2A). The muscle mass of the biceps can limit flexion. Extension is accomplished by straigthening the elbow. Most males can achieve 0°, but occasionally this is limited by biceps muscle tension. Females can often hyperextend to +5°. Perform tests for flexion and extension in one continuous motion and do both arms simultaneously.

The head of the radius articulates both with the distal humerus and proximal ulna. The articulation with the humerus is formed by the capitellum and with the ulna by the radial notch. The head of the radius is entirely covered by articular cartilage. The motion that occurs in this joint is pre-

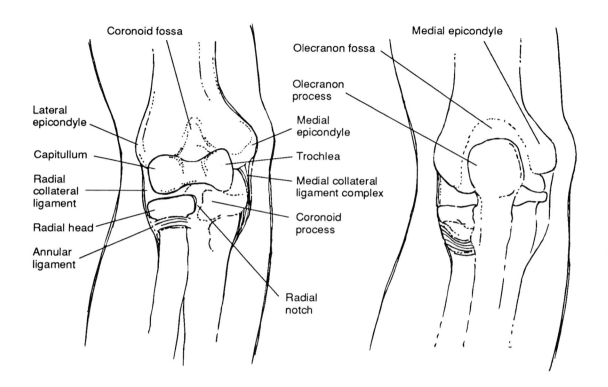

Figure 11.1. Anterior (A) and posterior (B) view of bony architecture and ligaments of the elbow joint.

dominantly rotation. Together with the distal radioulnar joint it provides approximately 80° to 90° supination as well as 80° to 90° pronation. Supination and pronation are tested with the elbow flexed to 90° (Figure 11.2B) and tucked in tightly to the side. A pencil is placed in the clinched fist (Figure 11.2C) and the fist is rotated. Full supination is accomplished when the palm is facing directly upward. Full pronation is accomplished when the palm is facing the floor. There should be 180° rotation. Limits to pronation and supination are determined by the degree to which the radius can rotate around the ulna.

Although the bony architecture of the elbow joint provides significant stability, the elbow ligaments still are of crucial importance for additional stability. The majority of the stresses during sports activity are laterally directed, valgus-producing stresses. This places the medial collateral ligaments under tension. The medial ligaments are therefore thought to be of more importance and are also better defined than the lateral collateral ligament complex (see Figure 11.1). Anteriorly and posteriorly the joint is covered by synovium and joint capsule, but no specific ligaments have been identified in these areas. Apart from the collateral ligaments, the annular ligament provides stability for the proximal radioulnar joint.

Although many muscles cross the elbow joint, only a few of them are prime elbow

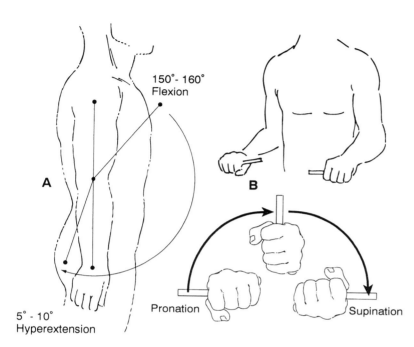

150°- 160°
Flexion

A

B

Pronation   Supination

5° - 10°
Hyperextension

Figure 11.2. Range of motion of the elbow. *A.* Flexion-extension. *B.* and *C.* Pronation-supination. (Modified from S Hoppenfeld. Physical Examination of the Spine Extremities. Norwalk, CT: Appleton & Lange, 1976: 50–51.)

movers. Many muscles also cross the shoulder or wrist and only exert a weak action on the elbow. The prime elbow movers are the brachialis, the biceps, the brachioradialis, and the triceps. The prime elbow flexors can be found anterior to elbow (Figure 11.3). The brachialis covers the anterior joint capsule and is a pure elbow flexor. Anterior to the brachialis is the biceps muscle and tendon, which is also a strong flexor of the elbow joint in addition to its action on the shoulder joint. Because of the biceps' insertion on the bicipital tuberosity of the radius, it is also a powerful supinator. Finally, there is the brachioradialis, which also flexes the elbow and supinates the forearm.

Elbow extension is primarily provided by the powerful triceps muscle (see Figure 11.3). Its three heads originate from the scapula and proximal humerus and insert together through the triceps tendon into the olecranon. The anconeus is a small elbow

extensor extending from the lateral side of the humerus to the ulna, but it has limited power.

In addition to the prime elbow movers, most of the wrist flexors and extensors as well as extrinsic finger flexors and extensors cross the elbow joint. Their effects on the elbow joint are minimal unless the prime elbow movers are not functional. On the lateral side of the elbow, the wrist extensors originate from the lateral epicondyle. On the medial side, the wrist flexors and pronator teres originate from the medial epicondyle.

The neurovascular structures that cross the elbow are of particular importance because they can be involved in pathology around this joint (Figure 11.4). The ulnar nerve crosses the elbow on the medial side between the epicondyle and the olecranon. This groove is covered by fibrous tissue and is often called the *cubital tunnel*. The radial nerve runs on the lateral side. It moves from

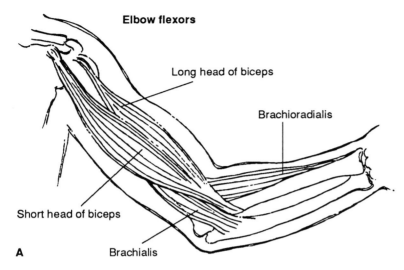

Figure 11.3. Prime flexors
(*A*) and extensors (*B*) of the
elbow.

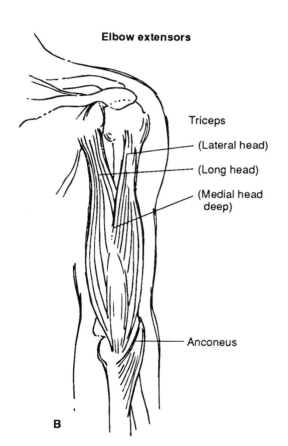

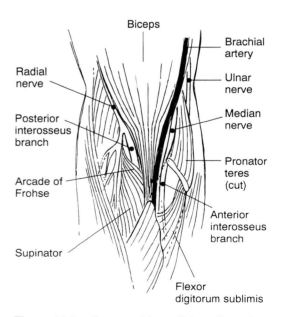

Figure 11.4. Course of the radial median, ulnar
nerve, and brachial artery across the elbow joint.

Table 11.1. Major Motor Innervation of Peripheral Nerves of the Upper Extremity

Nerve	Muscle
Radial nerve	Triceps wrist extensors Finger extensors Thumb extensors
Ulnar nerve	Ulnar wrist flexors Ulnar half of flexor digitorum profundus Intrinsic muscles of the hand
Median nerve	Radial wrist flexors All other finger flexors Thenar muscles

the posterior compartment of the upper arm around the radial neck into the extensor compartment of the forearm. The median nerve and brachial artery run anterior to the elbow joint superficial to the brachialis muscle. The major muscles with their nerve innervation are shown in Table 11.1.

HISTORY

In the evaluation of elbow injuries, a carefully obtained history can yield important diagnostic information. In acute, traumatic injuries it is important to obtain information about the mechanism of injury. If the direction of the deforming force is known, it becomes much easier to look for injured structures. For instance, if an athlete describes an injury that forced the elbow into valgus, then one can assume that the medial ligamentous structures were placed under tension and the lateral joint structures under compression. Therefore, the examiner is more likely to find a tear of the medial

(ulnar) collateral ligament or a compression fracture of the radiocapitellar joint (Figure 11.5) (5).

In chronic injuries it is important to question the patients regarding the onset of the problems. Was the patient involved in any unusual activities such as changes in sports, workout schedules, equipment, intensity, and duration of competition? This information is not only helpful in making the diagnosis but also is invaluable in designing a rehabilitation program once the diagnosis is made. Information regarding the nature of the pain in chronic injuries can also be helpful in determining the type of problem the patient is complaining of. Sudden elbow pain that is activity related and disappears rapidly with rest is often indicative of an intra-articular joint problem. Intra-articular loose bodies and osteochondritis dissecans can result in this type of pain. Elbow pain that worsens in the 24 hours following sports activities is generally associated with chronic soft-tissue inflammation such as tendinitis and bursitis. Pain that is associated with radiation into the wrist or hand

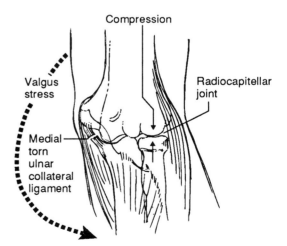

Figure 11.5. Valgus injury to the elbow, tension medially and compression laterally.

may be indicative of an injury to the nerves around the elbow.

Finally, we should always remember that elbow pain does not necessarily represent an intrinsic elbow problem. Cervical spine, shoulder, and hand pathology can all result in referred pain around the elbow. In addition, elbow pain can be a manifestation of a systemic disease such as rheumatologic disorders and malignancies. Therefore, every patient should be questioned regarding problems in other areas as well as their general health.

PHYSICAL EXAMINATION

The elbow joint is readily accessible for physical examination. Often the initial diagnosis can be made based on history and physical examination alone. Important information can be obtained from both inspection, palpation as well as some functional tests (6).

Inspection

Inspection of the elbow is particularly helpful if there is a contralateral, normal elbow for comparison. In acute injuries, gross deformity can be present due to fracture or dislocation. In more subtle injuries, inspection should include a careful evaluation of swelling and atrophy around the elbow joint. Swelling directly over the olecranon can be seen in olecranon bursitis as well as olecranon fractures. Swelling due to joint effusion is most easily detected and aspirated in the triangular space between the lateral epicondyle, radial head, and olecranon (Figure 11.6). Atrophy or depressions of the muscle mass around the elbow can sometimes be seen following tendon ruptures.

Palpation

The most obvious landmarks for palpation are the olecranon and the medial and

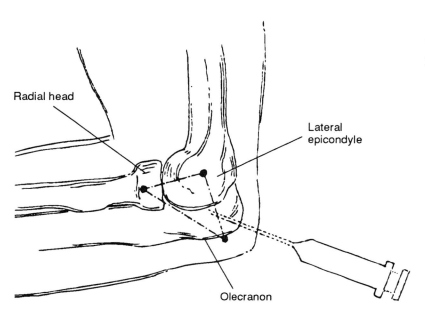

Figure 11.6. Lateral triangular space where joint effusion can be detected and aspirated.

Radial head

Lateral epicondyle

Olecranon

lateral epicondyles. Chronic tendinitis of the tendons attached to these areas is invariably associated with pain on palpation directly adjacent to these bony landmarks (Figure 11.7A). In addition, the radial head can generally be palpated on the lateral side of the elbow through the extensor muscles of the wrist and hand. This palpation is often facilitated by pronating and supinating the forearm during this palpation (Figure 11.7B). The radial head rotation can be clearly felt during this maneuver. Anteriorly the biceps tendon and brachial artery can be felt. On the medial side the ulnar nerve can often be palpated as it courses through the cubital tunnel (Figure 11.7C).

Functional Tests

If inspection and palpation have not revealed any clear evidence of displaced fractures or dislocations, it is generally safe to test the function of various structures around the elbow. Both active and passive motion should be evaluated in the injured and normal elbow. Less active motion than passive motion generally indicates marked muscle weakness or muscle inhibition due to pain. Most of our daily activities require motion from 30° flexion to 130° flexion. Therefore, flexion contractures of less than 30° may go unnoticed by the patient. In addition to flexion and extension, the range of pronation and supination should be evaluated. Following range of motion testing, the muscle strength around the elbow is evaluated. To test the elbow flexors, the elbow is placed in approximately 90° to 120° flexion. The examiner attempts to extend the elbow while the patient tries to resist this extension (Figure 11.8). In normal adults the flexor power can often not be overpowered by the examiner because of the strength of the biceps muscle. Extension strength is

measured with the elbow in approximately 45° in an opposite manner (see Figure 11.8). Pronation and supination are most easily tested with the elbow at 90° by the patient's side. The examiner can grip the patient's hand as if he or she is shaking hands. The patient is then asked to resist the pronation or supination movement by the examiner. Again, comparison with the normal side is helpful in detecting weakness.

Instability of the elbow joint due to ligamentous injury can be tested during a physical examination. Ligament injuries can result in varus or valgus instability depending on which collateral ligament was injured. Both varus and valgus instability are tested with the elbow flexed approximately 15° to 20° to "unlock" to olecranon out of the olecranon fossa. One hand of the examiner then stabilizes the distal humerus, whereas the other hand applies a valgus or varus stress to the distal forearm (Figure 11.9). A slight amount of varus and valgus motion can sometimes be appreciated in normal elbows but any increased motion compared to the normal side is considered a sign of instability.

A thorough neurologic examination should be part of every elbow evaluation. Both local neurologic abnormalities around the elbow as well as more distant nerve injuries can be responsible for pain around the elbow. More distant problems in upper and lower motor neurons can be detected through deep tendon reflexes. The biceps (C5), brachioradialis (C6), and triceps (C7) jerks are easily obtained and yield important information. Local and distant nerve problems can result in sensory changes distal to the elbow. Figure 11.10 shows the sensory distribution of peripheral nerves in this area. Local nerve problems such as excessive pressure can also result in hypersensitivity of the nerve. In those cases, light tapping over the compressed nerve seg-

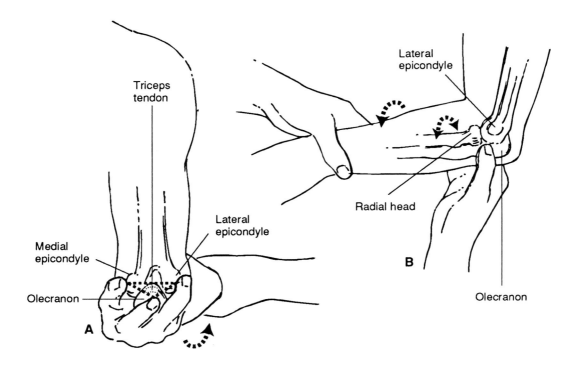

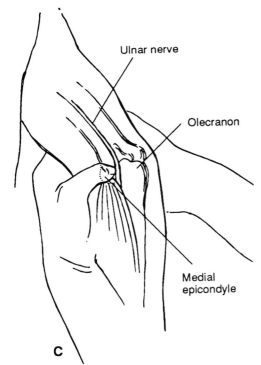

Figure 11.7. Palpation of the elbow. *A.* Bony land-marks. *B.* Radial head. *C.* Ulnar nerve.

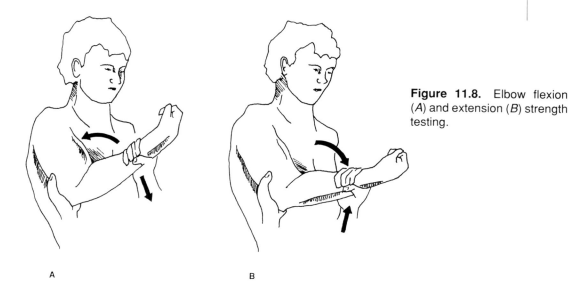

A   B

Figure 11.8. Elbow flexion (*A*) and extension (*B*) strength testing.

ment will result in paresthesias into the sensory distribution of the nerve. This so-called Tinel's sign should be looked for over the course of the ulnar, median, and radial nerves as they cross the elbow into the proximal forearm.

ACUTE CONDITIONS AND TREATMENT

This section on specific conditions describes injuries that are generally due to a single traumatic event in a previously normal elbow. These injuries often result in immediate disability and inability to continue the sports activity. Evaluation generally occurs on the field or shortly after the injury in the emergency department or office. A thorough history and examination will often yield important information. Most patients will require radiographic examination to rule out fractures or dislocations. Patients who can actively move their elbow through a full range of motion without pain or patients who were able to continue their sports activity despite the acute injury are exceptions to this rule. These pa-

tients can often safely be observed for 7 or 10 days to see if the symptoms resolve spontaneously.

Ulnar Collateral Ligament Tears

The repeated, rapid acceleration phase of throwing sports, such as baseball, tennis, and the javelin throw, subject the medial (ulnar) collateral ligament complex of the elbow to substantial stress. This stress may result in tears of the ligament complex.

The athlete will present with acute or subacute pain and swelling along the medial elbow. Valgus stressing with the elbow flexed 30° will reveal any laxity of the joint (see Figure 11.5). Stress x-ray views may be helpful in delineating laxity of the medial ligament complex.

In all but the most high-performance athletes initial treatment should be rest, protection from valgus stress, and gradual rehabilitation, followed by a slow return to throwing sports. In highly competitive athletes, with substantial laxity, consideration for early surgical treatment should be given. These athletes should have early referral to a sports oriented orthopedist.

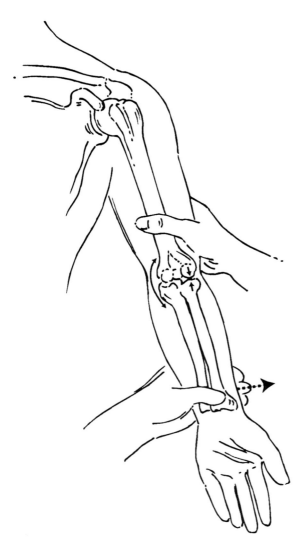

Figure 11.9. Valgus stress testing of the elbow in slight flexion.

Hyperextended Elbow

Clinical Case #1

A 17-year-old cross-country runner fell while running in the woods 3 hours before coming to your office. She tried to break the fall with her left arm. She complains of swelling and pain in the left elbow and increasing difficulty in completely extending the elbow.

Many elbow injuries occur as the athlete loses his or her balance while running, riding, or jumping. As a reflex most of us will stretch out one or both arms in an attempt to break the fall on contact with the ground. At the time of impact the elbow is often in the fully extended position. The outstretched hand will be slowed by the contact with the ground but because of the momentum of the body the elbow can be forced in hyperextension. Often, wrist and shoulder injuries can occur in a similar situation. If the hyperextension force is large enough an elbow dislocation will occur. It is possible that some hyperextension injuries are actually spontaneously reduced elbow subluxations or even dislocations.

The hyperextended elbow is predominantly a soft-tissue injury. Hyperextension is mainly restrained by the anterior elbow capsule and anterior part of the medial collateral ligament. On physical examination most of the tenderness will be found on the anterior aspect of the joint. Range of motion is often normal immediately after the injury but diminishes after swelling has occurred. At that time the athlete is often unable to fully extend the elbow, whereas full flexion is often still possible. The remainder of the examination is essentially normal. Radiographic evaluation is not mandatory if the initial evaluation indeed revealed a full or near-full range of motion. If no immediate evaluation was done and the range of motion is limited due to swelling, radiographic evaluation should be considered, especially if the range of motion does not improve significantly in the first 5 to 7 days following the injury. In the case of a hyper-

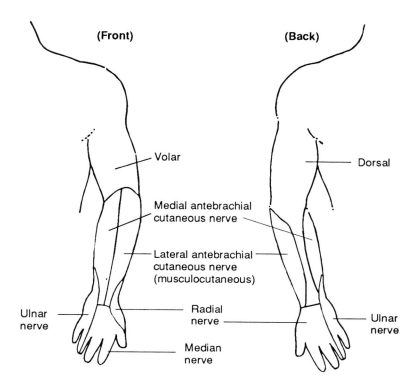

Figure 11.10. Distal sensory distribution of the peripheral nerves of the upper extremity.

(Front)   (Back)

Volar
Medial antebrachial cutaneous nerve
Lateral antebrachial cutaneous nerve (musculocutaneous)
Ulnar nerve
Radial nerve
Median nerve
Dorsal
Ulnar nerve

extended elbow the radiographs should be normal (Figure 11.11). The differential diagnosis includes fracture, dislocation, and an acute, distal biceps tendon rupture. In a biceps tendon injury there also will be swelling and pain at the anterior aspect of the elbow. The biceps tendon will not be palpable in the antecubital fossa as it is in a normal elbow. When testing biceps strength an abnormally bulging muscle mass will be seen in the upper arm. This injury is most commonly seen in weight lifters, football and gymnastics.

The elbow joint will still be a stable joint following an anterior capsular injury due to the bony contours of the joint surfaces and remaining ligaments. Therefore, prolonged immobilization is not necessary and may even be detrimental. A short period (24 to 48 hours) of immobilization in a sling

can be used in conjunction with icing and nonsteroidal anti-inflammatory drugs (NSAIDs) to improve comfort. However, as soon as comfort allows, active range of motion exercises should be started. The exercises should be focused on regaining full extension. Once full extension is regained, strengthening exercises can be added with an emphasis on elbow flexors (see section on elbow exercises). Full recovery without pain and normal strength and motion can take as much as 4 to 6 weeks. The athlete can return to participation once full extension and strength return.

Elbow Dislocation

A dislocation of the elbow can occur during a fall onto an extended arm as described in the previous section. However,

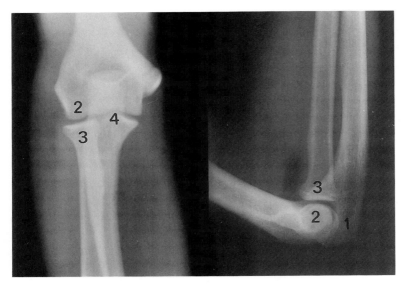

Figure 11.11. Normal anteroposterior and lateral radiographs of an adult elbow with olecranon (*1*), capitellum (*2*), radial head (*3*), and coronoid process (*4*). (Notice how the radial head points to the capitellum in both views.)

it can also occur while the elbow is in the flexed position. The vast majority of elbow dislocations are posterior or posterolateral dislocations. During extreme hyperextension the olecranon can lever itself out of the trochlea and result in a dislocation. If the elbow is flexed, a posterior-directed force can be large enough to push the olecranon posterior to the humerus. The athlete will complain of severe pain and generally is unable to actively move the elbow. In all cases there is a gross deformity with swelling that develops quickly. Because of traction on the nerves and swelling, there may be a change in the neurologic status distal to the elbow. Sensory changes in the ulnar and radial nerve distribution are particularly common. Radiographic evaluation is mandatory to determine the exact direction of the dislocation and rule out associated fractures.

Treatment consists of closed reduction followed by a short period of immobilization. Reduction of posterior dislocation is usually obtained by gentle traction in a slight degree of flexion. Following reduction, radiographs should be obtained to ascertain a concentric reduction of the joint. The elbow is immobilized in a posterior splint and sling for 1 to 2 weeks to allow the swelling to subside. In the second week following the injury, the splint is removed and active range of motion exercises are instituted similar to the rehabilitation of a hyperextended elbow. Return to full activities can take 6 to 10 weeks. Some patients will be left with a permanent flexion contracture. This is more likely to occur if the elbow has been immobilized for more than 2 weeks following the injury (7).

Elbow Fractures

Fractures around the elbow can occur in many different situations. A fall on an outstretched arm, direct impact on the elbow, and a sudden pull on the arm can all result in fractures. Children are particularly prone to fractures during athletics because of the presence of weaker, cartilaginous growth plates. The evaluation and management of fractures in the pediatric population is quite different from treatment of adult fractures and therefore will be addressed separately.

Pediatric Fractures

Clinical Case #2

A 10-year-old Little League outfielder fell while chasing a fly ball. He was unable to complete the game because of pain in the elbow. He comes to your office 2 hours later and you find that he does not want to move his elbow out of a 90° flexed position and he becomes tearful when you palpate over the lower humerus.

Fractures in and around the elbow joint are common injuries in children (8). Direct impact and falls on an outstretched upper extremity are the usual mechanisms of injury. In older children the pain, swelling, and sometimes deformity are often obvious. Occasionally in younger children the only sign of injury is the inability or unwill-

ingness to move the elbow joint due to pain. During the physical examination it is important to allow the child to relax and settle down. Gentle palpation will often reveal a point of maximum tenderness. In the case of a fracture, this is directly over the fracture itself. In all these cases, radiographic evaluation is needed. Radiographs will often lead to a correct diagnosis. However, elbow radiographs in children can be difficult to interpret because of the presence of multiple ossification centers around the elbow (Figure 11.12). The cartilaginous areas that separate the ossification centers from the metaphysis are often involved in the fracture. The fracture line through the cartilaginous area will not be visible on plain radiographs. Therefore, fractures can only be diagnosed when they involve the ossified part of the bone as well, or when there is displacement of the ossification center(s) compared to the normal elbow. In most cases a skilled interpreter is needed to evaluate elbow radiographs in children. Frequently films of the normal elbow are required. Good quality anteroposterior and

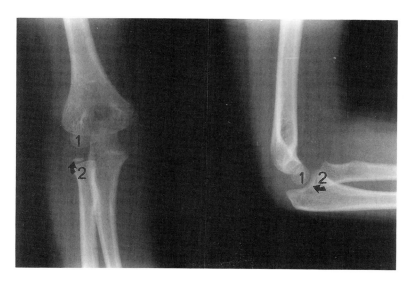

Figure 11.12. Normal anteroposterior and lateral radiographs of a pediatric elbow with ossification centers of capitellum (*1*) and radial head (*2*), which points to capitellum in both directions.

lateral views require an experienced radiologic technician but are essential for a good radiographic evaluation. The most common pediatric elbow fractures are briefly discussed.

Supracondylar Humerus Fracture

Some of these fractures have the elevated fat pad sign as the only radiographic evidence of fracture. About one third of these fractures have minimal to no displacement and offer minimal difficulty in treatment. They can be treated symptomatically with a supporting splint. On the other hand, a displaced supracondylar fracture requires considerable thought and skill in treating (9). Brachial artery injury due to the sharp edge of the proximal fragment with resulting ischemic contracture of the forearm muscles is a dreaded complication (Figure 11.13). Most children with this fracture are under 10 years old and fall on an outstretched arm at the time of injury. Immediate swelling and extension deformity are usually obvious. Emergency splinting and transport to a hospital for evaluation and treatment are needed. An emergency splint in slight extension is preferable because it is less likely to impair circulation. Rapid transport to a facility with experience in these types of fractures is needed. Reduction of displaced fractures becomes even more difficult when the treatment is delayed and the swelling has increased. Often percutaneous pinning under general anesthesia is needed to avoid vascular complications and late deformity. Admission to the hospital for observation is generally recommended. Following the reduction a long arm cast is used for 4 to 5 weeks before immobilization is discontinued. Although significant postimmobilization stiffness often develops, most children will be able to regain this motion without formal physical therapy if the fracture was reduced anatomically initially.

Distal Humerus Physeal Fractures

Fractures involving the cartilaginous physis of the distal humerus are often less dramatic injuries than supracondylar humerus fractures. Generally there is some mild swelling and limitation of motion but no gross deformity. Careful radiographic evaluation is needed to rule out such injuries because they are often associated

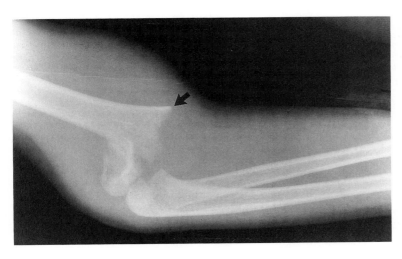

Figure 11.13. Supracondylar humerus fracture in a child. Arrow points to fragment that can injure brachial artery.

with subtle findings. Comparison anteroposterior and lateral views may be needed to find small degrees of displacements. If the fracture is entirely in cartilaginous tissue, an arthrogram may be needed to visualize the intra-articular fracture line. Arthrographic dye will leak into intra-articular fractures and outline the injury. Displaced intra-articular fractures are more prone to cause complications such as deformity and posttraumatic arthritis. If displaced physeal fractures are found, often surgical treatment is needed to accomplish a satisfactory reduction and eventual normal elbow function (10).

Proximal Radius and Ulnar Fractures

Proximal radius and ulnar fractures are less common than distal humerus fractures (10). Radial neck and head fractures can significantly impair pronation and supination if they are displaced. Reduction or excision of small displaced head fragments may be needed in such cases. Ulnar fractures can be associated with a radial head dislocation (Monteggia fracture). Radiographs can rule out such an injury. The radial head is reduced if the radial head in both the anteroposterior and lateral views points to capitellum or its corresponding ossification center of the distal humerus (see Figure 11.12).

Adult Fractures

Fractures in and around the elbow in adults are rare in athletes. Perhaps the most commonly encountered fractures in adult athletes are medial epicondylar avulsion fractures and radial head fractures.

Medial Epicondylar Avulsion Fractures

These injuries are common in the young adult who sustains a traumatic valgus stress to the elbow. Instead of tearing the medial collateral ligament, the bony epicondyle is avulsed. Physical findings include pain and swelling on the medial elbow, with limited motion. Often the joint will be lax to valgus stressing. Plane radiographs are indicated in any substantial injury to the medial side of the elbow.

Treatment of these injuries depends on the degree of displacement of the bony fragment. If the displacement is a few millimeters or less, then immobilization followed by bracing is appropriate. Fragments displaced more than 5 mm require surgical repair.

Radial Head Fractures

As in the child, the adult athlete may fracture the radial head with a fall on the outstretched hand. Due to the intra-articular location of the radial head, even minimally displaced fractures often result in the joint filling with blood and substantial limitation of motion.

If the fracture fragment is minimally displaced and elbow motion (particularly pronation-supination) is full, then symptomatic treatment is all that is required. Early mobilization is helpful to limit stiffness. Displaced fractures, if they limit elbow motion, should be treated surgically.

Other Elbow Fractures

Supracondylar humerus fractures and olecranon fractures are rare athletic injuries in adults. Both fractures usually displace due to muscle forces and typically require early surgical treatment.

Distal Biceps Tendon Ruptures

Although uncommon in athletes, distal avulsions of the biceps tendon from its attachment to the radial tuberosity may occur. The mechanism is usually forced elbow extension or forearm pronation against resistance, typically in weight lifters. The athlete will feel a tear or pop associated with pain and swelling in the antecubital fossa. There is usually no bunching of the biceps muscle belly, as seen in proximal ruptures of the long head.

The physical examination will reveal swelling and ecchymosis in the antecubital fossa. Although partial ruptures of the tendon may occur, more commonly there is complete avulsion of the tendon from bone. This distinction is made by palpation. The tendon of the biceps should be palpable in the antecubital fossa with resisted flexion of the elbow, with the arm in supination. If the tendon cannot be palpated, then the avulsion is complete. Marked weakness of supination will be noted as well. If the examiner can palpate a biceps tendon with this maneuver, then the diagnosis is a partial tear.

The treatment of distal biceps tendon injuries depends on the extent of the injury. Complete avulsions need early surgical repair because the athlete will be left with a marked weakness of supination without repair. Partial ruptures can be treated conservatively, with early protection in a sling, followed by gradual mobilization and strengthening.

CHRONIC CONDITIONS AND TREATMENT

This section reviews the more common elbow injuries that develop gradually and often present to the physician as a chronic condition. Many patients suffering from chronic elbow injuries are unable to clearly remember the time of onset. Pain is generally the first and often only symptom. At first the pain is only present during or after the sports activity. If the condition fails to correct itself, the pain becomes more severe

and often is present both during and after the activity. At that point many patients will seek medical attention.

Lateral Epicondylitis ("Tennis Elbow")

Clinical Case #3

A 38-year-old tennis player comes to your office with a 3-week history of elbow pain. The pain began after he played a match using his 9-year-old son's tennis racket. The pain is aggravated by anything that requires full elbow extension, lifting, shaking hands and following long periods of using his computer. Resisting wrist extension while the elbow is fully extended reproduces the pain.

Lateral epicondylitis or tennis elbow is the most common chronic injury resulting in elbow pain. It was first recognized as an elbow injury caused by racquet sports in the nineteenth century. It continues to be an extremely common injury among tennis players. Although it has been clearly associated with racquet sports, many patients who are never involved in these sports can present with this elbow condition. Use of the upper extremities in other sports such as weight lifting and pitching can be associated with lateral epicondylitis.

Despite its frequent occurrence, the exact pathophysiology of lateral epicondylitis remains unclear. It is universally agreed that lateral epicondylitis results in chronic pain near or at the common origin of the wrist extensor muscles at the lateral epicondyle (11). Repetitive, forceful activities such as racquet sports and weight lifting are associated with high loads within the extensor muscles of the wrist. Actual wrist motion is not needed to cause these high loads within the wrist extensor muscles. When the ball hits the racquet during a backhand stroke, the wrist will tend to be forced into palmar flexion. The wrist extensor muscles will fire, dampen the impact of the ball, and stabilize the wrist. The action is associated with a high tension within these muscles. Similarly the wrist extensors will fire during weight lifting to stabilize the wrist. Repeated forceful contractions possibly cause small microinjuries in the form of small tears within the extensor muscle-tendon mass. It appears that this preferentially occurs near or at the common tendon insertion into the lateral epicondyle. Small injuries can be repaired by the body itself. However, if repeated microtrauma exceeds the rate of healing, the cumulative effect of these injuries results in a macroinjury with clinically detectable symptoms. An inflammatory response is thought to occur at the site of injury, which results in pain. Several other factors may play a role in the development of this injury. It is possible that some age-related degeneration allows this injury to occur more quickly because most patients are over the age of 35 years. Faulty techniques and equipment have also been associated with an increased incidence of lateral epicondylitis. Excessive, active wrist dorsiflexion during the backhand swing (using only one hand) and failure to hit the ball on the "sweet spot" of the racquet are forms of faulty technique. Improper racquet size and stiff and tightly strung racquets are possible examples of equipment problems relating to lateral epicondylitis.

The typical patient with lateral epicondylitis will present with a several week history of chronic, intermittent elbow pain. The pain is often most severe during the initial sports activity but sometimes actually improves after a warm-up. The pain generally worsens during the rest period following the sports activity, even into the next morning. Most patients can clearly identify the area of pain around the lateral epicondyle.

The physical examination should reveal a markedly tender area directly over the lateral epicondyle (see Figure 11.7*B*) or slightly distal to it. However, if the tender area is more than 1 to 2 in. distal to the epicondyle, a different diagnosis should be considered. The pain can also be elicited by resisted wrist flexion or stretching the extensor muscles (Figure 11.14). In the resisted wrist flexion test, the patient is asked to maintain a dorsiflexed position of the wrist while the examiner exerts a force directed toward palmar flexion of the wrist. Passive stretching of the extensor muscles is done by forced palmar flexion of the wrist while the elbow is fully extended. Range of motion in the elbow is usually full and a neurovascular examination should be normal. Radiographs generally do not show any abnormalities unless the condition has been extremely chronic. In chronic cases sometimes a small spurlike projection can be seen at the lateral epicondyle analogous to a heel spur in plantar fasciitis. In first-time, uncomplicated cases a radiograph is generally not needed unless initial treatment has failed. If the symptoms are not typical of lateral epicondylitis, other tests should be performed to rule out other causes of lateral elbow pain. Abnormal neurologic findings may indicate a cervical radiculopathy or local compression neuropathy (see following sections). Loss of motion is more often associated with intra-articular elbow joint abnormalities such as osteochondritis dissecans or osteoarthritis.

If the history and physical examination are indicative of lateral epicondylitis, usually initial treatment can be instituted without further diagnostic procedures (12). Treatment follows the principles of management of most overuse injuries. Initially the offending stress should be removed or minimized to avoid further microtrauma. Generally, complete rest is not recom-

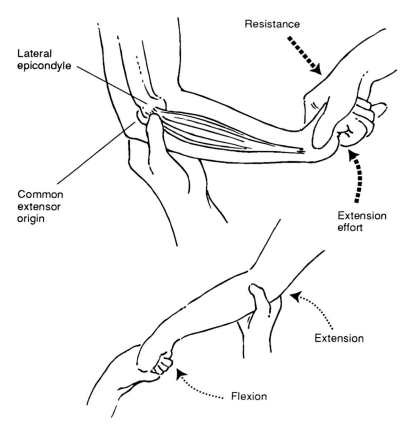

Figure 11.14. Provocative tests for pain at the lateral epicondyle in lateral epicondylitis.

mended because careful, protected motion is also a stimulus for healing of the soft tissue. Therefore, only relative rest is needed to maintain some load but overload should be avoided in the injured tissues. Relative rest may take different forms in different patients depending on the degree of injury and level of sports activity. Sometimes a decrease in the frequency and intensity of the sports activity suffices. Pain is the main guide in determining the degree of relative rest that is needed. Continued pain indicates excessive activities. Light workouts without pain can be beneficial. Equipment, technique, and workout schedules should be evaluated. The racquet should be appropriately sized and strung

and not be too heavy or stiff. Proper grip size can be determined (Figure 11.15) by measuring from the proximal palmar crease to the tip of the ring finger. The ruler should be placed on the radial side of the ring finger. If needed, use of the entire body and not just the wrist and elbow should be taught for the backhand stroke. It is often beneficial to switch to a two-handed backhand. Novice players should have adequate periods of rest between workouts and competition. Proper flexibility, endurance, and strength exercises should be done by all athletes.

In addition to activity modification some other therapeutic measures can be taken. A structured program of stretching and

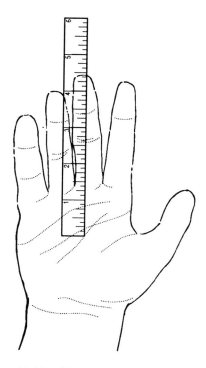

Figure 11.15. Measure from proximal palmar crease to the tip of the ring finger to determine proper grip size for racquet sports.

strengthening can stimulate the extensor muscles to heal without causing further injury. Strengthening is also important to avoid recurrence once normal activities are resumed. The stretching and strengthening should concentrate on the wrist extensors but should not ignore the wrist flexors as well as proximal musculature. Surgical tubing or dumbbells can be used approximately 20 minutes a day to perform most exercises (see section on exercises). NSAIDs can be used to alleviate some of the pain in lateral epicondylitis. Surgical specimens of lateral epicondylitis do not always show that inflammation is a predominant, histologic feature. Therefore, it is not clear whether NSAIDs will truly affect the pa-

thology of this injury. It is possible that early in the course of the injury, inflammation is a more important part of the lesion, making NSAIDs more effective at that point.

Physical modalities are thought to decrease inflammation and promote healing. Application of ice and ice massage directly after the sports activity may decrease some of the inflammation, if present. Heat, ultrasound, and electrical stimulation are thought to promote healing, although scientific evidence for this is lacking. The local use of a corticosteroid has been advocated in resistant cases. Although it can be administered through phonophoresis, it is often directly injected into the tender area using a parenteral preparation. If the pain recurs, a second or even third injection can be tried at 3-month intervals. Side effects include skin depigmentation and local subcutaneous atrophy. A therapeutic exercise program should be maintained following injections.

Bracing is occasionally helpful to alleviate the pain. In patients with severe pain, a short period of splinting of elbow and wrist may be needed to improve the pain and allow therapeutic exercises. Many athletes experience improvement with a tennis elbow strap (Figure 11.16). This is a commercially available strap or pneumatic splint that is applied just distal to the lesion directly over the extensor muscle mass. It is thought to decrease the forces in the tendon proximal to the strap. A wrist splint can be helpful for athletes who often work at a keyboard.

If after 6 to 12 months of combined intensive treatment no improvement occurs, surgical therapy can be considered. Various procedures have been described but most of them involve a release of the common wrist extensor tendon off the lateral epicondyle (13). Although the surgical procedure is relatively short and performed in

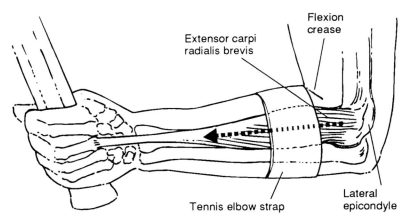

Extensor carpi
radialis brevis

Flexion
crease

Tennis elbow strap

Lateral
epicondyle

Figure 11.16. Tennis elbow strap placed distal to the flexion crease supports the exterior carpi radialis brevis to reduce the forces on the extensor origin.

an outpatient setting, the rehabilitation generally takes 2 to 4 months before full activities are resumed. Stretching and strengthening exercises are important after the surgery to reverse the disuse atrophy, promote healing, and prevent recurrence.

Medial Epicondylitis ("Golfer's Elbow")

Chronic pain on the medial side of the elbow can be due to an injury similar to lateral epicondylitis. The common origin of the wrist flexors at the medial epicondyle can also sustain repeated microtrauma due to repetitive forceful contractions. The resulting overuse injury can be a medial epicondylitis (14). This injury is not as common as lateral epicondylitis for reasons that are not clear. The onset and character of the pain is similar to lateral epicondylitis but is more often associated with a forearm stroke than a backhand stroke. Other sports activities associated with medial epicondylitis are pitching, weight lifting, and any other repeated forceful use of the wrist and finger flexor muscles.

Physical examination will reveal tenderness at or just distal to the medial epicondyle. Provocative tests include resisted wrist flexion and wrist flexor stretch-

ing performed in a reverse manner as described for lateral epicondylitis. The remainder of the examination is generally within normal limits.

Confusion and overlap with other causes of elbow pain on the medial side is much more common than with lateral elbow pain. Ulnar nerve compression neuropathy at the cubital tunnel can give similar findings upon examination. Usually some abnormal neurologic findings can be detected in this condition. Medial tension overload syndrome is a possible cause of medial-sided elbow pain. This syndrome is primarily caused by repeated valgus forces and can involve injury to the medial collateral ligament complex but sometimes also includes an element of medial epicondylitis. Both cubital tunnel syndrome and medial tension overload syndrome will be discussed in the following sections. In addition, cervical radiculopathy, elbow osteoarthritis, and median nerve compression neuropathy should be considered in the differential diagnosis.

Treatment of medial epicondylitis follows essentially the same principles as those outlined in the section on lateral epicondylitis. The main difference is the emphasis on the forearm flexor mass instead of extensor muscles. In addition, the forearm stroke or overhead pitching technique should be evaluated and corrected if needed. Corticosteroid injection and surgical release can also be considered in recalcitrant cases following similar guidelines.

Medial Tension Overload Syndrome

Clinical Case #4

A right-handed 34-year-old coach who participates in a summer softball league complains of recurrent right medial elbow pain. The pain is worse after a game and he notes some numbness and tingling from his elbow down to his little finger. Your examination reveals laxity with valgus stress of his right arm.

Repeated valgus-directed force on the elbow can result in a variety of overuse injuries often termed *valgus extension overload* or *medial tension overload syndrome*. Valgus-directed forces are extremely common in most overhead activities such as baseball pitching, football throwing, tennis ball serving, and volleyball spiking. In most of these motions the athlete goes through a cocking phase, acceleration phase, and follow-through phase. A marked valgus-directed stress is placed on the elbow, especially during the acceleration phase. The structures that have to resist this force are at risk for repeated microtrauma and resulting overuse injury. These structures include the medial collateral ligament complex and forearm flexor muscles on the medial side and the radiocapitellar joint on the lateral side (15). The radiocapitellar joint is placed under compressive stress while the former two are subjected to tensional loads (Figure 11.17). These tensile overloads on the medial side can lead to injury and gradual laxity of the medial ligament com-

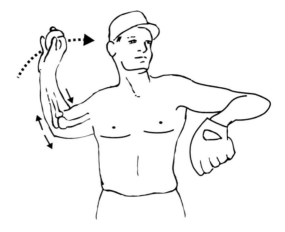

Figure 11.17. Mechanism of injury for medial tension overload syndrome due to throwing.

plex. The resulting instability can eventually lead to abnormal shear forces within the joint and subsequent osteophyte formation, particularly in the olecranon and coronoid area of the ulna. On the lateral side osteochondral injuries due to excessive compression can also lead to joint degeneration and loose bodies within the joint.

The throwing athlete with medial tension overload syndrome can present with a variety of symptoms and complaints. Repeated traction injuries to the medial collateral ligament complex will result in medial-sided pain during and after throwing activities. If the injury has progressed to instability, it is possible that the athlete also experiences ulnar nerve symptoms due to traction on the nerve as the elbow is forced in valgus. Once the joint is affected with osteochondral fragment or osteophyte formation the complaints may include limited range of motion and occasional locking or catching of the joint due to loose bodies.

Physical examination can reveal medial-sided tenderness, but unlike classic medial epicondylitis the tenderness is often not exclusively located at the epicondyle. Valgus stress on the elbow, as described previously, will increase the pain and may even reveal some instability compared to the nonsymptomatic side. In advanced stages a flexion contracture due to scarring and osteophyte formation in the joint can be found. Repeated traction on the ulnar nerve during throwing can lead to injury of the ulnar nerve with a positive Tinel's sign over the course of the ulnar nerve. Light tapping of the nerve around the elbow will result in paresthesias into the ulnar nerve sensory distribution of the forearm and hand.

In the early stages, when there is no limitation of motion, locking or catching, radiographic evaluation is not immediately needed prior to institution of initial treatment. In later stages radiographs can be helpful to determine the amount of joint involvement and thereby the treatment and prognosis of the injury. In the case of ulnar nerve symptoms, electromyography and nerve conduction velocity measurements can determine the extent of nerve involvement.

Initial treatment is aimed at diminishing or eliminating the offending forces. Proper throwing techniques can be helpful in diminishing the stress on the elbow. Side arm throwing should be discouraged because it places more valgus stress on the elbow than overhead throwing. Adequate warm-up, stretching, and strengthening routines should be part of the workout and competition (16). Besides rehabilitation involving the muscle around the elbow, particular attention should be paid to the shoulder and upper body strength and flexibility. Weak and tight muscles in these areas may lead to excessive stress on the structures around the elbow joint. During the symptomatic stage a decrease of the offending activities is mandatory. The number of full-speed pitches should be recorded and limited to a degree where the elbow is not painful. Several days of rest in between competition is needed to recover from excessive load on the elbow.

Icing following activities and NSAIDs can decrease pain. In more severe cases complete rest is necessary. Once the pain has subsided slow pitches can be performed. If these do not cause pain the activities are slowly increased. An aggressive strengthening and flexibility program should be continued during this increase in activities. The athlete should be advanced slowly over several weeks from going to the throwing motion without the ball to slow pitches over increasing distance to eventual fast pitches over the desired distances. During rehabilitation taping of the elbow can be helpful in decreasing hyperextension and valgus forces.

In athletes in advanced stages, surgical treatment may be needed (17). Loose bodies can be removed during arthroscopic surgery. Marked medial collateral ligament laxity can be improved by open reconstructive surgery. However, many elbows that require surgical intervention for this condition do not return to full and unlimited use despite some improvement after the surgery.

Little League Elbow

Little League elbow is the pediatric equivalent of medial tension overload syndrome. However, because of the presence of cartilaginous growth plates the injury tends to occur in a different location (18). The excessive medial tension can result in an injury to the medial epicondylar epiphysis. This is associated with pain and tenderness at the medial epicondyle in these immature but often highly competitive pitchers.

Radiographs are initially not mandatory but can show a widened growth plate on the medial side and fragmentation of medial epicondylar epiphysis. Excessive compression on the lateral side may also be able to trigger osteochondritis diseccans of the radial head or capitellum or osteochondrosis, resulting in lateral pain as well (see next section). If the osteochondritic fragment becomes detached, locking and catching can also occur.

Treatment follows the same principles as described for medial tension overload syndrome. In these young children emphasis should be placed on proper throwing technique, adequate rest, and decreasing the number of fast pitches thrown. Relief of pain usually occurs after 2 to 3 weeks of relative rest. Return to regular throwing activities is possible in 6 to 8 weeks.

Osteochondritis Dissecans and Osteochondrosis

Although not universally accepted, it seems that osteochondritis dissecans and osteochondrosis (Panner's disease) are two separate entities. Both involve bone and sometimes cartilage lesions on the lateral side of the elbow (19). Osteochondritis dissecans usually develops insidiously in children during the teenage years. A small island of subchondral bone usually in the capitellum separates and can become completely detached (Figure 11.18). Surgical treatment is necessary if detachment with locking and catching of the elbow occurs. Long-term deformity with late osteoarthritis is possible in advanced cases. Fortunately, the condition is rare.

Osteochondrosis appears to start much more acutely in children under 10 years of age. Radiographs reveal fragmentation of the entire capitellum suggesting that this is a form of osteonecrosis. Surprisingly, fol-

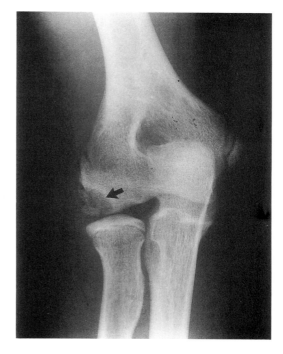

Figure 11.18. Osteochondritis dissecans of the capitellum. Arrow points to the osteochondritic fragment.

lowing a period of rest gradual recovery is often complete without long-term sequelae. Detachment and loose bodies do not usually occur.

Both conditions will result in lateral elbow pain often accompanied by a flexion contracture. Radiographs are generally recommended for lateral elbow pain in children to diagnose these conditions.

Compression and Entrapment Neuropathy

As the three major peripheral nerves cross the elbow they are susceptible to injury. Most nerve injuries in the elbow region are chronic injuries associated with low-level but persistent compression or entrapment, hence, the term *compression* or *entrapment neuropathy* (20). The chronic

compression results in demyelinization
with subsequent nerve dysfunction. Initial
signs of dysfunction are usually sensory in
nature—paresthesias and decreased sensation in the area supplied by and distal to the
affected nerve. For reasons that are not always clear the sensory symptoms tend to
vary significantly in intensity during the
day and night. Sometimes they can be particularly pronounced at night. The sensory
changes are described in many ways by the
patient, ranging from tingling to altered
sensation and even frank numbness.

The nerve is usually sensitive to additional external pressure at the site of
compression. Light tapping will cause
"electrical shocks" or paresthesias in the
sensory course of the nerve distal to the
lesion (Tinel's sign) (Figure 11.19). Objective evaluation is most commonly done by
determining two-point discrimination test-

ing. One inexpensive and easy way is to use
an unfolded paper clip. This is done by
lightly pressing the two ends simultaneously against the distal aspect of the finger
and asking the patient whether he or she
feels one or two points of the paper clip
without looking at the finger being tested.
At the volar, distal pad of the fingers the
patient should be able to distinguish two
separate points if the two ends of the paper
clip are brought together to about 3 to
5 mm. Smaller distances than that will be
felt as one single point. If the compression
neuropathy progresses it can also affect the
motor fibers of the nerve supplying the
distal musculature. Weakness and atrophy
of the distal muscles supplied by the affected nerve can be found at that time. It is
believed that the presence of weakness and
atrophy is an indication for surgical release
of the compression, whereas those athletes

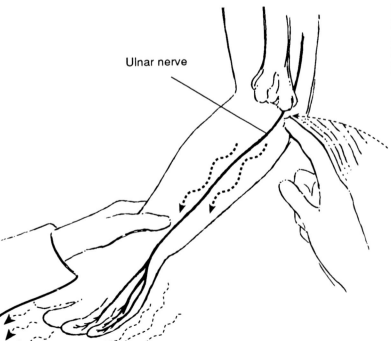

Ulnar nerve

Figure 11.19. Provocative test (Tinel's sign) for
cubital tunnel syndrome.
Percussion of the nerve reproduces distal symptoms.

with sensory changes only can usually be managed nonoperatively.

If a compression neuropathy is suspected but the history and physical examination findings are equivocal, additional diagnostic tests can be helpful. Electrodiagnostic studies can yield objective data to support the diagnosis of a compression neuropathy. Usually both electromyography (EMG) and nerve conduction studies are performed for this purpose. Significant compression of a peripheral nerve will result in a slowing of the electrical impulse across the site of compression with resulting abnormally low conduction velocities. Dysfunction of the motor nerve will result in abnormal EMG signals from the distally innervated muscles such as decreased recruitment on active contraction. These studies can also be helpful in distinguishing more proximal nerve lesions such as cervical radiculopathy and upper motor neuron lesions from compression neuropathy.

It is generally not recommended to obtain electrodiagnostic studies in every case of compression neuropathy. Mild cases can be managed nonoperatively; severe cases may be obvious and need surgical release irrespective of the results of electrodiagnostic studies. These studies can be of help when the clinical symptoms are unclear or confusing. However, one should remember that even in these cases electrodiagnostic data can yield both false-positive and false-negative results. Referral to an experienced neurophysiology laboratory can minimize this problem.

Ulnar Nerve Compression Neuropathy

The ulnar nerve is the most common peripheral nerve around the elbow affected by compression neuropathy. The ulnar nerve crosses the elbow through the cubital tunnel and can be compressed at various sites in and around the cubital tunnel (21). Proximally it can be compressed by the medial intermuscular septum as the nerve courses from the anterior to the posterior compartment of the upper arm. Within the cubital tunnel it can be affected by scar, synovitis, or even osteophytes. Excessive valgus due to an old malunited elbow fracture or valgus instability associated with medial tension overload syndrome can result in excessive traction and signs of entrapment neuropathy. Similar symptoms occur when the ulnar nerve is not well contained within the cubital tunnel. This is the most frequent cause of ulnar neuritis in athletes. Upon flexion the nerve can dislocate on top or even anterior to the medial epicondyle. Repeated flexion and extension with snapping of the ulnar nerve back and forth can also result in ulnar nerve injury. Distally it can be compressed by the head of the flexor carpi ulnaris.

During physical examination one should look for Tinel's sign over the course of the ulnar nerve (see Figure 11.19). A careful neurologic examination should focus on two-point discrimination in the ulnar one and one half digit and weakness or atrophy of the dorsal interosseous muscles. This results in weakness of finger abduction. In addition, hypothenar atrophy can be noted.

Treatment depends on the severity and cause of the symptoms. Compression associated with inflammatory changes can improve with anti-inflammatory measures such as rest, ice, and NSAIDs. If this fails, a local injection with corticosteroids around the nerve can be tried. Ulnar nerve symptoms associated with medial tension overload syndrome are best managed by decreasing the valgus-directed forces on the elbow. Symptoms due to a dislocating ulnar nerve can be improved by altering sports activities and decreasing repeated flexion and extension of the elbow. Many athletes with cubital tunnel syndrome improve subjectively with a medially placed elbow pad during sports activities. They minimize additional external impact on an already sensitive nerve.

If symptoms persist, and especially if objective motor nerve abnormalities develop, surgical treatment should be considered. Generally this consists of an exploration of the ulnar nerve along its entire course across the elbow with release of all compressive structures. Most surgeons will then transpose the nerve to a position anterior to the medial epicondyle. This decreases the tension in the nerve and puts it in a less vulnerable position. Postoperatively the elbow is often kept flexed in a splint or sling to allow the nerve to maintain its new position. Range of motion and strengthening exercises are subsequently started. Rehabilitation after surgery takes 2 to 4 months.

Median Nerve Compression Neuropathy

Entrapment and compression of the median nerve or its branches is also possible around the elbow. The most common sites of compression are just proximal to the elbow by a congenital fibrous structure (ligament of Struthers') or just distal to the elbow by the pronator teres or the edge of the flexor digitorum sublimis muscle (22). Symptoms usually involve vague pain in the anterior forearm and hand with sensory changes in the median nerve distribution. The compression distal to the elbow by the pronator teres or sublimis muscle involves the anterior interosseous branch of the median nerve, which does not contain cutaneous innervation. Therefore, the objective findings only include motor abnormalities such as difficulty in performing tip-to-tip pinch with the thumb and index finger, due to weakness of the flexor profundus muscle to the index and flexor pollicis longus to the thumb. Electrodiagnostic studies can be helpful to distinguish this condition from cervical radiculopathy or carpal tunnel syndrome.

Initial treatment is aimed at rest and decreasing any inflammatory changes if present. If not successful, or objective weakness is present, surgical exploration and release may be considered.

Radial Nerve Compression Neuropathy

Similar to the ulnar and median nerve, the radial nerve can be injured due to entrapment and compression around the elbow in various places. The most common site is just distal to the elbow as the posterior interosseous branch runs underneath the proximal edge of the supinator (arcade of Frohse). Other potential sites are the area around the radial head, a leash of vessels (leash of Henry) in the proximal forearm, and by the tendon of the extensor carpi radialis brevis (23).

The symptoms usually include lateral elbow pain occasionally radiating down to the wrist. On physical examination there is often tenderness at the site of entrapment. Most of these symptoms and findings are similar to lateral epicondylitis. Therefore, a careful examination is needed. Tenderness in radial nerve entrapment is usually more distal to the epicondyle than in lateral epicondylitis. Some authors feel that resisted supination or middle finger extension causes more pain in radial nerve compression neuropathy than the resisted wrist extension used as a test for lateral epicondylitis. Electrodiagnostic studies can be helpful if the distinction is not clear. A simpler test is an injection with local anesthetic at the lateral epicondyle, which will relieve the pain of lateral epicondylitis but not the pain of a compression neuropathy.

If rest and anti-inflammatory treatment do not relieve the symptoms, a surgical decompression may be needed.

Olecranon Bursitis

The contour of the posterior aspect of the elbow is predominantly formed by the olecranon process of the ulna. No protective muscle layer is present in this area. The olecranon bursa covers the tip of the olecranon and allows skin mobility over the olecranon during flexion and extension. Because of the lack of a protective soft-tissue layer this area is easily injured. Injuries to the olecranon bursa can be due to excessive friction, as in wrestlers or even basketball players as they use their elbow while trying to post up. The excessive friction can lead to increased fluid production by the lining of the bursa with subsequent pain and swelling (Figure 11.20). Injury may also be due to a direct blow or blows, as in hockey players. The differential diagnosis of posterior elbow pain includes triceps tendinitis and olecranon spurs. Triceps tendinitis usually occurs at its insertion into the olecranon. It is associated with local tenderness but generally little or no swelling. Olecranon spurs are most commonly seen in elite pitchers as part of medial tension overload syndrome.

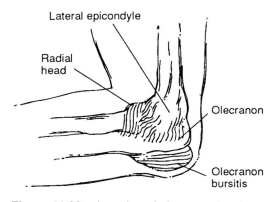

Figure 11.20. Location of olecranon bursitis.

The aseptic olecranon bursitis due to friction or impact is treated appropriately with protection and anti-inflammatory measures. A protective elbow pad can decrease additional friction and injury. Rest, ice, and compression can alleviate the acute symptoms. NSAIDs can be helpful for pain relief and resumption of athletic activities.

In addition to aseptic bursitis, a septic olecranon bursitis is sometimes seen. This is usually due to a direct inoculation through a break in the skin overlying the olecranon. Besides swelling, there is usually marked pain and redness, which is generally more pronounced than in aseptic bursitis. Sometimes the route of inoculation is evident if there is a small laceration or abrasion. However, often this is not directly obvious. Therefore, if there is any doubt as to whether the swelling represents a septic or an aseptic process it should be aspirated under sterile conditions. Antibiotics can be started while awaiting culture results. In those cases where a septic olecranon bursitis is clear a decision regarding drainage needs to be made. Drainage through needle aspiration may suffice in cases where the infectious fluid is thin and can be easily removed through aspiration. Repeated aspiration may be needed in the first few days to keep the fluid from reaccumulating. If the bursa is filled with thick pus, formal incision and drainage may be needed to clear the infection. Antibiotic coverage should be given in addition to a drainage procedure. The choice of antibiotics needs to be guided by culture results but should be focused on gram-positive organisms if culture results are still pending.

ELBOW EXERCISES

This final section reviews several commonly used elbow exercises for general

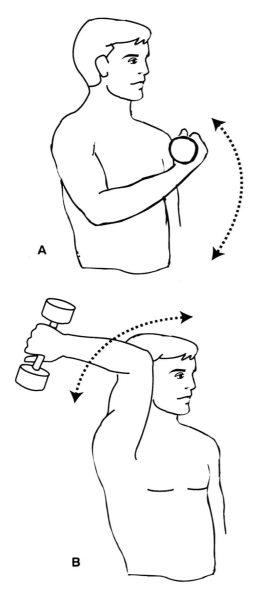

Figure 11.21. Biceps curls (*A*) and triceps extension exercises (*B*).

maintenance and rehabilitation. All stretching exercises should be done gradually without rocking or bouncing. Most stretches are held for 3 to 5 seconds each in

sets of 10 to 20. The strengthening exercises should be started with low resistance (1 to 5 lb) in two to three sets with a relatively high number of repetitions (10 to 20/set). If needed the resistance can be gradually increased over several weeks to improve both strength and endurance (24).

Biceps Curls

In a standing position the weight is lifted from full extension to full flexion of the elbow and subsequently lowered again to the resting position (Figure 11.21*A*).

Triceps Extensions

While standing or sitting the upper arm is fully forward flexed to 180°. The elbow is flexed maximally with a handheld weight. The exercise is started by bringing the elbow to full extension while maintaining the same position at the shoulder. The weight is then lowered again to the resting position (Figure 11.21*B*).

Wrist Curls

With the forearm supported on a bench or thigh a handheld weight is brought up from full wrist extension to full wrist flexion. The palm is facing up during this exercise. Subsequently the weight is lowered to its resting position (Figure 11.22*A*).

Wrist Extension

This exercise is similar to wrist curls except that the palm should be face down (Figure 11.22*B*).

Stretching Exercises

Stretching of the elbow and wrist flexors and extensors can be done with the elbow

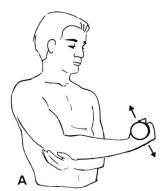 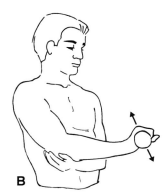

Figure 11.22. Wrist curls (*A*) and wrist extension exercises (*B*).

in full extension. In this position, pressure of the opposite hand is used to gradually stretch the muscles beyond the resting position in flexion or extension for 3 to 5 seconds before this pressure is released.

References

1. Nirschl RP. The etiology and treatment of tennis elbow. Am J Sports Med 1974;2:308–323.

2. Larson RL, Singer RM, Thomas S. Little League survey: the Eugene study. Am J Sports Med 1976;4:201–209.

3. Snook GA. Injuries in women's gymnastics. A 5-year study. Am J Sports Med 1979;7:242–244.

4. Hollingshead WH. Anatomy for surgeons, vol 3. The back and limbs. New York: Harper & Row, 1969.

5. Conway JE, Jobe FW, Glousman RE, Pink M. Medial instability of the elbow in throwing athletes. J Bone Joint Surg 1992;74A:67–83.

6. Hoppenfeld S. Physical examination of the spine and extremities. New York: Appleton-Century-Crofts, 1976.

7. Mehlhoff TL, Noble PC, Bennett JB, Tullos HS. Simple dislocation of the elbow in the adult. Results after closed treatment. J Bone Joint Surg 1988;70A:244–249.

8. Wilkins KE. Fractures and dislocation of the elbow region. In: Rockwood CA, Wilkins KE, King RE, eds. Fractures in children. Philadelphia: JB Lippincott, 1984:363–575.

9. Dameron TB. Transverse fractures of the distal humerus in children. Instr Course Lect 1981;30:224–235.

10. Rang M. Childen's fractures. Philadelphia: JB Lippincott, 1982.

11. Nirschl RP. Elbow tendinosis/tennis elbow. Clin Sports Med 1992;11:851–870.

12. Legwold G. Tennis elbow: joint resolution by conservative treatment and improved technique.

13. Coonrad RW, Hooper WR. Tennis elbow its course, natural history, conservative and surgical management. J Bone Joint Surg 1973;55A:1177–1187.

14. Leach RE, Miller JE. Lateral and medial epicondylitis of the elbow. Clin Sports Med 1987;6:259–272.

15. Dehaven KE, Evarts CM. Throwing injuries of the elbow in athletes. Orthop Clin North Am 1973;4:801–808.

16. Wilson FD, Andrews JR, Blackburn TA, McCluskey G. Valgus extension overload in the pitching elbow. Am J Sports Med 1983;11:83–86.

17. Indelicato PA, Jobe FW, Kerlan RK, Carter US, Shields CL, Lombardo SY. Correctable elbow lesions in professional baseball players. Am J Sports Med 1979;7:72–75.

18. Torg JS, Pollack H, Sweterlitsch P. The effect of competitive pitching on the shoulders and elbows of preadolescent baseball players.

Pediatrics 1972;49:267–272.

19. Singer KM, Roy SP. Osteochondrosis of the humeral capitellum. Am J Sports Med 1984;12:351–360.

20. Eversmann WW. Entrapment and compression neuropathies. In: Green DP, ed. Operative hand surgery, 3rd ed. New York: Churchill Livingstone, 1993:1341–1385.

21. Craven PR, Green DP. Cubital tunnel syndrome. J Bone Joint Surg 1980;62A:986–989.

22. Hartz CR, Linscheid RL, Gramse RR, Daube JR. The pronator teres syndrome: compressive neuropathy of the medial nerve. J Bone Joint Surg 1981;63A:885–890.

23. Roles NC, Maudsly RH. Radial tunnel syndrome. J Bone Joint Surg 1972;54B:499–508.

24. Roy S, Irvin R. Throwing and tennis injuries to the shoulder and elbow. In: Sports medicine. Prevention, evaluation, management and rehabilitation. Englewood Cliffs, NJ: Prentice-Hall, 1983:211–227.

THE WRIST

DONALD K. BYNUM, JR

12

Anatomy and Radiography
Evaluation of the Sprained Wrist
Ligamentous Instabilities
Distal Radioulnar Joint and Triangular
  Fibrocartilage

This chapter primarily discusses evaluation of the "sprained wrist" to help the primary care physician distinguish a minor wrist sprain from a more significant injury. Wrist sprains and hand sprains are extremely common. Most are indeed minor sprains requiring nothing more than symptomatic treatment. Unfortunately, it can be difficult to distinguish minor sprains from some of the more serious varieties in which the physical examination and radiographic findings are subtle. A high index of suspicion is necessary to recognize serious sprains or fractures not grossly obvious on physical examination.

A minor sprain should resolve within a week or two. If pain or swelling persists after 2 weeks, an in-depth examination is warranted as soon as possible. At that point the primary care physician should initiate presumptive care, specifically a splint or cast. If the problem involves the area around the distal radioulnar joint or triangular fibrocartilage, immobilization should control rotation of the forearm at neutral pronation-supination by means of a long arm splint or cast. Of course, if a significant problem is suspected at the time of injury the primary care physician should institute treatment immediately.

This chapter attempts to clarify some of the nuances of the physical examination that help distinguish major injuries from minor ones. It also points out some extremely helpful radiographic features. Only a few fractures are discussed.

ANATOMY AND RADIOGRAPHY

Accurate physical examination of the wrist requires the examiner to view the wrist radiographically in the mind's eye while performing the examination. Several features about normal x-rays give helpful hints to correlate with physical examination and to recognize abnormal pathology both on physical examination and abnormal x-rays.

On the normal anteroposterior x-ray (Figure 12.1), the radius has an oblique inclination from the distal radial styloid curving concavely to the edge of the distal radioulnar joint. The head of the ulna should be level with the articular margin of the distal radius or at most 2 mm proximal or distal to the distal radius. There are two facets in the distal radius, one for the scaphoid and one for the lunate. A slight ridge separating these two facets is normal and should not be misinterpreted as representing step-off of a fracture line. An increase of the normal step-off between scaphoid and lunate fossae suggests the possibility of a dye-punch or impaction fracture. Lister's tubercle, a bony prominence on the dorsum of the radius, is palpable on examination and lies almost directly in line with the scapholunate junction (Figure 12.2). Tenderness a few millimeters distal to Lister's tubercle should alert the examiner to the possibility of a scapholunate ligament rupture. The waist of the scaphoid lies in the anatomic "snuffbox" on physical examination (Figure 12.3). The dorsal lip of the radius extends distally as a slight shadow beyond the apparent articular margin of the radius.

There is uniform spacing of the cartilage space between the carpals. One can draw three smooth unbroken arcs through the carpals. The proximal arc traces the proximal bony margins of the scaphoid, lunate, and triquetrum. The middle arc traces the distal bony margins of the scaphoid, lunate, and triquetrum. The third arc is formed by the articular margins of the hamate and head of the capitate. These three arcs have different radii of curvature, but each one of them should represent a smooth unbroken

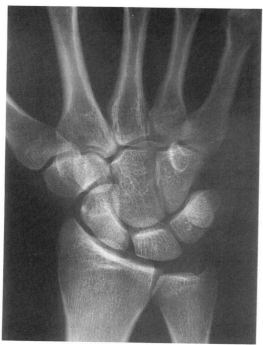

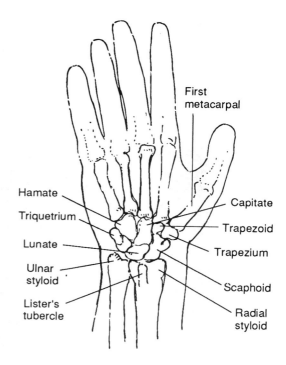

Figure 12.1. *A*. Normal anteroposterior x-ray of the wrist. Note the uniform spacing of the intercarpal joints. Any offset or break in the con- tour of any of the intercarpal arcs is highly suggestive of a significant injury. *B*. Schematic with bony structures labeled.

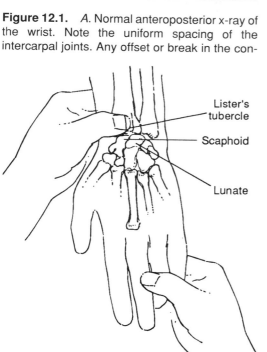

Figure 12.2. Lister's tubercle is a landmark for the scapholunate joint. Palpate 1 cm distal to Lister's tubercle.

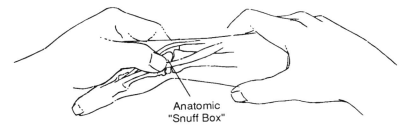

Figure 12.3. The anatomic "snuffbox" overlies the waist of the scaphoid. Tenderness here suggests a scaphoid fracture.

Anatomic
"Snuff Box"

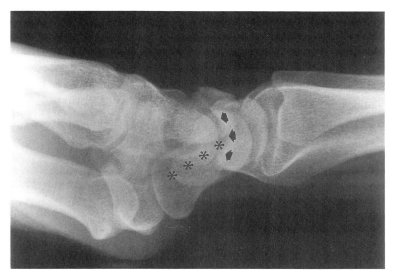

Figure 12.4. Normal lateral x-ray of the wrist. The long axis of the third metacarpal should be colinear with the radius. The concave cup of the lunate faces straight distally, neither dorsiflexed nor volar flexed (*arrows*). The long axis of the scaphoid (*stars*) is oblique (flexed). Compare the relationships of radius, scaphoid, lunate, and capitate to Figures 12.6 and 12.8*B*.

line with no step-offs or diastasis. A step-off or diastasis is highly suggestive of a clinically significant rupture of intercarpal ligaments (1). In the normal x-ray, the dorsal and volar poles of the lunate, especially the volar pole, may slightly overlap the head of the capitate, but this is seen as a faint projection of bone superimposed on the head of the capitate while the middle intracarpal arc and the distal intracarpal arc remain unbroken. The hook of the hamate shows as a **V** superimposed on the body of the hamate. The spacing of the carpometacarpal joints is similar to that of the carpal joints.

On the normal lateral x-ray (Figure 12.4), one can usually make out the slope of the radius, which angles from distal-dorsal to proximal-volar measuring approximately 11°. The metacarpals should be lined up in neutral flexion or extension relative to the longitudinal axis of the radius. In that position, the concave cup of the lunate should be directly in line with the radius. The head of the capitate should line up in the cup of the lunate colinear with the long axis of the radius. The scaphoid is positioned oblique to the long axis of the radius with its proximal pole being frequently obscured by or superimposed on the lunate and its distal pole coarsing distal and volar to articulate with the trapezium. On physical examination the distal pole (volar tubercle) of the scaphoid is the first bony prominence distal to the radius on the volar aspect of the wrist (Figure 12.5). Pain in the snuffbox provoked

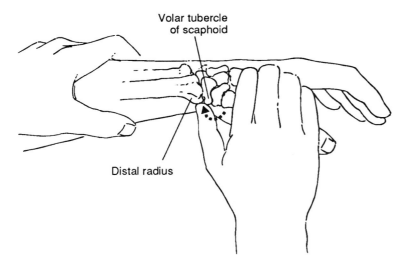

Volar tubercle
of scaphoid

Distal radius

Figure 12.5. Palpation of
distal pole (volar tubercle) of
the scaphoid.

by palpating the volar tubercle suggests a
scaphoid fracture. In pathologic conditions,
the cup of the lunate may appear to be tilted
facing dorsal or volar. Normal angles between the axes of the radius, scaphoid,
lunate, and capitate have been defined (2)
(Figure 12.6). Deviations from these normal
angles are highly suggestive of intercarpal
ligamentous disruption.

The oblique view of the wrist is more
helpful to detect small chip fractures or
erosions rather than to judge the alignment of the carpals. The pisiform may
come into profile in the oblique view,
whereas in the anteroposterior view it is
superimposed on the triquetrum such that
bony details of the two are often obscured.
True fractures of the pisiform are rare,
but occasionally avulsion fragments or calcific tendonitis can be seen on the oblique
view.

The normal anteroposterior, lateral, and
oblique views may not be sufficient to show
a fracture of the scaphoid. Thus, there is a
special view, the "scaphoid view," which is
taken with the wrist ulnarly deviated.
Ulnar deviation elevates the distal pole of

the scaphoid, bringing the full length of the
scaphoid and its waist into better radiographic profile (Figure 12.7).

The hook of the hamate is not well visualized on the routine wrist series and requires
either a special oblique view, carpal tunnel
view, or computed tomography (CT) scan
for thorough evaluation.

EVALUATION OF THE
SPRAINED WRIST

Physical examination and x-ray examination of the sprained wrist are done in an
attempt to distinguish the truly minor
sprained wrist from the one in which there
is a more significant occult injury. This is
not always easy. The focus of the examination is taken partly from the mechanism of
injury and partly from the location of pain.
Blatantly minor sprains need not be x-
rayed. If at any time the sprain is bad
enough to cause swelling the wrist should
be x-rayed. When pain is provoked by palpation of the anatomic snuffbox or the volar
tuberosity of the scaphoid, the special

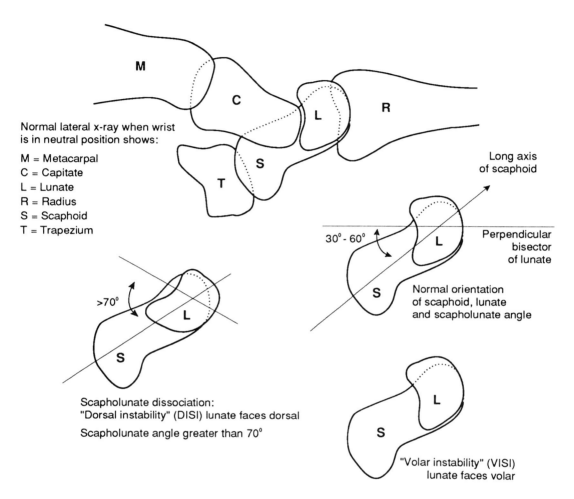

Normal lateral x-ray when wrist
is in neutral position shows:

M = Metacarpal
C = Capitate
L = Lunate
R = Radius
S = Scaphoid
T = Trapezium

Long axis
of scaphoid

30° - 60°

Perpendicular
bisector
of lunate

Normal orientation
of scaphoid, lunate
and scapholunate angle

>70°

Scapholunate dissociation:
"Dorsal instability" (DISI) lunate faces dorsal

Scapholunate angle greater than 70°

"Volar instability" (VISI)
lunate faces volar

Figure 12.6. Interpreting the lateral wrist
x-rays.

"scaphoid view" should be obtained in addition to the routine radiographic series.

Physical Examination

As with most musculoskeletal injuries, the physical examination is intended to localize pain at the injured structure. In the wrist, this is not always possible because the pain may be dispersed or diffused in the wrist and also may be referred to areas other than the actual injury. Precise palpation using the tip of the examiner's digit or a pencil eraser may help localize the injury. When swelling is localized to the carpal compartment and does not involve the distal radius, one should be suspicious of an intra-articular fracture or carpal ligament disruption. Extra-articular fractures of the distal radius present a more diffuse swelling. The character of the swelling will also depend on how soon after the injury the evaluation is performed. Areas of discrete swelling such as the ganglionlike swelling of an intra-articular injury will be-

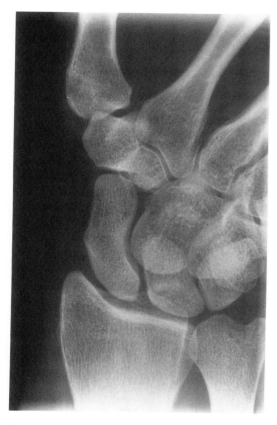

Figure 12.7. The scaphoid view. Ulnar deviation of the wrist pulls the scaphoid into more
extension, thus providing a more longitudinally
oriented profile, that is, a better view.

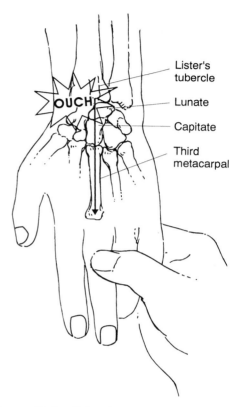

Figure 12.8. Pain distal to Lister's tubercle
suggests schapholunate ligament tear.

come more diffuse with the passage of time.
Swelling localized around a specific tendon
may likewise dissipate but will remain in
the vicinity. Maximum tenderness will usually localize at the site of injury.

Palpation of the wrist is carried out to
help localize pain. For instance, tenderness
to direct palpation in the anatomic snuffbox
should alert the examiner not only to the
possibility of a scaphoid fracture but also to
the possibility of a scapholunate ligament
tear (scapholunate dissociation). Deep palpation of the volar tubercle of the scaphoid

would also provoke pain suggestive of a
fracture or ligamentous injury. If palpation
of the tubercle is painless while palpation of
the anatomic snuffbox shows tenderness, a
contusion or minor sprain is more likely
rather than a more severe injury. Pain
just distal to Lister's tubercle suggests a
scapholunate ligament tear (Figure 12.8).
This is also the site of pain from small occult
dorsal ganglion cysts. Palpation of specific
carpal bones while attempting to move the
wrist through a range of motion either passively or by palpating as the athlete moves
the wrist should give the examiner clues as
to possible instabilities of carpal bones such
as a scaphoid, triquetrum, or capitate. The
examiner can also attempt ballottement or

translocation of these carpal bones past each other or past the radius. Tenderness at the insertion site of specific tendons or along their course would suggest acute injury or chronic tendinitis.

Radiographs frequently show no major fractures or dislocations but will show minor chips or avulsions off the dorsal aspect of carpal bones. These fractures represent capsuloligamentous avulsions. Most of the time they are not significant except as markers of a sprain; however, on occasion they may herald a more significant ligamentous disruption. The degree of ligamentous injury might need to be evaluated with stress views such as a wrist instability series or fluoroscopy before finalizing the diagnosis as a "minor sprain." It is appropriate to immobilize the wrist while awaiting a definite diagnosis.

LIGAMENTOUS INSTABILITIES

Almost every combination of carpal ligamentous instability has been reported. Even the more common varieties are sometimes difficult to diagnose, so this chapter discusses only two basic patterns.

Scapholunate Dissociation

Dorsal Intercalated Instability

This is an injury that usually occurs with a fall onto the outstretched hand and wrist. All of the ligaments connecting the scaphoid to the lunate get torn, resulting in painful symptomatic intercarpal instability. The mechanism of injury is identical to that of a scaphoid fracture so that a ligamentous dissociation should always be considered when the degree of swelling, mechanism of injury, or examination findings suggest scaphoid fracture. Unfortunately, the ma-

jority of these injuries are not recognized acutely, thus compromising the ultimate outcome.

Physical Examination. Tenderness and swelling are located in the radial and midportions of the wrist. Tenderness may only be present in the middorsal aspect of the carpus just distal to the radius. Tenderness would not be present distally over the base of the capitate. Most examiners would have difficulty distinguishing between pain at the head of the capitate and pain at the dorsal scapholunate ligament area. Acute injury pain in the dorsal midportion of the wrist, which does not lateralize to the anatomic snuffbox, should always be considered suspicious for a scapholunate dissociation. In the case of chronic pain, the differential diagnosis would also include an occult dorsal wrist ganglion. In severe cases, the examiner may be able to palpate the scaphoid as it snaps back and forth in the scaphoid fossa while the patient actively deviates the wrist radially and ulnarly or actively flexes and extends the wrist. Pronation and supination are less likely to provoke the clicks or clunks. The instability may be provoked by having the athlete clench the fist, thus providing axial load, while moving the wrist. Occasionally, the examiner may be able to palpate the proximal pole of the scaphoid as it rides dorsal to the adjacent lunate. This can be accentuated by flexing the wrist and then bringing the wrist back to extension. The examiner should exert direct dorsal pressure on the volar tubercle of the scaphoid. This pressure tends to correct the malalignment of the scaphoid and the examiner may feel the scaphoid click or clunk back into place in the scaphoid fossa. The same phenomenon may occur while moving the wrist from full radial deviation to full ulnar deviation (Figure 12.9).

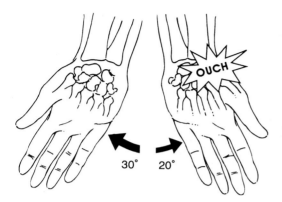

Figure 12.9. Painful click or clunk with scapholunate instability. (Modified from S Hoppenfeld. Physical Examination of the Spine Extremities Norwalk, CT: Appleton & Lange, 1976: 84.)

Radiography. There are several radiographic signs of scapholunate dissociation (Figure 12.10). These include: 1) increased scapholunate gap greater than 3 mm (Terry-Thomas sign [3]) (see Figure 12.10A), 2) cortical ring sign of the scaphoid, 3) prominence of the volar pole of the lunate under the head of the capitate, 4) increased scapholunate angle as seen on the lateral x-ray, and 5) dorsiflexed attitude of the lunate as seen on the lateral x-ray (see Figure 12.10B). The term "dorsal intercalated segmental instability" derives from the dorsal tilt of the lunate.

Treatment. This condition should be treated within the first 2 weeks if at all possible. By 3 weeks, the patient is entering the gray zone where treatment becomes less successful. Treatment requires surgical reduction and fixation of the carpals into their proper alignment so that the ligaments are reapproximated. This requires prolonged immobilization and should be considered a season-ending injury. Left untreated the end result is severe degenerative arthritis.

Volar Intercalated Instability

This type of intercarpal ligament sprain usually results from a torquing injury to the wrist or a fall onto the outstretched hand combined with torsion. The torn ligaments include combinations of lunate-triquetral, triquetral-hamate, and ulnar collateral ligament complex. The carpal instability may exist between the lunate and triquetrum or proximal and distal carpal rows.

Physical Examination. The findings may only be generalized pain and swelling on the ulnar side of the wrist. The precise structure injured is frequently difficult to localize. Sometimes the triquetrum can be translocated dorsal and volar past the lunate by stabilizing the lunate with one hand and attempting to push/pull the triquetrum with the other hand. The examiner should specifically palpate the hook of the hamate for possible fracture and the pisiform for strain injuries of the flexor carpi ulnaris (Figure 12.11). A painful clunk or even a visible shift of the bones in the wrist can sometimes be provoked by having the examiner radially deviate and flex the wrist approximately 20°, and with the patient relaxed the examiner should attempt to compress the hand and forearm together while moving the hand into ulnar deviation. If a painful clunk or shift occurs, the patient should be thoroughly evaluated by a knowledgeable hand surgeon. This same phenomenon can be provoked painlessly in loose-jointed persons and, when painless, it has no significance.

The examiner should attempt to distinguish distal radioulnar joint pain from ulnar-sided carpal pain. Pain can sometimes be localized to the dorsal or volar limbs of the triangular fibrocartilage by precise eraser-tip palpation. Distal radioulnar joint sprain should be suspected if pain is more intense when attempting to

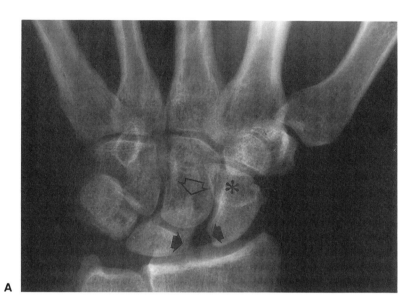

A

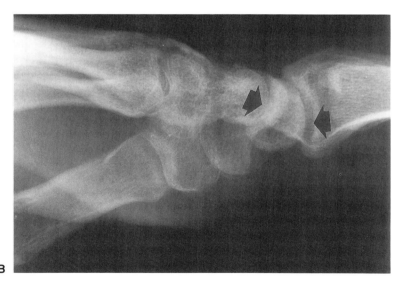

B

Figure 12.10. Anteroposterior and lateral x-rays of scapholunate dissociation (dorsal intercalated segmental instability). *A.* Note the increased scapholunate space (*solid arrows*), the cortical ring around the distal scaphoid (*as-* *terisk*), and the triangular appearance of the lunate extending into the head of the capitate (*open arrows*). *B.* Note the dorsal facing lunate (*arrows*) and the increased scapholunate angle. Compare to normal in Figures 12.1*A* and 12.4.

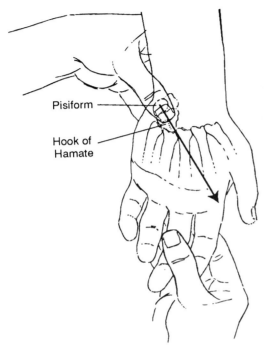

Figure 12.11. Palpation of volar aspect of the ulnar side of the wrist to locate prominent pisiform and much less prominent hook of hamate.

translocate the distal radioulnar joint or when rotating it, than if the pain occurs when performing wrist motions.

Radiography. In most instances, ligamentous injuries to the ulnar side of the wrist do not show well on plain x-rays. When present, x-ray findings would include: 1) volar tilt of the lunate as seen on the lateral x-ray, 2) disruption of one of the three carpal arcs, and 3) dorsal capsular avulsion fragments. These are frequently present with minimal displacement in minor sprains. They are important in the sense that they raise the examiner's index of suspicion.

Treatment. An acute injury should be treated within the first 2 weeks if at all possible.

This would require operative reduction and stabilization of the grade III injuries. Lesser degrees of injury can be treated with short-term (2 to 3 week) casting or splinting. Cases with recognizable radiographic abnormalities probably represent more significant injuries and should be evaluated and treated more aggressively.

Distal Radius Fractures

Most minor wrist sprains do not have significant swelling. If swelling is present in the distal radius or wrist, x-rays should always be obtained to evaluate possible fractures. This chapter does not expound on the treatment of distal radius fractures except to say that minor nondisplaced fractures can be treated symptomatically with splints or casts and should be protected from reinjury. Continued participation in athletics depends on the exact nature of the sport and whether or not the fracture can be adequately protected. Treatment of displaced fractures and intra-articular fractures requires decision-making and treatment beyond the scope of this chapter.

Scaphoid Fractures

The usual mechanism of injury is a fall onto the outstretched hand ("foosh"), which results in forceful dorsiflexion and impaction of the scaphoid against the dorsal rim of the radius. This mechanism of injury explains why snuffbox tenderness is so common even in the absence of a scaphoid fracture. In many wrist sprains, the dorsal rim of the radius and the waist of the scaphoid abut, resulting in a contusion of the scaphoid or even of the capsule with the result that pain can be provoked by deep palpation in the anatomic snuffbox. Conventional medical wisdom dictates that snuffbox tenderness should be equated with a scaphoid fracture unless x-rays prove otherwise. In fact, if the initial x-rays do not show a fracture, follow-up x-rays should be obtained in 7 to 14 days because the fracture line may be more visible after some resorption. I have found a reliable correlation of scaphoid fracture with pain provoked by deep palpation at the volar tubercle of the scaphoid. The examiner can palpate the volar distal radius and then move distally to the first bony prominence, which is the volar tubercle of the scaphoid. Exerting direct pressure against the tubercle tends to rotate the scaphoid into dorsiflexion, thus provoking motion and pain at the fracture site. When both snuffbox tenderness and volar tenderness are present, there is a high positive correlation with fracture. When tubercle palpation does not provoke pain in the snuffbox there is very little chance of a scaphoid fracture.

Radiography. When a scaphoid fracture is suspected on physical examination, a scaphoid series should be ordered because routine wrist anteroposterior lateral and oblique may not show the fracture (Figure 12.12).

If the x-rays are equivocal and it is important to return the athlete to competition without waiting 7 to 14 days for repeat x-rays, a bone scan of the wrist can be obtained after 24 hours and will almost always settle the issue.

Treatment. Treatment should be instituted as soon as possible. The old wisdom still applies! If a scaphoid fracture is highly suspect on physical examination but initial x-rays are "negative," treat as if a fracture is present and x-ray again at a later date. The

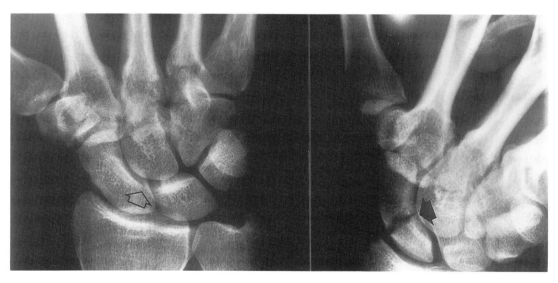

Figure 12.12. Scaphoid fracture. The routine anteroposterior view (*left*) appears almost normal. The slight disruption of the proximal tip of the scaphoid along the middle carpal arc adjacent to the head of the capitate could easily be overlooked (*open arrow*). The scaphoid view of the same wrist (*right*) emphasizes the advantage and necessity of obtaining this view to diagnose a scaphoid fracture (*solid arrow*).

nonunion rate in scaphoid fractures goes up dramatically with a delay in diagnosis and treatment regardless of which region of the scaphoid is fractured. There is a higher incidence of aseptic necrosis and nonunion with fractures of the proximal third of the scaphoid, but even fractures that would typically heal with immediate mobilization will have a higher nonunion rate if treatment is delayed. Some controversy exists as to whether or not a long arm thumb spica cast versus a short arm thumb spica cast is needed for nondisplaced fractures. There may be a slightly higher union rate when a long arm cast is used first as the primary treatment for 3 weeks. With such a small difference between the two treatment regimens, most athletes are probably treated satisfactorily with a short arm thumb spica cast. The cast can be plaster, fiberglass, or even rubberized so that the athlete may continue participation if rules allow. For instance, a quarterback with a scaphoid fracture in his nonthrowing hand could probably return to action. *Displaced fractures are highly suspicious for associated ligamentous tears and require thorough evaluation, treatment, and follow-up.*

Hamate Fracture

Fractures of the body of the hamate are particularly uncommon and would normally be associated with very severe injury to the wrist. A more common fracture is the hook of the hamate. The exact incidence of this fracture is unknown because it is usually not recognized acutely and is only brought to the physician's attention when a "wrist sprain" fails to resolve. It is possible that there are patients who have hamate hook fractures that do not heal but result in asymptomatic nonunions.

The mechanism of injury of the hook of the hamate fracture is usually a blow to the base of the palm by an implement held in the hand. The most common scenario is probably that of the golfer who strikes a tree root during a swing or similarly forcefully grounds the golf club. This fracture is also seen from the handle of a bat or from a direct fall onto the palm. It can occur in racquet sports.

Physical Examination. Examination would show pain localized to the ulnar side of the wrist. Frequently the pain cannot be well localized to the hamate and, in fact, it is not uncommon to have the pain referred to the dorsum of the wrist on the ulnar side. Deep palpation of the hook of the hamate (see Figure 12.11), even though it is on the volar side of the hamate, may result in pain on the dorsal side. This is probably explained on the basis of referred pain because the dorsal cutaneous branch of the ulnar nerve runs directly over the hamate and probably contains some articular fibers. Signs or symptoms of ulnar nerve paresthesias, ulnar nerve innervated intrinsic muscle weakness, or injury of flexor digitorum profundus tendons can be elicited in some cases. These structures pass immediately adjacent to the hook.

Radiography. The hamate hook typically fractures at or near its base so the fracture site may be difficult to see on plain x-rays. Plain x-rays should include a carpal tunnel view as well as a specially positioned lateral view of the hook. This view is not part of a routine wrist series and should be requested as an additional special view when the history or physical examination raise the possibility of a hook fracture. If these views do not adequately show the base of the hook, a CT scan with 1.5-mm cuts will show the base of the hook quite well and either confirm or rule out fracture. Although a bone scan may suggest a hook of the hamate fracture, the details in the scan are not sufficiently precise to rule out other osteochondral or nondisplaced fractures. In such cases, it is necessary to proceed with a CT scan after a bone scan.

Treatment. Most experience with hook of the hamate fractures is in the treatment of nonunions. Few fractures are recognized acutely. The natural history is thought, but not proven, to be that most of these fractures result in nonunion. Simple excision of the ununited fragment almost always results in return to normal function. Successful screw fixation of both acute fractures and nonunions has been reported but does not appear to offer any particular additional benefit over simple excision. Therefore, the primary care physician in conjunction with the athlete can exercise wide discretion in choosing whether or not to proceed with acute treatment of this fracture or to delay treatment and continue competition, selecting elective treatment at a later date. If deferred treatment is elected, the athlete should be warned about signs and symptoms of irritation of the motor branch of the ulnar nerve, which is adjacent to the hook, and about symptoms of tendinitis of the flexor tendons to the small and ring fingers because ruptures of these tendons have been reported in association with nonunions of the hook.

DISTAL RADIOULNAR JOINT AND TRIANGULAR FIBROCARTILAGE

Injuries of the distal radioulnar joint and triangular fibrocartilage complex may occur from either a fall on the outstretched hand or from a twisting, torquing injury (Figure 12.13). It is quite common to have minor ligamentous avulsions from the ulnar styloid with or without a small bone chip whenever a Colles' or similar fracture is sustained. Because some of the damaging force is dissipated through the fracture, the ligamentous injury may not be so severe.

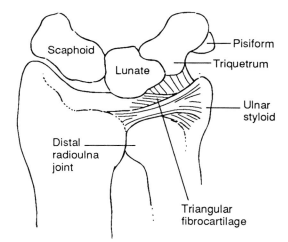

Figure 12.13. Distal radioulnar joint and triangular fibrocartilage.

There are some severe fractures in which dislocations of the distal radial ulnar joint accompany the fracture (Galeazzi's fracture) and these are usually easily recognizable. In other instances the injury may be primarily ligamentous tears on the ulnar side of the wrist or a significant fracture displacement of the ulnar styloid. When the majority of the styloid is fractured or a fragment is displaced more than 5 mm, this usually represents a significant ligamentous disruption of the distal radioulnar joint or triangular fibrocartilage complex. One should always bear in mind that ligamentous injuries occurring without bony avulsion fragments cannot be as easily recognized on x-ray and special attention during the physical examination should be directed toward ruling out such injuries.

Pain from an ulnar-sided wrist sprain, distal radioulnar joint, or triangular fibrocartilage injury is usually felt diffusely on the ulnar side of the wrist, and when great care is taken to pinpoint the most intensive locus of pain by palpating with a fingertip or pencil eraser, it is frequently possible to localize the injured structure.

The examiner should also attempt to demonstrate distal radial ulnar joint instability by one of the following three criteria:

1. Placing the forearm in full pronation may bring out dorsal instability of the distal ulna and will manifest by the head of the ulna appearing more prominent dorsally on the injured side than on the uninjured side.
2. Placing the forearm in full supination and viewing the distal radioulnar joint from the volar aspect can demonstrate volar instability of the distal ulna. In these situations, the head of the ulna may appear slightly more prominent in an ulnar direction more so than in a volar direction. There may appear to be an extra bulge on the ulnar edge of the wrist when viewing the silhouette of the wrist in supination.
3. By placing the forearm in neutral rotation with the injured limb resting on a table so it will be relaxed, the examiner can attempt to translocate (shuck, push/pull) the distal radius and ulna past each other in opposite directions.

If any of these maneuvers is asymmetrical to the uninjured side or demonstrates the suspected abnormality, the limb should be placed in a long arm cast or splint in neutral rotation until surgical consultation can be obtained.

Treatment

Any ulnar-sided wrist injury severe enough to result in swelling should be evaluated radiographically and by very focused physical examination. Minor injuries which have no associated swelling can probably be treated symptomatically and followed for 1 to 2 weeks for spontaneous resolution. If the examination is abnormal or swelling is present, the limb should be placed in a long arm splint or cast in neutral rotation. This provides presumptive treatment for either distal radioulnar joint, triangular fibrocartilage, or ulnar-sided carpal ligament injuries until reassessment by either the primary care physician or a specialist can be performed. If symptoms persist for more than 2 weeks, the athlete should be referred for surgical evaluation. These suggestive guidelines are dogmatic because these ulnar-sided injuries can result in chronic disabling pain, and because they are so difficult to identify on physical examination and because x-rays may appear totally normal, it is best to institute presumptive treatment in any but the most minor sprains. Having made that statement, I still think that most ulnar-sided sprains are minor and it is only the ones with visible swelling or any radiographic abnormality that are likely to be the problematic injuries. Because the exact proportion of minor to significant sprains is unknown, prudence dictates that the primary care physician have a high index of suspicion for these injuries and institute protective treatment whenever any serious concern exists.

References

1. Bellinghausen H-W, Gilula LA, Young LE, Weeks PM. Post-traumatic palmar carpal subluxation. Report of two cases. J Bone Joint Surg 1983;65A:998–1006.

2. Linsheid RL, Dobyns JH, Beabout JW, Bryan RS. Traumatic instability of the wrist: diagnosis, classification and pathomechanics. J Bone Joint Surg 1972;54A:1612–1632.

3. Frankel VH. The Terry-Thomas sign. Clin Orthop 1977;129:321–322. Letter.

THE HAND AND FINGERS

13

DONALD K. BYNUM, JR

General Considerations in the Jammed
  Finger
Flexor Tendon Injuries
Dislocations and Sprains
Fractures

Injuries of the hand are ubiquitous in athletic endeavors. Most amount to minor sprains or contusions. In fact, most are probably never even evaluated by a trainer or physician because the athlete recognizes them as minor injuries. The minor nature of most hand injuries leads to the common occurrence of underestimating the extent of a significant injury, resulting in a delayed diagnosis or misdiagnosis. This chapter will help the primary care physician understand the nuances of the mechanisms of injury, physical examination, and radiographic findings of "real injuries" as opposed to minor sprains and contusions.

GENERAL CONSIDERATIONS IN THE JAMMED FINGER

The term "jammed finger" is a nondiscriminating term in the context of mechanism of injury. Whether the finger is hit by a ball, twisted, pulled, crushed, kicked, or stomped, the following guideline is useful. To be considered a minor injury, the patient should have full active extension at all joints and should have at least 75% of normal active flexion with no joint instability or angular deviation of the finger. A finger injury that meets these criteria is probably a minor injury and can be safely observed. Any injury not meeting these criteria is suspicious for a significant injury and should be further evaluated by x-ray and clinical examination. The structures to be considered in a jammed finger include the extensor mechanism, flexor tendons and pulleys, joint capsule and ligaments, bones, and even the fingernails (Figure 13.1). The joint above and the joint below an area of injury should be examined as well as the structures circumferentially at the site of injury. It is important to remember that multiple injuries can coexist in the same finger. Also,

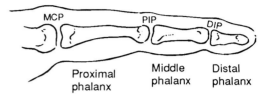

Figure 13.1. Bones and joints of the finger. DIP, distal interphalangeal; MCP, metacarpophalangeal; PIP, proximal interphalangeal.

because of the interconnections among the various structures in the digits, an injury of one structure may secondarily affect function of another. Thus, it is important to examine the entire digit to appreciate the full extent of injury.

In general, early motion is desirable whenever possible. This minimizes tendon adhesion and usually maximizes the range of motion achieved at recovery. Buddy-taping is an extremely useful technique to allow early active motion and continued participation in sports while still protecting an injured finger. Most minor injuries and some major injuries can be effectively treated by buddy-taping. The risk of early motion is that a partially ruptured tendon or ligament may subsequently rupture, or a nondisplaced fracture may be displaced; therefore, sequential reassessment is an important aspect of treatment. Splinting, when necessary, should be limited to the minimum number of joints or bones needed to achieve adequate immobilization. The caveat is that some athletes have to be splinted or casted more than the customary degree simply to inhibit them from overdoing activity.

Extensor Injuries

If an athlete with a jammed finger does not have full, active extension at the metacarpophalangeal (MCP), proximal interphalangeal (PIP), or distal interphalangeal (DIP) joints, an extensor tendon injury should be suspected. Fractures, subluxations, and dislocations may also cause extension lag. Their occurrence underscores the need for radiographic evaluation. If excessive swelling obscures the bony anatomy, it is doubly important for the finger to be x-rayed or at least reexamined less than a week from the time of injury. Delayed treatment of significant injuries usually results in a poorer outcome than early treatment.

Anatomy of the Extensor Mechanism

The functional anatomy of the extensor mechanism is actually more complex than that of the flexor mechanism (Figure 13.2). At the MCP joints, the central extensor tendons cross directly over the joint and are maintained in this centralized position by sagittal fibers of the extensor hood. There is no direct extensor insertion into the dorsal cortex of the proximal phalanx. Rather, the proximal phalanx is lifted by the hood fibers' insertions into the volar plate and volar aspect of the phalanx. The central tendon passes distally and inserts as the central slip at the base of the middle phalanx, thus contributing to PIP extension. Extension of the PIP joint is also provided by the lateral bands that originate from the lumbrical and interosseous muscles in the hand. The lateral bands pass volar to the MCP joint and course obliquely out the finger to pass to the dorsal aspect of the PIP joint. In the region of the PIP joint the central slip and lateral bands exchange interdigitating fibers, thus helping to tether each other into proper position and providing duplicate extensor power. Some of the fibers from the central slip pass distal to the PIP joint and join with fibers from the lateral band and these in turn unite over the middle phalanx with a similar contribution from the opposite side of the finger to form the terminal extensor. The terminal extensor courses distally to finally insert at the base of the distal phalanx.

Mallet Finger (Baseball Finger or Drop Finger)

Clinical Case #1

A 28-year-old male tennis player reached up casually to catch an out-of-bounds ball. Instead, the ball struck the end of his long finger, causing the finger to feel somewhat "numb." He noticed that he could not straighten the tip of the finger. His 55-year-old neighbor sustained a similar injury 20 years ago playing softball. He never had this treated and the finger never regained full motion. The tennis player is concerned that this might happen to his finger. Examination reveals that the MCP and PIP joints are nontender. The distal phalanx is flexed 70° and can be actively flexed further to about 80°. When

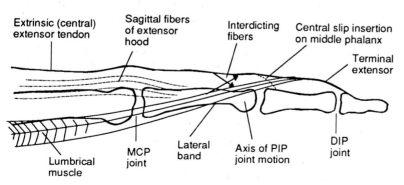

Figure 13.2. Extensor mechanism, lateral view.

Extrinsic (central) extensor tendon

Sagittal fibers of extensor hood

Interdicting fibers

Central slip insertion on middle phalanx

Terminal extensor

Lumbrical muscle

MCP joint

Lateral band

Axis of PIP joint motion

DIP joint

the patient relaxes, the tip of the finger returns to the 70° position but cannot be actively extended beyond that. The DIP joint is stable to radial and ulnar deviation and can be placed back into normal full extension during the examination but falls back into flexion when released.

Fortunately, the physical findings in mallet finger are obvious and thus the condition is easy to diagnose. The most common mechanism of injury is a direct blow to the end of the finger by a ball while the finger is being actively held in extension. Any lack of full, active extension at the DIP joint should be considered a mallet finger. Occasionally a patient with a nailbed injury or distal phalanx fracture will be unable to fully extend the DIP joint due to pain, but in those cases there is some partial active extension. Rarely, a mallet injury will occur in combination with a distal phalanx fracture or nailbed injury.

Physical Examination. The hallmark of the mallet injury is the inability to actively extend the DIP joint. This is almost always an all-or-none situation—that is, either the patient has full extension at the DIP joint or has no active extension at the DIP joint (Figure 13.3). Slight incomplete extension rebound secondary to skin elasticity should not be mistaken for active extension. Collateral instability or dorsal or volar dislocation of the distal phalanx disqualifies the injury from being called a mallet finger and will usually require more extensive evaluation and treatment. The examiner should, of course, examine the remainder of the finger for concomitant injuries.

Anatomy. The pathologic anatomy is complete rupture of the terminal extensor or avulsion of the extensor from its insertion along with a fragment of bone. In the case of

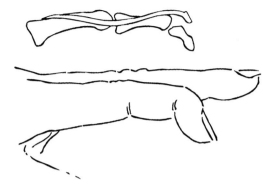

Figure 13.3. Mallet finger.

the jammed finger, the retinacular ligaments are also usually disrupted, resulting in no extension of the DIP joint. In the case of a small laceration it is possible to cut the terminal extensor tendon without cutting the retinacular ligaments and still have weak extension at the DIP joint.

Radiography. Treatment decisions are influenced by the presence or absence of fractures, subluxations, and dislocations, so an x-ray is needed to ascertain their presence. The usual x-rays required are anteroposterior and lateral views of the digit.

Treatment. Treatment of the pure terminal extensor rupture or mallet finger is relatively straightforward. The DIP joint should be splinted in full extension—not hyperextension—full time, for about 8 weeks (Figure 13.4). If the PIP joint does not hyperextend it need not be splinted. If the patient has generalized ligamentous laxity, it may be desirable to splint the PIP joint flexed about 30° simultaneous with the DIP splinting to minimize the possible occurrence of a secondary swan-neck deformity. To minimize skin maceration the patient should be taught to change the splint once or twice daily without allowing the DIP joint to flex. The splint may be placed either

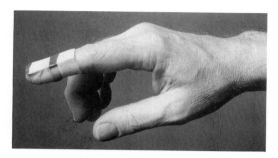

Figure 13.4. Dorsally placed aluminum splint used to treat a mallet finger. There should be minimal padding between the aluminum and the skin to prevent skin breakdown and to maintain full extension.

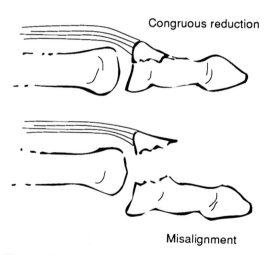

Congruous reduction

Misalignment

Figure 13.5. Mallet finger.

dorsal or volar on the finger. Most patients prefer the splint placement dorsal because this interferes with use of the finger less than if the splint is on the volar surface. If placed dorsal, the splint should be padded or contoured "ever so slightly" to prevent excessive pressure on bony prominences at the DIP joint.

If the mallet injury is associated with an avulsion fracture and a congruous reduction (Figure 13.5) can be obtained without

surgery, then simple splinting has been shown to be equally effective as surgical treatment for fractures representing up to 30% of the joint's surface and possibly even 50% of the joint's surface (1,2). Surgery is rarely necessary for a simple mallet finger. If a congruous reduction cannot be obtained or if the joint remains subluxed (partially dislocated), then a specialist should be consulted. There is no effective exercise or physical therapy treatment for mallet finger. Fortunately, most mallet fingers can also be treated effectively even in the face of a delayed diagnosis of several weeks. Treatment techniques are similar to acute cases but require longer periods of splinting. Surgical treatment is generally reserved for cases involving large fractures or cases having failed splint treatment.

The athlete may be allowed to return to sporting activities while wearing the splint if permitted by the rules of the sport. After 8 weeks, the splint is removed and motion exercises are begun. If an extension lag recurs, splinting is reinstituted for another 2 weeks. If the extension lag does not recur, the finger can be left out of the splint except during athletic participation that might engender reinjury, and at those times the finger should be protected with a splint or taping for 3 months from the time of injury.

Boutonniere Injury (Extensor Rupture at the Proximal Interphalangeal Joint)

Clinical Case #2

A 32-year-old nurse, an avid softball player, comes to your office complaining of pain in her knuckle. She was hit by a softball 4 days ago and has noted progressive decrease in her ability to straighten the finger. Examination reveals pain on the dorsal surface of the PIP joint and inability to fully extend the PIP joint. The PIP joint rests in 30° flexion and is stable to radial and ulnar deviation. You can manually extend the

PIP joint to full extension. The patient can actively flex the PIP joint to 95° and can actively extend it to 30°. The DIP joint does not flex quite as far as those in the adjacent fingers but has full active extension. The MCP joint is normal.

Incomplete extension at the PIP joint should make the examiner suspicious of a boutonniere injury, although again articular fractures, dislocations, and capsuloligamentous sprains may be the cause of incomplete extension. The insidious thing about a boutonniere injury is that the initial physical examination may be normal or near normal in the case of a partial rupture of the extensor mechanism, but then it may progress to a more abnormal condition over the following days or weeks. Thus, the athlete should be cautioned about progressive deformity or scheduled to return for re-evaluation of PIP joint injuries.

Physical Examination. The boutonniere injury results in incomplete active extension of the PIP joint coupled with incomplete flexion of the DIP joint or even an extension contracture or hyperextension contracture of the DIP joint. In severe cases, there may be complete loss of any active extension at the PIP joint and, in fact, attempts to actively extend the PIP joint may result instead in flexion. The distinction to be made on physical examination is between a primary flexion deformity of the PIP joint due to an injury of the joint itself and extension lag due to the boutonniere injury. In acute boutonniere injuries without concomitant joint injury, the examiner can usually fully extend the PIP joint. If there is a joint injury such as a collateral ligament tear, interposition of lateral bands or joint fragment fracture, it may not be possible to manually place the joint in full extension. In chronic cases, the distinction may not be made

as easily. Frequently in the chronic boutonniere injury the displaced lateral bands act as a fixed tether holding the joint in some degree of flexion. A joint injury per se may also result in chronic flexion contracture. If the DIP joint has full mobility, the injury is more likely limited to the PIP joint per se and does not involve the lateral bands or extensor mechanism. If the DIP joint has an extension contracture, the most likely problem is a boutonniere injury that has resulted in fixed deformity.

Anatomy. The interdigitating fibers of the central extensor and the lateral bands at the PIP joint become disrupted, allowing the lateral bands to slip volar to the extension axis of the joint (Figure 13.6). This is not an all-or-none phenomenon. The extension lag may be slight at first and become

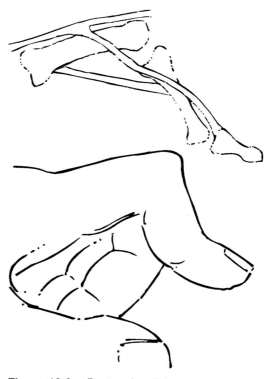

Figure 13.6. Boutonniere injury.

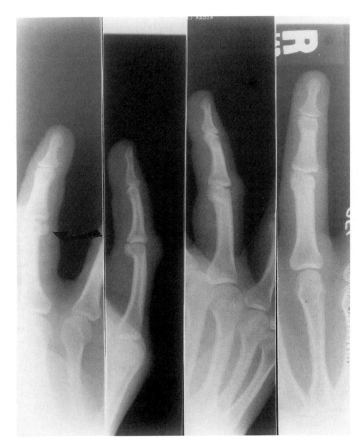

Figure 13.7. The full extent of an injury may not be appreciated unless both medial and lateral oblique x-rays are obtained. In this case, the patient could only flex the PIP joint 45° following a "jamming injury." The displacement of the fractured condyle was seen only on the medial oblique view (*arrow*). Anteroposterior and lateral views alone did not show the extent of injury. The loss of active flexion at the PIP joint suggested the need for the additional x-ray views. This case emphasizes the importance of both physical examination and x-rays and the fact that neither can stand alone in the evaluation of finger and hand fractures. Surgical excision of the fragment was successful in restoring full motion 6 months after the injury.

more severe as progressive subluxation of the lateral bands occurs.

The extension contracture at the DIP joint is a secondary deformity due to altered force vectors and is not part of the primary injury. The contracture can develop rapidly and become severe so that the athlete cannot flex the DIP joint.

Radiography. Radiographic evaluation of the acute extension lag at the PIP joint or the chronic boutonniere appearance should always be performed to rule out bony causes of the deformity. Anteroposterior, lateral, and oblique x-rays are usually sufficient to determine if there is a significant bone in-

jury. Occasionally both medial and lateral obliques may be necessary to determine the full extent of an injury (Figure 13.7).

Treatment. Treatment should be instituted as soon as possible because a delay in treatment greatly prolongs the necessary period of treatment and may result in permanent impairment. Treatment usually consists of splinting the PIP joint in full extension while simultaneously allowing active flexion of the DIP joint (Figure 13.8). A simple aluminum splint taped over the dorsum of the PIP joint is usually sufficient. Splint initially for 3 to 4 weeks. Reinstitute splinting if the deformity recurs. *Indiscrimi-*

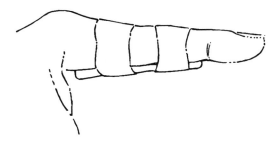

Figure 13.8. An aluminum splint to treat extensor disruption at the PIP joint. A simple splint such as this may be effective in preventing a boutonniere deformity but is ineffective for treating an established boutonniere deformity. Do not splint the entire digit in full extension or excessive stiffness may occur. Splint may also be placed dorsally.

nate splinting of a jammed finger with all joints in full extension can easily lead to a stiff finger. Fingers are meant to move and thus should be splinted only for the minimal amount of time necessary for tendon healing or to achieve joint stability from a sprain. Significant finger stiffness can result from as little as 2 or 3 weeks of inappropriate splinting. Thus, it is important to establish an accurate diagnosis as soon as possible and allow those uninjured parts to move freely. Allowing motion at the DIP joint in the boutonniere injury not only maintains mobility at that joint but maintains some gliding of the lateral bands around the PIP joint as they heal. Flexion of the DIP joint while the PIP joint is fully extended may actually help to draw the yoke formed by the converging lateral bands back to their normal dorsal position. If both joints are splinted in extension, the beneficial effects of DIP motion are lost.

Delayed treatment of boutonniere injuries is possible but is usually much more prolonged than early treatment, is more fraught with residual impairment, and may require surgical intervention. Hence, con-

tinued participation in sports without fully protective splinting is unadvisable.

Sagittal Band or Extensor Hood Rupture at the Metacarpophalangeal Joint

Clinical Case #3

A 40-year-old hospital administrator complains of a snapping feeling over the MCP joint of the long finger of his left hand. He is learning karate with his son and he tried to break a piece of wood with his fist. Examination reveals tenderness over the MCP joint and decreased ability to extend the finger at the MCP joint. When the examiner manually extends the joint for him he is able to hold it there against force but after he flexes it he is again unable to fully extend. When he flexes the finger there is a slight sideways "jump" of the extensor tendon at the MCP joint.

The mechanism of injury of the extensor apparatus at the MCP joints is different from that of the interphalangeal (IP) joints. The extensor tendons as they cross the MCP joint are quite stout and not directly anchored to bone; thus, they are not easily injured by an axial blow (jamming injury) to the digit. Furthermore, injury is much less common at this level than at the IP joints. When injury occurs, it is usually a rupture of the sagittal fibers of the extensor hood. The mechanism of injury seems to be a sudden forceful grip, possibly combined with some torsional force, that results in rupture of the anchoring sagittal fibers from their volar attachments. For example, the patient may be hitting a strong tennis backhand or lifting weights and feel a sudden pop around the MCP joint. The injury may also occur from a direct blow, such as when performing karate maneuvers or hitting objects with the bare knuckles. Frequently the athlete will not be aware that a significant injury has occurred because the pain may not be severe. Initially there may be no extension lag and no deformity. In addition to tenderness, the athlete may notice two symptoms. The first is snapping or subluxation of the extensor tendon. The second, inability to extend the MCP joint, may not occur in all cases or may develop progressively.

Physical Examination. The physical examination may show one of two things. In milder cases the extensor tendon may visibly sublux or snap off the metacarpal head and fall to one side during active flexion of the MCP joint. The most common rupture is the radial sagittal bands of the index finger resulting in the tendon subluxing to the ulnar side of the metacarpal head. When the patient actively extends the finger, the tendon may pop back up into its normal location centralized over the MCP joint. In more severe cases the patient may not be able to actively extend the MCP joint. If the joint is passively extended and the tendon relocates to its normal position, the patient may then be able to hold the MCP joint extended against resistance. In contradistinction to the boutonniere and mallet injuries, there is usually no associated extensor imbalance or contracture of the adjacent joints.

Radiography. Unless there has been a direct blow to the hand raising the possibility of a fracture, x-rays are usually not necessary to make this diagnosis. Associated injuries such as spontaneous avulsion of a collateral ligament are so incredibly rare as to make x-rays unwarranted unless the presentation is highly atypical.

Treatment. There is some disagreement as to whether surgical or nonsurgical treatment is preferable in acute cases. Both approaches have been used successfully (3). When recognized acutely this injury has been successfully treated by extension splinting of the MCP joint for 4 to 6 weeks. Splinting of the MCP joint in extension is best accomplished with either a hand cast or hand-based molded plastic splint held on with Velcro straps (Figure 13.9). It is hard to properly stabilize a narrow aluminum splint using tape alone. Using a cast with the aluminum splint incorporated into the cast or using the hand-based molded plastic splints is much more reliable than attempting to simply tape on an aluminum splint. Splint treatment is not uniformly successful for the athlete so the primary care physician may wish to consult a surgeon immediately.

There has even been limited experience treating chronic cases with splinting in nonathletes. However, in chronic cases surgical reconstruction of the extensor hood is usually required. Fortunately, reconstruction of the extensor hood is a reasonably successful operation, and although results can never be guaranteed, this does raise the possibility of an athlete continuing to compete at a crucial time without undergoing surgery acutely. The decision to delay treatment should not be undertaken

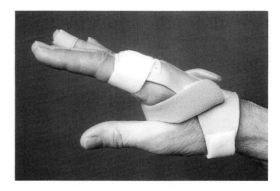

Figure 13.9. A hand-based splint used to hold the MCP joint in nearly full extension. It can also be used to treat extensor hood ruptures and collateral ligament ruptures.

lightly. If definitive treatment is delayed the finger should be buddy-taped to an adjacent digit.

FLEXOR TENDON INJURIES

Jersey Finger

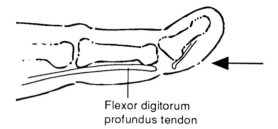

Flexor digitorum
profundus tendon

Figure 13.10. "Jersey finger" injury mechanism.

Clinical Case #4

A 17-year-old high school football player injured his right ring finger while attempting to tackle an opponent by grabbing the jersey and shoulder pads. He was treated with buddy-taping for 1 week. He now complains of inability to move the tip of the finger.

Jersey finger, rupture of the flexor digitorum profundus from its insertion on the distal phalanx (Figure 13.10), occurs most commonly when a football or rugby player is trying to tackle an opponent and a fingertip becomes entangled in the opponent's jersey. Other mechanisms include a sudden extension force of the fingertips caused by the pullaway of a horse's reins or catching the fingertip in a basketball net. The common pathway of these and other mechanisms is that there is a sudden force attempting to extend the fingertip against the resistance of the actively flexing profundus tendon.

Physical Examination. Findings are straightforward. The athlete will be unable to actively flex the DIP joint. The flexor digitorum profundus is the only active means of flexing the DIP joint. Inability to actively flex this joint should lead to immediate consideration of flexor digitorum profundus rupture. Other possibilities for inability to flex the DIP joint would include fracture, dorsal subluxation or dislocation, and inhibition due to the pain of a partial

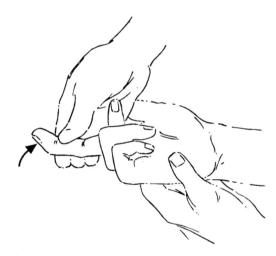

Figure 13.11. A "Jersey finger" injury. The DIP joint cannot be actively flexed with the MCP and PIP held in extension.

rupture. If the examiner holds the MCP and PIP joints in full extension manually and isolates the athlete's attempts to flex the DIP joint, some motion will usually be evident if the profundus is not ruptured (Figure 13.11). If there is no active flexion of the DIP joint, the athlete should be referred for definitive diagnosis and treatment as soon as possible.

Radiography. X-rays are advisable to rule out fracture, subluxation, or dislocation of the DIP joint and to determine if the tendon avulsion occurred with a large fragment of bone. Occasionally a large enough fragment will be avulsed that the tendon does not actually retract proximally into the finger because the bone fragment will not pass through the flexor pulley system. In such a case, there may actually be some active flexion of the DIP joint as the bone fragment pulls against the distal flexor pulley, although this flexion would be weak.

Treatment. The window of opportunity for a good repair and best functional result with this injury is "the sooner the better." It is extremely important that the diagnosis be made early. There is no physical therapy treatment for this condition. Unfortunately, this injury is easily and frequently overlooked because most of the hand function appears normal and there is no obvious deformity. It is assumed that the distal joint is just sprained or jammed, and it is not until several weeks later when joint motion has not returned that the real diagnosis is made. In such cases the decision regarding surgical repair, tendon grafting, or acceptance of the functional deficit and rehabilitation is more complex because achieving good results with a late repair is certainly less reliable than with an acute repair.

Flexor Digitorum Superficialis Rupture

This is an extremely uncommon injury without a definitely recognized athletic mechanism of injury. It can occur during forceful grip, resisted flexion, or attempted flexion during forced hyperextension (4).

Physical Examination. Examination would reveal, of course, tenderness at the site of injury, but would be positive only for lack of isolated active flexion of the PIP joint (Figure 13.12). The maneuver is the same one used to test for laceration of the flexor digitorum superficialis when the profundus is intact. If the athlete is asked to

simply close the hand and make a fist or close the finger without eliminating flexor digitorum profundus function, the PIP joint would still flex and the diagnosis could be missed. To isolate superficialis function at the PIP joint, the examiner must allow the injured digit to move freely while immobilizing all the other fingers and the wrist in full extension (see Figure 13.12). This effectively eliminates contribution of the flexor digitorum profundus to the PIP joint of the injured finger and all flexor power should occur only through the superficialis. Lack of PIP flexion would be diagnostic of flexor digitorum superficialis rupture. One exception to this rule is that sometimes the superficialis of the small finger cannot act independently of the ring finger and examination of the small finger must be performed with the ring finger also free to move. Resistance is then placed against the PIP joint of the small finger to determine if there is any active power. PIP dislocations and fracture-dislocations also result in inability to flex the joint. In those injuries, however, the joint cannot be flexed by the profundus, the superficialis, or passively by the examiner without significant difficulty and pain.

Rupture of the Annular Flexor Pulleys

Clinical Case #5

A 23-year-old back-packing enthusiast comes to your office for evaluation of a progressive flexion contracture of the left ring finger. Approximately 3 months ago he was at his local outfitter's shop and took a lesson on rock climbing. While on the practice wall one foot slipped and he was barely able to hang on with his hands. He did feel a slight burning, tearing sensation in his left ring finger at the time, but the finger seemed to function normally when he examined it after getting off the wall. He developed

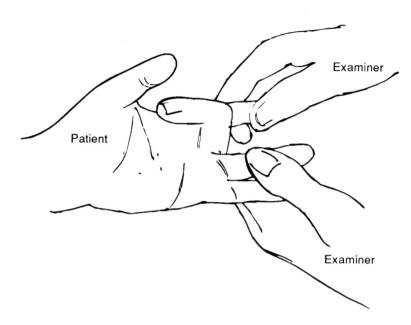

Figure 13.12. Superficial isolation testing—two-handed technique.

a slight flexion contracture over the next few days, which he assumed would resolve. Instead, it has become progressively worse. Examination reveals a 60° flexion contracture of the PIP joint, no altered motion of the DIP joint, and no joint instability of either joint to collateral stress. It seems as if the flexor tendons crossing the PIP joint are more palpable in this finger compared to his other fingers.

This is an uncommon injury that has only recently been recognized. The one sport in which this may occur with some frequency is in rock climbing or wall climbing (5–7). This injury has not been recognized to occur from a simple jamming episode or hyperextension injury. As best as can be determined from interviews with patients with this injury, it results from exerting extremely forceful flexion power while the fingers are already partially flexed.

Anatomy. The function of the annular pulleys is to hold the flexor tendons adjacent to the bones and prevent bowstringing. If suf-

ficient force is exerted, a pulley can rupture. The resultant bowstringing of the flexor tendons across the PIP joint results in a greater moment arm of flexion (leverage), which the much weaker extensors have a difficult time overcoming. In the untreated injury, the patient may suffer progressive flexion contracture of the PIP joint due to this imbalance of flexor and extensor forces.

Physical Examination. Findings include flexion contracture of the PIP joint and palpable or visible bowstringing of the flexor tendons across the PIP joint. It might be difficult to distinguish a chronic flexion contracture due to a flexor pulley rupture from those caused by a joint injury or boutonniere injury solely on the basis of physical examination. The distinction of this injury from the boutonniere injury on physical examination is that DIP joint motion would be normal in this injury, whereas DIP joint flexion is restricted in the boutonniere injury. In acute injuries where there is a strong tendency for a flexion attitude of the PIP joint or if the examiner can feel bowstring of the flexor tendons, the athlete should be referred as soon as possible for evaluation by a hand surgeon. In chronic cases of PIP joint flexion contracture, rupture of an annular pulley would be low on the list of the differential diagnoses but should be considered.

Radiography. Plain x-rays have not been helpful in diagnosing this condition. A magnetic resonance imaging (MRI) scan showing hemorrhage, edema, or bow-stringing at the site of injury, a tenogram, or possibly an ultrasound demonstrating bowstringing of the tendons could supplement the physical examination in difficult cases. However, as with other forceful injuries, x-rays are probably warranted in acute cases to rule out avulsion fractures.

Treatment. Treatment of this injury should consist of surgical repair of the flexor pulley. If left untreated, patients suffer progressive flexion contractures of the PIP joint. This injury is uncommon enough that there is no experience with physical rehabilitation as a primary treatment, but given the altered mechanical forces across the PIP joint it is unlikely that therapeutic modalities alone could fully restore active extension at the PIP joint.

DISLOCATIONS AND SPRAINS

Skier's Thumb or Gamekeeper's Thumb

This common injury occurs in nonathletic trauma as well as sporting trauma. Originally described as a chronic condition of those who suffered the injury by pulling the heads off small game, the acute form most often seen in modern society stems from a ski pole hyperabducting the thumb during downhill skiing. It can also occur from a fall on the outstretched thumb or from bicycle handlebars, steering wheels, parallel bars, and from balls hitting the thumb. Basically any mechanism of injury that results in hyperabduction or torsion of the thumb MCP joint can cause this injury. There is no age or gender predilection.

Anatomy. The ulnar collateral ligament of the MCP joint is ruptured from its insertion on the base of the proximal phalanx of the thumb (Figure 13.13). The dorsal capsule is usually also torn and the attachment of the volar plate to the proximal phalanx may be injured to varying degrees. The volar plate attachment is much stronger than that of the dorsal capsule so the disruptive forces tend to propagate dorsally more than volarly. In severe cases, the thumb may be abducted so far that the stump of the collateral ligament is pulled out from under the aponeurosis of the adductor pollicis muscle and then cannot go back under this

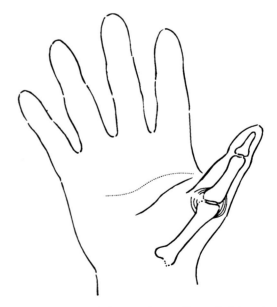

Figure 13.13. Injury to ulnar collateral of thumb MCP joint gamekeeper's or skier's thumb.

aponeurosis when the thumb has returned to normal position. This lesion is called the Stener lesion (8). The significance of the Stener lesion is that the ligament cannot heal back to its normal attachment at the base of the proximal phalanx. When the Stener lesion is not present, there is a much better chance at satisfactory healing.

Physical Examination. This is directed at distinguishing the minor injuries from those in which the Stener lesion is present. Grade I injuries in which there are micro-tears of the ligament resulting in pain but no discernible instability and grade II injuries in which the ligament is actually torn off the bone but not fully displaced can heal satisfactorily with nonoperative treatment. The grade III injuries in which the ligament is completely ruptured and the joint is unstable due to the associated capsular injuries are more likely to have a Stener lesion.

Examination reveals tenderness to palpation along the ulnar border of the MCP joint of the thumb, usually some tenderness around the dorsal aspect of the thumb and variable degrees of tenderness on the volar aspect. On occasion, one might be able to palpate the stump of the displaced collateral ligament adjacent to the metacarpal head. The proximal phalanx usually sags toward the volar aspect of the joint, but this is difficult to discern due to swelling. Collateral stability of the joint should be tested both with the MCP joint held in extension and in flexion. With the metacarpal stabilized, the examiner should exert radial deviation pressure against the proximal phalanx (Figure 13.14). When this is done with the MCP joint in extension, the volar plate, if intact, will be tight at the ulnar corner and will confer stability to the joint. This is favorable evidence for a grade I or II injury. *If the joint is unstable in extension, allow-*

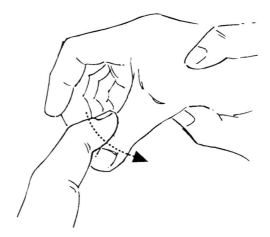

Figure 13.14. Stress testing of ulnar collateral ligament of the thumb.

ing more than 30° radial deviation, the injury is most certainly a grade III. When the MCP joint is flexed during examination, the volar plate is relaxed and if the joint is still stable to collateral testing, this is good evidence for a grade I injury, whereas a grade II injury may or may not be stable in flexion. The grade III injury would be unstable in both flexion and extension. The distinction between grades II and III is not always clear-cut and may compound treatment decisions.

Radiography. Anteroposterior, lateral, and oblique films of the thumb are recommended routinely because frequently the ligament avulses a piece of bone that may range in size from very small to one representing a significant articular surface of the joint (Figure 13.15). Significantly displaced fragments (≥3 mm) should probably be fixed surgically. In cases without a bony avulsion, volar subluxation of the proximal phalanx past the metacarpal head would indicate a more severe injury and might mitigate toward surgical treatment. The degree of subluxation is difficult to deter-

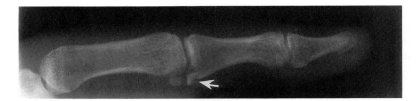

Figure 13.15. Gamekeeper's thumb, skier's thumb. Although the small bone fragment is slightly malrotated, it is not significantly displaced. This represents a grade II injury, which can be treated nonoperatively. Displacement of the fragment 3 mm or more should raise suspicion of a Stener lesion, probably best treated surgically.

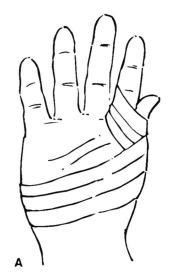

A

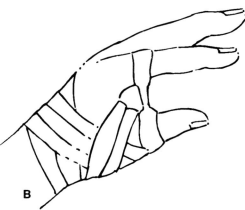

B

Figure 13.16. Taping of ulnar collateral ligament injuries for sports.

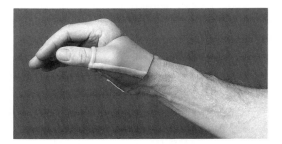

Figure 13.17. A hand-based splint used to treat minor skier's (gamekeeper's) thumb.

mine on physical exam so x-ray is often helpful although not totally diagnostic of grade III injuries.

Treatment. Grade I injuries can usually be treated by continued participation in sports with or without the use of a strapping or taping technique to prevent reinjury, depending on the nature of the sport (Figure 13.16). Grade II injuries, likewise, can usually be treated with strapping, taping, or a thumb spica splint or cast, depending on individual circumstances (Figure 13.17). In the case of splinting or casting, 3 weeks of immobilization would be all that is necessary in most instances. Grade III injuries present more of a dilemma. The degree of thumb instability and pain itself may preclude continued sports participation. If a satisfactory nonoperative treatment technique can be individualized to the athlete, the option does exist to delay surgical treatment. Although some surgeons feel the best treatment is early surgical treatment, evidence also indicates that some patients with grade III injuries will ultimately heal satisfactorily without surgery although the course may be protracted. Some patients, however, will not heal satisfactorily without surgery and delayed treatment can be performed. The distinction between early surgical treatment and late surgical treatment is mainly one of speeding the time course of recovery and possibly improving the ultimate joint motion in those patients treated acutely. Unfortunately, there is no standard in the physical examination or in x-ray or other imaging studies that is predictive of which patients with grade III injuries will heal satisfactorily without surgery. It is generally thought that the presence of a displaced avulsion fracture portends a bad outcome without surgical repair. The general trend in treatment of this injury has been toward surgical repair of the grade III injuries and nonoperative treatment of the grade I and II injuries. However, because delayed surgical repairs generally have a satisfactory but not identical outcome as acute repairs, the athlete is presented with the option of continued participation while deferring surgery to a more convenient later date.

The Proximal Interphalangeal Joint

Dislocations of the PIP joint are common injuries in a jammed finger. The distinction to be made on clinical examination and for treatment purposes is whether the joint is stable or unstable once it is reduced (relocated). The most common dislocation is straight dorsal, does not involve collateral ligament injury, and is stable once it is re-

duced. Collateral ligament injuries usually render the joint unstable. Associated fractures may or may not result in instability. In general, x-rays are advisable to rule out fractures and subluxations.

Volar Plate Avulsion

A common PIP joint injury is the volar plate avulsion or sprain. The mechanism of injury is hyperextension with resultant detachment of the volar plate from its insertion on the middle phalanx.

Physical Examination. The finger should have essentially full active extension and flexion. Examination will usually reveal localized tenderness on the volar aspect of the PIP joint. When collateral stress shows no instability of the collateral ligaments and attempts to fully extend the joint do not result in unstable hyperextension, the diagnosis should be considered a grade I or II PIP volar plate disruption. If the joint hyperextends on examination (Figure 13.18), the injury should be considered serious enough to require treatment. The examiner should also specifically perform the flexor digitorum superficialis isolation test to rule out a rupture of the flexor digitorum superficialis. The points of tenderness of these two injuries are very close together so that discerning between the two injuries on the basis of tenderness alone is difficult. The distinction is important. Whereas a minor volar plate sprain does

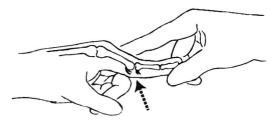

Figure 13.18. Volar plate injury showing PIP hyperextension.

not require aggressive treatment, a rupture of the flexor digitorum superficialis requires surgical repair as soon as possible.

Radiography. If the digit has full active extension and active flexion to 75% of the normal joint motion, x-rays are probably unnecessary. If the digit does not meet those criteria, then an x-ray should be obtained to rule out fractures or subluxations.

Treatment. If the joint is stable to collateral stress and does not hyperextend or subluxate dorsally when fully extended, it is basically an innocuous injury and should be treated with early active motion. Buddy-tape this finger to the adjacent finger. Do not flex this finger in a splint for a prolonged period of time or the patient may develop a flexion contracture. If the joint hyperextends, treat with an extension block splint for 1 to 2 weeks (Figure 13.19), followed by buddy-taping for a few weeks during participation.

Dorsal Dislocation or Coach's Finger

The straight dorsal dislocation is essentially a variant of the volar plate rupture. It can be treated by closed reduction and usually is . . . by the coach. If the joint is stable after reduction, it can be treated with early motion and buddy-taping. The important distinction in this instance is the difference between a straight dorsal dislocation and one associated with a collateral ligament tear. If the mechanism of injury includes rotation or collateral stress, one or both collateral ligaments may be torn. The collateral ligament injury in combination with the volar plate injury is not stable and needs to be protected.

Physical Examination. While the joint is dislocated, it is usually quite easy to palpate the base of the middle phalanx riding dorsal to the head of the proximal phalanx. Prior to attempting reduction, the examiner should

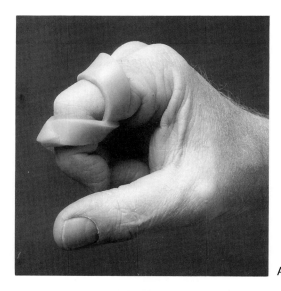

A

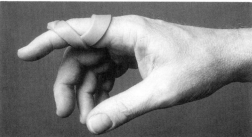

B

Figure 13.19. An extension block splint used to treat a PIP joint injury. This type of splint allows active motion (*A*) but prevents hyperextension (*B*).

perform a neurovascular examination of the digit both for purposes of documenting the neurovascular status and the therapeutic reason that if the examination changes for the worse after the reduction, entrapment of the neurovascular bundle in the joint should be considered (rare). If this occurs, the finger should be redislocated and the patient referred for emergency surgical treatment. If the dislocation is straight dorsal, the collateral ligaments (Figure 13.20*A*)

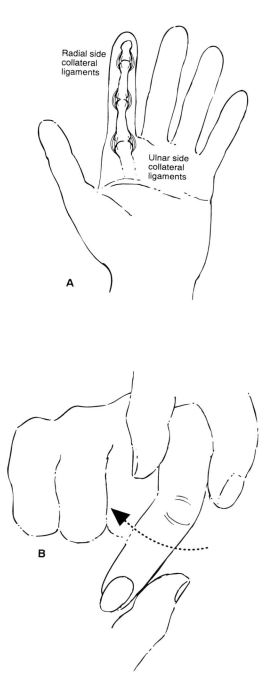

Radial side
collateral
ligaments

Ulnar side
collateral
ligaments

A

B

Figure 13.20. Collateral ligaments of PIP (A) and stress testing (B).

are usually not completely ruptured and the joint is stable to collateral stress. If the collateral ligament is completely ruptured, the dislocation will probably not rest in the straight dorsal position but will be off to one side or rotated. Collateral stress testing should be gentle while the finger is dislocated and should be repeated more vigorously after the reduction (Figure 13.20B).

Radiography. If the joint is reduced on the field and is totally stable and has full range of motion, x-rays are probably unnecessary. If the joint tends to hyperextend, this may signify a volar rim fracture so x-rays should be obtained. If the dislocation is not easily reducible on the field, x-rays should be obtained before further reduction attempts to ascertain if the injury is more complicated than a simple dislocation.

Treatment. If the joint is dislocated, reduction should be attempted as soon as possible because reductions of dislocated joints are usually much less traumatic, easier to perform, and much less painful if performed quickly. When this injury is recognized on the field, it is common for a coach, trainer, or other player to "pop it back into joint." Straight longitudinal traction possibly with some thumb pressure pushing the middle phalanx distally is all that is usually required for a reduction immediately after injury. If reduction is performed after the finger becomes swollen, it may be necessary or desirable to perform digital nerve blocks to anesthetize the finger before the reduction. After reduction, the finger should be checked again for collateral stability, active flexion and extension, and instability in hyperextension. If the joint tends to hyperextend, the finger should be put into a splint at 30° PIP joint flexion for 1 to 2 weeks. If the joint does not hyperextend, it should be buddy-taped to an adjacent finger. Buddy-taping will allow early active motion of the joint while preventing

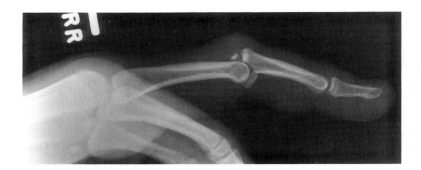

Figure 13.21. A dorsal fracture dislocation of the PIP joint in a collegiate coach. The extent of injury went unappreciated for a week. The x-rays were obtained because of inability to flex the PIP joint.

reinjury. By instituting a short period of splinting, at most 2 weeks, followed by buddy-taping, the finger with a hyperextensible joint can usually be rehabilitated without surgery. If an immobilizing splint is used, only the PIP joint should be included in the splint so that DIP motion can be allowed to help maintain mobility of the flexor and extensor tendons past the healing area of scar tissue. The joint should be held flexed only as far as necessary to achieve a congruous reduction as confirmed by x-ray. Excessive flexion will result in permanent residual flexion contracture. Dislocations with collateral ligament injuries generally take a minimum of 3 months and up to 6 months to heal satisfactorily. Buddy-taping should be maintained during strenuous activities for 3 months.

Fracture Dislocation

Clinical Case #6

A 26-year-old women's field hockey coach was playing a pick-up game of basketball and sustained a jamming injury to the left ring finger. She initially treated this with ice and a dorsal aluminum splint. After 1 week, she still could not flex the PIP joint so she sought the advice of the team physician. Examination showed mild swelling and ecchymoses, an irregular feeling of the bony contour on the dorsal side of the PIP joint, and active flexion of only 20° at the PIP joint. The MCP joint was normal and the DIP joint appeared normal but would only flex 50°. Radial and ulnar deviation collateral testing was normal within the limits of the patient's pain tolerance. X-rays showed the base of the proximal phalanx was partially dislocated dorsally (subluxed) and the volar half of its articular surface was fractured and displaced (Figure 13.21).

In some instances when axial load or jamming is applied along with hyperextension forces, the base of the proximal phalanx will fracture. The degree of fracture varies and must be assessed by x-ray. If the fracture is large enough, the base of the middle phalanx will tend to sublux dorsally off the head of the proximal phalanx. The athlete will then be unable to flex the joint enough to meet the criteria for the "it's ok" minor jammed finger.

Physical Examination. The finger rests near full extension, but the patient will be unable to achieve good flexion. Collateral instability is usually not part of this injury but when present would indicate a much more guarded prognosis for recovery. The dorsal subluxation of the middle phalanx may or may not be palpable or visible depending on swelling. DIP joint flexion will be mildly reduced due to excessive tension on the extensor caused by the displacement.

Radiography. Anteroposterior, lateral, and oblique x-rays are helpful here, not only to make the diagnosis but to help determine treatment. If the articular fragment is small enough, it may be possible to perform a closed reduction and splint the joint and achieve a good result without surgery. Larger fragments require surgical treatment.

Treatment. If x-rays show a small volar lip fragment and a congruous reduction can be obtained, the finger can be treated with either a PIP flexion splint or an extension block splint for about 2 to 3 weeks. If a stable congruous reduction cannot be obtained as confirmed by postreduction x-rays in the splint, some type of surgical treatment will be necessary. This injury is not compatible with continued participation in most instances. The recuperative period before return to participation varies depending on the type of surgical repair. It may be as short as 4 weeks but is more likely to be as long as 3 months.

The Metacarpophalangeal Joint

Dislocation of the MCP joint with or without collateral ligament injury is fairly uncommon but important. The mechanism of injury is usually a jamming-type injury with axial load rather than pure hyperextension. If this injury can be reduced nonoperatively, it is usually stable and is compatible with continued participation in sports. It is important, however, to distinguish between the simple dorsal dislocation and the complex dorsal dislocation. They both basically represent degrees of severity of the same injury.

Anatomy and Physical Examination. When the finger is hyperextended at the same time axial load is applied, the volar plate ruptures at its origin on the metacarpal neck and rides dorsally with the proximal phalanx. The collateral ligaments usually elevate as a sleeve but one or both may rupture. In a simple dislocation, the proximal phalanx comes to rest on the dorsal aspect of the metacarpal head, but the volar plate has not come completely around far enough to become interposed between the base of the phalanx and the metacarpal head. In the complex dislocation, the displacement has occurred slightly further and the trailing edge of the volar plate displaces sufficiently to become entrapped (Figure 13.22). The simple dislocation can be reduced manually. The complex reduction requires surgery. The appearance of the finger can be important in making the distinction. With the simple dislocation, the finger will tend to appear hyperextended at an angle, whereas with the complex dislocation, there may be more of a tendency for the finger to appear parallel to the metacarpal.

Radiography. If one or two attempts at closed reduction are unsuccessful, anteroposterior, lateral, and oblique x-rays should be obtained to assess any possible fracture component of the injury. It is not uncommon to find an avulsed fragment representing a collateral ligament attachment or to find an osteochondral fragment off the metacarpal head.

Treatment. As with most dislocations, the best treatment is to get the joint reduced as soon as possible. It is theoretically possible to convert a simple dislocation to a complex dislocation if reduction is performed im-

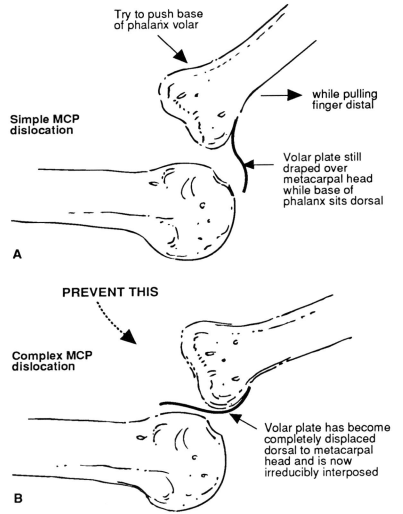

Try to push base
of phalanx volar

while pulling
finger distal

Volar plate still
draped over
metacarpal head
while base of
phalanx sits dorsal

**Simple MCP
dislocation**

A

PREVENT THIS

**Complex MCP
dislocation**

Volar plate has become
completely displaced
dorsal to metacarpal
head and is now
irreducibly interposed

B

Figure 13.22. Treatment
of MCP joint dislocation.

properly. *Do not hyperextend the finger further.* The proper reduction maneuver is to apply volar-directed pressure to the base of the proximal phalanx while at the same time applying longitudinal traction in line with the metacarpal. The goal is really to push the base of the phalanx back volarly around the metacarpal head rather than to apply traction while inadvertently hyperextending the finger further. Once re-

duction is achieved, the joint is usually stable and can be treated with buddy-taping. If reduction cannot be achieved after one or two attempts, there is probaby a complex dislocation and the athlete should be referred for surgical treatment. In the complex dislocation, the flexor tendons and lumbricals have been carried so far dorsally that the metacarpal head is buttonholed between them. Traction actually tends to tighten the entrapment, much like the action of a Chinese finger trap, so that traction actually impedes the closed reduction.

Regardless of whether treatment is by simple closed reduction or surgery, the best correlation of a good outcome is early motion. Prolonged splinting of this injury results in significant loss of motion at the MCP joint. Immobilize the joint for a week or less and use buddy-taping as soon as comfort allows. Continue buddy taping for 6 weeks.

FRACTURES

A few general principles must be considered regarding fractures of the phalanges and metacarpals. First, one of the main functional attributes of the hand is that it is highly mobile. Unfortunately, there is very little soft tissue between the tendons and underlying bone. This results in a strong tendency to develop restrictive adhesions between the tendons and bones. Thus, even though fractures may require some splinting or immobilization, it is desirable to resume motion as soon as safely possible. Some minor fractures, in fact, do not require immobilization and an athlete's option to continue participation would depend on pain and ability to prevent further injury.

Second, most but not all nondisplaced fractures tend to remain nondisplaced unless re-exposed to a deforming force. This is because in the fingers there are many small cutaneous ligaments and fibers that anchor the glabrous skin of the palm and fingers to the underlying bones, and this in turn tends to help splint the bones in position if those fibers are not ruptured with the initial fracture. In the metacarpals the transverse metacarpal ligament can help

prevent displacement of a single metacarpal fracture.

Third, neither x-ray evaluation nor physical examination can stand alone without the other in evaluating hand fractures. Many fractures cannot be accurately assessed and may even be missed on physical examination. Radiographs alone may not be sufficient to evaluate rotary malalignment in the tubular bones of the hand. Specific physician examination for rotational assessment in the fingers is essential to complement the x-rays.

Fourth, fractures of the metacarpals and phalanges tend to heal more quickly than other fractures of the appendicular skeleton. Thus, when immobilization is required, it may be discontinued and rehabilitation begun earlier than for other fractures.

Finally, x-ray evidence of union tends to lag behind clinical union. Many fractures are clinically stable and suitable for re-entry into participation before the fracture line is completely obliterated on x-rays.

Mechanisms of Injury

Finger fractures are very common. Most of them, amazingly enough, are not debilitating. There are of course, exceptions. Mechanically, the mechanisms of injury are bending, torsion, and axial load or combinations of these. There are no particular associations between specific sports and specific fractures.

Metacarpal Neck Fractures

The most common and trivial of these is the fracture of the fifth metacarpal neck, the so-called boxer's fracture. Much less common but potentially more troublesome are fractures of the second and third metacarpals. The injury occurs from a direct blow, usually the fist striking an object or person.

Physical Examination. Localized swelling and possibly loss of the prominence of the metacarpal head are seen. The metacarpal head is usually flexed or depressed in relationship to the shaft. The examiner should palpate the palm to determine if the metacarpal head is depressed far enough to present a palpable lump in the palm. Specific attention should be directed at making certain the athlete has full active extension to at least neutral at the MCP joint and has active flexion of at least 70°. Malrotation is assessed by checking for involuntary crossing or overlap of the fingers when the fist is closed (Figure 13.23).

Radiography. X-rays are obtained to confirm the fracture, to be certain it is extra-articular, and to measure the displacement of the distal fragment. Occasionally the degree of

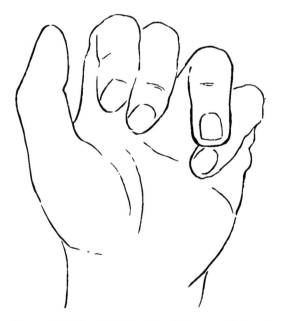

Figure 13.23. Rotational malalignment is best assessed by flexing the fingers. Moderate rotational malalignment of phalangeal or metacarpal fractures may not be noticeable if the fingers are extended.

displacement or flexion of the fracture is severe enough to warrant treatment.

Treatment. Treatment is usually nonsurgical, consisting of either splinting, bracing, or casting. The fracture rarely goes to nonunion and could actually be treated without any immobilization; however, immobilization greatly reduces the pain. Whether to attempt closed reduction or surgical pinning of the fragment depends on the amount of flexion. In general, if the patient has full active extension of the MCP joint and the carpometacarpal joint is mobile enough to prevent the metacarpal head from presenting a prominent lump in the palm, the fracture can be treated without surgical reduction. The second and third metacarpals have very little motion in the dorsal-volar plane and thus can accept very little residual flexion of the distal fragment without the metacarpal head presenting a prominent lump in the palm. Ten degrees flexion of the distal fragment is probably the maximum safe limit for most patients. Angulation greater than 10° in the second or third metacarpal should be referred for surgical evaluation. The fourth and fifth metacarpals, however, have more motion through their carpometacarpal joints than the second and third and so are able to compensate for more displacement of the metacarpal head. As much as 45° residual flexion is acceptable, whereas 45° to 60° is in the equivocal zone and anything greater than that may be unacceptable and should be evaluated by a surgeon. Any rotational malalignment resulting in involuntary crossing of the fingers sufficient to impair use of the hand would require surgical treatment.

Most athletes are unable to continue participation with the injured hand if it involves gripping an implement. Fortunately, this fracture heals enough within 3 to 4 weeks to allow return to participation in most instances.

Metacarpal Shaft Fractures

When these fractures are nondisplaced they can usually be treated with a compressive dressing, splint, short arm cast, or even no immobilization if the patient's pain is not severe. The limits of acceptability for shaft displacement in the finger metacarpals is much less than for metacarpal neck fractures. This is because a lesser angle in the shaft will portend a greater displacement of the metacarpal head than does a similar degree of angulation at the metacarpal neck. Metacarpal shortening of up to 1 cm is acceptable. Malrotation is unacceptable and should be sought out on physical examination by observing the alignment of the fingers in flexion.

Physical Examination. The most important aspect of the physical examination in metacarpal fractures is to determine the rotational alignment of the fracture. This should be assessed by having the patient flex the MCP joints and fingers as much as possible (see Figure 13.23). If the fingers show any tendency for crossing over or under each other (malrotation), it will be more easily recognized with the MCP joints fully flexed than with them extended. When the joints are extended, there is more laxity of the collateral ligaments and capsule as well as a narrower profile of the metacarpal head. This results in the joint being looser and more able to accommodate or obscure malalignment and malrotation.

Any functional impairment due to malrotation will be more of a problem for the patient when the fingers cross during grip. By examining rotation with the joints flexed, simulating grip, the potential functional impairment is more evident.

The thumb has much more rotary motion at its carpometacarpal joint than do the fingers and is therefore able to accommodate much greater degrees of fracture malalignment. It would be important to check the athlete's ability to oppose the thumb to each of the fingertips and to the base of the small finger. Clinical assessment of thumb function is more important than any radiographic criteria such as angular alignment, comminution, obliquity of the fracture line, or locale of the fracture within the metacarpal shaft. If the athlete is unable to touch the thumb tip to all four fingertips, surgical consultation should be obtained.

Intra-articular Fractures of the Base of the Thumb (Bennett's Fracture or Rolando's Fracture)

Whereas stable extra-articular fractures of the thumb's metacarpal shaft and metaphyseal regions are usually of little consequence, intra-articular fractures of the base of the thumb can be disabling (Figure 13.24). The mechanism of injury is any kind of a jamming injury or fall onto the thumb. The symptoms are usually pain, swelling, and limited motion.

Physical Examination. Pain, swelling, decreased motion, and occasionally crepitance are apparent. The thenar eminence frequently swells considerably following any trauma to the area so the degree of swelling is a poor guide of the degree of injury. During the first day or two after deep contusion, thenar eminence swelling alone may limit motion but the swelling of a contusion resolves fairly rapidly. Pain may be difficult to localize as to whether located in the shaft region or intra-articularly at the carpalmetacarpal joint. One cannot exclude intraarticular fractures of the base of the metacarpal just because the thumb metacarpal seems stable to examination or tender-

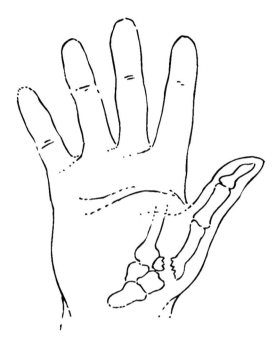

Figure 13.24. Bennett's fracture of thumb MCP joint.

ness seems to be located more toward the shaft than the carpometacarpal joint. The swelling may be tense enough to splint a fracture and prevent the examiner from feeling motion at the fracture site or the fragments may be impacted enough that motion of the fracture fragments is not detectable. If sharp pain or limited motion persists beyond 48 hours, one should seriously consider a fracture and obtain radiographic evaluation.

Radiography and Treatment. Anteroposterior and lateral and oblique views of the thumb are usually sufficient to determine whether or not there is a significant injury. Any fracture with a fracture line extending into the joint should be evaluated for possible surgical treatment. If a fracture shows 1 mm or less intra-articular displacement it can usually be treated by short arm thumb spica casting alone. Place the thumb in position to touch the tips of the long and index fingers (tripod pinch), not in the simian position! Any displacement greater than 1 mm will probably require surgical treatment. The distinction between a Bennett's fracture (single fracture line) and a Rolando's fracture (multiple fracture lines) is important for the primary care physician. A Rolando fracture can appear nondisplaced to the inexperienced observer when in fact the multiple fragments have shifted in such a way as to camouflage the displacement. The safest approach is that any basilar thumb fracture with multiple fracture lines should be considered excessively displaced and evaluated accordingly. Any fracture with a single fracture line showing more than 1 mm displacement should also be evaluated for possible surgical treatment. The minimally displaced Bennett's fracture can be treated using a short arm thumb spica splint or cast with the thumb placed into the position of tripod pinch. Fractures such as these in cancellous bone heal quickly so only 3 to 4 weeks of immobilization is necessary before beginning rehabilitation. Protect from a reinjury for an additional month.

References

1. Green DP, Rowland SA. Fractures and dislocations in the hand. In: Rockwood CA, Green DP, eds. Fractures, 3rd ed, vol 1. Philadelphia: JB Lippincott, 1991:446–453.

2. Stark HH, Boyes JH, Wilson JN. Mallet finger. J Bone Joint Surg 1962;44A:1061–1068.

3. Burton RI. Extensor tendons—late reconstruction. In: Green DP, ed. Operative hand surgery, 3rd ed, vol 2. New York: Churchill Livingstone, 1993:1955–1988.

4. Gibson CT, Manske PR. Isolated avulsion of a flexor digitorum superficialis tendon insertion. J Hand Surg 1992;12A:601–602.

5. Bollen SR. Soft tissue injury in extreme rock climbers. Br J Sports Med 1988;22:145–147.

6. Bollen SR. Hand injuries in competition climbers. Br J Sports Med 1990;24:16–18.

7. Tropez Y, Menez D, Balmat P, Pem R, Vichard PH. Closed traumatic rupture of the ring finger flexor tendon pulley. J Hand Surg 1990;15A:745–747.

8. Stener B. Displacement of the ruptured ulnar collateral ligament of the metacarpophalangeal joint of the thumb. A clinical and anatomical study. J Bone Joint Surg 1962; 44B:869–879.

PELVIS, HIP, AND THIGH INJURIES IN SPORTS

ERIC T. SHAPIRO

14

Epidemiology
Anatomy
History
Physical Examination
Specific Traumatic Injuries
Overuse Injuries

EPIDEMIOLOGY

The most common injuries to the hip and thigh regions in athletes are muscular. Treatment is usually conservative and recovery is often complete. Time lost from athletic participation, however, may be frustratingly long for both the athlete and physician. The importance of conditioning, flexibility, and warm-up cannot be overstressed in preventing these muscle injuries. The inherent stability of the ball-and-socket configuration of the hip joint, as well as its vast muscular envelope, make it resistant to athletic injuries. The hip is much less frequently injured in athletes than the knee or ankle.

The nerve supply to the hip joint is from three nerves: gluteal, femoral, and obturator. The obturator nerve is also the motor nerve to the adductor or medial thigh muscles and the sensory nerve to this area as well. For reasons that remain unclear, particularly in the child and adolescent, injury to the hip will lead to pain, referred in the distribution of the obturator nerve, and the youngster with hip problems often will present with complaints of medial knee pain. The sports medicine practitioner must keep this in mind and always examine the hip when medial thigh or knee pain is part of the young athlete's symptoms.

ANATOMY

The pelvis is subjected to many forces while absorbing the stresses of muscular activity. The pelvic girdle is composed of three joints: the hip joint, the sacroiliac joint, and the pubic symphysis (Figure 14.1).

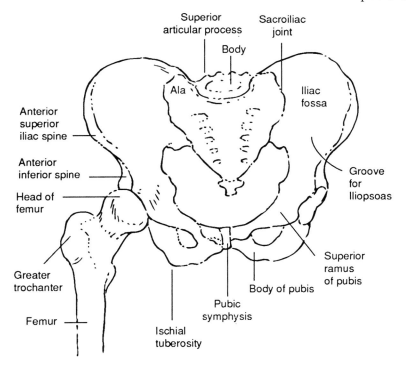

Figure 14.1. Pelvis and hip joints.

The pelvic ring, made up of the pelvis and sacrum, is the platform for support of the trunk and upper body. Muscles, attached to the bony pelvis, are a source of power for locomotion but also a source of injury. The muscles of the thigh are divided into four groups based on location: anterior, posterior, medial, and lateral. The anterior muscle group consists of the quadriceps femoris and the sartorius (Figure 14.2). The quadriceps femoris is a combination of four muscles: rectus femoris, vastus lateralis, vastus medialis, and vastus intermedius. The rectus femoris crosses the hip joint and arises from two tendons, one from the anterior inferior iliac spine and the other from the groove above the acetabulum. The others arise from the shaft of the femur. They all insert via the quadriceps tendon, patella, and patella tendon onto the tibial tubercle. The sartorius muscle arises from the anterior superior iliac spine and inserts with the gracilis and semitendinosus onto the tibia to make up the pes anserinus.

The hamstring muscles comprise the posterior group, which consists of three muscles that span both the hip and knee on the posterior aspect of the thigh. The three muscles are the semitendinosus, semimembranosus, and the biceps femoris (Figure 14.3). All three originate from the tuberosity of the ischium while a portion of the biceps also takes origin from the femur. The posterior portion of the adductor magnus is functionally considered a hamstring due to its shared origin with the other hamstrings and its vertical line of pull (1,2).

The medial muscles of the thigh are the gracilis, pectineus, adductor longus, adductor brevis, adductor magnus, and obturator externus (Figure 14.4).

The lateral group muscles are in the buttock. They consist of the gluteus maximus,

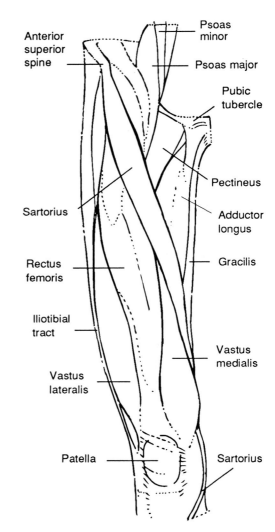

Figure 14.2. Muscles of the anterior thigh.

gluteus medius, gluteus minimus, tensor fascia lata, and short external rotators (Figure 14.5).

HISTORY

As in all other anatomic areas, overuse injuries usually present with an insidious

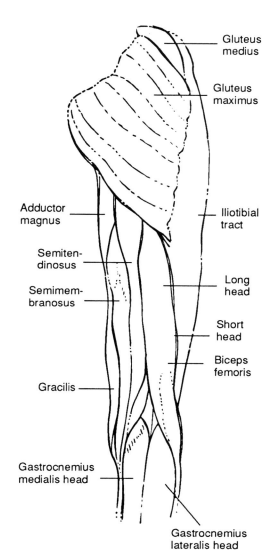

Figure 14.3. Muscles of the buttock and the posterior thigh.

onset, whereas traumatic injuries have a definite time of onset. Superficial injuries may be well localized by the athlete; injuries deep in the muscular envelope may be vague and difficult for the athlete to pinpoint. Due to the referral of pain from hip pathology along the sensory distribu-

tion of the obturator nerve, the practitioner must always think of hip pathology when the athlete reports medial thigh or knee pain.

Pain can also be referred to the groin or buttock region from pathology in the back, abdomen, or pelvic region. If one cannot identify a local cause of the athlete's symptoms, look for a source of referred pain.

Muscle Strain Injuries

Stretch-induced muscle injuries or strains are cited as the most frequent injury in sports (3). Muscle strain injuries are painful and keep athletes from participating in their sport. If not diagnosed, treated, and rehabilitated properly, return to their sport can be delayed and injuries can recur.

A *strain* is a tearing or stretching of a musculotendinous unit. Strains are classified as first, second, and third degree. A *first-degree strain* consists of minimal stretching of the musculotendinous unit without permanent injury. A *second-degree strain* indicates a partial tear of the musculotendinous unit. When complete disruption of a portion of the musculotendinous unit occurs, it is classified as a *third-degree strain.*

Muscle strain injuries occur most often in sprinters or speed athletes. They are most common in sports in positions requiring bursts of speed or rapid acceleration. Sports that require these actions include track, football, soccer, field hockey, and basketball (4). Most of these injuries are indirect strain injuries. A distinction must be made between these indirect injuries, direct-contact muscle injuries, and exercise-induced muscle soreness. Indirect or strain injuries are failures of the muscle or tendon in response to excessive tension or stretch in the musculotendinous unit. Strain injury typically occurs near the musculotendinous

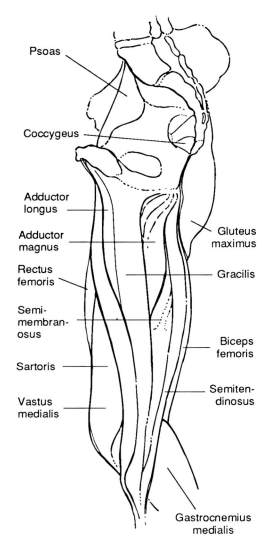

Figure 14.4. Muscles of the medial thigh.

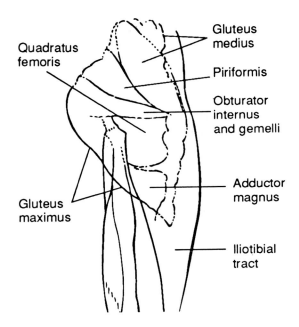

Figure 14.5. Lateral group of muscles (buttock).

tractions, the muscle can be considered to be controlling or regulating motion. Much of the muscle action involved in running and sprinting is eccentric (6). The hamstrings act not so much to flex the knee as to decelerate knee extension during running. Likewise, quadriceps serve to prevent knee flexion as much as to power knee extension in running (7). These muscles are acting to control joint motion or to decelerate the joint and are therefore acting eccentrically (8).

Direct-contact muscle injuries occur with a direct blow to the involved muscle area. This injury is associated with pain and swelling and decreased motion of the area involved. Muscle strain injuries can be distinguished clinically from exercise-induced muscle soreness. A strain injury is an acute and usually painful event that is recognized by the athlete as an injury. *Muscle soreness* is

junction and is characterized primarily by inflammation and edema, and to a lesser extent by hemorrhage (5). Often indirect injury occurs during eccentric action of the muscle, meaning that the muscle is activated while lengthening and is attempting to resist being stretched. With eccentric cona condition characterized by muscle pain often 12 to 24 hours after exercise and usually without a simple identifiable injury (9–11). The conditions are alike in that they are more prone to occur with eccentric exercise, and passive stretching and active contraction will cause discomfort.

Tendon and muscle injuries around the pelvis, hip, and thigh account for a significant loss of time from sport and are a common source of pain and impaired performance following return to competition. It is important to understand and know which muscles are prone to strain injury. Muscles at risk for injury usually include the two-joint muscles. These are muscles that cross two or more joints and are subjected to stretch at more than one joint (8,12). A frequent characteristic of the injured muscles is their ability to limit range of motion of a joint because of the intrinsic tightness in the muscle. For example, the hamstring muscles can limit knee extension when the hip is flexed.

PHYSICAL EXAMINATION

Inspection

Observe the athlete walking or running to note any gait abnormalities. These abnormalities may give a clue to any underlying muscle or joint pathology. Examine the athlete for any sign of abrasion, laceration, bruising, or swelling in the pelvic, hip, and thigh regions.

Palpation

With the athlete supine or standing, the examiner palpates the bony prominences of the pelvis, hip, and thigh. Local tenderness will help define the athlete's injury. The examiner should palpate the anterior superior

iliac spines, the iliac crests, the pubic symphysis, the ischial tuberosities, and the greater trochanters (Figure 14.6). All are easy to palpate except the ischial tuberosity. To palpate the ischial tuberosity, the hip is flexed, which moves the gluteus maximus upward and the tuberosity is then easily palpable (Figure 14.7A).

Tenderness to palpation over the greater trochanter may indicate trochanteric bursitis (Figure 14.7B). The area of the bursa may feel boggy to palpation. Although rare, ten-

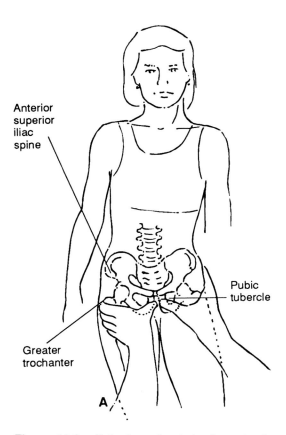

Figure 14.6. Palpation of anterior bony landmarks. *A.* Anterior superior iliac spines and iliac crests. *B.* Pubic symphysis.

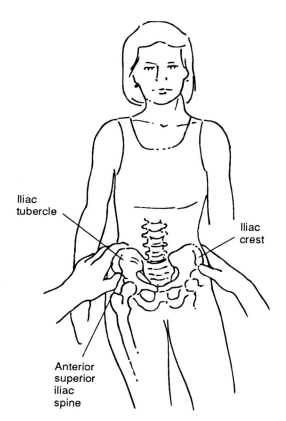

Figure 14.6. *Continued*

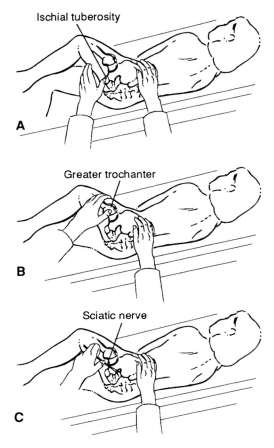

Figure 14.7. Palpation of posterior bony landmarks (*A* and *B*) and sciatic nerve (*C*).

derness over the ischial tuberosity may be due to ischial tuberosity bursitis. Next palpate between the greater trochanter and the ischial tuberosity in the area of the sciatic nerve (Figure 14.7C). Pain in this area can be discogenic in origin. Tenderness to palpation over the anterior superior iliac spine and anterior inferior iliac spine may be due to an injury to the sartorius or rectus femoris origins, respectively. Tenderness over the crest in a young athlete can be caused by iliac apophysitis.

The hamstring muscles can be palpated from their origin to insertion. Both limbs should be examined for comparison. Tenderness at their origin can be due to ischial bursitis. Tenderness along their length can be from trauma or muscle strain. The hamstrings are examined with the athlete prone or in the lateral position. Direct pressure as well as motion at the hip and the knee can elicit sore areas.

The rectus femoris muscle is the only two-joint muscle of the quadriceps, making it more

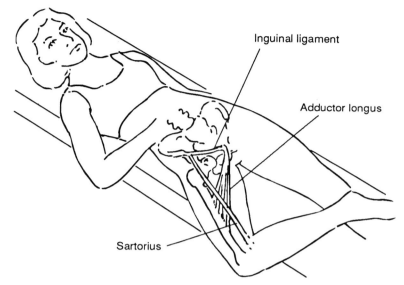

Figure 14.8. Palpation of adductor longus muscle.

Inguinal ligament

Adductor longus

Sartorius

susceptible to injury. Neither head is easily palpated because the muscle lies in a depression proximally between the tensor fascia lata and the sartorius. With avulsion at its attachment site, however, tenderness can be elicited.

The adductor longus is superficial within the adductor group and is accessible to palpation. For examination, the leg is abducted away from the midline with the hip and knee flexed (Figure 14.8).

The iliopsoas muscle is the primary hip flexor. It is not palpable due to its deep position. When injured or when a psoas bursitis occurs, pain will be evident with active hip flexion, especially to resistance.

Range of Motion

The athlete's hip should be examined for range of motion. When standing, the athlete should be able to actively abduct the hip at least 45° and adduct the leg at least 20°; flexion should be at least 135°. With the ath-

lete supine, passive range of motion is performed in flexion, abduction, adduction, internal rotation, and external rotation (Figure 14.9). To check for hip extension, the athlete is laid prone with knees slightly bent and the leg passively extended. The normal value for hip extension is 30° (Figure 14.10).

To properly examine an injured athlete, the examiner must have a grasp of the anatomy and function of each muscle group. With this knowledge, a treatment plan can be instituted.

SPECIFIC TRAUMATIC INJURIES

Hamstring Strains

Statistics show that the hamstrings are the most commonly strained muscle of the thigh (13). The hamstring muscle group is intricately involved in both stability and locomotion of the lower extremity. *It is often neglected in the weight room, as compared to its*

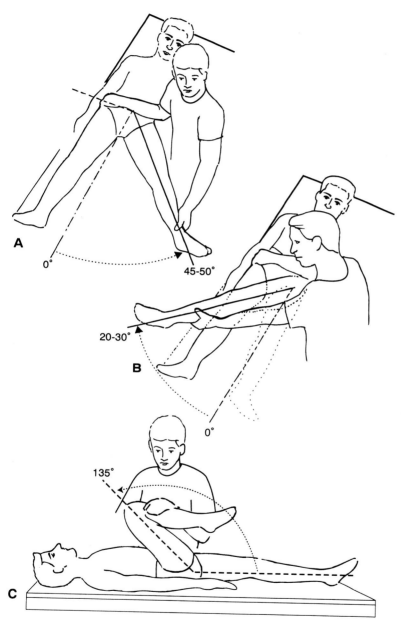

Figure 14.9. Normal limits
of hip motion. *A.* Abduction
45° to 50°. *B.* Adduction
20° to 30°. *C.* Flexion
135°. (Modified from S
Hoppenfeld. Physical Examination of the Spine
Extremities. Norwalk, CT:
Appleton & Lange, 1976:
156–157.)

*antagonist muscle group, the quadriceps, and
frequently insulted with improper stretching
exercises.* The end result of this neglect and
abuse is often a strain of one or more of the
hamstring muscles. The sensation of a sud-

den tearing or popping that one experiences with a hamstring strain carries with
it the uncertainty of a quick return to the
sport and a future of possible recurrence of
injury. Most hamstring strains occur early

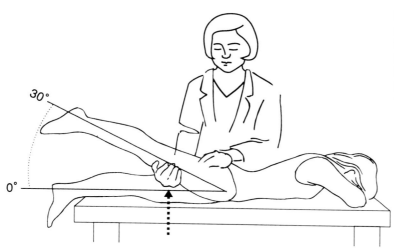

Figure 14.10. Normal limit of hip extension 30°. (Modified from S Hoppenfeld. Physical Examination of the Spine Extremities. Norwalk, CT: Appleton & Lange, 1976: 156.)

in training and are linked to poor conditioning and preparation for their intended sport.

Clinical Case #1

A 40-year-old office worker who plays racquetball once a week comes to your office the morning after an injury. He had been a little late for his weekly game the night before. He began playing hard without warm-up. Ten minutes into the match he felt a "pull" in the back of his thigh; he continued to play, with only a little soreness. This morning he is limping and has significant stiffness and pain in the back of his thigh. On examination, he is locally tender in the midportion of his medial hamstrings and has pain with passive straight leg-raising.

Proximal musculotendinous injuries most often occur in the biceps femoris muscle. Distal injuries occur most often in a semimembranosus (14). Hamstring strains occur in speed athletes when they are starting with a sudden, violent hamstring contraction as in a sprinter accelerating out of the starting blocks, a jumper on his take-off

leg, or a baseball player running to first (Figure 14.11*A*).

Risk factors in hamstring injuries include a previously incompletely healed injury, which can predispose to a subsequent injury. Fatigue is thought to increase the risk for hamstring injury. Hamstring strains are associated with inadequate warm-up, poor flexibility, fatigue, deficiency in reciprocal actions of opposing muscle groups, and imbalance between quadriceps and hamstring strength (15).

Immediate *treatment* follows the RICE principle: rest, ice, compression, and elevation. Crutches should be used by athletes with a limp. Athletes must be prohibited from returning to play until completion of a rehabilitation program that includes a progressive running program. Running is resumed gradually, with a player first jogging, then increasing speed, and if free from pain, progressing to sprinting. Further treatment modalities include physical therapy for range of motion and functional strengthening exercises, bandaging, and medications. Nonsteroidal anti-inflammatory drugs (NSAIDs) help reduce inflammation and edema. Neoprene sleeves can

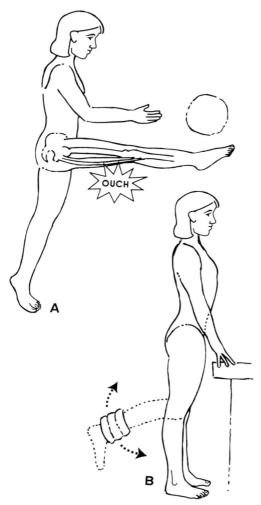

Figure 14.11. *A.* Hamstring strain. *B.* Hamstring strengthening should concentrate on eccentric contraction (lowering the weight).

be worn when returning to competition. These sleeves provide support, which adds to the player's confidence, and they keep the muscles warm during activity. Long term, the athlete should concentrate on flexibility and strengthening the hamstrings. Use of eccentric-strengthening (muscle lengthening while contracting, such as lowering a weight) exercises may

reduce the risk of recurrent strains (Figure 14.11*B*).

In children and adolescents, indirect injuries involving the musculotendinous unit can disrupt the origin or insertion of the tendon at its attachment to bone. This injury can be a tendinous avulsion or more commonly an avulsion fracture of the attached bone. Examples of avulsion fractures include the anterior superior iliac spine by the pull of the sartorius muscle (Figure 14.12), the anterior inferior iliac spine by the rectus femoris muscle, and the ischial tuberosity by the common action of

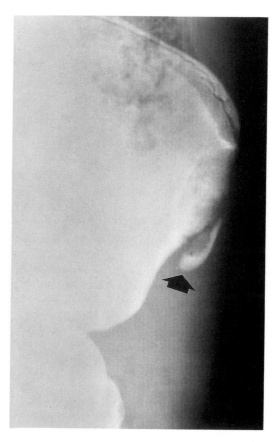

Figure 14.12. Avulsion of the anterior superior iliac spine (*arrow*).

the hamstring muscles. Tendon injuries are common, but avulsion fractures are rare. Surgical repair of tendon or bone is rarely indicated. Athletes with rectus femoris avulsions typically present with sudden, severe anterior hip pain while running. The pain occurs at push-off with an extended hip and moderately flexed knee. On physical examination, pain is localized to the anterior inferior iliac spine and is exacerbated by active *extension* of the knee against resistance. Avulsions are treated like strains.

Quadriceps Strains

The rectus femoris muscle is the most prone to strain of the quadriceps muscles because it is the only one that crosses two joints. This strain is particularly common with running, jumping, and kicking activities. It may partially or completely disrupt from its musculotendinous junction and retract, creating a bulge in the anterior thigh, which enlarges with quadriceps activation. The bulge may be confused with a muscle hernia. The athlete will develop a change in contour of the thigh, but rarely will develop any permanent functional deficit. Their strength and function in the extremity are compensated for by the other muscles of the quadriceps femoris group.

Acute treatment follows the RICE principle. Conservative treatment works well and the athlete is helped with rehabilitation. This includes range of motion and progressive resistive exercises following the initial stages of healing in an effort to restore the size and strength of the quadriceps femoris mechanism. As in the hamstring strain, eccentric strengthening is stressed (Figure 14.13).

Groin (Adductor Longus) Strains

An athlete can strain the adductor longus with running and cutting activities often

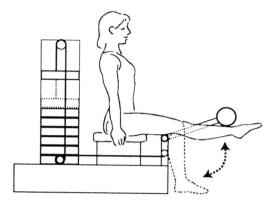

Figure 14.13. Eccentric srengthening of the quadriceps muscle; athlete concentrates on lowering the weight.

seen in soccer, baseball, football, and hockey players (Figure 14.14). Hockey players forcefully abduct their thigh in push-off and rapidly shift their weight to the opposite leg to initiate the glide stroke (16). This motion can cause groin strain. Athletes who

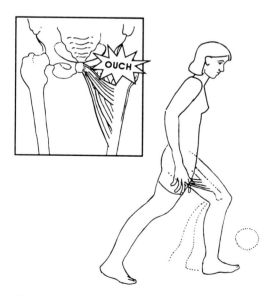

Figure 14.14. Adductor longus (groin) strain.

slip on muddy fields are also prone to groin strains.

These strains usually involve the adductor longus muscle and occur as incomplete tears from the proximal tendon and infrequently as complete tears from their distal insertion. The complete tears may produce a prominent mass near the origin of the adductor longus that may be mistaken for a soft-tissue tumor. The strain is usually first or second degree and in most cases occurs at the attachment to the pelvis. These injuries can be severely disabling on a temporary basis but rarely produce chronic disability.

An adductor strain is especially painful when the athlete adducts the thigh against resistance. The best treatment of adductor strains is prevention. Proper warm-up and stretching are important. Gentle stretching is performed with abduction of the thighs with the knees bent and the soles of the feet together (Figure 14.15). Stretching may be done with a partner. There is no need for reattachment of the injured tendon. Conservative methods are the treatment of choice because of the lack of disability. RICE, NSAIDs, stretching and time work well.

Quadriceps Contusions

Contusion of the thigh is a common injury in contact sports. There is a tendency to undertreat it or not treat it at all. At the community and high school level, the athletes may be told to run it off. This inadequate treatment can result in prolonged recovery and permanent disability from loss of muscle strength, flexibility, or myositis ossificans.

Quadriceps contusion (charley horse) is defined as an external blow to the thigh causing bleeding and soft-tissue damage to the thigh (Figure 14.16). The development of increasing pain, swelling, and impairment of the quadriceps function and knee

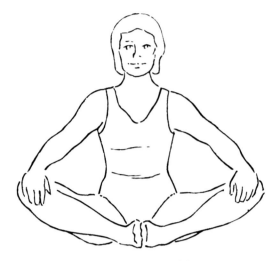

Figure 14.15. Adductor stretching.

stiffness constitute a quadriceps contusion. The muscles of the anterior thigh are vulnerable to external blows because they lie in contact with bone throughout the length of the thigh. Blunt trauma causes transmission of force through the fluid compartment of all muscles, but damage usually occurs only in the layer next to the bone (17).

As in all athletic injuries, prevention of a thigh contusion is the preferred method of management. The athlete who participates in a collision sport, such as football, is somewhat protected by a thigh pad. Unfortunately, in sports such as basketball and soccer, the thigh has no protection. In football, the injury usually results from a direct blow by the opponent's helmet. In soccer and basketball, the opponent's knee is usually driven into the athlete's unprotected thigh. Trauma to the thigh usually occurs anterior and anterolateral because the medial part of the thigh is protected by the athlete's other leg. If the thigh is struck in the center of the thigh pad, the injury is usually prevented. However, if the blow occurs at the periphery of the pad, the pad

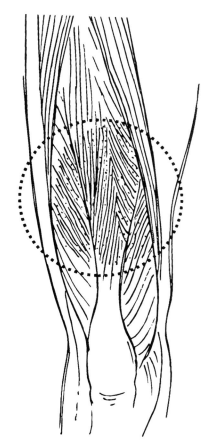

Figure 14.16. Quadriceps contusion or charley horse.

edge can be driven into the thigh creating a contusion.

Clinical Case #2

The high school trainer calls you about one of the soccer players. She took a knee to the thigh in this afternoon's game. She sat out the rest of the game with an ice pack, and now the trainer wants to know what to do. She is already developing stiffness and cannot bend her knee to 90°.

Classification of quadriceps contusions follows the West Point study in which knee range of motion was assessed at 12 to 24 hours after injury. Mild contusions had active knee motion greater than 90°, moderate contusions 45° to 90°, and severe contusions less than 45° (18,19). Ryan and colleagues (18) proposed a three-phase treatment plan for quadriceps contusion. The purpose of phase I treatment is to limit hemorrhage. RICE principles are used, usually for 24 hours in mild contusions and up to 48 hours in moderate to severe contusions. Initially the hip and knee are immobilized in flexion, which increases tension-limiting hematoma formation (Figure 14.17). Crutches are used for walking, and isometric quadriceps exercises are performed. Phase II begins when the thigh is comfortable and pain free at rest and has a stabilized thigh girth. At this point, mobilization is initiated. Motion is increased using a stationary bicycle. The athlete is advanced to phase III, functional rehabilitation, which increases strength and endurance. The athlete should wear a thick pad over the thigh for 3 to 6 months when returning to contact sports.

The differential diagnosis of quadriceps contusion must eliminate muscle rupture and arterial bleeding (20). Although rare in the thigh, acute compartment syndrome can occur. The early signs are progressive pain, tense thigh, and pain with passive motion. Delayed signs of a thigh compartment syndrome are decreased sensation in the distribution of the femoral nerve and marked quadriceps weakness (21).

Ruptures of the rectus femoris usually occur by direct trauma combined with a stretch to a contracted muscle. Due to pain and hematoma, muscle bulge and weakness are difficult to evaluate. These injuries are best treated conservatively.

Myositis Ossificans

Despite careful treatment, our high school soccer player (Clinical Case #2) con-

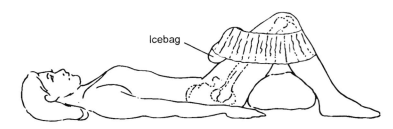

Figure 14.17. Icing of a quadriceps contusion in flexion will limit hemorrhage and speed recovery.

tinued to have significant pain and disability 4 weeks after her injury. The area of injury was much less swollen, but it still felt warm and firm.

Quadriceps contusion can result in myositis ossificans, a condition of benign heterotopic bone formation (Figure 14.18). When athlete sustains a quadriceps contusion or quadriceps strain, hemorrhage into the muscle substance occurs. The athlete complains of pain, swelling, increased warmth to the thigh, and decreased motion. As mentioned, the most common cause of a contusion is a blow to the thigh by an opponent's helmet or knee. Treatment for the contusion or strain was outlined in the section on quadriceps contusion. This protocol should be followed to reduce the incidence of myositis ossificans.

Ryan's West Point study (18) cited five risk factors associated with development of myositis ossificans: previous quadriceps injury, injury occurring during football, knee motion less than 120°, delay in treatment greater than 3 days, and ipsilateral knee effusion. The incidence of myositis ossificans in their study was 9% overall as compared to 20% reported by Jackson and Feagin (19). There was a 17% incidence of moderate and severe contusions in Ryan's study and a 72% incidence in Jackson and Feagin's.

Myositis ossificans must be differentiated from osteosarcoma. History of trauma

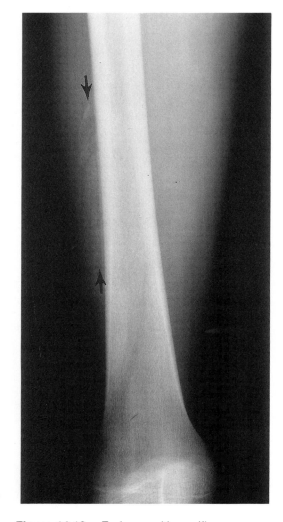

Figure 14.18. Early myositis ossificans.

helps distinguish the two entities, but 40% of osteosarcoma patients note a history of trauma to the affected limb (22). Myositis ossificans is usually located about the shaft of the femur, whereas osteosarcoma is typically located about the end (metaphysis). Myositis ossificans differs from osteosarcoma in that it causes no bony destruction, and once matured the myositis ossificans lesion decreases in pain and size. The alkaline phosphatase level in the myositis ossificans patient is at most mildly elevated.

Surgical intervention for myositis ossificans is rarely necessary. The West Point group did not use aspiration, injectable or oral medications, femoral nerve blocks, or radiation therapy in their initial treatment of quadriceps contusions. They felt the risks and side effects to be higher with these treatments as compared to the course of quadriceps contusion and myositis ossificans. Surgery is only indicated in rare instances. With appropriate nonoperative management, conservative treatment yields excellent results without significant impairment. Surgery is performed only when mature myositis ossificans causes pain, decreases knee motion, or is frequently reinjured due to its location. This surgery should not be considered until full maturation of the myositis ossificans, usually at 6 to 12 months (23). Myositis ossificans is usually apparent on x-ray at 4 weeks. By 4 to 6 months, the mass has stopped expanding, and full maturation with laminar bone occurs at the 6- to 12-month period (Figure 14.19). Aggressive early attempts at knee motion, early return to competitive physical activity, and deep massage to the thigh should be avoided because these may delay recovery.

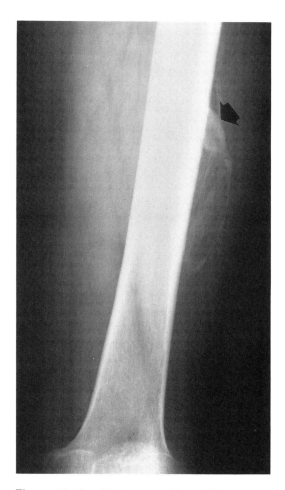

Figure 14.19. Mature myositis ossificans.

Greater Trochanteric Bursitis

Greater trochanteric bursitis is an inflammation of the bursa overlying the greater trochanter. There are two main causes for this entity. Blunt trauma to the greater trochanter can cause injury to the soft tissues overlying the greater trochanter with resulting inflammation of the bursa. Another cause is the rubbing of the tensor fascia lata and the iliotibial band over the greater trochanter.

This condition is seen in runners and is more common in female athletes. Predisposing factors are a high Q angle (see page 397) and a broad pelvis. Training and competing on banked surfaces increases the incidence of greater trochanteric bursitis.

Treatment is rest, ice, NSAIDs, and soft-tissue physical therapy modalities. If refractory to these treatments, a steroid injection can help reduce the inflammation. Differential diagnosis for trochanteric bursitis is lumbar radiculopathy and lumbar facet syndrome. These should be considered if symptoms do not improve.

Iliopsoas Bursitis

Although iliopsoas bursitis is usually seen in patients with underlying degenerative or inflammatory arthropathies of the hip joint, it may occur as a result of trauma or overuse activities in athletes. Its clinical features include groin pain, local tenderness beneath the inguinal ligament, or a palpable mass. Symptoms may be exacerbated during hip extension, which will shorten an athlete's stride (24). Treatment is conservative initially using NSAIDs and rest. A corticosteroid injection can be helpful in refractory cases.

Hip Pointer

A hip pointer is a contusion of the athlete's iliac crest (Figure 14.20). It occurs from a blow to this region. The hip pointer can occur in any contact sport. A direct helmet blow to the iliac crest in football or a slash of a stick to the crest in hockey are common causes.

Initially the pain is minor, but once bleeding occurs, the area is very painful. The athlete may have trouble getting out of bed

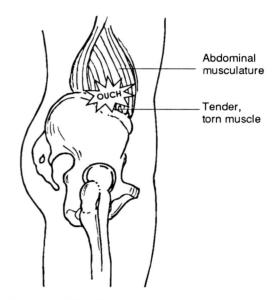

Figure 14.20. Hip pointer.

because since the abdominal musculature attaches to the crest, and sitting up is painful. Initial treatment is ice, rest, and NSAIDs. On return to sporting activities, the athlete requires additional protection over the iliac crest (25).

OVERUSE INJURIES

Iliac Apophysitis

Overuse injuries in young athletes are on the rise due to increased distance training in these athletes. Distance runners and hurdlers tend to be prone to iliac apophysitis. It is caused by the repetitive contractions of the muscular attachments to the iliac apophysis. These continued contractions can lead to iliac apophysitis or a stress fracture of the iliac apophysis (26). This condition occurs more in the anterior half of the crest in the 14- to 16-year-old distance runner. Symptoms include pain over the crest with running, which is gradual in onset. The athlete may be tender to palpation at the origins of the tensor fascia lata, gluteus medius, and the abdominal obliques. Pain is exacerbated when the hip is abducted against resistance. Treatment is ice, rest, and NSAIDs. Stretching should be resumed when pain decreases; decreased mileage is recommended on return to running.

Osteitis Pubis

Osteitis pubis occurs often with high-mileage running programs and in soccer players. Forces centered at the pubic symphysis include tension from the rectus abdominis and adductor musculature. There appears to be a fatigue failure of the ligaments and tendons at their insertion onto the symphysis. The athlete usually presents with an insidious onset of groin pain and occasionally pain at the sym-

physis pubis. Palpation of the symphysis pubis causes pain. X-rays should be obtained and checked for bone resorption (Figure 14.21) or stress fracture. Films may be negative, and if symptoms warrant further study, a bone scan is indicated. Treatment involves rest from training, NSAIDs, and stretching. Gradual return to running will help decrease the recurrence rate.

Stress Fractures

Stress fractures are occurring with increasing frequency in athletes. Nearly 10% of all sports-related injuries seen in sports medicine clinics are stress fractures (27). A stress fracture is most often a partial biologic breakdown of bone. Rarely will a stress fracture go on to a true fracture. Femoral neck stress fractures are, however, one of several locations where this may occur. These are overuse injuries that occur

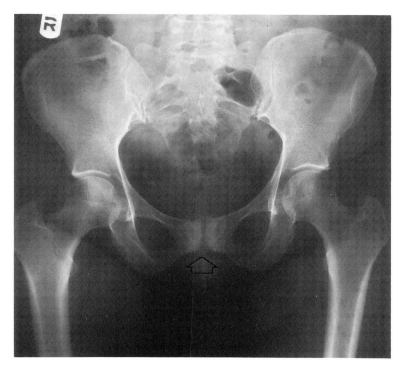

Figure 14.21. Osteitis pubis; note resorption and sclerosis at the symphysis.

from repetitive trauma to bone associated with running, jogging, or jumping. Stress fractures occur in the lower extremity 95% of the time (28). Although the tibia and metatarsals are the most commonly involved bones, the pelvis and femur are also involved. Stress fractures of the femur are most common in the femoral neck and in the proximal medial part of the femoral shaft (28,29). Running is the cause of most of these stress fractures (30). The cause is multifactorial and can be related to poor conditioning, changes in shoe wear or running terrain, gait abnormalities, or the athlete's training routine and mileage per week (28,31). Stress fractures occur 12 times more often in female athletes than their male counterparts in similar training conditions (30). The reason for the higher incidence in women is unknown, but possible explanations include gait differences, bone size, and running biomechanics, training errors, as well as a high incidence of amenorrhea in the female athlete. Clinical implications of amenorrhea center on loss of bone mass when estrogen levels are low for a prolonged time (32). Peak incidence for stress fractures occur between the ages of 18 and 25 years old (33).

Femoral Neck Fractures

Clinical Case #3

An aerobics instructor from the local health club comes to the office. She teaches up to five high impact aerobics classes per week and recently has developed pain in her groin, which is vague and poorly localized. Examination shows her to be slightly tender over the anterior hip and medial thigh. She has minimal discomfort on the extremes of hip motion. Should you be concerned?

Femoral neck fractures are seen most commonly in distance runners. Athletes complain initially of groin or thigh pain and aching hip pain during or after running. With continued running, pain occurs with ambulation and daily activities.

On physical examination, the athlete will have pain with extremes of hip motion and pain to palpation in the inguinal area. Often diagnosis of femoral neck stress fractures is delayed due to a presumed diagnosis of groin or thigh muscle strain. There must be a high index of suspicion in runners. Initially x-rays will be negative for a stress fracture and it can take weeks to months to show the new bone formation associated with a stress fracture (Figure 14.22). A technetium bone scan, with coned down views of the hips, should be performed if the diagnosis of femoral neck stress fracture cannot be made with plain x-rays. The scan will show increased uptake in the femoral neck region.

Devas described two types of femoral neck stress fractures (34). The more com-

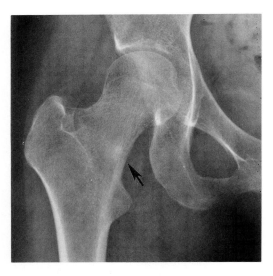

Figure 14.22. Stress fracture of femoral neck (*arrow*).

mon type, which occurs in the young runner, is the compression type. It occurs in the inferior medial portion of the femoral neck. The second type occurs on the lateral border of the femoral neck and is called a tension fracture. The tension type usually occurs in an older population. The compression type is a stable fracture, whereas the tension type is less stable and can displace (Figure 14.23).

Conservative treatment has been successful in most cases of compression type, but if a femoral neck stress fracture displaces, open reduction and internal fixation are necessary. Athletes with femoral neck fractures must be monitored closely to ensure proper healing. The principle of treatment is to reduce the athlete's activity *below the level of pain*. Initially the athlete is placed on crutches and touch-down weight bearing. Then partial weight bearing with periodic x-rays to check healing and anatomic alignment follows. The athlete will then progress to full weight bearing when pain resolves. Prior to return to a running sport, the athlete begins bicycle riding and running in water. Femoral neck stress fractures that are located on the superior neck (tension) are at significant risk to displace and may require bed rest or surgery to prevent this. Early consultation with an orthopedic surgeon should be obtained. For the more common compression type, if symptoms have not resolved after 6 weeks of appropriate treatment, then consultation with an orthopedic surgeon is appropriate.

Subtrochanteric Stress Fracture

Subtrochanteric stress fractures present with vague pain in the upper thigh and hip. Deep palpation over the bone distal to the greater trochanter may cause pain. The athlete's pain is progressive until running becomes intolerable. Diagnosis is similar to

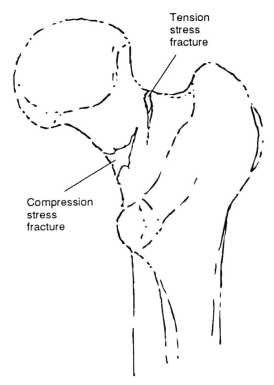

Figure 14.23. Stress fractures of the femoral neck can occur on the compression or tension side of the femoral neck.

femoral neck stress fractures, but often relies on a bone scan, because plane films are rarely diagnostic (Figure 14.24). Treatment consists of partial weight bearing on crutches until resolution of the pain. The athlete can progress to bicycling and walking at this point with gradual return to running.

Femoral Shaft Stress Fractures

Typical presentation of a femoral shaft stress fracture would be a 16-year-old female, cross-country runner who complains of insidious onset of thigh pain with no history of injury to the thigh. The symptoms

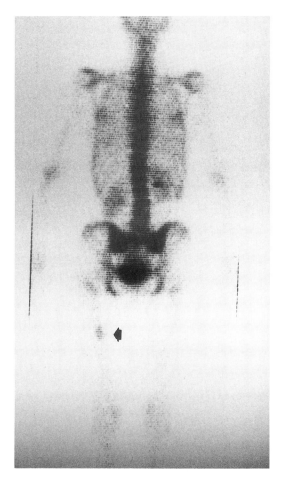

Figure 14.24. Technetium bone scan demonstrates subtrochanteric stress fracture (*arrow*).

are a diffuse thigh aching. The athlete believes she strained a quadriceps muscle and continues competing. The pain worsens and occurs with normal ambulation. On physical examination, pain to bony palpation occurs in the midthigh. X-rays should be taken. If early in course, x-rays may be negative. If symptomatic for 4 to 6 weeks, a stress fracture may be evident on x-ray. If x-rays are negative, a bone scan should be obtained. Treatment is conservative, consisting of relative rest, including bicycling and swimming during the early treatment time. Impact-loading sports are avoided for at least 2 months (29).

Pubic Rami Fractures

Although rare, stress fractures of the inferior pubic rami do occur in female runners and occasionally in soccer players. There is usually a long history of pain in the pelvic region. On physical examination, there is pain to palpation at the junction of the inferior pubic ramus and the pubic symphysis. Treatment consists of rest until pain free. Activity such as bicycling or swimming is allowed if it does not cause pelvic discomfort.

Other Conditions

Piriformis syndrome is an uncommon cause of hip pain or sciatic-type pain in running athletes. The athlete will usually have insidious onset of buttock pain with radiation down the back of the thigh. Rarely will the athlete complain of true sciatica. Palpation of the sciatic nerve between the greater trochanter and ischial tuberosity will be painful and often reproduces the symptoms (see Figure 14.7C).

Piriformis syndrome results from either a direct irritation and inflammation of the sciatic nerve by a contracted piriformis, or by an anatomic variant. The normal course of the sciatic nerve is just below the piriformis. In 5% or less of the population, the nerve passes through or over the piriformis, making irritation of the nerve much more likely (Figure 14.25). Treatment consists of NSAIDs, backing off on exercise frequency or intensity, and piriformis stretching (Figure 14.26). Recalcitrant cases may benefit from local steroid injection. Rarely is surgery required.

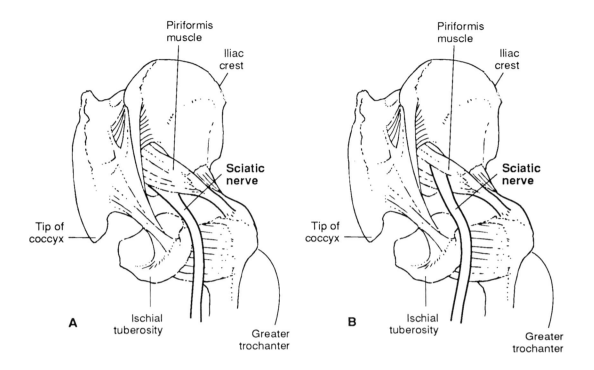

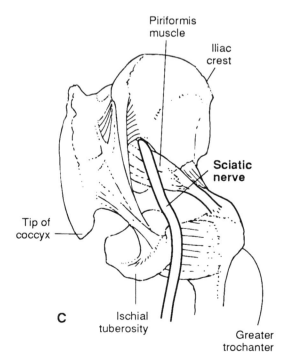

Figure 14.25. Relationship of sciatic nerve to piriformis muscle. *A.* Normal—nerve below muscle. *B.* Abnormal—nerve through muscle. *C.* Abnormal—nerve above muscle.

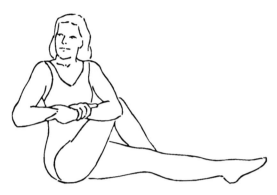

Figure 14.26. Piriformis stretching.

Clinical Case #4

A 10-year-old boy is active in karate. He has recently been complaining of knee pain, and his mother has occasionally noted him limping. No specific injury can be recalled. His knee examination is unremarkable except for a little pain when you forcibly internally rotate his leg. Careful examination of his hip demonstrates a little loss of rotation. Should you obtain x-rays? If so, should these be hip films, knee films, or both? Yes, you obtain radiographs of the hip because that is the location of your physical findings.

Adolescent athletes may present with knee, thigh, hip, or groin pain with an associated limp. Several conditions not usually associated with athletics must be considered while treating these young athletes.

Slipped capital femoral epiphysis is a common disorder found in adolescents characterized by posterior inferior displacement of the femoral capital epiphysis on the femoral neck. The adolescent usually presents with knee, thigh, or groin pain. A limp is usual but not universal. The condition can be acute, chronic, or acute on chronic. Acute slips behave like fresh fractures with extreme pain with movement and the inability to bear weight. Chronic slipped capital femoral epiphysis is more common with a gradual onset and progression of signs and symptoms lasting more than 3 weeks in duration. Acute on chronic is an acute progression of a chronic slip. On physical examination, there is limited internal rotation. The hip rides into external rotation as it is flexed. Usually a limp is present. Bilateral anterior posterior and lateral x-rays are necessary to confirm the diagnosis (Figure 14.27). Up to 25% of cases are bilateral. The athlete should be referred to the orthopedic surgeon. Recommended treatment for this condition is surgical fixation.

In the younger athlete, Legg-Calvé-Perthes disease must be considered. This disorder is most common in boys. Age of onset is 3 to 12 years old with average age of 6. Only 10% to 15% of cases are bilateral. This disease is an idiopathic disorder of the proximal epiphysis of the femur characterized by osteonecrosis of the proximal femoral epiphysis. Symptoms include hip or *knee pain*. Physical examination shows restriction of motion of the affected hip especially extension, abduction, and internal rotation. A positive Trendelenburg gait and generalized muscle atrophy of the affected side are typical. Consultation with an orthopedic surgeon is appropriate. Treatment is conservative with an attempt to contain the femoral head in the acetabulum. X-rays are essential to identify and classify the stage of this disorder (Figure 14.28).

In any age athlete, the primary care physician must consider other courses when conservative measures fail. An x-ray should be obtained to rule out bony neoplasm or any type of fracture.

References

1. Caperson PC. Groin and hamstring injuries. Athl Training 1982;17:43–45.

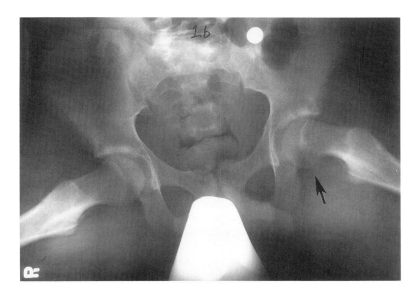

Figure 14.27. Frog lateral radiograph of both hips shows slipped capital femoral epiphysis on left (*arrow*).

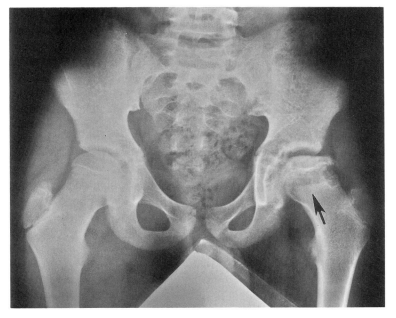

Figure 14.28. Anteroposterior radiograph demonstrates Legg-Calvé-Perthes disease of left hip (*arrow*).

2. Hollinshead WH, Jenkins DB. Functional anatomy of the limbs and back, 5th ed. Philadelphia: WB Saunders, 1971:270.

3. Glick JM. Muscle strains, prevention and treatment. Physician Sports Med 1990;8:73–77.

4. Peterson L, Renstrom P. In: Granna WA, ed. Sports injuries: their prevention and treatment. Chicago: Yearbook Medical Publishers, 1986:465.

5. Garrett WE Jr. Injuries to the muscle-tendon unit. Instr Course Lect 1988;37:275–282.

6. Bosco C, Montanari G, Tarkka I, et al. The

effect of prestretch on mechanical efficiency of human skeletal muscle. Acta Physiol Scand 1987;131:323–329.

7. Mann RA, Hagy J. Biomechanics of walking, running, and sprinting. Am J Sports Med 1980;8:345–350.

8. Garrett WE Jr. Muscle strain injuries: clinical and basic aspects. Med Sci Sports Exercise 1990;22:436–443.

9. Armstrong RB. Mechanisms of exercise-induced delayed onset muscular soreness: a brief review. Med Sci Sports Exercise 1984; 16:529–538.

10. Asmussen E. Observations on experimental muscular soreness. Acta Pneumatol Scand 1956;2:109–116.

11. Schwane JA, Johnson SR, Vandenakker CB, Armstrong RB. Delayed-onset muscular soreness and plasma CPK and LDK activities after downhill running. Med Sci Sports Exercise 1983;15:51–56.

12. Brewer BJ. Mechanism of injury to the musculotendinous unit. Instr Course Lect 1960; 17:354–358.

13. Klafs CE, Arnheim DD. Modern principles of athletic training, 4th ed. St. Louis: CV Mosby, 1977:370–372.

14. Speer KP, Lohnes J, Garrett WE Jr. Radiographic imaging of muscle strain injury. Am J Sports Med 1993;21:89–96.

15. Kulund DN. Hamstring strain. The injured athlete, 2nd ed. Philadelphia: JB Lippincott, 1988:431–432.

16. Merrifield HH, Cowan RF. Ice hockey groin pulls. Am J Sports Med 1979;1:41–42.

17. Walton M, Rothwell AS. Reactions of thigh tissues of sheep to blunt trauma. Clin Orthop 1983;176:273–281.

18. Ryan JB, Wheeler JH, Hopkinson WS, Arciero RA, Kolakowski KR. Quadriceps contusions. West Point update. Am J Sports Med 1991;19:299–304.

19. Jackson DW, Feagin JA. Quadriceps contusions in young athletes. J Bone Joint Surg 1973;55A:95–105.

20. Rooser B. Quadriceps contusion with compartment syndrome: evacuation of hematoma in two cases. Acta Orthop Scand 1987; 58:170–171.

21. Winternitz WA, Metheny JA, Wear LC. Acute compartment syndrome of the thigh in sports-related injuries not associated with femoral fractures. Am J Sports Med 1992;20:476–478.

22. Ray MJ, Bassett RL. Myositis ossificans. Orthopaedics 1984;7:532–535.

23. Norman A, Dorkman H. Juxtacortical circumscribed myositis ossificans: evolution and radiographic features. Radiology 1970;96:301–306.

24. Toohey AK, LaSalle TL, Martinez S, Polisson RP. Iliopsoas bursitis: clinical features, radiographic findings, and disease associations. Semin Arthritis Rheum 1990;20:41–47.

25. Butler JE, Eggert AW. Fracture of the iliac crest apophysis: an unusual hip pointer. Am J Sports Med 1975;3:192–193.

26. Clancy WG, Foltz AS. Iliac apophysitis and stress fractures in adolescent runners. Am J Sports Med 1976;4:214–218.

27. Matheson GO, Clement DB, McKenzie DC, Taunton JE, Lloyd-Smith DR, MacIntyre JG. Stress fractures in athletes: a study of 320 cases. Am J Sports Med 1987;15:46–58.

28. McBryde AM Jr. Stress fractures in runners. Clin Sports Med 1985;4:737–752.

29. Hershman EB, Lombardo J, Bergfeld JA. Femoral shaft stress fractures in athletes. Clin Sports Med 1990;9:111–119.

30. Hulkko A, Orava S. Stress fractures in athletes. Int J Sports Med 1987;8:221–226.

31. Orava S, Puranen J, Ala-Ketola L. Stress fractures caused by physical exercise. Acta Orthop Scand 1978;49:19–27.

32. Drinkwater BC, Nilson K, Chestnut CH, Bremner WJ, Shainholtz S, Southworth MB. Bone mineral content of amenorrheic and eumenorrheic athletes. N Engl J Med 1984; 311:277–281.

33. Gudas CJ. Patterns of lower-extremity injury in 224 runners. Compr Ther 1980;6:50–59.

34. Devas MD. Stress fractures of the femoral neck. J Bone Joint Surg 1965;47B:728–738.

THE KNEE

JOHN C. RICHMOND

15

Epidemiology
Anatomy
History and Physical Examination
Radiographs and Special Studies
Traumatic Knee Injuries
Overuse Knee Injuries
Rehabilitation
Prevention

It is difficult to read a sports page in any major newspaper these days and not see a report dealing with an athlete sidelined by a knee injury. Knee injuries are occurring with alarming frequency at all levels of athletic participation, from "pee-wee" to adult, from recreational to professional.

The knee joint differs significantly from the other joints of the lower extremity in that there is little, if any, inherent bony stability to the knee. Although the hip and ankle are exposed to similar stresses in our athletic society, neither joint presents the practitioner with the problems encountered in dealing with knee injuries. The hip joint, due to the inherent stability of its ball-and-socket design, rarely sustains significant injury. The ankle, although frequently injured, has a bony anatomy that often functions well despite significant injury. The knee, with the complexity of menisci, multiple ligaments, and the patellofemoral joint, faces both frequent injury and an unforgiving reliance on many structures. When injured, the knee often fails to function adequately for continued athletic participation.

As a physician dealing with an athletic knee injury, one often faces the challenges of a difficult diagnosis. The emotions of a competitor who must take time from his or her sport are commonly encountered and must be appropriately addressed. It remains difficult for both the athlete and the treating physician to cope with the major change in life-style that a severely injured knee brings in the short term, and perhaps permanently. The enjoyment experienced by an athlete who has returned to sports following the accurate diagnosis and treatment of a knee injury is a substantial reward for the practitioner.

EPIDEMIOLOGY

The true risk of knee injury in sports remains in question. That knee injuries are common is well known; various studies have documented high frequencies in many common sports. Due to the many different methods used in these studies, range of injury rates varies widely. The percentages of knee injuries in some common sports are given in Table 15.1.

Some common themes are apparent in knee injuries, even with the varied methodology used in the studies (1–3). Younger athletes, before their teenage years, have a much lower injury rate than teenagers. This is true across many different sports, including soccer, football, and gymnastics. The rate of knee injuries also increases from the teenage years, with collegiate and senior athletes having rates higher than their younger counterparts. Unfortunately, insufficient data exist to be able to scientifically explain these differences, although various authors have implicated the increasing size and speed of older athletes, as well as the increased time they devote to sports. The flexibility of the younger athletes has also been noted as a possible factor in their lower injury rates.

When one looks at gender as a predilection for knee injury, there are slightly higher rates for females than males, with

Table 15.1. Percentages of Knee Injuries in Common Sports

Soccer	12–20%
Football	13–36%
Running	20–40%
Basketball	14–21%
Wrestling	5–20%
Skiing	14–24%

one study noting a substantially higher percentage of knee injuries in women (20%) than in men (11%) in various intercollegiate sports (4).

Injuries in most sports are more likely to occur in competition than in practice, with the exception of the early season when injury rates during practice are higher.

ANATOMY

The knee is much more than a simple hinge. It is a large and complex joint. The complexity arises from articular surfaces that have multiple radii of curvature, four main ligaments with varied fiber length and attachment sites, and the dynamic extensor apparatus that must be finely balanced. For the knee to function normally, particularly when exposed to the rigors of athletics, all components need to be working in concert. Any major disruption of normal anatomy, whether genetic, developmental, or through injury, may lead to problems. These can range from the trivial to the severe, including early degeneration of the joint.

The Extensor Mechanism

The three main components of the extensor mechanism are the quadriceps muscle, the patella, and the tendinous expansions (Figure 15.1). They extend the leg, stiffen the knee, and protect the articular surface of the femur. The quadriceps muscle, the largest muscle in the body, envelops the femur and is composed of four muscle groups—the rectus femoris, vastus intermedius, vastus lateralis, and vastus medialis. The first three function to extend the knee, whereas the main function of the vastus medialis is to balance the patella and maintain its tracking within the femoral trochlea

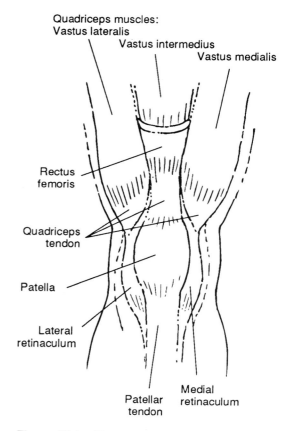

Figure 15.1. Extensor mechanism of the knee.

(5). The quadriceps tendon forms as a fusion of these four muscles. The superficial fibers from the rectus femoris continue over the patella anteriorly to join the patellar tendon. The deep fibers of the quadriceps tendon insert directly onto the patella. The vastus medialis and lateralis blend into the static soft-tissue stabilizers of the patella—the medial and lateral patellofemoral ligaments—to form the medial retinaculum and the lateral retinaculum of the patella.

The patella is basically triangular and can be divided into anterior and posterior surfaces (Figure 15.2). The anterior surface is rough and covered by the insertions of the

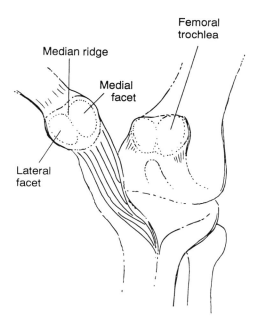

Median ridge

Medial facet

Femoral trochlea

Lateral facet

Figure 15.2. Patellofemoral joint.

quadriceps tendon, its anterior expansion, and the patellar tendon. The anterior surface is striated by numerous vascular channels and the tendinous insertion, leading to a bristled appearance on the tangential x-ray.

The posterior surface naturally separates into the ovoid articular surface and the inferior nonarticulating portion, which is one fourth to one third of the patellar height. The articular surface is divided into the medial and lateral facets by the median ridge. The lateral facet is usually somewhat larger. The medial facet has a secondary ridge of articular cartilage, which subdivides into the medial facet proper and a small "odd" facet. The "odd" facet, although covered with articular cartilage, does not normally contact the femur.

The articular surface of the femur can be divided into the trochlea and tibiofemoral articulations. The patella articulates with

the trochlea in all but the extremes of motion. The femoral trochlea is normally slightly higher on the lateral facet, resisting the forces that tend to push the patella laterally.

In full extension, the patella articulates with the synovial surface of the femur. As the knee is flexed, the patella will slide onto the articular surface of the femoral trochlea. This begins at about 10° of knee flexion and is determined by the length of the patellar tendon. A long patellar tendon leads to patella alta and requires more knee flexion before the patella is seated within the relative stability of the femoral trochlea. In early flexion, the lower one third of the patellar articulating surface contacts the femur. As flexion increases, the contact area moves more proximal on the patella.

The patellar tendon runs from the patella to insert on the tibial tubercle. The quadriceps angle (Q angle) is the angle between the rectus femoris and the patellar tendon and is increased with a more laterally placed tibial tubercle (see Figure 15.8).

Synovial Space

Synovium lines the entire interior of the knee that is not cartilaginous (the articular surfaces and menisci). Folds in the synovium are called *plicae* (see Figure 15.33). Several plicae are common. These include the ligamentum mucosum, medial patellar plica, and the suprapatellar plica. When the plicae occur, they present potential sites for inflammation caused by repetitive trauma.

Tibiofemoral Articulation

This is the weight-bearing portion of the knee joint (Figure 15.3). Its main bony components are the femoral condyles and the tibial plateaus. Because the femoral condyles are flatter anteriorly and more

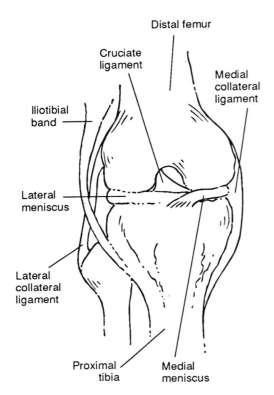

Figure 15.3. Tibiofemoral joint.

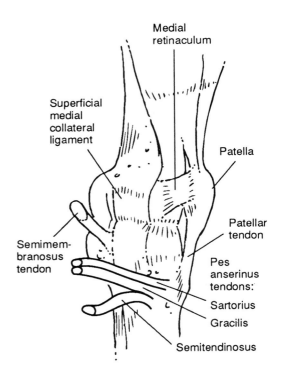

Figure 15.4. Medial aspect of the knee.

curved posteriorly, the ligaments from femur to tibia must be complex to retain stability through the range of motion. The tibial articular surface is nearly flat medially, whereas the lateral plateau is actually convex. Due to this shape, the integrity of the collateral and cruciate ligaments is crucial for stability of the knee. The menisci contribute to stability by creating a concave tibiomeniscal surface to articulate with the femur.

The capsule envelops the knee joint in a fibroligamentous sleeve. It extends medially and laterally from the patella and patella tendon as the medial or lateral retinaculum. Within the capsule, specialized ligamentous condensations add to the stability of the joint. These include the medial and lateral collateral ligaments.

The medial (tibial) collateral ligament (MCL) and lateral (fibular) collateral ligament (LCL) are the main valgus and varus stabilizers of the knee. The MCL has both a superficial and deep portion. The superficial MCL is continuous with the medial retinaculum anteriorly (Figure 15.4) and runs from the femoral epicondyle to insert on the tibia, three fingerbreadths below the joint line. The superficial MCL fans out posteriorly as the posterior oblique ligament (posteromedial capsule). The deep MCL is much shorter than the superficial and its fibers blend into the meniscus. It can be separated into meniscofemoral and meniscotibial segments.

The LCL is a thin, ropelike structure running from the femoral condyle to the fibular head (Figure 15.5). Deep to it, the lateral capsule has meniscofemoral and menis-

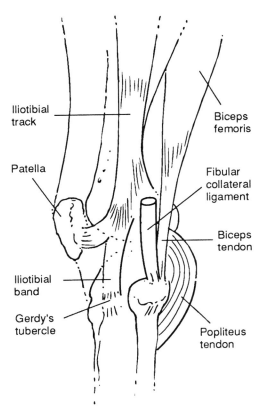

Figure 15.5. Lateral aspect of the knee.

cotibial segments and blends posteriorly into the posterolateral capsule (arcuate complex).

The static collateral ligaments are dynamically supported by secondary stabilizers. On the medial side, these are the medial retinaculum with the medialis muscle, the pes anserinus tendons (sartorius, gracilis, and semitendinosus) and the semimembranosus tendon. Laterally the dynamic stabilizers include the iliotibial band, popliteus muscle, and biceps muscle.

The cruciate ligaments (anterior and posterior) are so named because they cross within the femoral notch. They are intracapsular but are enveloped in synovium, so they are topographically extrasynovial.

The anterior cruciate ligament (ACL) is perhaps the most important ligament for the knee in athletes. This is due to its main function, which is to stabilize the joint during deceleration, and to the high risk of ACL injury in sports. The ACL arises from the posterior aspect of the lateral wall of the intercondylar notch of the femur and inserts in a broad area between the tibial spines. The posterior cruciate ligament (PCL) arises from the anterior aspect of the medial wall of the intercondylar notch of the femur and inserts on the posterior aspect of the proximal tibia. In more than 95% of knees, there is an accompanying posterior meniscofemoral ligament (either ligament of Humphrey or Wrisberg) that runs from the posterior horn of the lateral meniscus to blend with the PCL at its femoral attachment.

The fibrocartilaginous medial and lateral menisci cover two thirds of the tibial articular surface (Figure 15.6A). The medial meniscus has a larger radius of curvature and is firmly attached to the capsule throughout its periphery. Its outer few millimeters are vascularized. The lateral meniscus is more circular. The popliteus tendon separates the lateral meniscus from the posterolateral capsule, leading to increased mobility and decreased vascular supply in this portion of the meniscus.

HISTORY AND PHYSICAL EXAMINATION

Unfortunately, unless you happen to be the team physician at the site of an athletic event, you rarely see a traumatic knee injury at the time it occurs. Much more commonly, you are confronted with the problem several hours or days later, when the athlete has a swollen, painful knee and the physical examination is limited at best. The history is crucial and will often allow one to make the diagnosis.

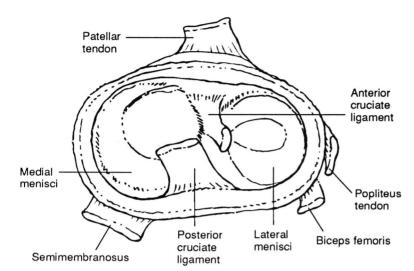

Figure 15.6. Tibial articular surface and menisci.

Patellar tendon

Anterior cruciate ligament

Medial menisci

Popliteus tendon

Semimembranosus

Posterior cruciate ligament

Lateral menisci

Biceps femoris

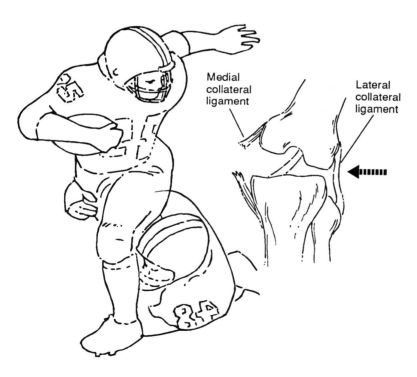

Medial collateral ligament

Lateral collateral ligament

Clinical Case #1

A 17-year-old female soccer player is injured during a high school soccer away game on Saturday afternoon. It was a noncontact (she was not struck by another player) injury that happened as she cut to avoid a defender. She felt a "pop" in her knee as it buckled. She was able to walk to the sidelines shortly after the injury, but she felt her knee was unstable. She remained on the bench, icing her knee, for the remainder of the game. By the time of the bus ride home, her knee was swollen and stiffening. Saturday night she was seen in the emergency department, where pain and swelling prevented an adequate examination; x-rays were "negative," and she was given crutches and an Ace bandage. Monday afternoon she arrives in your office.

History

The basic mechanism of injury is best divided into two main categories, *traumatic* and *overuse*. This generalization allows easy separation of most athletic injuries and is most helpful in establishing a diagnosis and treatment plan. As we think of our 17-year-old soccer player, key historical points come into focus for a *traumatic injury*. These include 1) the mechanism of injury, 2) the presence of a "pop" associated with the injury, 3) the timing of swelling, 4) the ability to continue play on the injured knee, and 5) the ability to walk on the leg.

The mechanism of injury should be ascertained in as much detail as possible. The mechanisms may be separated into contact and noncontact injuries. A contact injury occurs when the athlete's knee is struck by another athlete or strikes a hard surface. By careful questioning, the examiner should find out whether the athlete's foot was firmly planted on the ground and the direction of the force applied (e.g., a football player blocked from outside the knee has

been subjected to a *valgus* force) (Figure 15.6*B*). In a fall on a flexed knee, the tibial tubercle will often strike the ground first, leading to a *posterior* force on the tibia. A noncontact injury typically occurs when the athlete cuts to change direction or lands awkwardly from a jump. Typically, noncontact injuries result in damage to the ACL, whereas contact injuries result in damage to the collateral ligaments. The PCL is infrequently injured in sports; when injured, often a fall on the tibial tubercle is the most common mechanism.

When the athlete feels a "pop," or it is heard by other participants or spectators, this has a high likelihood of being an ACL injury (6). As many as 90% of injuries associated with a "pop" include an ACL injury.

The timing of swelling following the injury helps determine whether an intra-articular vascularized structure has been injured because blood will rapidly fill the joint in such a case. If the athlete notes swelling within the first 4 hours following injury, then a hemarthrosis has formed. This is indicative of a substantial injury, as noted by Noyes and colleagues (7), where they carried out arthroscopic examination on knees with acute hemarthrosis and identified a multiplicity of injuries (Table 15.2). Most knees with a hemarthrosis will have more than one injured structure. In this study it averaged two.

If the athlete is able to continue to play following an acute injury, then this is often, but not always, a relatively trivial injury. For example, contusions, mild sprains, and meniscal tears in the avascular portion of the meniscus can permit the athlete to finish the contest. The inability to bear weight on the injured knee implies the opposite, that the injury is substantial (e.g., complete collateral or cruciate ligament tears or displaced meniscal tears).

Table 15.2. Findings in Knees with
Hemarthrosis

Injury	Percentage
Partial ACL tear	28
Complete ACL tear	44
Minor ligament sprain	41
Major ligament tear	21
Complete meniscal tear	70
Partial meniscal tear	21
Femoral chondral fracture	20

ACL = anterior cruciate ligament.
SOURCE: Noyes FR, Bassett RW, Grood ES, Butler DL.
Arthroscopy in acute traumatic hemarthrosis of the
knee. J Bone Joint Surg 1980;62A:687–695.

From the history alone, of a noncontact
injury, a "pop," and the early swelling of a
hemarthrosis, we can have a high suspicion
of an ACL injury. Other injuries, although
less likely, are also possible with this history. These include peripheral meniscal
tears, articular surface injuries, collateral
ligament tears, and patella subluxation.

In the chronic state, following a traumatic
injury, one should attempt to identify those
athletes who are suffering from "mechanical symptoms." These are best defined as
symptoms that cause the knee to buckle
(give way), either partially or completely,
or to lock (resulting in a block to motion).
The mechanical symptoms result from
some impediment to the smooth gliding of
the joint's articular surfaces (e.g., an abnormally lax ligament, unstable meniscal fragment, or loose body). The mechanical
symptoms themselves are not preceded by
pain, but often lead to pain or swelling after
the event. This is in contradistinction to
painful buckling or locking, which often occurs in overuse conditions, and pain is the
inciting event. These athletes are much
more likely to have an anatomic anomaly or

training error than a mechanical disruption
of the joint.

The predictability of the buckling episodes by the athlete is also a helpful bit of
historical information. The buckling associated with chronic ligamentous insufficiency
is often predictable, and the athlete can
learn to avoid those activities that lead to
giving way. Buckling associated with a
meniscal tear or patellofemoral problems is
usually not predictable.

Clinical Case #2

*A 35-year-old man has been a runner for
many years, usually running 20 miles per week.
He has been an occasional competitor in short
races. Eight weeks ago, he began to increase the
intensity and distance of his running to train for
a marathon. This has included more hill running, as well as raising his distance to 40 miles
per week 3 weeks ago. That is when he developed
the insidious onset of lateral knee pain. Initially
the pain came on after a mile or so of running
and he could "run through it." Of late the pain
is more severe, it has forced him to cut down on
his speed and mileage, and frequently makes him
stop running. He has not noted any swelling
and has had no prior problems with either knee.
He has recently bought new running shoes, to
no avail.*

Pain can be a symptom of virtually any
traumatic or overuse injury in the knee.
Therefore, unless one can identify the
anatomic cause of the pain, it is not particularly helpful in making the diagnosis. As
part of the history, careful localization of
pain, particularly in overuse injuries, will
be helpful in identifying the anatomic structure that is causing pain.

In overuse injuries, a very detailed history of the symptoms, their relation to activity, and changes in activity or equipment

will be necessary to diagnose the problem. The most common causes of overuse injuries are training errors or anatomic anomalies. A detailed exercise history, including distance, speed, surface, and equipment, will reveal the training errors. A careful physical examination will be necessary to identify anatomic predispositions for injury.

This athlete has an overuse syndrome, probably related to his overzealous sudden increase in athletic stress. A common condition with these symptoms is iliotibial band friction syndrome (discussed later in the chapter), although patellofemoral problems often present with a similar history. Physical examination will help differentiate the various diagnoses.

Physical Examination

The examination of any injured knee should be broken down into five categories as follows: observation, palpation, range of motion, stability testing, and special testing (meniscal and patellofemoral). Our ability to assess all aspects of each of these categories may well be limited by the athlete's injury. The examination is best performed with the athlete in loose-fitting shorts with the skin bare from upper thigh to toes.

Observation

Observation includes the athlete's gait and use of assistive devices (e.g., brace or crutches). The gait examination may be widely varied due to the severity of the athlete's injury. In chronic or overuse injuries, it may even require the examiner to observe the athlete running or jumping. The overall alignment should be noted (Figure 15.7), whether varus (bowlegged), valgus (knock-kneed), or neutral (ankles and knees touch together). Patellofemoral alignment standing and supine, including the quadriceps angle (Q angle), should be recorded. The Q angle is a measure of the vector of pull of the quadriceps muscle (Figure 15.8). It is formed by the intersection of two lines at the center of the patella. These lines connect the anterior superior iliac spine to the midpoint of the patella and the midpoint of the patella to the tibial tubercle. The higher the Q angle, the greater the lateral force vector on the patella with quadriceps muscle activity. The normal Q angle is 12° or less in males and 14° or less in females. Q angles greater than these norms contribute to pa-

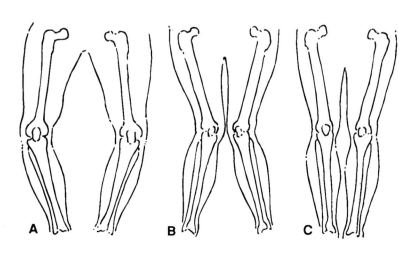

Figure 15.7. Alignment of the knee: varus (A), valgus (B), neutral (C).

A   B   C

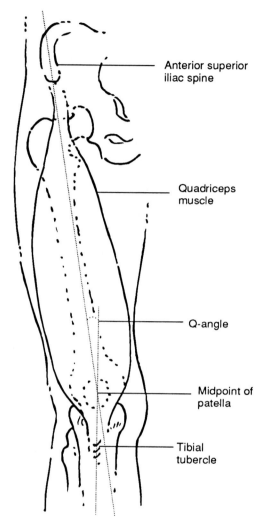

Figure 15.8. Quadriceps angle (Q angle) determines the vector of pull of the quadriceps muscle on the patella.

tellar malalignment and increase the risk of symptoms. Any deformity of the joint and swelling, either localized or diffuse, should be observed. Any areas of ecchymosis or abrasions should be noted. These will help identify the mechanism and the injured structures.

Palpation

Palpation is used in several ways in the knee examination. These include localizing areas of tenderness, establishing the integrity of anatomic structures, and identifying pathologic conditions (e.g., effusion or crepitation). After the athlete identifies any areas of pain, palpation should be used to try to identify which structures are injured. This is sensitive for most structures (notable exceptions being the cruciate ligaments and the articular surfaces) but is not specific. In many areas several structures overlap, and the examiner must use a detailed knowledge of anatomy to differentiate the injured structure.

Many subcutaneous structures can be carefully palpated to establish their integrity. The LCL can be felt with the leg in the figure-four position (Figure 15.9), beginning at the fibular head and tracing it proximally to the femur. The patella and quadriceps tendon are easily felt, as are the hamstring tendons. The medial patellar plica, when present, can often be rolled un-

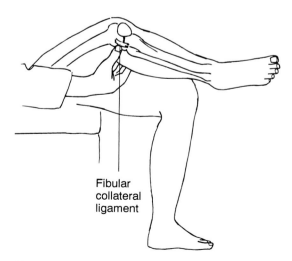

Figure 15.9. Palpation of the lateral collateral ligament.

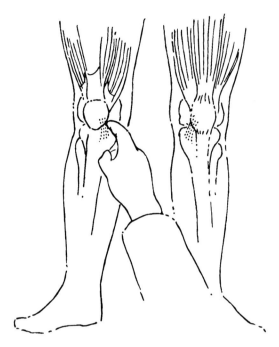

Figure 15.10. Palpation of medial patellar plica.

fusion is large, the patella can be balloted (Figure 15.11). This is done by pushing the patella posteriorly when the knee is extended. With a large effusion, the patella will move back to hit the femur, and then float forward when the pressure is released. In cases of a smaller effusion, a fluid wave should be sought (Figure 15.12). Fluid within the joint is a very nonspecific finding, but a sign that, whatever the problem is, it is more than trivial.

Crepitus is the sound or vibration produced by the movement of irregular joint surfaces or soft tissues within the joint. The two most helpful ways to elicit crepitus are illustrated in Figure 15.13 (8). The quality of the crepitus helps to determine its cause. A fine grinding, similar to a fine grit sandpaper against wood, is typical of the bone-on-bone of advanced arthritis. A somewhat coarser grinding is typical of the roughened cartilage of chondromalacia patella. Finally, clicking and snapping often represent thickened soft tissues or large flaps of damaged cartilage.

Range of Motion

The knee normally has a range of motion from 0° extension to 135° of flexion (Figure 15.14). It is not unusual to have some hyperextension (recurvatum) as a normal

der one's fingers palpating along the femoral condyle, medial to the patella (Figure 15.10). An effusion, fluid within the synovial space, is identified by a combination of palpation and observation. If the ef-

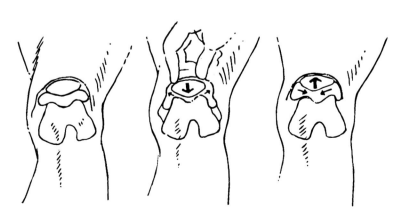

Figure 15.11. A large effusion makes the patella ballotable. (Modified from S Hoppenfeld. Physical Examination of the Spine Extremities. Norwalk, CT: Appleton & Lange, 1976: 195.)

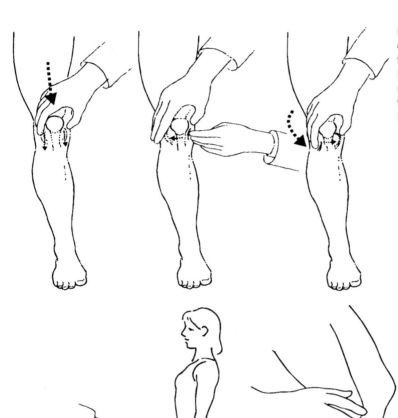

Figure 15.12. A moderate effusion is identifiable by a fluid wave. (Modified from S Hoppenfeld. Physical Examination of the Spine Extremities. Norwalk, CT: Appleton & Lange, 1976: 196.)

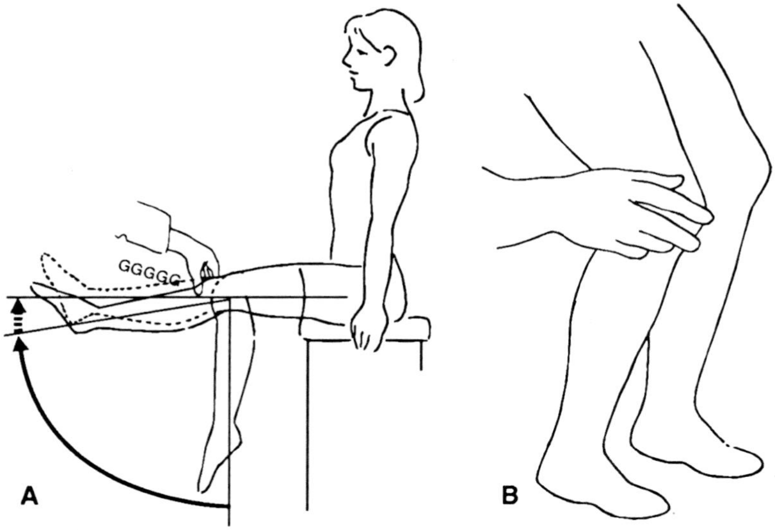

Figure 15.13. Crepitus from the patellofemoral joint (*A*) with resisted extension and (*B*) the more sensitive squatting test.

finding. Very flexible athletes, such as gymnasts, may have 150° to 160° of knee flexion. As always, comparison to an uninjured opposite knee will reveal the range of motion that is normal for that athlete. A "locked knee" is one that has a mechanical block to full motion caused by a displaced meniscal fragment. When this initially occurs, the loss of motion may be large, with extension to −20° to −30° and flexion to about 90°. If untreated, there will be gradual deformation of the displaced fragment and motion may return to the normal range, although it will always be a few degrees less in both flexion and extension than the athlete's other knee.

Stability Testing

Stability testing is performed to ascertain the integrity of the ligaments in the knee. The tests have been developed so that individual ligaments are isolated by a given test. In performing each test, due to the wide variability in normal ligamentous laxity between people, you must *always* compare to the opposite knee as a control. As with any ligament injury (sprain), there are three severity grades as shown in Table 15.3. When the injury is acute, there is local tenderness, swelling, and ecchymosis to assist in our assessment. In the chronic state, we must depend on laxity alone.

Patient *relaxation* is key to performing a good assessment of knee stability because any muscle guarding will overcome the examination. This is particularly true in the acutely injured knee, where pain increases the athlete's propensity to guard the joint. The examination is best performed with the athlete supine on the examination table, with his or her hands resting comfortably on the abdomen (to promote muscle relaxation). With an acute injury, placing a pillow behind the injured knee will allow the patient to relax the thigh muscles and be comfortable. It is best to examine the injured knee first to decrease the anticipation of pain.

For an athlete with an acutely injured knee, the examiner should perform the Lachman test (Figure 15.15) first to assess anterior-posterior stability. This is done with the knee in 20° to 30° of flexion. While stabilizing the femur with one hand, the examiner alternately draws the tibia forward and backward with the other hand. The hand holding the thigh should be proximal enough to avoid compressing the suprapatella pouch, which is often distended and painful to pressure. Any increased translation of the tibia compared to the opposite knee is indicative of injury to the ACL or PCL. If the examiner has small hands, or the athlete has a large leg, the Lachman can be performed without having to grasp the leg, by placing the fingers behind the tibia and femur and alternating lifting tibia and femur while looking for increased translation. With athletic injuries, and a positive Lachman test, almost all (>95%) are ACL injuries, but the physician must be on guard to pick up the rare PCL injury. In this case, the tibia often lies in a subluxed position (already translated posteriorly) before examination begins. This is identified by noting if the tibial tubercle is less prominent on the injured side with both knees flexed 50° to 60° and observing from the side with the athlete relaxed.

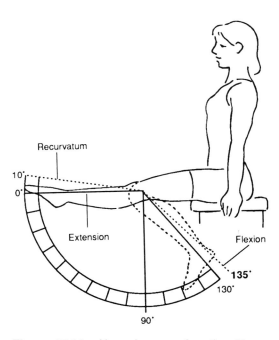

Figure 15.14. Normal range of motion 0° extension to 135° of flexion. Up to 15° of hyperextension (reservation) can be normal.

Table 15.3. Grading Ligament Injury

Grade	Tenderness	Laxity	End Point	Structural Damage
Normal (0)	–	–	Firm	None
Minimal (I)	+	–	Firm	Interstitial Fiber tear
Moderate (II)	++	+	Firm	Partial tear
Severe (III)	+	++	Soft	Complete tear

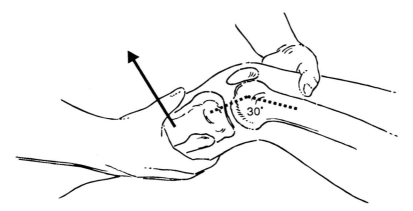

Figure 15.15. Lachman test. Increased translation of the tibia is diagnostic of a cruciate ligament injury. The feel of the end point of translation is important. A "soft" end point also indicates cruciate ligament injury.

The anterior-posterior drawer test is similar to the Lachman but is performed with the knee flexed 80° to 90° (Figure 15.16). This often cannot be done with an acute injury (because the athlete cannot flex the knee this far comfortably), but is very helpful in chronic cases. Again, the examiner needs to note the starting position of the tibia by the relative prominence of the tibial tubercle. Any increase in translation of the tibia will feel anterior, but the starting position will reveal the true injury. If the tibia starts posterior (tibial tubercle less

prominent), then the PCL is injured (see Figure 15.16*B*). If the tibia starts in its normal position (tibial tubercles of equal prominence), increased anterior translation indicates ACL injury.

The quality of the end point for the drawer and Lachman tests is very important, particularly in an acute injury, when the overall increase in translation from the injury will be lessened by swelling and muscle guarding. With the drawer or Lachman tests, the normal cruciate ligament has a "ping" sensation as its firm end point. The loss of this normal "ping" often indicates a complete cruciate ligament tear, either anterior or posterior, depending on which "ping" is absent.

The MCL and LCL are also assessed with the knee in 20° to 30° of flexion, for comfort

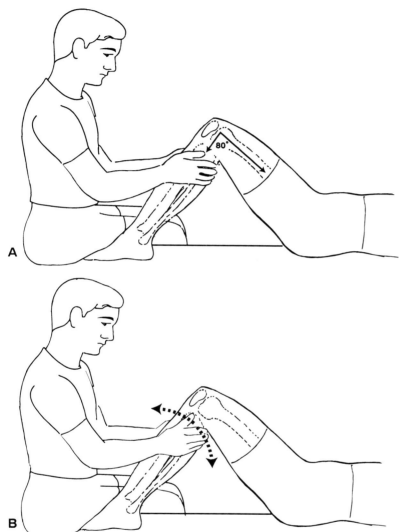

Figure 15.16. Anteroposterior drawer testing. (Modified from S Hoppenfeld. Physical Examination of the Spine Extremities. Norwalk, CT: Appleton & Lange, 1976: 186.)

and to relax the posterior capsule of the joint (Figure 15.17). The athlete should remain supine, with hands crossed on the abdomen to keep both quadriceps and hamstring muscles relaxed. The valgus stress test is used to assess the MCL. During this examination, the examiner stands on the same side of the table as the injured knee, uses the opposite hand (e.g., left hand to test right knee) to support and act as a fulcrum while a laterally directed force is applied at the ankle (using the right hand on the right ankle or left hand on the left ankle). When performing a valgus stress test, the examiner's palm is lateral as the fulcrum while the fingers support the knee in the popliteal space. When performing a varus stress test, the examiner's palm is in

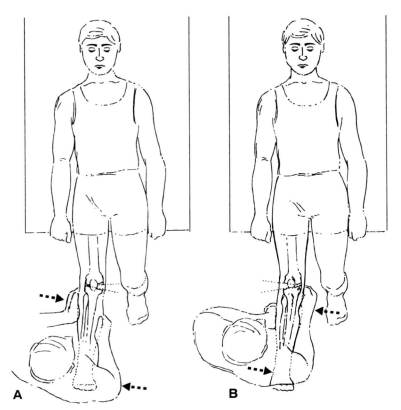

Figure 15.17. Valgus (*A*) and varus (*B*) testing in 30° of flexion assesses the integrity of the collateral ligaments.

A   B

the popliteal space and the fingers are medial to act as a fulcrum. With the knee flexed 20° to 30°, the collateral ligaments are assessed; if any laxity is found, the test should be repeated with the knee fully extended to assess the posterior capsule. Both laxity and feel of the end point must be assessed.

Injury to the ACL or the posteromedial or posterolateral capsule leads to more complex rotational laxities.

Injury to the ACL, which has resulted in it being nonfunctional, leads to anterolateral rotatory instability of the knee. This is a complex rotation of the knee that often leads to buckling when the athlete attempts to stop or change direction. Multiple tests have been described to identify this insta-

bility; they all produce an anterior subluxation of the anterolateral tibia near full extension, with a subsequent sudden reduction of the tibia under the femur at about 20° to 30° of flexion. This sudden reduction has been termed the "pivot-shift" phenomenon. It is best elicited using the flexion rotation drawer test described by Noyes and colleagues (Figure 15.18) (9).

Posteromedial capsular stability is evaluated with the Slocum test (10). The knee is flexed 70° to 80°, with the examiner sitting on the athlete's foot, to stabilize rotation of the leg (Figure 15.19). The anterior drawer test is performed first with the leg in neutral rotation and then in comfortable external rotation. In the externally rotated position, the anterior tibial excursion with drawer

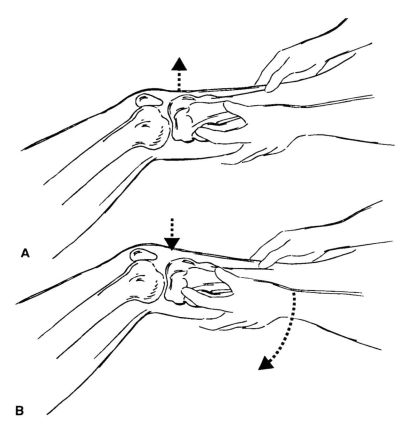

Figure 15.18. Flexion-rotation drawer test. *A.* With the knee near full extension gravity causes the femur to subluxate posteriorly into external rotation. *B.* Flexion of the knee with an axial load will cause a sudden shift as the tibia reduces. This is the "pivot-shift" phenomenon.

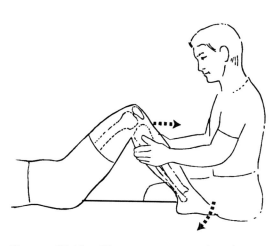

Figure 15.19. Slocum test, anterior drawer with the tibia held in external rotation.

testing should be substantially decreased over the excursion in neutral rotation. If the excursion is not decreased, then the Slocum test is positive, and the posteromedial capsule has been injured.

Posterolateral rotatory instability results from injury to the posterolateral or arcuate ligament complex. It is most easily demonstrated with the external rotation recurvatum test or the posterolateral drawer test, illustrated in Figure 15.20.

Included in the stability examination is the assessment of patellofemoral mechanics. Patella stability and tracking are dependent on the complex interaction of the dynamic forces of the quadriceps muscle, the static restraint of the medial and lateral

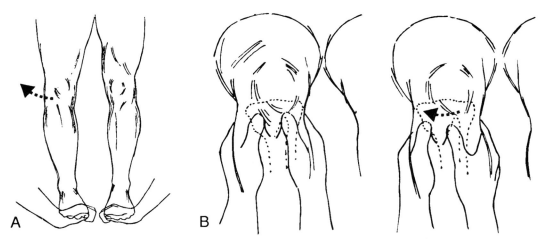

Figure 15.20. *A.* External rotation recurvatum test. Lifting the leg by the great toe results in recurvatum of the knee and increased external rotation of the tibial tubercle (*arrow*). *B.* Posterolateral drawer, increased external rotation of tibia with posterior drawer (*arrow*).

retinaculum, and the articulation of the patella and femoral trochlea. There is a consistent valgus alignment of the patellofemoral joint, which leads to the potential for lateral maltracking of the patella. Three common tests for patellofemoral stability are the apprehension test, the patella tilt test, and the Sage test.

The patella apprehension test is performed with the athlete's knee in full relaxed extension by applying a laterally directed force on the medial edge of the patella (Figure 15.21). The test is positive when the athlete appears apprehensive or notes the sensation that the kneecap is about to "go out." The patella tilt test is also performed with the knee fully extended. With both thumbs under the lateral border of the patella, and with the examiner's index fingers stabilizing the medial patella, an attempt is made to tilt the patella medially. The inability to tilt the patella is indicative of an excessively tight lateral retinaculum. The Sage sign is a test to identify a tight lateral patellar retinaculum and tilt (11). The athlete is supine with the knee

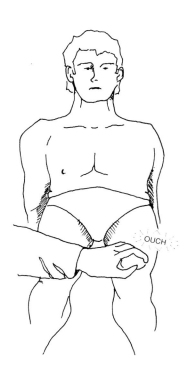

Figure 15.21. Patella apprehension test.

relaxed and supported at 15° to 20° of flexion. The patella is medially displaced by the examiner. The test is positive when the medial excursion is less than one fourth of the greatest width of the patella, indicating an excessively tight lateral patellar retinaculum.

Special Testing

Special tests for patellofemoral and meniscal pathology have evolved as means of identifying injury to these structures. Some tests are specific to the condition involved and quite sensitive; their routine use is encouraged. Other tests have a low accuracy (the combination of specificity and sensitivity for the given condition), and although they are listed here, their routine use is discouraged because they are misleading.

The patella grind (or compression) test is performed with the knee flexed 20° to 30°. As the athlete contracts the quadriceps muscle, extension is prevented by resisting knee motion at the lower leg, thus increasing patellofemoral compressive forces. This test is positive for patellofemoral pathology when it reproduces the athlete's pain. This is a reliable test.

The patella inhibition test is performed with the knee in full extension with the quadriceps muscle relaxed. The examiner applies firm, posteriorly directed pressure to the quadriceps mechanism at the proximal pole of the patella and has the athlete simultaneously contract the quadriceps muscle vigorously (Figure 15.22). This test is positive when the athlete feels pain or is inhibited from contracting the quadriceps muscle due to anticipation of pain. This test is not very helpful due to a high number of false positives caused by pain in any condition that leads to synovitis of the knee.

McMurray's test for medial meniscal tearing is performed with the patient supine (Figure 15.23). The examiner then acutely flexes the athlete's hip and knee and internally rotates the foot while palpating the posteromedial joint line. Simultaneously, the examiner extends the knee and externally rotates the foot. A "truly" positive McMurray's test elicits a loud clunk, which is felt under the examiner's fingers. This is rare, even in proven meniscal tears, but has a nearly 100% correlation with meniscal tearing when present (12). More commonly, the test causes pain and a click may or may not be palpated. This is a "mildly" positive McMurray's test and

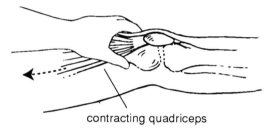

Figure 15.22. Patella inhibition test.

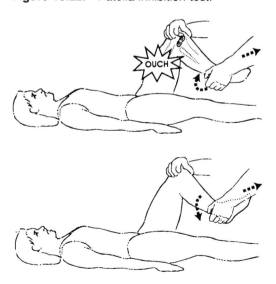

Figure 15.23. McMurray's test for meniscal tear. *A.* Medial. *B.* Lateral.

should be so noted because it suggests a meniscal tear. The lateral meniscal McMurray test is performed by acutely flexing the hip and knee with the foot externally rotated. The examiner then simultaneously extends the knee and internally rotates the foot while palpating the posterolateral joint line, and the results are reported as "truly" or "mildly" positive by the presence of clunk or pain with or without a click.

The forced flexion test has the best overall accuracy in identifying a meniscal tear (13). It is performed with the athlete supine while the examiner gently forces the knee into maximal hyperflexion. It is positive when the athlete notes pain *and* localizes the pain to the posteromedial or posterolateral joint line.

"Duck walking" is another meniscal test that has a similar mechanism (forced flexion). The athlete is asked to squat and take a few steps forward in this position. The test is only positive if it causes pain localized to the posteromedial or posterolateral joint line, or the athlete is unable to perform due to a feeling that the knee would lock or give way.

Apley's grind test is mentioned only to note its major inaccuray rate (Figure 15.24). Performed with the athlete prone and the knee flexed 90°, the examiner rotates the foot internally and externally, first with a distraction force, then with a compression force. The test is called positive when pain is elicited only with compression. It has little or no correlation with meniscus tearing and is not recommended as part of the routine knee examination.

RADIOGRAPHS AND SPECIAL STUDIES

Plain radiographs are an important diagnostic tool in the examination of the

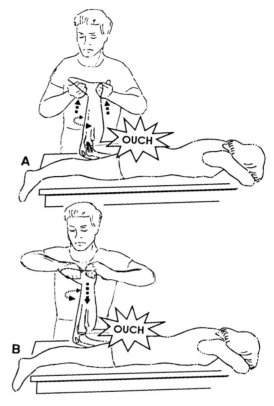

Figure 15.24. *A.* Apley's distraction test to identify ligamentous injury. *B.* Apley's compression test to identify meniscal injury.

knee, but they are not universally necessary. They should be reserved for certain specific indications. The standard knee series for athletic injury should include anteroposterior, lateral, tunnel, and skyline views. These studies should be ordered for any of the circumstances listed in Table 15.4. If you are working in a training room setting, you must be sure to get x-rays when indicated and not overlook them due to inconvenience.

Arthrography of the knee has become less frequent due to the widespread availability magnetic resonance imaging (MRI). This is due to the need for injection of contrast material into the joint for arthrog-

Table 15.4. Indications for Routine
Radiographs

Hemarthrosis
Suspected loose body
Grade II or III ligament injury
Suspected osteochondritis dissecans
Patellofemoral malalignments, not responsive
   to conservative treatment
Patella dislocation
Inability to reach clinical diagnosis

---

raphy, with its attendant morbidity, and the
additional information about ligamentous,
bony, and extracapsular structures available from MRI.

Although MRI scanning of the knee (and
other joints) for athletic injuries has become
widespread due to the soft-tissue imaging
of this technique, its cost ($800 to $1200 per
study) means clear-cut indications are required for ordering it, particularly when
several recent reports have noted its inaccu-
racy (14–16). We have developed a list of
specific indications for MRI in our clinic
(Table 15.5), which hopefully controls the
cost of diagnosing knee injuries. There are
other instances where you might order
an MRI scan of the knee, but you should
carefully think through the diagnosis and
resort to the scan only after exhausting less
expensive techniques.

TRAUMATIC KNEE INJURIES

The primary care physician will encounter traumatic knee injuries both in the office
or clinic, training room situation, and on the
field. An acute knee injury on the field
presents the physician with the additional
challenge of diagnosing potential limb-
threatening conditions at the time of occurrence. The number one priority is to rule
out vascular injury or major fracture or
dislocation. Following this, as the initial

examiner, you will have the opportunity to
examine the knee within several minutes of
the injury, at a time when there is little or no
swelling, and often very little pain.

On the field, the initial assessment of a
knee injury should be of alignment or deformity, indicative of displaced fracture or
dislocation. If there is substantial deformity, immediate transport to an emergency department is necessary. Appropriate splinting and neurovascular assessment
must be performed before the injured athlete is transported. If the alignment of the
leg is normal, proceed with a brief history
and physical examination of the field, before moving the athlete. At all times the
safety of the athlete is of primary concern,
and he or she is moved only when the physician has determined it is safe to do so. The
on-the-field history can be very brief, limited to short questions such as, "What happened? What did you feel? Where does it
hurt? Can you move your foot? Can you
move your knee?" Examination can be limited to assessing bony and ligamentous integrity. Fractures of the femur or tibia may
occur and require splinting and emergency
transport. Likewise, "near dislocations"
(three or more major ligamentous structures torn) require splinting before the athlete is moved. In this situation emergency
transport is appropriate.

For lesser injuries, with one or two ligaments injured, the athlete can be assisted,
not weight bearing on the injured leg to the
sidelines, where a more thorough examination should be performed before the pain
and swelling increase. In injuries that
seem to be least severe, with no disruption
of any of the four major ligaments, an intact
quadriceps mechanism, and full range
of motion, it is appropriate to allow the
athlete to leave the field under his or her
own power. The athlete is often very anxious at the time of knee injury. We are all
aware of athletic careers ended by knee

Table 15.5. Indications for MRI of the Knee

Hemarthrosis, cause unknown	Unable to make diagnosis by repetitive examinations
ACL tear, limited indications	Planning nonoperative treatment, to assess menisci
Possible meniscal tear	When diagnosis is unlikely, but symptoms persist (will decrease negative athroscopies)
? Spontaneous osteonecrosis	Older patients with atraumatic pain
Third-degree MCL sprain	To assess status of ACL/PCL

ACL = anterior cruciate ligament; MCL = medial collateral ligament; PCL = posterior cruciate ligament.

injury; this is particularly accentuated if a teammate or friend has had a severe knee injury. Reassurance of the athlete is important and will help him or her relax for the examination.

Allowing an athlete to return to the game after a knee injury is a difficult decision. Complete the examination on the sideline or locker room before deciding. Do not allow the decision to be swayed by pressure from coaches, family, or the athlete. Returning to play can only be allowed when there is *no* increased risk of further injury. Therefore, the injury must be minor (e.g., contusion or grade I sprain), the knee must have full range of motion, and the athlete must be able to run full speed and cut without a limp. If you have concerns, even in trivial injuries, it is appropriate to ice the knee for 10 to 15 minutes after the initial sideline examination. Then re-examine the athlete, looking for effusion or subtle laxities. If any question remains, err on the side of safety.

Ligamentous Injuries

Ligamentous injuries of the knee represent a major and increasing problem in athletics because of the high frequency of ligament injury arising from the increasing size and speed of our athletes, the aggressive nature of our play, and the use of artificial surfaces (17). Increased sophistication in diagnosing ligamentous injuries may also be contributing to an apparent rise in ligament injury rates. The dependency of the knee on ligamentous restraint for athletic stability only accentuates the problem.

Grading

The severity of any ligament injury should be defined, using the American Medical Association classification schema (see Table 15.3). This system is based on the degree of ligamentous injury (mild, moderate, and severe) and the accompanying symptoms and signs. A first-degree sprain is by definition an injury to the ligament, in which there is *no* increased laxity of that ligament. If there is laxity present then there is either a second- or third-degree sprain. A second-degree sprain is differentiated clinically from a third-degree sprain by the feel of the "end point" on examination and the amount of laxity. A second-degree sprain has a "firm" end point on stressing, as the ligament fibers that were not torn in the injury become taut. A third-degree sprain has a "soft" end point, as translation is gradually stopped when other ligament and tendon fibers (secondary restraints) become taut.

Healing

The healing of an injured ligament depends on two main factors: the presence of a vascularized bed for the formation and maturation of scar and protection from excessive stress. The healing of a ligament is stimulated by lesser amounts of stress (18). Information from laboratory and clinical studies has radically altered the way we treat ligament injuries over the last 10 years. Our treatment principle will be to treat nonoperatively those ligament injuries that are well vascularized and can be protected from excessive stress. Those injuries that are not well vascularized (e.g., ACL injuries) or cannot be protected from excessive stress (e.g., combined ligament injuries) often require early surgical intervention.

In virtually all cases, we can safely allow motion and some protected stress to the ligament. This will promote healing of the ligament and nutrition to the articular cartilage.

Medial Collateral Ligament

The MCL remains the most commonly injured knee ligament in sports. This is due to it being at risk from contact on the outside of the leg or knee when the foot is planted or in twisting injuries.

Clinical Case #3

A 26-year-old recreational softball player presents to your office the day after she injured her left knee in a collision at second base. She is using crutches that she has borrowed from a friend.

In obtaining further history you should pursue the five important questions for a traumatic injury: 1) mechanism of injury? 2) presence of a "pop"? 3) timing of swelling? 4) continue to play? and 5) able to walk?

In response to these you find that she was struck on the lateral aspect of the left leg with her foot planted. She felt pain but no "pop." She was able to continue to play that inning, but stiffness prevented her from finishing the game.

She was able to walk with only a mild limp until she got up this morning, when the knee was slightly swollen and painful along the medial joint line.

Your suspicion prior to examining the patient should be that of a first- or second-degree sprain of the MCL, but a careful examination is necessary. The first test should be the Lachman, best done in an acute injury with the knee supported at 20° of flexion by a pillow (see Figure 15.15). Important is not only the translation, but the feel of the end point. If a "ping" is present, then the ACL is intact. (She has a "ping.") Valgus stress testing can also be carried out with the knee supported by a pillow (see Figure 15.17). No matter what the degree, a valgus stress will cause some pain in an MCL injury. If there is no increased laxity at 20° to 30° of flexion (compared to the other knee), the injury is first degree. If there is some increased laxity, but a "firm" end point, then the injury is second degree (partial tear). If there is significantly increased laxity with valgus stress, with a "soft" end point, then there is a complete tear (third-degree sprain) of the MCL. (She has some laxity but a "firm" end point.)

You should continue with the laxity examination to assess all of her ligaments (PCL and LCL). Palpation should be used to define any area of tenderness, and therefore, the anatomic structures injured. (She has pain on the femoral epicondyle.) Finally you should check for an effusion by balloting the patella (see Figure 15.11). If it is not ballotable (the patella does not rise up after you push it down against the femur), you should check for a fluid wave (see Figure 15.12). Regardless of the degree of MCL sprain, there is rarely a large (ballotable) effusion unless another structure is injured. (She only has a small fluid wave.)

The superficial MCL is a long structure stretching from the medial epicondyle of the femur to insert three fingerbreadths below the joint line on the tibia. A tear of the MCL at its tibial insertion will cause pain a significant distance from the joint line. The deep MCL includes the short menisio-femoral and menisiotibial ligaments.

With the diagnosis of MCL injury confirmed through history and physical examination, and the isolated nature of the injury confirmed through the remainder of the physical examination, routine radiographs are indicated only in second- or third-degree sprains. Radiographs are obtained only to rule out associated bony injury (e.g., avulsion fracture, physeal fracture in a child with open growth plates, or tibial plateau fracture in older athletes).

For first-degree MCL sprains we can expect rapid recovery with minimal treatment. The general treatment program for isolated MCL injuries is presented in Table 15.6. The use of crutches or a knee immobilizer for comfort is very helpful for the athlete for a few days after injury. Regular icing for 15 minutes three to four times a day is appropriate until pain and swelling have resolved. The exercises listed here are described in detail in the rehabilitation section of this chapter. Efforts should be made to maintain muscle tone with quadriceps setting and straight leg lifts (out of the knee immobilizer) early on after a first-degree MCL sprain. The athlete may be rapidly progressed to more aggressive strengthening and endurance work as comfort allows. Return to athletics is only based on the function of the knee (full pain-free range of motion, with normal strength, and resolving effusion). There are no arbitrary times necessary because ligamentous strength is retained. No support is needed to return to athletics, but for several weeks the athlete may feel more secure with an elastic or neo-prene sleeve (patella cutout recommended) or just an Ace wrap.

Recovery from a second-degree MCL sprain is longer and its management somewhat more complex. Because some ligament fibers remain intact, the torn fibers are internally splinted from excessive stress and the use of a knee immobilizer or crutches is only for comfort. This is usually necessary for 7 to 10 days. Because pain and effusion persist for a significant time, muscle atrophy and stiffness are likely to be a problem. Early rehabilitation should consist of isometric quadriceps strengthening and range of motion exercises. These can be increased to isotonic and endurance exercises as the athlete tolerates them. More aggressive athletes benefit from the early return to sport, which can be obtained from working with a physical therapist or athletic trainer.

It takes up to 6 weeks for full return of ligamentous strength following a significant second-degree MCL sprain (19). Often, the competitive athlete is ready to go back to athletics 2 to 3 weeks after injury. It is appropriate to prescribe an off-the-shelf functional sports brace for this situation and have the athlete use the brace for up to 8 weeks after injury. In the higher-risk sports (e.g., football, soccer, and basketball) encourage the use of that brace throughout the season in which the injury occurred.

For "isolated" third-degree MCL sprains nonoperative treatment has recently become the treatment of choice, but requires that one be exacting in establishing the "isolated" nature of the ligamentous injury (20). To do this, the ACL and PCL must be proven intact. This can be done with MRI scanning and instrumented laxity testing (see ACL section), but may require examination under anesthesia and arthroscopy. Unless the examiner has extensive experience dealing with significant knee ligament

Table 15.6. Treatment of Isolated Medial Collateral Ligament Injuries

Grade	Residual Strength	Healing Potential	Healing Time	Early Protection	Rehabilitation	Brace for Sports
I	Virtually 100%	Good	Few weeks	Knee immobilizer (few days)	Aggressive early on	None
II	Substantial decrease	Good	6 wk	Knee immobilizer (7–10 days)	Aggressive as swelling decreases	Hinged sports brace for this season
III	Little or none	Good, if protected	10–14 wk	Hinged protective brace (6 wk)	See Table 15.9	Hinged sports brace for 4–6 mo

injuries, it is recommended that all third-degree MCL sprains be evaluated by a sports-oriented orthopedic surgeon to confirm the isolated nature of the injury, before embarking on the nonoperative treatment. In the best study of the nonoperative treatment for isolated third-degree MCL sprains, Indelicato and colleagues (20) demonstrated less than 5 mm of increased valgus laxity and excellent functional result at 2 years and longer follow-up in all patients treated nonoperatively. The nonoperative program is complex and is presented in Table 15.7. The thrust of the nonoperative program is to limit the stress on the completely torn MCL early on, to allow some healing to begin. Then, to gradually increase in a protected fashion, the stresses applied to the ligament, while gradually rehabilitating the thigh musculature.

Anterior Cruciate Ligament

Injury to the ACL has become epidemic in our young sports-minded society. This injury has become so common and its sequelae so serious that many sports-ori-

ented magazines have featured articles on the subject. The ACL is at risk in sports when the athlete is cutting or pivoting (often it is torn in a noncontact injury) and also when the athlete is struck on the knee with the foot planted. The anatomy of the ACL is such that its fibers are "nearly isometric." This means that they normally are all under about equal tension in any knee position. This often results in complete tearing (third-degree sprain) of the ACL when it is injured. The importance of the ACL lies in its biomechanical function, which is to coordinate the rotation of the femur on the tibia. When the ACL is nonfunctional from injury, activity-related buckling will ensue when the athlete tries to cut or pivot on the involved leg.

More has been written on the ACL in the last 15 years than on any other subject in sports injury. This is not only due to its alarming frequency, but also to the severe consequences of the chronic ACL insufficiency and to the complexity of treatment for ACL injury. There is *no* correct treatment for all athletes with ACL tears; rather, we must "tailor the treatment" to the pa-

Table 15.7. Detailed Nonoperative Treatment Isolated Third-Degree
Medial Collateral Ligament Sprains

	0–2 Wk	*2–6 Wk*	*>6 Wk*
Range of motion	Long leg orthosis locked at 30° flex	Long leg orthosis 30°–90° flex	Full range of motion out of brace
Weight bearing	Crutches, partial weight bearing	Weight bearing as tolerated	Full weight bearing
Strengthening	Isometric quad/hamstring	Isometric and isotonics in brace	Full isotonic stress closed chain
Return to sport			Quad strength > 60%, begin running Quad strength > 80%, agility drills Quad strength > 90%, full athletics in brace

tient. We need to develop a treatment plan for each individual athlete based on age, activity level, degree of laxity, and willingness to modify athletic activities (6,21).

Clinical Case #4

A 42-year-old salesman presents to your office 1 week after a knee injury sustained in a touch football game with his teenaged boys. He was injured in a collision and is unable to identify the mechanism. He did not feel a pop but was unable to continue and noted early swelling. The swelling is improving, but his knee feels "weak." Examination reveals only a moderate effusion (fluid wave present) and a minimally increased anterior Lachman test with a "soft" feeling for the end point. The pivot shift cannot be assessed due to pain. Should you obtain plain x-rays? Yes, this is by history a hemarthrosis and small bony avulsions may reveal the nature or extent of the injury.

In the face of an acute ACL injury diagnosis will be based largely on history and a subtly increased Lachman test with a soft end point. Instrumented laxity testing is a technique that can be helpful in confirming or ruling out ACL injury (Figure 15.25). Several devices are commercially available, which allow identification, to the nearest

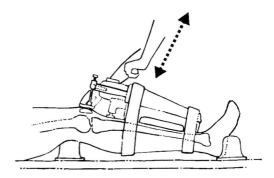

Figure 15.25. Instrumented laxity testing can be a more sensitive way of identifying and quantitating cruciate ligament damage.

millimeter, of any increase in anterior or posterior laxity of the knee. Daniel and coworkers confirmed the sensitivity of these devices in detecting ACL injury in acute cases (22).

If you have the luxury of being on the sidelines during an athletic contest, you will often be able to elicit a pivot shift using the flexion rotation drawer maneuver early on, before pain and swelling develop. Within a few hours of the injury, this is often impossible to assess due to guarding of the knee by the athlete.

As alluded to earlier, most fibers of the ACL are under equal tension throughout the range of motion. Therefore, it is more frequent that all fibers are torn (third-degree sprain) than just a partial tear, although second-degree sprains of the ACL do occur. Also, because any ACL fiber failure requires major force, first-degree ACL sprains are not of clinical import.

Because the functional instability and disability from ACL injury results from "giving away" episodes (which are the equivalent of the pivot), it is best to define third-degree ACL sprain as one that results in a pivot (ACL-deficient knee), even if some fibers remain in continuity. A second-degree ACL sprain is one that leads to increased anterior tibial translation but no rotational instability (absent pivot).

There is an approximately 50% chance that the athlete will tear a meniscus at the time of ACL injury. This is more likely to be the lateral meniscus than the medial meniscus. The medial meniscus is also at high risk of injury with any subsequent pivoting episode. We have established that the meniscus is the key to successful functional outcome following ACL injury (23). Therefore, goals of treatment should be prevention of buckling episodes, by either surgery or nonoperative means and identification of meniscal pathology for early repair if possible. The definitive treatment of acute ACL injuries is not emergent, as has been established by Shelbourne and colleagues (24). In fact, very early operative treatment of ACL injuries may lead to an increased risk of postoperative stiffness.

With the luxury time for definitive treatment planning, any athlete with an acute third-degree ACL sprain, or hemarthrosis with presumed ACL tear, should be placed in a knee immobilizer, with crutches for comfort for the first few days. Range of motion and isometric quadriceps strengthening should be started. Repetitive icing and nonsteroidal anti-inflammatory drugs (NSAIDs) will help reduce the swelling. The options for treatment are surgical or nonsurgical. (It is best not to term nonsurgical as conservative because for an aggressive athletic teenager performing pivoting sports, the most conservative course of action for ACL injury is reconstruction.) (25) Current surgical techniques entail an arthroscopic-assisted reconstruction, most often using an autologous tendon to substitute for the ACL. Nonsurgical treatment begins with aggressive rehabilitation of thigh musculature, both quadriceps and hamstring. Proprioceptive and agility exercises as well as endurance training follow. The use of functional bracing for the ACL-deficient knee remains controversial. This is due to no demonstrable laboratory effect of the braces on rotational laxity, although the majority of patients feel that the braces help. In clinical trials, buckling episodes are reduced, but 60% of athletes still had giving way episodes in the brace (21). Our recommendation has been to use functional bracing, since the cost ($600 to $1000) is substantially less than the morbidity of a meniscal tear that may happen when the knee pivots. More than 25 functional braces are on the market, with no clear-cut advantage for any brand (26). Because fit and comfort are crucial if the athlete is to use the brace (instead of leaving it in the closet), it is wise to use a brand that your bracemaker or orthotist is familiar with and can reproducibly get to fit well. Request that it be set up for an ACL injury.

The mainstay of nonsurgical treatment in the athlete with a positive pivot is activity modification. This will substantially reduce the athlete's exposure to injury, if he or she is willing to stop or reduce the time at sports that have frequent stopping, cutting, or turning. Maturity does factor into this, in that the younger athlete is much less likely to modify athletic activities. Age is *not* a contraindication for surgical treatment. With today's high activity levels of people in their fifties, it is not uncommon to see ACL injury in this group and occasionally to reconstruct the ligament if they are unwilling to modify their athletic endeavors.

The athlete with an acute ACL injury should be started on rehabilitation and given an early referral to the sports-oriented orthopedic surgeon. For the athlete to make an appropriately informed decision, he or she must be advised of the details, including the risks, of both operative and nonoperative treatments. For the athlete favoring nonoperative treatment, we recommend an MRI scan to assess meniscal status. In the case of a meniscal tear that could be repaired by suturing, this may tip the decision toward early ACL reconstruction. The long-term success of meniscal repair is better than 90% in ACL stabilized knees but less than 70% if the knee remains unstable (positive pivot shift) (27).

For the second-degree ACL sprain (negative or trace pivot with mildly positive Lachman), nonsurgical treatment is an attractive alternative for the nonstrenuous athlete and a reasonable approach in any athlete. The program should follow general rehabilitation guidelines, and follow-up must be careful, to resort to early surgery if instability develops.

Not all ACL-injured athletes are encountered early on. The treatment of chronic ACL insufficiency can also be surgical or nonsurgical. Unfortunately, by 2 years from the initial injury 80% of ACL-deficient knees will have meniscal tearing. This reduces the functional outcome of any treatment if partial meniscectomy must be performed. Any patient with symptoms or findings of a meniscal tear and ACL insufficiency should see the orthopedist before embarking on a nonoperative treatment program. The nonsurgical program outlined above can be considered in the lower demand athlete, particularly one not involved in cutting sports. ACL reconstruction is the treatment of choice for the athlete involved in cutting or pivoting sports, who is unwilling to modify activities and has a pivot.

Younger athletes are also sustaining ACL injuries as early as age 7 or 8 years, although this is uncommon. More often, the prepubescent athlete will sustain a tibial spine avulsion, which leads to ACL deficiency. The young athlete will have even more troubles with an ACL-deficient knee than older athletes (28). Any suspicion of an ACL tear in a prepubescent athlete mandates consultation with an orthopedic surgeon. Tibial spine fractures require near anatomic reduction to restore stability and surgical techniques must be specialized in the knee with open growth plates. A sports-oriented orthopedic surgeon or one with experience in treating children is recommended.

Posterior Cruciate Ligament

The PCL is infrequently injured in athletes. Estimated as occurring one twentieth to one fiftieth as often as ACL injury in some studies, the frequency of PCL injury may be higher than we think. This is because PCL injury is associated with less pain and swelling when it occurs and because it presents much less symptomatology in the chronic state. The PCL is truly extrasynovial in the knee and when torn, usually does not lead to a large hemarthrosis, but rather a small effusion with only moderate pain. The most common mechanism of the PCL injury is a direct blow on the tibial tubercle when the knee is flexed. In athletes, this is most likely to occur when the athlete falls onto the knee on a hard surface. If the athlete's foot is dorsiflexed, the gastrocnemius muscle protects the PCL. If the athlete's foot is plantar flexed, then the PCL is more likely to be torn.

As a result of the mild pain and swelling with PCL injury, athletes with acute PCL injury may not present to the physician for many days, if at all. They typically have only a small effusion. The physical examination may be confusing, in that you may detect an increased translation on the drawer or Lachman tests but the knee begins in the subluxed position and the translation (although anterior) reduces the tibia. A firm end point ("ping") on the anterior drawer or Lachman, with a soft end point on the posterior test, is helpful in identifying PCL injury. The diagnosis is confirmed when the tibial tubercle can be seen to drop back with a gravity posterior drawer.

Partial PCL tears (first- or second-degree sprains) are tolerated very well in athletes if no other ligament is torn. Athletes with increased posterior translation, who have a firm end point to posterior drawer testing, can be expected to do well when rehabilitated in a nonoperative approach. Rehabilitation should stress quadriceps muscle strength and endurance. Functional bracing has little role in PCL injuries because there

is no clinical benefit or biomechanical evidence for the use of a sports brace in the PCL injured knee.

The treatment of a third-degree PCL sprain remains controversial because the natural history of the PCL-deficient knee has not been fully worked out. In the only truly prospective study of PCL injuries, Parolie and Bergfeld reported little functional disability and no signs of osteoarthritis (29). Others have noted deterioration of the medial femoral articular surface in some athletes with PCL-deficient knees (30). This is more likely in athletes with combined injuries.

The surgical treatment of complete PCL tears has been unreliable at best (31). Weighing this, and the satisfactory function of most athletes with isolated PCL injuries, we reserve surgical reconstruction of the PCL for specific indications. For acute injuries, these are the knees with combined laxities (e.g., medial and posterior). In the chronic cases, PCL reconstruction is indicated for persistent symptoms (largely pain and weakness) and combined instabilities.

Lateral Collateral Ligament

The LCL is the least frequently injured in sports of all the knee ligaments because the knee is usually protected from a blow to the medial side by the athlete's other leg. Because the LCL is subcutaneous it can be easily examined in the figure-four position (see Figure 15.9). Sprains of the LCL are graded on the same system used for MCLs. Isolated third-degree sprains of the LCL always result in injury to the lateral capsule as well.

Treatment for first- and second-degree LCL sprains follows the same program and a very similar time frame that was used for MCLs (see Table 15.6). By and large these injuries do well and early recovery and return to athletics can be anticipated using this schema. Nonoperative treatment of third-degree LCL sprains does not work as well as medial side injuries (32). It is therefore recommended that complete LCL tears be referred for early surgical treatment.

Combined Knee Ligament Injuries

The most frequent combined knee ligament injury is to the ACL and MCL. This is particularly common in contact sports such as football and soccer, where pivoting and collision can occur simultaneously. One must always be thorough in examining any knee injury and perform as complete an examination that the athlete can tolerate. Do not be trapped by identifying only one of several ligaments injured. In the 1950s, O'Donoghue wrote extensively about ligament injuries occurring in athletes (33). The injury complex of MCL, ACL, and medial meniscus tear is often termed the "O'Donoghue triad" or "unhappy triad." Shelbourne and Nitz in an extensive study have shown that combined MCL and ACL tears are much more likely to be associated with a lateral meniscal tear (34). This is six times more likely to occur than with medial meniscal tear and should probably carry the title of "unhappy triad."

Because the functional stability of the knee is so dependent on the ligamentous support, combined injuries will often result in substantial morbidity and permanent disability. Therefore, any combined ligament sprain, which is more than first degree, should receive early evaluation by an orthopedic surgeon.

Knee Dislocations and Near Dislocations

A *knee dislocation* is defined as dislocation of the tibiofemoral joint. These are rare in athletics but do occur. They represent a potentially catastrophic injury for an athlete, because not only are two or three major ligaments torn completely, but there is also substantial risk of neurovascular injury. When encountered on the athletic field, these require urgent transport to the emergency department and emergent reduction by an orthopedic surgeon. Neurovascular status should be carefully assessed and documented. There is a 5% risk of vascular injury with athletic knee dislocations (much lower than with high velocity dislocations) (35). Therefore, vascular assessment with ultrasound is appropriate. Operative treatment is necessary to address the ligament injuries.

A *near dislocation* occurs when three of the four major ligaments are torn completely, without a dislocation requiring reduction being identified. The typical patterns are ACL, PCL, and MCL or ACL, PCL, and LCL. The risk of vascular injury is less than with a dislocation, but careful assessment of the distal pulses is appropriate, as is urgent orthopedic evaluation, because early surgical treatment is necessary.

The Patellofemoral Joint

The patella is at constant risk for traumatic lateral subluxation or dislocation due to the consistent valgus of the Q angle (see Figure 15.8). With this alignment, quadriceps contraction leads to a lateral force vector on the patella, which is resisted by the shape of the femoral trochlea, the medial retinaculum, and the vastus medialis obliquus (VMO) fibers. The combination of this alignment, with a lateral traumatic force on the patella, may result in lateral subluxation or dislocation (36). Although this may occur in a normal knee, it is much more likely to occur in a joint that has an anatomic predisposition such as excessive Q angle, deficient bony anatomy, inadequate VMO, or laxity of the medial retinaculum.

Patellar Dislocation

Patellar dislocation is defined as having the patella completely displaced from the femoral trochlea. Due to the valgus Q angle, almost all patellar dislocations are lateral, unless the athlete has had prior patellofemoral reconstructive surgery. Three common mechanisms lead to lateral patellar dislocation. The most common is an external rotation stress, followed by valgus force, and least likely, a direct blow. Dislocation may occur with or without contact.

Clinical Case #5

A 17-year-old high school soccer player injured his knee while playing recreationally with his friends. He thinks he was hit on the kneecap but is unsure. He had previously dislocated this patella at age 15, requiring reduction in the emergency department. He was able to "put it back" with this new injury but had significant pain and rapid swelling. As you examine him the day after the current injury, you note a large effusion, tenderness at the medial epicondyle, and a normal (although limited) ligamentous examination.

Initial patellar dislocation is painful due to tearing of the medial retinaculum in its substance or from its origin at the medial epicondyle. If encountered on the athletic field, the diagnosis is obvious due to the laterally displaced patella. The knee is usually held in some flexion by the athlete. It is appropriate to perform one gentle attempt at reduction on the field, to reduce pain. An early reduction may be much easier than one performed an hour or so later in an emergency department where substantial amounts of sedation may be required. The reduction maneuver is to extend the knee while applying a medially and anteriorly directed force to the lateral border of the patella. If reduction does not occur easily, urgent transport to the emergency department is required.

Routine radiographs are necessary following any patellar dislocation because osteochondral fracture to either the patella or the lateral side of the femoral trochlea may occur with the injury.

Definitive treatment for initial patellar dislocation can be either operative or nonoperative. In athletes who have one or more of the significant anatomic predispositions (Table 15.8), consider relatively early surgery (after joint mobilization and muscle strengthening to reduce the risk of postoperative stiffness). In athletes with anatomic predisposition or previous patellar dislocation, the success of nonoperative treatment is 50% or less, whereas appropriate surgical treatment should have better than 85% success (37). Because the injured knee is usually significantly swollen, it is helpful to examine the opposite knee for anatomic predispositions. If the athlete has normal anatomy, then nonoperative treatment will be successful in at least 75% of cases (38).

The nonsurgical treatment begins with the use of a knee immobilizer for ambulation for several days to weeks, with gradual weaning from the immobilizer as the effusion resolves, strength returns, and motion

Table 15.8. Anatomic Predisposition for Patellar Instability

Excessive Q angle
 Males, >12°
 Females, >14°
Atrophic vastus medialis obliquus
Shallow femoral trochlea
Hypermobile patella
Tight lateral retinaculum

is possible beyond 90° of flexion. Isometric strengthening and range of motion exercises are instituted from the beginning. More aggressive quadriceps strengthening and endurance exercises are added when the patient is free from the immobilizer. Return to athletics is not permitted until the effusion and pain have completely resolved and the musculature is fully rehabilitated. Agility training should be completed before return to athletics, and it is often helpful to use a patellar stabilizing support made from elastic or neoprene for sports.

Patellar Subluxation

Patellar subluxation is the painful shifting of the patella in the femoral trochlea, without dislocation. It is almost always lateral. It may occur as a single traumatic event with a similar mechanism as patellar dislocation. Much more commonly, patellar subluxation is repetitive, following a traumatic injury or more often as the atraumatic sequelae of patellar malalignment.

In the case of an initial traumatic subluxation, even with anatomic predisposition, definitive treatment should be nonoperative, following the program for patellar dislocation. The rate of success in this case approaches 85%. If recurrent patellar subluxation is present and does not respond to the nonoperative treatment regimen presented for atraumatic patellar malalignment, outlined in the overuse section, then consideration should be given to the operative approach.

Meniscal Injury

The menisci have several functions. Most importantly they increase the contact area between the femur and tibia, reducing the stress on the articular surfaces. The menisci are also secondary stabilizers of the joint, contributing to stability when there is ligamentous laxity. The menisci also help to circulate synovial fluid, important for the nutrition of articular cartilage.

As part of the aging process, the water content of the menisci decreases and a gradual weakening occurs. This leads to a decrease in the force necessary to tear a meniscus. A *traumatic* meniscal tear occurs in a normal (or nearly normal) meniscus and will be considered in this section. A *degenerative* meniscal tear is one that occurs with little or no trauma (in an abnormal meniscus) and will be considered in the section on overuse and degenerative conditions of the knee.

Clinical Case #6

A 27-year-old recreational tennis player was injured when he slipped and hyperflexed his knee. He felt a "give" that was not particularly painful and after a few minutes, he was able to continue the match, with minimal discomfort. By the next morning, he had some swelling and was aware of clicking when he climbed stairs. With tennis the next week, he had his knee "give way." At examination several days later, mild tenderness at the posteromedial joint line and pain in the same location are the only positive physical findings.

There are many patterns of meniscal tearing (Figure 15.26). Tears may occur in association with ligamentous injury or as an isolated injury. The most common mechanisms of isolated meniscal injury involve rotation, flexion, or a combination of flexion and rotation. The meniscus is largely avascular and aneural with only the peripheral few millimeters at its capsular attachment having a blood and nerve supply. The large majority of meniscal tears occur centrally in the avascular portion and are often relatively nonpainful when they

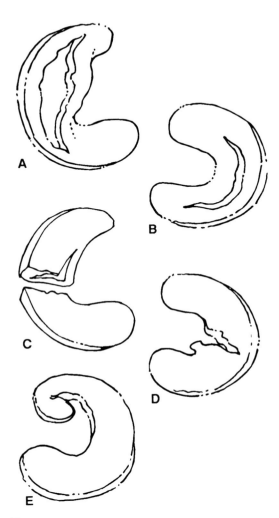

Figure 15.26. Five common patterns of meniscal tearing. *A.* Bucket handle. *B.* Longitudinal. *C.* Horizontal or cleavage. *D.* Radial. *E.* Parrot beak.

occur. Swelling following the tear takes many hours and may not be noticed by the athlete because it may only be a mild to moderate effusion, leading to a feeling of stiffness.

For acute meniscal tears the physical findings are an effusion with joint line ten-

derness over the involved meniscus. Pain at the meniscus (not just diffuse discomfort) with forced flexion is a helpful diagnostic sign. As noted in the section on physical examination, the traditional tests, Mc-Murray's and Apley's, are often not helpful, particularly with an acute injury, because they will be painful with almost any injury. Careful ligamentous examination is indicated.

"Locked" Knee

A "locked" knee is one that has a mechanical block to full flexion and extension, most commonly from a displaced bucket handle meniscal tear. This must be differentiated from a knee that lacks motion due to pain. In a true "locked" knee, there is a springy end point when the knee is gently forced into maximum flexion or extension. When the injury is acute, the athlete may lack 20° to 30° of full extension. After several weeks, the athlete will gain significant motion even if the meniscus remains "locked," and just lack 5° to 10° of full extension and flexion. Whenever a "locked" knee is recognized, early surgical treatment is indicated to limit articular surface damage from the displaced meniscus and to preserve as much meniscus as possible.

Traditional treatment of meniscal tears 20 years ago was total meniscectomy (39). The unfortunate consequence of this was a significant risk of osteoarthritis, which increases with time. Even today's most common treatment for meniscal tears, arthroscopic partial meniscectomy, leads to early evidence of excessive articular surface stress and the risk of osteoarthritis (40). This makes the goal in the treatment of meniscal injuries the retention of as much meniscal tissue as is possible. For those suspected acute meniscal injuries associated with a hemarthrosis, it is appropriate to be aggressive diagnostically, with either early MRI scanning or arthroscopy. Acute peripheral tears have a 90% or better chance of healing (and therefore preserving the entire meniscus) if treated appropriately. Small peripheral tears (1 cm or less in length) will heal nonoperatively if they are stable. Longer, unstable tears often require surgical stabilization to promote healing.

For central meniscal tears in a younger athlete, it is often temptimg to allow the athlete to finish the current season before definitive treatment (arthroscopic partial meniscectomy). This, unfortunately, is not without risk, because an unstable meniscal segment may displace, causing the knee to "lock" or buckle. This may cause substantial irreparable articular surface damage. Even for the athlete in season, we encourage very early arthroscopy with partial meniscectomy (or meniscal repair if feasible) because the athlete may be able to return to sports as early as 2 to 3 weeks after partial meniscectomy. In the chronic state, many meniscal tears will lead to *mechanical symptoms* with locking or buckling. Often an effusion and joint line tenderness are noted on physical examination. Smaller tears, particularly lateral radial tears, do not cause mechanical symptoms, but do give local tenderness and pain.

Several studies have confirmed the accuracy of a careful history and physical examination for meniscal tears. MRI scanning should *not* be ordered routinely, but rather reserved for diagnostic dilemmas. For the younger athlete with a traumatic meniscal tear, especially if accompanied by a hemarthrosis, early evaluation by an orthopedic surgeon is appropriate.

Articular Surface Injuries

These injuries mainly consist of "fractures" of the articular cartilage or osteochondral injuries. This includes osteo-

chondritis dissecans (OCD). When the injury involves only cartilage, a piece of hyaline cartilage is either raised as a flap or broken free within the joint. Rarely, the injury occurs at the "tidemark" (the junction of hyaline cartilage and bone) and a hemarthrosis will develop following the initial injury. More commonly the injury is within the cartilage and no bleeding occurs, only a gradual effusion.

Clinical Case #7

A 26-year-old woman biker comes to your office several weeks after an injury when she landed wrong, coming down a slope in the hills. She felt pain in the knee, but she was able to get home without much difficulty. Since then her knee has not felt "right" and she has had a sensation of swelling. She has a feeling that the knee might give way, but it has not buckled.

Recognizing articular surface injuries is exceedingly difficult when there is no bony fragment. The history is only of an injury followed by swelling. The mechanism of injury may be a direct blow or twist. Mechanical symptoms often ensue with repetitive effusions. Physical findings are nonspecific and routine radiographs are not helpful when there is no bony fragment. In chronic cases, calcification of the loose pieces may occur. This leads to calcified "loose bodies" on radiographs.

If there is no bony fragment, it is appropriate to treat suspected articular surface injuries nonoperatively, with rest, isometric strengthening, range of motion exercises, and observation as the athlete returns to function. If persistent pain, effusion, or mechanical symptoms occur, then surgical treatment is indicated. When a bony fragment is present early, surgical intervention is indicated, because there is a possibility of surgical repair and restoration of the hyaline articular surface.

Osteochondritis dissecans primarily involves the subchondral bone (Figure 15.27). There is a cleavage through the bone, while the articular cartilage remains intact (at least early on). Although the etiology is not clearly established, trauma is felt to be the principal cause. There is also a familial predisposition, perhaps implicating hormonal or local vascular anomalies that contribute to the development of OCD. The basic pathology is a flat to conical area of avascular bone immediately adjacent to the articular surface. In acute lesions there is no separation from the surrounding normal bone. In more chronic cases, a fibrous plane develops separating the lesion from sclerotic bone surrounding it.

Osteochondritis dissecans occurs in adolescents and young adults. Although it may occur anywhere in the knee, the classic location is on the lateral aspect of the medial femoral condyle. The cause in this location is probably from impingement against the medial tibial spine in extension or against the odd facet of the patella in hyperflexion. Rarely is OCD recognized as an acute injury. Typically, the athlete presents with chronic pain, usually activity related. Early on, the articular cartilage (nourished by synovial fluid) remains intact and the fragment does not separate. Later, if the lesion does not heal, the articular cartilage will fracture and the fragment may break free forming a loose body. In the later stages, mechanical symptoms (locking or buckling) will ensue.

The physical findings of OCD are subtle. They include tenderness over the lesion and often muscle atrophy from disuse. With OCD in the classic location, the athlete may walk with the foot in external rotation, to prevent tibial spine impingement against the lesion. Routine radiographs are the

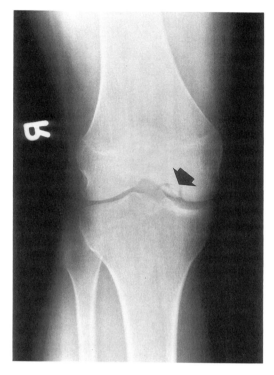

Figure 15.27. Osteochondritis dissecans (OCD) involving the medial femoral condyle (*arrow*).

mainstay in diagnosing OCD. Because the diagnosis cannot be made without x-rays, routine radiographs should be obtained in any athlete with knee pain in whom a diagnosis is not clear by history and physical examination. Often a tunnel view of the knee improves the radiographic visualization of the lesion.

Healing of the lesion should be the treatment goal in all cases of OCD, except where displacement and loose body formation have already occurred. In children, with wide open growth plates, nonoperative treatment is usually successful (unless the lesion has been present for a long period of time). This nonoperative treatment consists of protection, by either crutches or knee immobilizer, and restriction of athletic activity. If, after 4 months, there are no signs of clinical *and* radiographic healing, then surgery should be considered. In the athlete with closed (or closing) growth plates, nonoperative treatment will *not* work and early surgery is indicated. Surgery is directed at promoting healing through drilling or internal fixation of the lesion, if the articular surface is in good repair. Removal of the lesion (or loose body) is performed only if there is no chance of maintaining the articular cartilage. Unfortunately, removal leads to early posttraumatic arthritis.

Fractures

A detailed discussion of all fractures occurring about the knee is beyond the scope of this text. Certain fractures, however, are common in sports injuries and are worthy of discussion. These are tibial spine fractures, tibial plateau fractures, and physeal (growth plate) fractures.

Tibial Spine Fractures

The medial tibial spine, with surrounding articular cartilage, can be avulsed (Figure 15.28). The mechanism of injury is similar to an ACL injury, often being noncontact through deceleration. An immediate hemarthrosis will ensue. These injuries usually occur with open growth plates, although they may occur in teenagers, whose physes have recently closed.

Physical examination is usually limited by the hemarthrosis. If the spine is displaced, then the anterior Lachman and drawer tests will be positive (often with only a subtle increase in laxity, with a "soft" end point). In nondisplaced fractures, there will be no increased anterior laxity.

The diagnosis of a tibial spine fracture requires at least anteroposterior and lateral radiographs, with additional oblique views sometimes necessary.

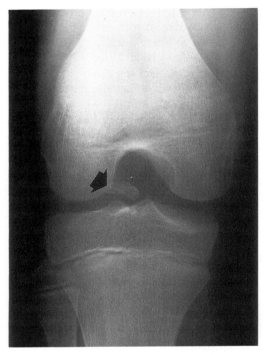

Figure 15.28. Displaced avulsion fracture of the tibial spine (*arrow*). Surgery is required to restore tension to the anterior cruciate ligament.

The treatment of nondisplaced fractures is with extension casting for 6 to 8 weeks, depending on the age of the patient. Displaced fractures must be reduced to restore tension to the ACL. This is sometimes possible by extension casting but often requires surgery. In the child with open growth plates, surgery may be complex to prevent injury to the physis.

Tibial Plateau Fractures

As the benefits of exercise have become widely recognized, older people are participating in athletics, including more strenuous and violent sports. With aging, particularly in postmenopausal women, but to a lesser extent in men, there is a loss of bone mass. This leads to a loss of bone strength. Like a chain, the musculoskeletal system will fail at its weakest link. In the older athlete, this may be with a fracture, as opposed to a ligamentous injury (Figure 15.29). This is particularly true with a valgus injury, where the older athlete may sustain a lateral tibial plateau fracture, instead of an MCL sprain.

The physical findings will be of a hemarthrosis due to the intra-articular fracture, with lateral joint line tenderness. If the fracture is depressed, then there will be some valgus laxity due to the loss of the lateral tibial height. Routine radiographs in this case should include a 10° caudad anteroposterior view and two obliques, to have the best chance to visualize the fracture.

If you have a high suspicion of a fracture,

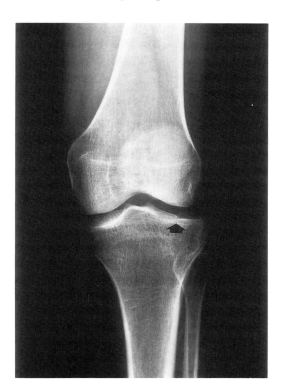

Figure 15.29. Fracture of the lateral tibial plateau (*arrow*).This injury resulted from a valgus stress in a 44-year-old woman skier.

but are unable to identify one with routine radiographs, aspiration of the joint can be helpful diagnostically. If there is blood and fat (from the marrow cavity) in the joint fluid, then a fracture of some kind has occurred, and further radiographic tests (e.g., tomograms, computed tomography scan, or bone scan) is warranted.

The treatment of tibial plateau fractures may be operative if they are significantly displaced or depressed, or nonoperative with immobilization and the use of crutches if displacement/depression is minimal. Assessment by an orthopedic surgeon is indicated if the fracture is displaced or depressed.

Injuries to the Growth Plate

Through the principle of "weak link failure," a child exposed to trauma at the knee may injure the growth plate. Where the cartilage of the growth plate becomes calcified, before it is remodeled to bone, is called the zone of provisional calcification. This is the weak link in a child's musculoskeletal system and a point of potential failure.

At the knee, the distal femoral physis is most at risk for injury. This is because the MCL spans the tibial physis and, therefore, protects it. The femoral origin of the MCL is distal to the physis. With less support, it is exposed to greater forces.

In a child with potentially open growth plates (14 or less in a boy and 12 or less in a girl) and tenderness over the femoral physis following injury, it is prudent to x-ray the knee, prior to performing a vigorous ligamentous examination. Any widening or displacement of the growth plate indicates a physeal fracture. Tenderness localized to the growth plate should be assumed to indicate a nondisplaced physeal injury, and immobilization for 3 to 4 weeks is indicated. Stress x-rays are not indicated because further injury to the physis is possible.

Treatment of physeal fractures requires

anatomic alignment and displaced injuries may require closed or open reduction. Immediate evaluation by an orthopedic surgeon is appropriate if a physeal fracture is displaced.

Tendon Ruptures

The patellar and quadriceps tendons are at risk of rupture due to the high forces generated by the quadriceps muscle. These injuries are not common, particularly in the young athletic population. Often, when they occur, there is an underlying metabolic disease, such as diabetes or uremia. Rarely a vigorous, otherwise healthy athlete will rupture either the patella or quadriceps tendon. A complete tear is a major injury with substantial early swelling, pain, and the inability to bear weight on the injured extremity. The mechanism of injury may be jumping, a direct blow, or weight lifting.

The diagnosis is confirmed by physical examination. The athlete is unable to straight leg lift or extend the knee against gravity. When the patellar tendon is ruptured, the patella migrates several centimeters proximally, and a defect can be palpated in the tendon through the hematoma. When the quadriceps tendon ruptures, the patella will migrate a centimeter or so distally, and the defect will be palpable just proximal to the patella.

Occasionally, a partial rupture of either occurs, but the athlete is unable to straight leg lift, secondary to pain. In these cases the patella will not migrate. A helpful test is to infiltrate the area with lidocaine to alleviate the pain. If a substantial portion of the tendon is intact, then the athlete will be able to straight leg lift with the pain relieved. In performing the straight leg lift test, be sure the athlete does not internally rotate the hip, which will enable him or her to lift the leg using the iliotibial band. Keep the athlete's toes pointing toward the ceiling.

Radiographs are indicated with either partial or complete tendon rupture to ascertain if a piece of patella has been avulsed. A knee splint and crutches as well as icing are the immediate treatment, until early surgical repair can be performed. Complete ruptures require surgery as do substantial partial tears in active athletes. Less substantial partial ruptures, particularly in the nonathlete population, may be treated with protection, followed by gradual rehabilitation.

OVERUSE KNEE INJURIES

The prior section of this chapter dealt with "macrotraumatic" events. These were caused by a single episode, which caused some structure (e.g., ligament, cartilage, tendon, or bone) to fail suddenly. This section focuses on repetitive overuse injuries. These result from "microtraumatic" events—small injuries to structures, which become significant by their number, resulting in chronic injury. This is often accompanied by inflammation, swelling, and pain.

Usually a cause of an overuse injury can be identified. The cause leads to stress on a structure, which exceeds the body's usual reparative processes. Typical causes include anatomic malalignment, which leads to excessive stress; training errors, which push training such that normal healing cannot occur; and aging, which reduces the normal resistance of tissues to injury. Another cause of overuse injury is the gradual scarring, which occurs with many small injuries, leading to inflexibility and the predisposition to further injury.

History and Physical Examination

Because no one episode leads to overuse injuries, certain details must be focused on when addressing these athletes. The onset of the problem is again key. How did symptoms (in the case of overuse injuries, almost always pain) first occur? What activity was the athlete participating in? Was there a change in activity (e.g., change in the intensity of sport or change in sport)? Changes in footwear (shoes getting old or new shoes) can also affect the knee. Finally, are there activities that exacerbate or reduce the symptoms?

The physical examination should not vary substantially from that performed in the case of a macrotraumatic injury, but careful palpation is even more important to identify the injured structure.

Anterior Knee

This is pain anterior to the collateral ligaments in the region of the patella and has often just been called "chondromalacia" by the less experienced examiner, but in actuality includes numerous specific diagnoses. The treatment of each is somewhat different and a careful approach will allow the physician to reach an accurate diagnosis and to proceed appropriately. Almost all anterior knee pain will be aggravated by those activities that increase pressure on the anterior structures, such as climbing stairs or hills, or prolonged sitting with a bent knee (often called the "movie theater sign").

The Patellofemoral Joint

As discussed earlier, some patellofemoral problems (patellar dislocation/subluxation) follow macrotrauma. Much more commonly, patellofemoral disorders result from overuse in the face of anatomic misalignments. These misalignments include lateral patellar tilt, lateral patellar subluxation, excessive Q angle (see Figure 15.8), and excessive quadriceps or hamstring tightness. These misalignments may

lead to one or several clinically separable patellofemoral conditions. These are lateral patellar compression syndrome, recurrent lateral patellar subluxation, true chondromalacia, and patellofemoral pain. It is of value to try to reach a specific diagnosis for every patient because certain subtleties of treatment may facilitate recovery.

In general the treatment of patellofemoral overuse problems in athletes is nonoperative and follows the format initially presented by DeHaven and colleagues (41). That treatment program is formalized and is broken into four phases: 1) symptomatic control, 2) muscle strengthening, 3) graduated running program, and 4) long-term maintenance.

Control of the symptoms is obtained by elimination or reduction of those activities that produce symptoms. NSAIDs are prescribed in dosages that will alleviate inflammation. Icing is used regularly. Physical therapy modalities to reduce inflammation can also be used. Return of flexibility is a major component in this phase, stretching both quadriceps and hamstring muscles.

The muscle strengthening program is one of *isometric* quadriceps and *isotonic* hamstring strengthening. It is begun as soon as pain has abated sufficiently. Performed daily, 5 days a week, the program consists of three sets of 10 repetitions each of straight leg lifts and hamstring curls using progressively increasing weights.

The running program is graduated from jogging, to half speed, three-quarter speed, and then to full speed and cutting. It is *not* begun until the symptoms are controlled, and the athlete is lifting 10 to 30 lb isometrically with the quadriceps, depending on the individual's size.

The final component of the program is maintenance, with strengthening 2 to 3 days a week. It also includes other supplemental measures, such as patella supports or taping, orthotics, and flexibility programs.

With this type of program, more than two thirds of athletes will be able to return to unrestricted sports participation, while only 11% in DeHaven's series were unable to return to some level of athletic activity.

Lateral patellar compression syndrome develops from excessive tension in the lateral retinaculum. Its primary symptom is pain, either on the medial or lateral facet of the patella, or in the lateral retinaculum. The cardinal physical findings are a positive Sage sign and a positive patella tilt test. This condition may coexist with lateral subluxation or true chondromalacia.

The treatment of lateral patellar compression syndrome includes not only our basic rehabilitation program but also stresses patellar mobilization as well as quadriceps and hamstring flexibility (36).

Lateral patellar subluxation may begin without trauma. In such cases it is usually bilateral (although one side often becomes symptomatic first). The symptoms are of "giving way," followed by pain. The giving way often happens with pivoting on the affected knee or with stair climbing. During the time between buckling episodes, the athlete often has patellar pain.

Physical findings in recurrent subluxers often include not only the anatomic predisposing misalignments, but also a positive apprehension sign (see Figure 15.21). Treatment includes our usual program, stressing the dynamic stabilization of the patella by improving quadriceps strength. The use of an elastic or neoprene support, which has a horseshoe pad to stabilize the patella, can be of substantial benefit, both early in the treatment, and also on return to athletics.

Chondromalacia patella describes the specific pathologic entity in which the hyaline cartilage of the patella becomes softened and fibrillated. The cardinal finding is crepitus with resisted extension, either sitting or with a deep knee bend (see Figure 15.13). It may be identified alone or as part of lateral compression or recurrent subluxation. The treatment program for symptomatic chondromalacia should include the treatment of underlying anatomic misalignments. The finding of chondromalacia, unfortunately, implies permanent damage to the joint, and appropriate long-term planning with the athlete is indicated. The athlete should be counseled about this and might consider avoiding activities that strain the patellofemoral joint and substituting less strenuous ones (e.g., switch from jogging to low-impact aerobics).

As a final category, there will be athletes with pain clearly coming from the patellofemoral joint that does not have a clearly identifiable cause. This is most commonly found in adolescent girls but may be found at any age in either sex.

It can be seen with athletes who are overtraining, particularly with activities that create large patellofemoral forces (42). Activity modification and a careful rehabilitation program are the treatments of choice. For the adolescent, once one is sure that there is no other problem, it is appropriate to reassure the athlete and the parents that recovery will ensue, but it may take a long time. The athlete must be diligent in the exercise program.

Athletes with excessive pronation of the feet (see Chapter 18) are predisposed to patellofemoral pain. This is particularly true in females with excessive Q angles and tibial torsion, who often have anterior knee pain. Orthotic shoe inserts to correct the excessive pronation are a critical part of the treatment of these athletes.

In the treatment of patellofemoral disorders, patience and persistence are required by the patient and the physician (43). Recovery is often delayed and continued conservative treatment should be followed for a minimum of 4 months before considering a surgical approach. In athletes failing to improve with a self-directed program or in whom the earliest possible result is desired, working with a physical therapist can be of great benefit.

Although the large majority of athletes with patellofemoral problems will be successfully treated with a nonoperative program, some athletes will continue to have symptoms. Treatment of these athletes should be directed at preventing the development of chondromalacia (41). Recurrent subluxations or persistently painful lateral overload may lead to articular surface damage. If 4 to 6 months of a regularly performed exercise program fails to alleviate symptoms and allows the athlete to return to sports, surgery can be considered (as can the cessation of athletic participation). A number of surgical procedures, both arthroscopic and open, are directed at correcting the underlying anatomic causes of the problem.

Patellar Tendinitis and Related Disorders

A number of conditions can lead to pain in the patellar tendon region in athletes. These include patellar tendinitis, quadriceps tendinitis, prepatellar bursitis, infrapatellar bursitis, Osgood-Schlatter disease, and Sinding-Larsen-Johansson disease. An accurate diagnosis of each condition will allow appropriate treatment.

Patellar tendinitis is often called "jumper's knee" because of its frequent association with jumping sports (e.g., basketball, volleyball, high jumping). It is caused by excessive stress in the patellar tendon (Figure 15.30). The symptoms are of activity-related pain in the tendon, most frequently at its origin from the patella, although they may occur anywhere within the tendon. Physical examination should reveal tenderness in the tendon and occasionally some swelling. A helpful finding is that the tenderness is usually greater when the athlete's knee is extended and lessened when the knee is flexed. Flexing the knee puts the tendon under stretch and the tenderness is harder to elicit. Occasionally, in an acute case, you will be able to elicit a fine crepitus from the tendon sheath as the athlete extends the knee. Many athletes with patellar tendon problems will have tight quadriceps muscles.

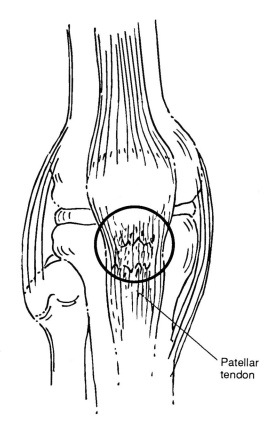

Figure 15.30. Site of inflammation, pain, and tenderness in "jumper's knee."

Patellar tendon

When patellar tendinitis occurs in children, there may be progressive calcification of the proximal tendon (44). This is called *Sinding-Larsen-Johansson* disease. Two thirds of the children who have symptoms of patellar tendinitis will have progressive calcification of the proximal tendon, which will often coalesce with the patella itself to give an elongated distal pole on lateral roentgenograms. X-rays are not routinely needed in an athlete with patellar tendinitis and should only be ordered when the individual does not respond to treatment.

In minor cases of patellar tendinitis, the athlete can continue to participate in sports during treatment. Icing before and after exercise, careful quadriceps stretching, and NSAIDs are the simplest treatment. Several commercially available patellar tendon supports can be helpful in alleviating symptoms. For athletes who do not respond to this simple treatment, the addition of an organized physical therapy program is helpful. This should include the use of ultrasound, transverse friction massage, and a supervised flexibility and quadriceps strengthening program. Strengthening should stress eccentric techniques and be instituted gradually after symptoms have been controlled.

Some athletes with patellar tendinitis will have had a traumatic onset. In these cases, conservative treatment will often fail due to mucoid degeneration at the site of the injury (45). Diagnostic ultrasound (or MRI) can be used to identify an area of mucoid degeneration. Surgical excision of this will usually return the athlete to participation.

In athletes with chronic patellar tendinitis who do not respond to conservative treatment, a single steroid injection can be beneficial. A mixture of long-acting corticosteroid and local anesthesia is injected superficially and deep to the tendon using a 25-gauge needle (this prevents injection of steroid under pressure into the tendon itself). An 18-gauge needle is then used with the bevel parallel to the tendon fibers. Twelve to 15 punctures are made in the tendon to allow the steroid to bathe the inflamed fibers of tendon.

Quadriceps tendinitis is much less common than patellar tendinitis. It is seen in jumping athletes but tends to occur slightly later in life (athletes in their late twenties, thirties, and forties). Symptoms are pain localized to the insertion of the quadriceps tendon into the patella. Treatment is basically the same as in patellar tendinitis, with the exception that if a support is used, it should have a silicon gel donut to encircle the patella.

Prepatellar bursitis also presents with pain at the inferior pole of the patella (Figure 15.31). Although the onset may be a single traumatic blow, it much more commonly arises from repetitive trauma as in wrestling. In acute cases the bursa may be fluid filled. In long-standing cases the bursa will be thickened and areas of chronic scarring will feel like "loose bodies" within it.

The mainstays of treatment for prepatellar bursitis are NSAIDs and protective padding to prevent recurrent trauma. Some acute cases with large amounts of fluid are best treated with aspiration followed by NSAIDs and padding. The aspirate is usually a dark red to brown fluid.

In some cases of chronic prepatellar bursitis, infection may develop from skin abrasion. In these athletes there is a sudden increase in pain, with localized warmth and erythema. Aspiration is indicated to identify an organism and get rid of the excess fluid. Appropriate antibiotics, as well as short-term immobilization, are also indicated.

In the adolescent athlete, swelling and pain at the tibial tubercle are the manifestations of Osgood-Schlatter disease (46). It

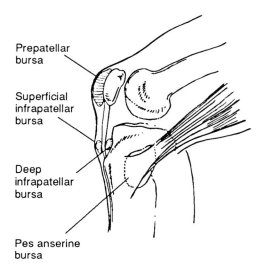

- Prepatellar bursa
- Superficial infrapatellar bursa
- Deep infrapatellar bursa
- Pes anserine bursa

Figure 15.31. The major bursae of the knee. Prepatellar bursitis is the most common in athletes.

typically occurs in athletes aged 9 to 13 years, particularly those who are active at more than one sport. It is more common in boys than girls and is bilateral in about one third of cases. Most cases are insidious in onset.

Physical findings are of localized swelling and tenderness at the tibial tubercle (Figure 15.32). Although the history and examination make the diagnosis, routine radiographs are indicated to rule out possible bone tumors, because this is the age group at risk for primary bone malignancy. The findings on x-ray are increased width of the apophysis of the tibial tubercle or fragmentation of the tubercle.

Treatment of Osgood-Schlatter disease is largely symptomatic. Activity should be reduced to a level that controls symptoms. Many athletes will have to temporarily give up some sports and limit participation to their favorite. Protective padding during, and ice after, athletics can help. The under-

lying pathology is a stress fracture in the physeal cartilage of the apophysis. The disease is usually self-limited and symptoms abate as the growth plate closes (typically by 12 years in girls and 14 years in boys).

In some cases, traumatic avulsion of the tibial tubercle can occur in adolescents who have Osgood-Schlatter disease (47). This typically occurs in a very active athlete with a history of pain in the region of the tibial tubercle. With a vigorous jump or sudden stop there is sudden pain and buckling of the knee. The athlete will not be able to stand or straight leg lift. Swelling about the tubercle develops quickly. The patella will be high riding (more proximal) than the normal side. Plain radiographs will demonstrate the avulsion of the tibial tubercle (often a large fragment). This will require surgical repair. Because the risk of this occurring is small, it seems appropriate to allow restricted athletics in these adolescents until the growth plate has closed.

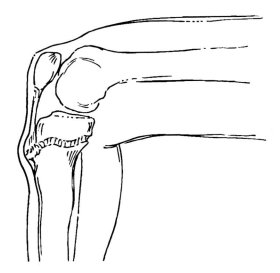

Figure 15.32. Prominent and painful tibial tubercle in Osgood-Schlatter disease.

Commonly, the fragmentation of the apophysis in Osgood-Schlatter disease results in an ossicle in the tendon or the deep infrapatellar tendon bursa after growth plate closure. This results in persistent irritation of the tendon and *infrapatellar bursitis* in the later teens or twenties. These athletes will have a prominent, tender tubercle, and radiographs will reveal an ossicle if present. The nonoperative treatment is the same as in patellar tendinitis. Frequently, however, nonoperative treatment fails if there is an ossicle, and surgical excision of the ossicle usually alleviates the condition.

Hypertrophic Mediopatellar Plica

Plicae are folds that normally occur in the synovium of the knee. Between 20% and 40% of people have a fold in the medial parapatellar area (Figure 15.33), which extends from the undersurface of the medial retinaculum to the fat pad. This is the medial patellar plica, which is exposed to injury with repetitive bending activities, including running, speed walking, or cycling. Much less frequently the medial patellar plica may be injured by direct trauma. Following injury, the plica may become thickened and fibrotic, leading to persistent pain with repetitive activities.

The symptoms of an inflamed medial patellar plica are pain, most often localized to the mediopatellar region, snapping, and marked intolerance to prolonged sitting with the knee bent (which stretches the plica). Rarely will it cause a painful giving way sensation. A hypertrophic medial patellar plica can often be palpated under the medial retinaculum as a band rolled under the examiner's finger (see Figure 15.10). If this is present and the athlete reports this as the source of symptoms, the diagnosis of a symptomatic medial patellar plica is confirmed. Often one will identify

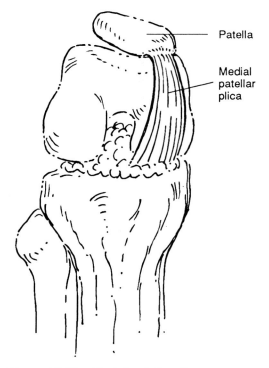

Figure 15.33. Medial patellar plica.

tight hamstrings in a patient with an inflamed plica.

The treatment of a symptomatic plica is directed toward reducing inflammation with icing and NSAIDs, while improving hamstring flexibility. If this fails, a local corticosteroid injection into the plica may help. Rarely is arthroscopic surgery indicated to confirm the diagnosis and remove the thickened band.

Iliotibial Band Friction Syndrome

The iliotibial band is a long tendon, stretching from its muscle of origin at the hip, the tensor fascia, to insert on both the lateral border of the patella, and anterolateral proximal tibia, at a location called Gerdy's tubercle (Figure 15.34). Separating the band from the underlying epicondyle of the knee is a bursa. With repetitive athletics, most often distance running or cycling, the iliotibial band will rub over the femoral epicondyle. This will cause bursitis or tendinitis. Pes planus (flat feet) are a predisposing factor to this in runners. The use of clipless pedals, with cleats that do not allow rotation of the foot, may cause this in cyclists. It is a common cause of lateral knee pain in triathletes.

The athlete will have pain over the lateral epicondyle, which may extend down toward Gerdy's tubercle. This area will be tender to palpation, and often it will feel thickened. There may even be crepitus with flexion and extension as the band slides over the thickened bursa.

The treatment for iliotibial band friction syndrome should include icing, NSAIDs, and correcting any footwear problems. Orthotics are indicated in athletes with flat feet. In athletes who do not respond, a formal physical therapy program of ultrasound, deep transverse friction massage, and stretching (Figure 15.34C) will often alleviate the symptoms. Rarely will a steroid injection be necessary. Surgical release of the iliotibial band can be considered in an athlete who fails to respond to all other treatments.

Other Bursae

Two other bursae about the knee that are not infrequently inflamed are the pes anserine bursa (see Figure 15.31) and the biceps bursa. The pes bursa lies between the pes tendons and the medial collateral ligament, approximately 2 cm below the medial joint line. The biceps bursa is between the biceps tendon and the fibular head, at the insertion of the fibular collateral ligament. Either one can become inflamed through repetitive exercise, causing localized pain, swelling, and tenderness.

Treatment for either pes anserine or biceps bursitis is icing, NSAIDs, and often local physical therapy modalities. The judicious use of local corticosteroid injection can be helpful in treating resistant cases.

Less Common Forms of Tendinitis

Other tendons about the knee may become inflamed in athletics. Included are the popliteus and semimembranosis tendons. These are uncommon and identified by

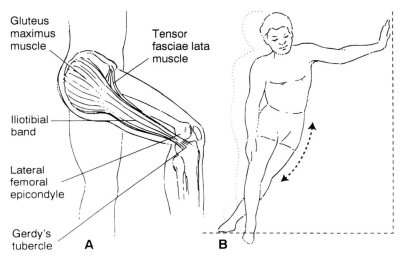

Gluteus maximus muscle

Tensor fasciae lata muscle

Iliotibial band

Lateral femoral epicondyle

Gerdy's tubercle

A

B

Figure 15.34. Iliotibial band friction syndrome. With repetitive extension (*A*) and flexion (*B*), the iliotibial band rubs over the lateral femoral epicondyle leading to a bursitis or tendonitis.

pain at or near these tendon insertions, usually in distance runners. Running hills, particularly downslopes, seems to be an inciting event. The diagnosis must be made by careful physical examination, localizing symptoms to the involved tendons. The general treatment program for overuse injuries is appropriate. Rarely, the differentiation of these conditions from an underlying meniscal tear may be a problem. In these cases, it is best to proceed with a trial of conservative treatment. If this fails, an MRI scan may be helpful in differentiating meniscal from tendon pathology.

Degenerative Joint Disease

We are often confronted with osteoarthritis in athletes in today's population. People are exercising at times when their articular surfaces and menisci have undergone degeneration, either due to previous trauma or aging. These athletes present some special problems, both in diagnosis, and in management.

With degenerative joint disease, there is deterioration of the articular surfaces. This begins as softening and proceeds to fibrillation and loss of joint cartilage. There may also be softening in the meniscus. The resulting cartilaginous debris leads to inflammation in the joint. Secondary changes develop with the formation of osteophytes, thickening of the capsule, and ultimately joint space narrowing.

It is common to encounter an older athlete, who presents with knee pain that follows minimal or no trauma. Clicking or catching sensations are often present. Often the athlete has an effusion or just swelling. Osteophytes may be palpable. Weight-bearing radiographs should be obtained, which may just show spurring (Figure 15.35), but may also demonstrate joint space narrowing (Figure 15.36).

It is frequently difficult to determine if the athlete is symptomatic from the degeneration or from a mechanically significant meniscal tear. The presence of substantial joint line tenderness and mechanical symptoms (buckling, locking, or giving way sensations) helps identify those with meniscal tearing. In the absence of mechanical symptoms, a protracted course of nonoperative treatment is appropriate. This should include reduced activity levels, isometric quadriceps strengthening, NSAIDs, and weight loss if indicated. The presence of mechanical symptoms, or a failure of nonoperative treatment, is an indication to consider arthroscopic or even open surgery (if joint space destruction is severe on x-ray). Arthroscopic treatment can be successful when the joint space remains well preserved. When the joint is extremely narrowed, the success of arthroscopic treatment is limited, but may still be worthwhile in the very active athlete.

Periarticular Cysts

There are three typical locations for cyst formation at the knee joint. The most common by far is the Baker (or popliteal) cyst. Meniscal cysts, from either the lateral or, rarely, medial meniscus, may also be found. Any of the cysts presents as a somewhat painful swelling, which may be firm and rubbery, or soft and fleshy. They can be diagnosed by the feel, their typical location, and transillumination to confirm their cystic nature.

Baker's cyst is located posteriorly in the popliteal space and represents fluid migration into the semimembranosis bursa (the bursa between the semimembranosis tendon and the medial head of the gastrocnemius muscle) from the joint. In 20% to 30% of people there is a connection between this bursa and the joint space, so any intra-

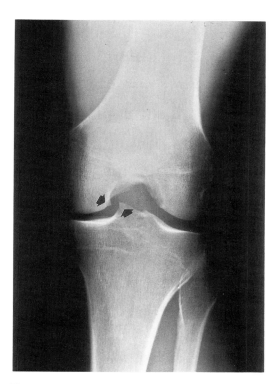

Figure 15.35. Spurring (*arrows*) about the knee indicative of early osteoarthritis.

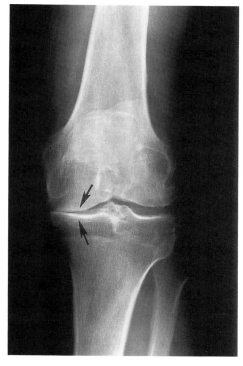

Figure 15.36. Medial joint space narrowing (*arrows*) indicative of advanced osteoarthritis.

articular fluid may accumulate in the bursa. Therefore, any intra-articular condition that causes an effusion can lead to a Baker's cyst. The athlete will usually appreciate this as a fullness or tightness in the back of the knee. The physical findings may be subtle, and palpation of the contralateral knee can be helpful in demonstrating the fullness in the involved knee. If you feel the mass is not typically cystic, ultrasound can be used diagnostically to confirm the fluid quality of the mass, and rule out tumors or an aneurysm. The treatment for a Baker's cyst is to treat the underlying intra-articular condition appropriately, and the cyst will usually resolve or shrink to a point where it is no longer symptomatic.

Rarely a Baker's cyst will rupture, spontaneously or through trauma. This leads to sudden popliteal and calf swelling, with pain, easily confused with thrombophlebitis. Ultrasound is the diagnostic tool of choice to differentiate the two. Treatment of a ruptured cyst includes local ice, stretching, and gradual return to function. Because the synovial fluid can be quite irritating to the soft tissues, NSAIDs are often helpful in speeding recovery.

Meniscal cysts may occur as a result of tearing in the body of the meniscus. This leads to channels through the meniscus that can act as one-way valves to accumulate the fluid in typical locations. Laterally, this is anterior on the joint line, while the medial meniscus cyst is posteromedial. The lateral cysts are 10 times more common than medial. Both are typically firm and rubbery. They vary in size from day to day, often related to activity levels. The treatment for a symptomatic meniscal cyst is arthroscopic surgical removal of the damaged meniscus, which usually results in resolution of the cyst. For cysts not significantly symptomatic to warrant excision, transillumination will confirm the diagnosis, and symptomatic treatment with icing and episodic NSAIDs is helpful.

REHABILITATION

Rehabilitative treatment of a knee injury should begin as soon as the physician sees the athlete for all but the most severe injuries (e.g., fractures, dislocations, and multiple ligament tears). If rehabilitation is delayed, even a few days, reflex inhibition of the quadriceps muscle in a swollen, painful knee will lead to rapid muscle atrophy and prolong recovery unnecessarily. Treatment of more severe injuries can be complex. For less severe injuries, a basic schema of rehabilitation will follow. Included in any rehabilitation program should be components of strengthening, range of motion, endurance, and agility.

Strengthening

There are three basic types of muscle strengthening exercises: *isometric, isotonic,* and *isokinetic*. An *isometric contraction* of muscle occurs when the athlete contracts against an immovable object, so the joint does not move. This is least stressful on the joint. The classic ways to do this in knee rehabilitation are quad sets and straight leg raises as illustrated in Figure 15.37. An *isotonic contraction* occurs when the athlete

moves the joint against a constant resistance, as in lifting a weight. This puts increased strain on the joint due to the shear of the joint surfaces. *Isokinetic contraction* occurs when the muscle moves the joint at a fixed rate, measured in degrees per second. This requires complex machinery (e.g., Cybex, Biodex, KinCom) and can be very stressful to the joint if not used judiciously.

Muscle exercising can be further divided into *closed* or *open* kinetic chain exercises (Figure 15.38). Closed chain occurs with the foot planted, as in a squat or leg press, whereas open chain occurs with the foot free, as in doing a resisted knee extension. Open chain exercises are very effective at isolating a given muscle, but allow unopposed contraction of that muscle, which may not be beneficial, because large stresses

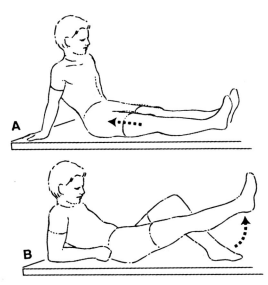

Figure 15.37. Quadriceps set. *A.* Athlete tightens quadriceps muscle and maintains concentration for 7 seconds. *B.* Straight leg raise, athlete lifts leg and maintains straight for 7 seconds.

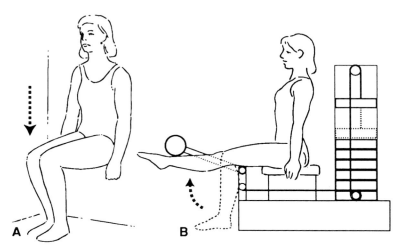

Figure 15.38. Closed kinetic chain quadriceps exercise (*A*) or squat. Open kinetic chain quadriceps exercise (*B*) or knee extension.

go unopposed. Closed chain exercises require co-contraction of opposing muscles, as in a squat, where both quadriceps and hamstring muscles contract. These have recently come into favor as being less stressful to both ligaments and tendons (48). They can also be done with less sophisticated equipment.

Another way to look at muscle exercising is whether the muscle shortens or lengthens while it is contracting. When the muscle shortens during an exercise, as in lifting a weight, this is a *concentric contraction*. When the muscle lengthens during the exercise, as in lowering a weight, this is an *eccentric contraction*. Eccentric strengthening has the advantage of being more effective in strengthening tendons and being helpful in reducing muscle pulls. Routine weight lifting has an equal mixture of concentric and eccentric contraction. It is easily possible to design a program where eccentric strengthening is stressed, by lifting the weight with both legs, and lowering with only one leg.

Any strengthening program type typically involves a progressive increase in the resistance against which the athlete is working. This is called a progressive resistance exercise program.

Range of Motion

Swelling and pain following injury may limit range of motion of the athlete's knee. The necessity of some form of immobilization or protection following injury will exacerbate this. Current thinking is to stress early range of motion following knee injury, using protection if necessary, in any case where motion will not compromise the outcome from the injury. There are three basic range of motion exercises: active, active-assisted, and passive.

In active range of motion exercises, the athlete moves the knee through a range of motion using only the muscles of the injured leg. With active exercises, pain will tend to limit mobilization, which may be good or bad. The inhibition of pain from a recent injury will slow return of motion and give time for healing. On the down side, pain may prevent regaining full motion. Another risk of active range of motion is that the muscle forces may strain an injured ligament and cause stretching during healing. This is most notable with the use of hamstring muscles stressing the PCL in regaining knee flexion.

In active-assisted range of motion exercises, the joint is mobilized by a combination of the muscles from the same leg and another force (e.g., a therapist or the opposite leg). This will improve range of motion more rapidly than active range of motion because the extra push will help overcome stiffness and the inhibition of pain.

In passive range of motion exercises, all force is supplied externally to the injured knee, either by a therapist or the other leg. This eliminates muscle forces that may strain an injured ligament, but must be carefully regulated to follow any limitations on motion.

Endurance

Recovery from any injury for an athlete must include full return of endurance both of the cardiopulmonary system but also the muscles of the involved extremity. Attempts should be made to minimize any loss of cardiopulmonary fitness by having the athlete work out with his or her other extremities from the beginning. This can be done with swimming or upper extremity cycling. Well-leg cycling, using an exercise cycle with a toe clip can also be used. The injured leg is propped out on a chair. This has the added advantage of giving a small, but measurable, effect on the muscle conditioning of the injured leg.

Most strenuous endurance exercises using the injured knee will lead to swelling early after a significant injury and should be delayed until swelling is resolved. With

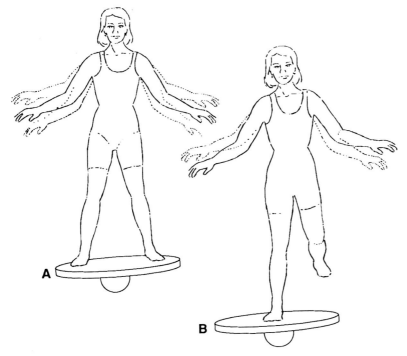

Figure 15.39. Use of balance board for proprioception is beneficial not just in knee injuries, but in any joint injury of the lower extremity.

Table 15.9. Basic Rehabilitation Following Knee Injury

Injury Phase	Protection	Strengthening	Range of Motion	Endurance	Proprioception
I. *Acute*	Knee immobilizer	Quad sets Hamstring sets	Gentle active only	Well-leg cycling	None
	Crutches	Straight leg raises		Upper extremity	
II. *Subacute*: Swelling and pain decreasing	Wean from immobilizer	Straight leg raises	Active and active assisted	Well-leg cycling	One-leg balance
	Gentle compression wrap	Short arc isotonic PREs	Increase as tolerated	Upper extremity	
III. *Recovering*: Swelling and pain resolving	Compression wrap	Increasing arc PREs	Full	Begin gentle cycling, stair climber	Begin balance board
		Stress closed			
IV. *Near full recovery*	Sports bracing, if necessary	Full arc PREs	Full pain free	Aggressive, return to running	Balance board to cutting program with running

PREs = progressive resistance exercises.

modern exercise equipment available, a program can be designed for the athlete that begins with the exercise cycle or rowing machine and progresses to the cross-country ski machine and stair climber, as the knee recovers. Swelling and pain can be used as signs of a too rapid progression. Finally, the athlete can return to running, progressing from a jog, to half speed, to three-quarters speed, and then full speed.

Proprioception

The nerve endings that sense joint position are located in the ligaments, capsule, and tendons about the knee. With injury, joint position sense is decreased and there is a predisposition to further injury (49). Any rehabilitative program following injury should include a proprioceptive re-education program. The program should begin with simple one leg balance, progress to a balance board (Figure 15.39), and involve practice in cutting, starting, and stopping.

General Rehabilitation Program

It is clear that there is no one program to return to athletics after a knee injury

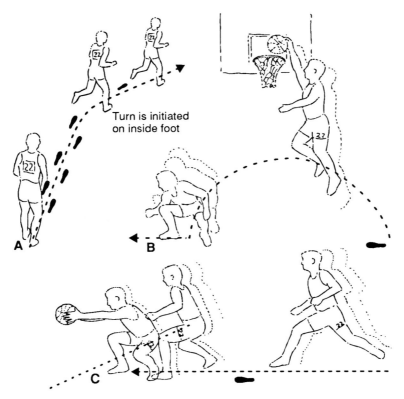

Turn is initiated
on inside foot

Figure 15.40. Prevention techniques to reduce the risk of anterior cruciate ligament injury in sport. *A.* Accelerated rounded turns: player #20 approaches the defender #15 at a slower speed and accelerates off the inside foot to go around the defender. *B.* Bent knee landing: avoid landing and immediately pushing off from an extended knee. *C.* Three-step stop: plan to stop, do not attempt to stop in one step.

because there are so many possible injuries and gradations. However, certain principles can be followed. This will promote early recovery and safe return to athletics.

Table 15.9 is a general outline for rehabilitation from most knee injuries. Icing immediately after the injury and for 15 minutes at least three times per day should continue through the acute phase. This phase ends when the pain and swelling begin to subside. Icing after exercises, which should be performed three times per day, continues through the subacute phase. As the swelling and pain resolve, the more aggressive "recovering" program takes over. If swelling or pain after exercise is a problem in the third or fourth phase, then the intensity or frequency of the exercise should be reduced. Return to athletics is not allowed until the athlete has completed the program.

PREVENTION

No evidence supports the theory that improved strength and conditioning will decrease the risk of knee injury. In fact, the improvement in both strength and conditioning in athletes, which has occurred over the last two decades, has been accompanied by an increase in knee injuries. The late Charles Henning, M.D., from Wichita, Kansas, identified many of the mechanisms of knee injuries, particularly ACL injury. Prior to his untimely death, he devised several valuable methods that can be incorporated into coaching techniques.

The high-risk mechanisms for ACL injury identified by Henning are: 1) the plant and cut, 2) the straight knee landing, and 3) the one-step stop. Each of these is common in athletics and puts the athlete at high risk for ACL injury. To prevent these injuries, coaches, beginning with young athletes, should teach three basic skills. These are: 1) accelerating rounded turns, 2) bent knee landings, and 3) two-step stops (Figure 15.40).

There has been much written about the use of "prophylactic" knee braces for football (50,51). These devices are hinge braces that have been designed to reduce the risk of knee injury. If one carefully evaluates this confusing and contradictory literature, the best interpretation is that the use of prophylactic knee braces in football decreases the severity of collateral ligament injury, but does not affect the frequency of these injuries. The use of prophylactic knee braces does not change the rate of cruciate ligament injuries. Football players, particularly linemen and linebackers, should be encouraged to wear them, and must be carefully instructed in how to apply them. If improperly applied, they can slip down the leg, and lead to ankle injury.

We must all work toward the reduction of injury in sport. This should include rules enforcement, coaching education, and medical care. Safety in athletics is a team effort.

References

1. Keller CS, Noyes FR, Buncher CR. The medical aspects of soccer injury epidemiology. Am J Sports Med 1987;15:S105–S112.
2. Halpern B, Thompson N, Curl WW, Andrews JR, Hunter SC, Boring JR. High school football injuries: identifying the risk factors. Am J Sports Med 1987;15:S113–S117.
3. Wroble RR, Mysnyk MC, Foster DT, Albright JP. Patterns of knee injuries in wrestling: a six year study. Am J Sports Med 1986;14:55–66.
4. Lanese RR, Strauss RH, Leizman DJ, Rotondi AM. Injury and disability in matched men's and women's intercollegiate sports. Am J Public Health 1990;80:1459–1462.
5. Lieb FJ, Perry J. Quadriceps function: an anatomical and mechanical study using amputated limbs. J Bone Joint Surg 1968;50A:1535–1548.
6. Noyes FR, Pekka AM, Matthews DS, Butler DL. The symptomatic anterior cruciate-deficient knee. Part I: the long-term functional disability in athletically active individuals. J Bone Joint Surg 1983;65A:154–162.
7. Noyes FR, Bassett RW, Grood ES, Butler DL. Arthroscopy in acute traumatic hemarthrosis of the knee. J Bone Joint Surg 1980;62A:687–695.
8. Waldron VD. A test for chondromalacia patellae. Orthop Rev 1983;12:103–104.
9. Noyes FR, Grood ES, Suntay WJ, Butler DL. The three dimensional laxity of the anterior cruciate deficient knee as determined by clinical laxity tests. Iowa Orthop J 1982;3:32–44.
10. Slocum DB, Larson RL. Rotatory instability of the knee. J Bone Joint Surg 1968;50A:211–225.
11. Gecha SR, Torg JS. Clinical prognosticators for the efficacy of retinacular release surgery to treat patellofemoral pain. Clin Orthop 1990;253:203–208.

12. Evans PJ, Bell D, Frank C. Prospective evaluation of the McMurray test. Am J Sports Med 1993;21:604–608.

13. Fowler PJ, Lubliner JA. The predictive value of five clinical signs in the evaluation of meniscal pathology. Arthroscopy 1989;5:184–186.

14. Polly DW Jr, Callaghan JJ, Sikes RA, McCabe JM, McMahon K, Savory CG. The accuracy of selective magnetic resonance imaging compared with the findings of arthroscopy of the knee. J Bone Joint Surg 1988;70A:192–198.

15. Glashow JL, Katz R, Schneider M, Scott WN. Double-blind assessment of the value of magnetic resonance imaging in the diagnosis of anterior cruciate and meniscal lesions. J Bone Joint Surg 1989;71A:113–119.

16. Kriegsman J. Negative MRI findings in knee injury: clinical implications. Contemp Orthop 1991;22:549–555.

17. Powell JW, Schootman M. A multivariate risk analysis of selected playing surfaces in the National Football League: 1980 to 1989. Am J Sports Med 1992;20:686–694.

18. Gomez MA, Woo SL-Y, Amiel D, Harwood F, Kitabayashi L, Matyas JR. The effects of increased tension on healing medial collateral ligaments. Am J Sports Med 1991;19:347–354.

19. Laws G, Walton M. Fibroblastic healing of grade II ligament injuries. J Bone Joint Surg 1988;70B:390–396.

20. Indelicato PA, Hermansdorfer J, Huegel M. Nonoperative management of complete tears of the medial collateral ligament of the knee in intercollegiate football players. Clin Orthop 1990;256:174–177.

21. Noyes FR, Matthews DS, Mooar PA, Grood ES. The symptomatic anterior cruciate-deficient knee. Part II: the results of rehabilitation, activity modification and counseling on functional disability. J Bone Joint Surg 1983; 65A:163–174.

22. Daniel DM, Stone ML, Sachs R, Malcolm L. Instrumented measurement of anterior knee laxity in patients with acute anterior cruciate ligament disruption. Am J Sports Med 1985; 13:401–407.

23. McConville OR, Kipnis JM, Richmond JC, Rockett SE, Michaud MJ. The effect of meniscal status on knee stability and function after anterior cruciate ligament. Arthroscopy 1993;9:431–439.

24. Shelbourne KD, Wilckens JH, Mollabashy A, DeCarlo M. Arthrofibrosis in acute anterior cruciate ligament reconstruction. Am J Sports Med 1991;19:332–336.

25. Clancy WG Jr, Ray JM, Zoltan DJ. Acute tears of the anterior cruciate ligament. J Bone Joint Surg 1988;70A:1483–1488.

26. Cawley PW, France EP, Paulos LE. The current state of functional knee bracing research. Am J Sports Med 1991;19:226–233.

27. DeHaven KE, Black KP, Griffiths HJ. Open meniscus repair. Technique and two to nine year results. Am J Sports Med 1989;17:788–795.

28. McCarroll JR, Rettig AC, Shelbourne KD. Anterior cruciate ligament injuries in the young athlete with open physes. Am J Sports Med 1988;16:44–47.

29. Parolie JM, Bergfeld JA. Long-term results of nonoperative treatment of isolated posterior cruciate ligament injuries in the athlete. Am J Sports Med 1986;14:35–38.

30. Keller PM, Shelbourne KD, McCarroll JR, Rettig AC. Nonoperatively treated isolated posterior cruciate ligament injuries. Am J Sports Med 1993;21:132–136.

31. Lipscomb AB Jr, Anderson AF, Norwig ED, Hovis WD, Brown DL. Isolated posterior cruciate ligament reconstruction. Am J Sports Med 1993;21:490–496.

32. Kannus P. Nonoperative treatment of grade II and III sprains of the lateral ligament compartment of the knee. Am J Sports Med 1989;17:83–88.

33. O'Donoghue DH. Surgical treatment of fresh injuries to the major ligaments of the knee. J Bone Joint Surg 1950;32A:721–738.

34. Shelbourne KD, Nitz PA. The O'Donoghue triad revisited. Combined knee injuries involving anterior cruciate and medial collateral ligament tears. Am J Sports Med 1991;19:474–477.

35. Shelbourne KD, Porter DA, Clingman JA, McCarroll JR, Rettig AC. Low-velocity knee dislocation. Orthop Rev 1991;20:995–1004.

36. Fulkerson JP, Shea KP. Current concepts

review: disorders of patellofemoral alignment. J Bone Joint Surg 1990;72A:1424–1429.

37. Cash JD, Hughston JC. Treatment of acute patellar dislocation. Am J Sports Med 1988; 16:244–249.

38. Hawkins RJ, Bell RH, Anisette G. Acute patellar dislocations. The natural history. Am J Sports Med 1986;14:117–120.

39. Sanchis M, Sanchis V, Torres J-I. Long-term results after conventional total meniscectomy: a point of reference. Arthroscopy 1988; 4:206–210.

40. Bolano LE, Grana WA. Isolated arthroscopic partial meniscectomy. Functional radiographic evaluation at five years. Am J Sports Med 1993;21:432–437.

41. DeHaven KE, Dolan WA, Mayer PJ. Chondromalacia patellae in athletes. Am J Sports Med 1979;7:5–11.

42. Messier SP, Davis SE, Curl WW, Lowery RB, Pack RJ. Etiologic factors associated with patellofemoral pain in runners. Med Sci Sports Exerc 1991;23:1008–1015.

43. Sandow MJ, Goodfellow JW. The natural history of anterior knee pain in adolescents. J Bone Joint Surg 1985;67B:36–38.

44. Medlar RC, Lyne ED. Sinding-Larsen-Johansson disease. J Bone Joint Surg 1978; 60A:1113–1116.

45. Scranton PE Jr, Farrar EL. Mucoid degeneration of the patellar ligament in athletes. J Bone Joint Surg 1992;74A:435–437.

46. Ogden JA, Southwick WO. Osgood-Schlatter's disease and tibial tuberosity development. Clin Orthop 1976;116:180–189.

47. Ogden JA, Tross RB, Murphy MJ. Fractures of the tibial tuberosity in adolescents. J Bone Joint Surg 1980;62A:205–215.

48. Baratta R, Solomonow M, Zhou BH, Letson D, Chuinard R, D'Ambrosia R. Muscular coactivation. The role of the antagonist musculature in maintaining knee stability. Am J Sports Med 1988;16:113–122.

49. Schutte MJ, Dabezies EJ, Zimny ML, Happel LT. Neural anatomy of the human anterior cruciate ligament. J Bone Joint Surg 1987;69A:243–247.

50. Sitler M, Ryan J, Hopkinson W, et al. The efficacy of a prophylactic knee brace to reduce knee injuries in football. Am J Sports Med 1990;18:310–315.

51. Grace TG, Skipper BJ, Newberry JC, Nelson MA, Sweetser ER, Rothman ML. Prophylactic knee braces and injury to the lower extremity. J Bone Joint Surg 1988;70A:422–427.

ANKLE INJURIES IN SPORTS

M. PATRICE EIFF

Anatomy and Biomechanics
Ankle Sprains
Chronic Ankle Instability
Peroneal Tendon Subluxation and
    Dislocation
Peroneal Tenosynovitis
Ankle Fractures
Transchondral Talar Dome Fractures
Ankle Rehabilitation

The ankle is the most frequently injured major joint in athletes, representing approximately 10% of all sports injuries (1). Ankle injuries constitute up to 25% of all time-loss injuries in every running and jumping sport (2). The top ankle-injury sports are basketball, soccer, hiking, gymnastics, volleyball, and skating. Ligamentous injuries or sprains of the ankle are commonly encountered by primary care physicians and represent over half of all ankle injuries (1). Other sports-related ankle conditions seen by primary care physicians include chronic ankle instability, ankle fractures, peroneal tenosynovitis, and peroneal tendon subluxations or dislocations.

ANATOMY AND BIOMECHANICS

Three bones make up the ankle joint: the distal tibia, the distal fibula, and the talus. They are bound together by a joint capsule and uniting ligaments that form a functional unit. The ankle is a modified hinge joint. Movement of the ankle mortise, the talus-distal tibia articulation bordered by the medial and lateral malleoli, results in dorsiflexion and plantar flexion (Figure 16.1A). Inversion and eversion of the ankle occur primarily at the subtalar joint, the articulation between the talus and the calcaneus.

Several features of the bones of the ankle

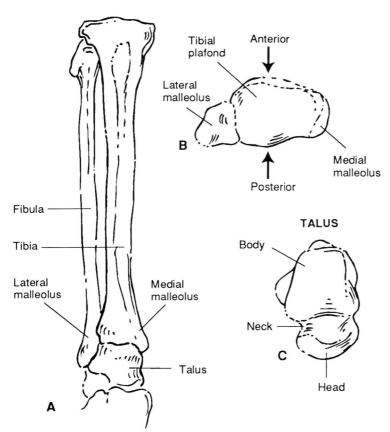

Figure 16.1. The bones of the ankle. *A.* Anterior view of the tibia, fibula, and talus. *B.* View of the underside of the tibial plafond demonstrates its wider anterior dimension. *C.* The corresponding articular surface of the talus.

relate to ankle biomechanics and injury patterns. The inferior surface of the distal tibia, articular and concave, is referred to as the "tibial plafond," or "ceiling" (Figure 16.1B). The talus, covered largely by cartilage, is interposed between the tibia and calcaneus. The talus fits more snugly under the tibial plafond during ankle dorsiflexion (Figure 16.1C). The plafond is broader anteriorly than posteriorly, which results in increased bony contact and stability in the dorsiflexed position. This anatomic relationship between the distal tibia and the talus explains why the plantar flexed ankle has the least amount of bony stability and is more vulnerable to ligamentous injury in this position.

The distal fibula forms the lateral malleolus and changes position to stabilize the ankle mortise in response to weight bearing. The posterior surface of the fibula has a sulcus for the peroneus longus and brevis tendons. A more shallow sulcus may predispose the individual to peroneal tendon dislocation.

The ligaments of the ankle include the medial deltoid ligament, three lateral ligaments (anterior talofibular, calcaneofibular, and posterior talofibular), and the distal tibiofibular ligaments. The deltoid ligament, a thick triangular band with superficial and deep fibers, originates from the medial malleolus and attaches to the navicular, calcaneus, and talus (Figure 16.2). It is crossed superficially by the posterior tibial and flexor hallucis longus tendons. The lateral ligaments arise on the lateral malleolus (Figure 16.3). The anterior talofibular ligament provides stability during plantar flexion. The calcaneofibular ligament stabilizes both the ankle and subtalar joints, especially during inversion. The common peroneal tendon sheath, which originates approximately 3 cm proximal to the tip of the lateral malleolus,

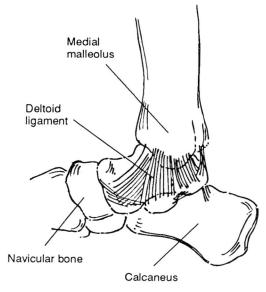

Figure 16.2. The deltoid ligament and its attachments.

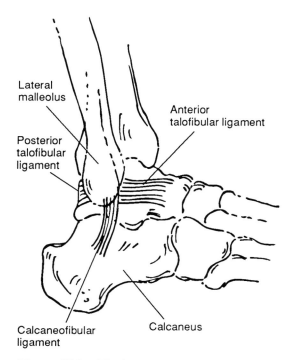

Figure 16.3. The lateral collateral ligaments.

crosses directly over this ligament. The posterior talofibular ligament protects against posterior displacement of the talus but is rarely torn unless the ankle becomes dislocated. The anterior and posterior tibiofibular ligaments, the inferior transverse ligament, and the interosseous membrane bind the tibia and fibula together just above the joint line (Figure 16.4). Together these ligaments form the ankle syndesmosis.

Two important anatomic findings explain why inversion injuries of the ankle are more common than eversion injuries. First, the medial malleolus is shorter than the lateral malleolus, allowing greater talar inversion than eversion. Second, the lateral ligaments consist of three discrete fascicular bundles oriented in different planes and are therefore not as strong as the broad, fanlike deltoid ligament.

Additional stabilization of the ankle joint is provided by the muscles of the lower extremity (Figure 16.5). The primary plantar flexors of the foot are the gastrocnemius and soleus muscles. The tibialis posterior and the peroneus longus and brevis

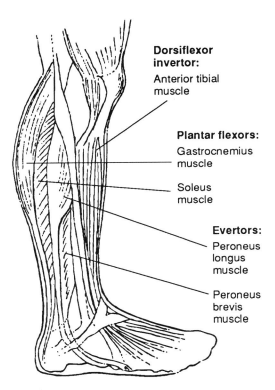

Figure 16.5. The muscles of the lower leg, lateral view.

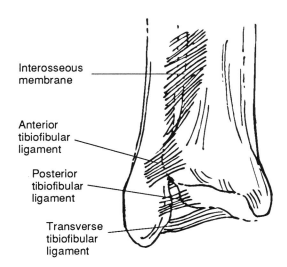

Figure 16.4. The syndesmotic ligaments.

muscles assist in plantar flexion. The peroneus longus muscle is the main evertor of the foot and provides protection against an inversion stress. The powerful tibialis anterior muscle produces dorsiflexion and inversion of the foot.

ANKLE SPRAINS

Description

Ankle sprains are among the most common acute injuries treated in physicians' offices and emergency departments (3). In his study at West Point Academy, Jackson found that one third of all cadets sustained an ankle sprain during their 4 years of study (4). Athletes with this injury lose time from sports and daily activities. Ankle sprains are a common athletic injury in basketball, volleyball, and soccer.

History

In the athlete with a twisting injury of the ankle, it is important to ascertain the position of the foot and the direction of stress to define more clearly the mechanism of injury. Over 80% of all ankle sprains involve the lateral ligaments. A lateral sprain occurs following an inversion injury often with the foot in some degree of plantar flexion. The lateral ligaments are usually injured in succession from front to back: anterior talofibular, then calcaneofibular, then posterior talofibular (Figure 16.6). A medial ankle sprain or injury to the deltoid ligament results from an eversion stress such as when a basketball player comes down from a rebound and steps on another's foot. A less common type of ankle sprain is a syndesmosis sprain, the so-called high sprain. Syndesmosis sprains are usually caused by an external rotation-eversion mechanism, for instance, when a football running back is tackled from the side with his foot in a toe-off position. This mechanism results in injury to the distal tibiofibular and interosseous ligaments.

Following an acute injury, the athlete will experience immediate pain, often a sensation of a pop, and decreased weight-bearing ability. Associated symptoms of swelling, bruising, and a feeling of instability should be elicited. A history of chronic ankle instability or prior ankle injuries or fractures may affect treatment and recovery time.

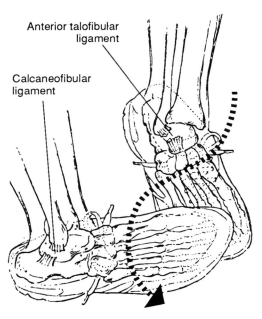

Figure 16.6. Injury to the lateral ligaments of the ankle. A tear of the anterior talofibular ligament occurs following inversion in the plantar flexed ankle. Further inversion force causes disruption of the calcaneofibular ligament.

Physical Examination

An examination done within a few hours of injury can be helpful in localizing specific ligamentous injuries before swelling and tenderness become more diffuse. Although most athletes with ankle sprains do not present to their primary care physician soon after an acute injury, team physicians and emergency room physicians often are the first to assess early injury. As a general rule, the uninjured ankle should be examined first to detect abnormalities in the injured ankle more easily.

The ankle should first be inspected for swelling and ecchymosis. The degree of swelling upon examination is not a reliable indicator of injury severity nor the presence of a fracture (5). Swelling is probably more related to the amount of time from injury to presentation and the patient's actions after the injury. Ecchymosis is often present several hours after injury in moderate and severe sprains.

The amount of range of motion limitation and the athlete's weight-bearing ability are useful guides to the severity of the injury. Active range of motion is most easily tested with the athlete seated on the examination table with both feet together. Plantar flexion, dorsiflexion, inversion, and eversion should be tested in both ankles simultaneously to detect asymmetries. The normal range of motion of the ankle is plantar flexion to 50° and dorsiflexion to 20° (Figure 16.7). Weight-bearing can be tested simply by asking the athlete to stand on both feet, then stand on the injured foot alone, and finally, raise up on the toes of the injured foot. Weight-bearing ability is also grossly assessed by observing the athlete's gait. Marked limitation of range of motion and impairment of weight-bearing ability indicate a more severe sprain.

Following inspection and assessment of range of motion and weight-bearing ability, the ankle should be palpated for areas of tenderness. Examination of the athlete with a painful and diffusely swollen ankle makes localization of the specific ligamentous injury more difficult, but looking for areas of *maximum* tenderness often aids in diagnosis. Following an inversion sprain, the athlete is usually maximally tender over one of the three lateral ligaments. Athletes with lateral ligament sprains often have medial tenderness too, due to the impact of the talus on the medial malleolus during inversion. Increased tenderness over the lateral malleolus or the base of the fifth metatarsal following an inversion stress indicates a higher likelihood of an avulsion fracture in these sites (Figure 16.8). A deltoid ligament sprain leads to marked ten-

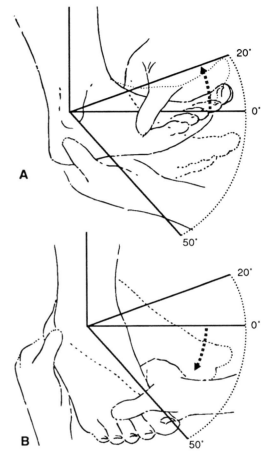

Figure 16.7. Normal range of motion of the ankle. *A.* Dorsiflexion. *B.* Plantar flexion. (Modified from S Hoppenfeld. Physical Examination of the Spine Extremities. Norwalk, CT: Appleton & Lange, 1976: 223.)

derness over this ligament as well as the medial malleolus because an associated avulsion fracture is not uncommon. Maximum tenderness over the anteromedial aspect of the ankle joint and increased pain with external rotation of the foot may indicate a syndesmosis sprain. With any ankle sprain, it is important to palpate along the length of the tibia and fibula to detect asso-

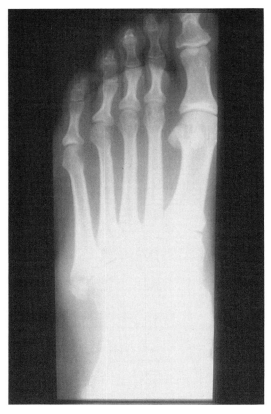

Figure 16.8. Avulsion fracture of the fifth meta-tarsal base at the site of attachment of the peroneus brevis tendon.

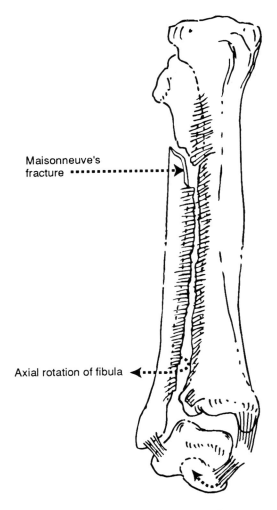

Maisonneuve's fracture

Axial rotation of fibula

Figure 16.9. Maisonneuve fracture. An external rotation force causes a deltoid ligament injury and a fracture of the proximal fibula.

ciated fractures. A fracture of the proximal fibula, called a *Maisonneuve fracture*, may accompany a medial and syndesmotic ankle sprain (Figure 16.9).

The final aspect of the physical examination of the athlete with an ankle sprain is determination of the degree of ligament laxity. Although tests of ligament stability are sometimes difficult to interpret in the presence of pain, muscle spasm, and swelling, valuable information can still be gained. Even if the athlete is unable to relax enough to allow an accurate assessment of ligament laxity, pain elicited with joint stressing usu-

ally indicates that the ligament has been injured.

Two other soft-tissue injuries may be mistaken for ankle sprains, but they can be readily distinguished by physical examination. These are ruptures of the Achilles tendon and rupture of the posterior tibial tendon. Both are described in Chapter 18. The key to differentiating these injuries from ankle sprains is that the location of tenderness and swelling is not over the ligaments. The Thompson test (Figure 16.10) will demonstrate a rupture of the Achilles tendon.

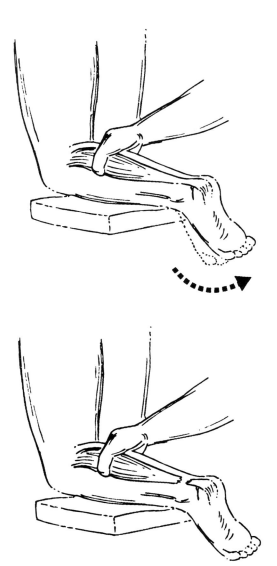

Figure 16.10. Thompson test. (Modified from S Hoppenfeld. Physical Examination of the Spine Extremities. Norwalk, CT: Appleton & Lange, 1976: 218.)

Following a lateral ankle sprain, the relative laxity of the ligaments is tested using the anterior drawer and inversion stress tests (Figure 16.11). The ankle should be in a neutral position and the knee flexed to 90° to perform these tests optimally. The uninjured ankle should be examined first. The anterior drawer test is performed by stabilizing the distal tibia and grasping the heel with the other hand and pulling forward. Significant forward translation of the injured ankle compared to the uninjured ankle indicates laxity of the anterior talofibular ligament. The inversion stress test is accomplished by stabilizing the tibia with one hand and grasping the heel with the other and inverting the foot. Excessive motion with this maneuver indicates laxity of the calcaneofibular ligament. As is the case with any test of ligament stability, it is important to note the degree of laxity as well as whether or not a firm end point is felt. A firm end point feels like pulling on a discrete length of rope, which holds the joint together as opposed to a "mushy" end point, which has more the feel of a rubber band. There are no specific physical examination techniques to detect laxity of the deltoid ligament or the syndesmosis but x-rays may reveal joint widening as a clue to ligament laxity.

Ankle Sprain Grades

Ankle sprains can be classified according to the following criteria:

Grade 1: Minimal stretch or tear of ligament. Mild pain and swelling. Full range of motion. Able to bear weight. No joint instability.
Grade 2: Partial tear of ligament. Moderate pain and swelling. Decreased range of motion. Difficulty with weight bearing. Some laxity on joint stability testing.

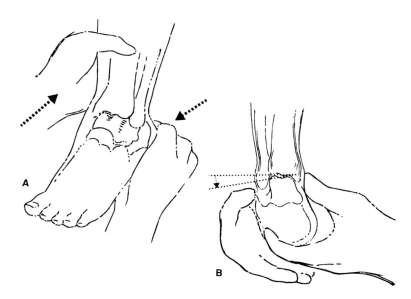

Figure 16.11. Techniques for performing the inversion stress test (*A*) and the anterior drawer test (*B*).

Grade 3: Complete tear of ligament. Severe pain and swelling. Minimal range of motion. Unable to bear weight. Definite laxity on joint stability testing.

Grading an ankle sprain using this classification is most useful in determining the expected length of disability when counseling athletes during their injury rehabilitation. Following early mobilization and supervised rehabilitation of all severities of ankle sprains, Jackson found the average length of disability to be 8 days for grade 1 injuries, 15 days for grade 2 injuries, and 19 days for grade 3 injuries (4). Although not well established in the scientific literature, those with a severe grade 2 or grade 3 sprain may be more likely to have problems with functional instability (sensation that the ankle "gives way") or recurrent sprains.

Diagnostic Tests

Ankle x-rays need not be obtained in all athletes with ankle sprains. Several studies have attempted to establish guidelines for the selective use of x-rays in the evaluation of ankle injuries (5–7). The findings from these studies have not been consistent, but there is general agreement about when it is safe *not* to obtain an ankle x-ray. Young adults with minimal swelling, no bony tenderness, and good weight-bearing ability do not require x-ray evaluation. Individuals over the age of 40 years are more likely to have a fracture following an inversion injury (5). An AP, lateral, and mortise view (anteroposterior with 15° of internal rotation) should be obtained in moderate to severe lateral sprains to rule out associated fractures or ankle instability as evidenced by widening of the ankle mortise (Figure 16.12).

All medial sprains should be x-rayed because these injuries often involve a fracture of the medial malleolus, which is more likely to give way than the very strong deltoid ligament complex. Several weeks after a syndesmosis sprain, radiographs of the ankle joint may reveal heterotopic ossification within the interosseous membrane (Figure 16.13). However, the presence of this finding has not been shown to relate to

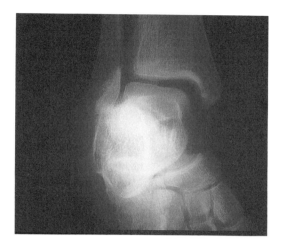

Figure 16.12. Widening of the ankle mortise on the medial side of the joint following a deltoid ligament tear.

ultimate ankle function (8). Stress views of the ankle are not useful in the primary care setting because of the large variation in the literature as to what constitutes abnormal laxity.

Treatment

Despite the frequency of this injury and the potential for significant morbidity, no accepted single method of treatment predominates. Proposed treatments include plaster immobilization, early mobilization, taping or strapping, elastic bandaging, functional bracing, and primary surgical repair. Despite this wide range of treatments, most physicians accept reduced time lost from work and daily activities, ankle stability, and prevention of recurrent sprains as treatment goals.

Most randomized controlled trials of nonoperative management compare immobilization to early mobilization (9–14). Proponents of immobilization emphasize that casting provides enhanced stability and

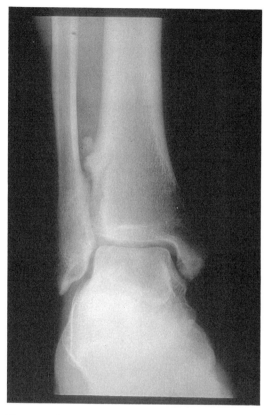

Figure 16.13. Heterotopic ossification of the interosseous membrane following a syndesmotic ankle sprain.

compliance with therapy. Physicians favoring early mobilization cite advantages of early return to function, less muscle atrophy, and better mobility. A growing body of evidence favors early mobilization because it has been shown to get patients back to work and daily activities faster than immobilization without any difference in long-term outcomes (9,10,15).

The acute treatment of ankle sprains is similar to that of other acute athletic injuries—rest, ice, compression, and elevation, or the RICE formula. Swelling is probably the leading cause of pain and may affect the rate of ligament healing. Therefore, measures to reduce swelling should be the primary objective of the initial treatment of ankle sprains. Early application and continuous use of external compression is the most effective deterrent to swelling (16). A U-shaped felt or foam pad around the periphery of the malleolus held in place by an elastic wrap greatly enhances swelling resolution. This form of compression combined with cryotherapy is very effective in the first 48 to 72 hours of ankle sprain treatment. Although many different protocols for cryotherapy exist, a commonly used method is draping an ice bag over the ankle for 20 minutes every 2 to 4 hours. Limited weight bearing and ankle elevation, with the ankle higher than the knee, also help minimize swelling by enhancing venous return. Even though the use of limited weight bearing is helpful, it is extremely important that the athlete maintain some weight bearing with ambulation from the time of the injury. This is best done by having the athlete use crutches and a heeltoe gait. This forces the foot into dorsiflexion with each step, maintaining ankle range of motion and limiting swelling. Wrapping the ankle to make the athlete *non–weight bearing* should be *condemned* because this will lead to significantly increased swelling and limited dorsiflexion. After the acute treatment phase, the athlete should begin ankle rehabilitation exercises (see section on Ankle rehabilitation later in the chapter). It is common for the athlete to have pain in the tendons about the ankle when recovering from a severe sprain. This is probably from edema or hemorrhage into the tendon sheath and responds well to nonsteroidal anti-inflammatory drugs (NSAIDs).

Eversion injuries not associated with fractures can be managed successfully using the same treatment guidelines as for in-

version sprains. Syndesmosis sprains are characterized by a prolonged healing time. In these types of sprains, symptoms of pain and stiffness especially during pushing off commonly persist for 2 to 4 months. For many athletes, these residual symptoms may limit their performance but usually do not prevent participation. Treatment of syndesmosis sprains should focus on ankle rehabilitation, in particular, restoration of pain-free range of motion.

Prevention

Adhesive taping as a protection against ankle sprains is used extensively in athletics. In recent years, more investigation has been done to determine the effectiveness of this practice. Several studies have shown that taping is effective in restricting joint range of motion (17–20). However, its usefulness in providing adequate support of the ankle during competition is questionable considering the consistent evidence that taping loses much of its support after just 10 minutes of exercise (17,21). The true test of the effectiveness of taping lies in its ability to prevent ankle injuries during exercise or competition. In the only randomized prospective study of the effect of taping on ankle injury rates, Garrick and Requa demonstrated that taping decreased the ankle sprain rate significantly in intramural basketball players (22). Taping appears to be more beneficial in preventing injuries in those with a history of prior ankle sprains (22,23).

Because the amount of support afforded by ankle taping decreases substantially during exercise, many athletes, athletic trainers, coaches, and physicians have begun to use functional bracing to prevent ankle injuries. The aim of these braces is to support the ankle without hindering athletic performance. Advantages of functional bracing over taping include: 1) the brace can be independently applied by the athlete, 2) a reusable brace is more cost effective than taping, and 3) bracing avoids the skin irritation caused by adhesive tape. The many braces available to prevent ankle injuries vary widely in their design, cost, construction, and support features.

Unfortunately, the effectiveness of most ankle braces has not been adequately tested. In a retrospective study in football players, ankle injuries occurred less often in those wearing lace-up supports than in those with taped ankles, confirming the advantages of braces over routine taping (24). Only one product, a pneumatic compression brace, has been tested in a large randomized prospective trial. This trial demonstrated the effectiveness of this brace in significantly reducing the ankle sprain rate in over 13,000 injury exposures (25).

CHRONIC ANKLE INSTABILITY

Clinical Case #1

A 15-year-old high school student is seen by her family physician following an inversion injury of her left ankle that occurred while playing basketball 2 days before. She has been able to bear minimal weight and complains of moderate pain and swelling. The athlete reports having sprained this ankle many times in the past. The first inversion sprain was approximately 2 years ago. At that time, x-rays were taken without evidence of fracture and she was casted for 1 week followed by a rehabilitation program and compression dressings. She has remained active in athletics but has had approximately five recurrent sprains since that initial injury, the last one being 8 months ago. She has no symptoms or functional instability with daily activities,

walking on uneven ground, or wearing high heeled shoes. The sprains have all occurred with high-level sports such as soccer or basketball. She wears a lace-up ankle brace during these activities. Examination of the left ankle reveals moderate swelling over the lateral malleolus and maximum tenderness over the anterior talofibular and calcaneofibular ligament. Range of motion is from 10° dorsiflexion to 30° plantar flexion. Assessment of ligament stability shows 1+ laxity with the anterior drawer test and 2+ laxity with the inversion stress test. Peroneal muscle strength is normal bilaterally. The athlete is able to stand on the left foot alone but is unable to raise up on her toes.

Description

The above case illustrates a common problem in athletics. Ankle instability can be described as either mechanical or functional. Mechanical instability refers to abnormal physical examination findings, such as balance deficit, a positive anterior drawer test, or evidence of joint opening on stress x-rays (Figure 16.14). Functional instability is usually described as a sensation of the ankle giving way, particularly on uneven surfaces. Unfortunately, a direct correlation between mechanical and functional instability is lacking. Studies show that those with mechanical instability do not necessarily have a higher rate of functional instability and vice versa (26–28). It appears that instability is a complex syndrome in which mechanical, functional, and neuromuscular factors such as peroneal muscle weakness or proprioceptive deficits may all play a role.

History

Athletes with chronic ankle instability usually seek care for their condition when

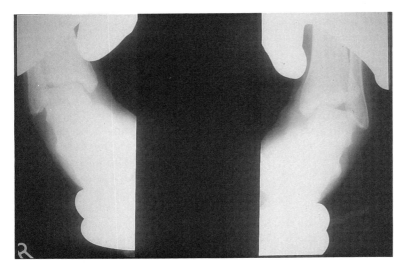

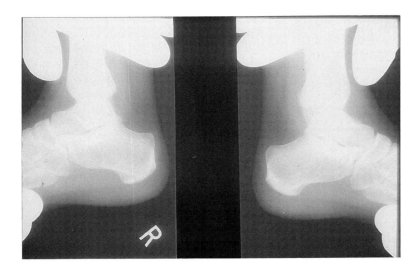

Figure 16.14. Stress radiographs of the ankle. *A.* Inversion stress applied to the ankle causes an abnormal talar tilt following a tear of the calcaneofibular ligament. *B.* Lateral view demonstrates anterior displacement of the talus following a tear of the anterior talofibular ligament.

their performance diminishes or they begin to lose more time from their sport due to recurrent injuries. The problem is usually unilateral. There may be a history of inadequate treatment or rehabilitation for prior injuries because athletes with this problem often self-treat or minimize the extent of injury.

Physical Examination

The athlete with chronic ankle instability usually has some objective evidence of mechanical instability. Laxity on ligament testing is the most common abnormality. Balance deficits and weakness of the ankle evertors are other physical findings associated with instability. Swelling is an inconsistent finding. Individuals who complain of functional instability may have a normal ankle examination.

Treatment

Most patients with chronic ankle instability (even those with mechanical laxity) should have a trial of rehabilitation and taping or functional bracing. To begin, the rehabilitative program should be directed toward obtaining a full range of motion of the ankle and subtalar joint. The main thrust of rehabilitation is detailed in the Ankle Rehabilitation section of this chapter and is directed toward strengthening and proprioceptive training.

Consideration for surgical joint reconstruction should be given for any athlete who continues to have functional instability after rehabilitation. Factors that should be considered in treatment decisions include the ongoing demands placed on the ankle during sports, prior success with rehabilitation, compliance and comfort with functional braces, and future exercise or sport involvement. Consultation with an orthopedic surgeon is advisable so that the athlete can be advised of the option of reconstructive surgery.

PERONEAL TENDON SUBLUXATION AND DISLOCATION

Description

The incidence of peroneal tendon dislocation varies in the literature. Although this injury was first reported in a ballet dancer, it occurs in several sports and represents slightly less than 1% of lower extremity injuries in skiers (29). The exact mechanism of

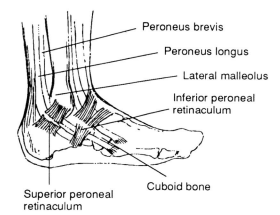

Figure 16.15. Three regions of stenosis of the peroneal tendons at sites of increased stress: (*1*) posterior to the lateral malleolus at the peroneal sulcus; (*2*) overlying the peroneal tubercle; and (*3*) under the cuboid as the peroneus longus tendon courses under it.

injury responsible for this injury is still controversial. Most agree that it involves a sudden, forceful dorsiflexion force at the ankle with a simultaneous powerful contraction of the peroneal muscles leading to a tear of the superior peroneal retinaculum (Figure 16.15). It occurs in both the inverted and everted foot. A flat or convex posterior distal surface of the fibula instead of a well-formed retromalleolar groove may predispose individuals to peroneal subluxation or dislocation.

History

A typical presentation for an acute tendon dislocation might be a skier who reports falling forward after catching a ski tip in the snow. A snapping sensation accompanied by pain felt in the posterior lateral ankle is often reported. Many individuals with this injury present weeks to months after the initial injury. They give a history of recurrent inversion injuries associated with pain and snapping in the area of the peroneal tendons and a feeling of instability.

Physical Examination

After an acute peroneal tendon dislocation, moderate swelling and ecchymosis are usually present in the lateral malleolar area. Maximum tenderness is felt posterior and superior to the lateral malleolus in contrast to an inversion ankle sprain, which causes tenderness over the lateral ligaments. Resisted dorsiflexion with eversion causes increased retromalleolar pain. The peroneal tendons generally relocate after the injury so when trying to diagnose this condition, an attempt should be made to redislocate them. This is especially important in the athlete with a history consistent with recurrent subluxation. The dislocation procedure is performed by dorsiflexion and eversion of the foot against resistance. After this maneuver, the tendons can be palpated lateral and anterior to the fibula and will spontaneously reduce when the foot is released.

Diagnostic Tests

An x-ray of the ankle following an acute peroneal tendon dislocation may reveal an avulsed cortical fracture of the peroneal groove. The presence of this finding may not alter therapy significantly unless the avulsed fragment is large and markedly displaced.

Treatment

The optimal treatment for this injury is undetermined. Operative and nonoperative therapies have been used with varying degrees of success. In the case of an athlete with a chronic symptomatic subluxating peroneal tendon, surgical repair is usually required. Several surgical approaches have been developed to hold the peroneal tendons in place including rerouting the tendons, constructing a new retinaculum, or deepening the peroneal groove on the lateral malleolus.

PERONEAL TENOSYNOVITIS

Clinical Case #2

A 36-year-old woman comes in for evaluation of right ankle pain. Her symptoms began 2 months ago following an ankle sprain. Initially she had good resolution of most symptoms following the injury but has continued to have recurrent pain. The pain is felt on the lateral aspect of the foot, anterior to the malleolus, and is described as an aching pain that waxes and wanes in intensity. She has noticed occasional mild swelling. Her symptoms became bothersome enough that she was unable to perform her usual work duties of operating a foot pedal on a sewing machine. She has been taking ibuprofen occasionally with some relief. Examination of the right ankle reveals no swelling or ecchymosis. Range of motion is from 20° dorsiflexion to 50° plantar flexion. There is increased pain with inversion. Moderate tenderness is noted anterior and inferior to the lateral malleolus. The ankle is stable to ligament testing. The patient walks with a slight limp favoring the right ankle.

Description

Tenosynovitis of the peroneal tendons is usually secondary to stenosis of the tendon sheath at regions of increased stress around fixed pulleys. This occurs in three anatomic sites: 1) posterior to the lateral malleolus at the peroneal groove; 2) at the peroneal tubercle on the lateral calcaneus; and 3) at the undersurface of the cuboid where the peroneus longus tendon passes. Stress in these areas leads to microtrauma and subsequent inflammation.

The two most common mechanisms resulting in peroneal tenosynovitis are chronic mechanical overuse and trauma such as inversion ankle injuries, lateral malleolar fractures, and calcaneal fractures. This condition occurs more commonly in athletes who participate in running sports, dance, or gymnastics. Overuse of the peroneal tendons occurs following training errors such as a sudden increase in running distance, speed, or sprinting. Athletes with cavus feet or bowlegs, who tend to run on the lateral aspects of their feet are predisposed to this condition. Direct pressure on the peroneal tendons secondary to ill-fitting shoe wear may also cause inflammation. A possible anatomic etiology leading to this condition is a congenital enlargement of the peroneal tubercle.

History

Typically, individuals with peroneal tenosynovitis report pain and swelling inferior to the lateral malleolus. Those with a history of prior ankle trauma relate symptoms that have not resolved since their initial injury. The chronicity of the symptoms is what distinguishes this condition from a ligamentous injury. If there is no history of trauma, the individual should be questioned about activities leading to repetitive microtrauma.

Physical Examination

Physical examination of the individual with peroneal tenosynovitis reveals an antalgic gait, limited subtalar joint motion, and point tenderness over the area of tendon stenosis. There may be associated swelling along the inflamed tendon sheath or, in the absence of edema, a thickened peroneal sheath may be palpable. Pain is often exacerbated by forced plantar flexion and inversion.

Treatment

The initial treatment of this condition consists of decreased activity (non–weight bearing, if severe), ice, and oral NSAIDs. Once the swelling and pain subside, the athlete should begin a rehabilitation program emphasizing peroneal strengthening exercises (see Ankle Rehabilitation section). Gradual return to activity is advisable. A lateral heel wedge may be helpful to relieve tension on the peroneal tendons. Steroid injections may be helpful but are rarely necessary.

ANKLE FRACTURES

In the evaluation of any traumatic or twisting injury to the ankle, a fracture of the fibula, tibia, or talus must be considered in the differential diagnosis. In general, fractures resulting from avulsion forces are transverse and fractures due to talar impact against the malleoli are oblique. Rotatory forces produce a spiral fracture pattern. In reviewing radiographs for fractures, the examiner should look for the following: 1) presence of a transverse distal malleolar fracture indicating avulsion of the corresponding ligament, 2) type and level of a fibula fracture, and 3) any displacement of the talus in the mortise. The clear space between the talus and the lateral malleolus, distal tibia, and medial malleolus should be equal. For a talar shift to occur, there must be a ligamentous injury or fracture in two places around the ankle joint (Figure 16.16).

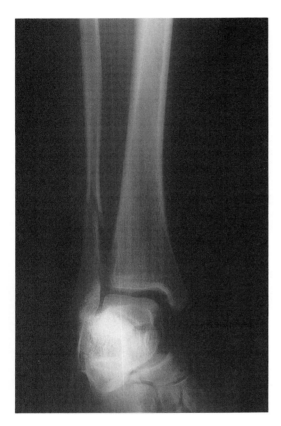

Figure 16.16. An unstable ankle following an eversion injury. A tear of the deltoid ligament combined with a fibular fracture disrupts the ankle joint in two places resulting in a shift of the mortise.

A number of classification systems have been developed to categorize ankle fractures based on the mechanism of injury or the level of the fracture of the fibula. The two most widely used are the Lauge-Hansen and Danis-Weber classifications. These classification schemes generally assist the orthopedic surgeon in comparing the results of treating similar injuries and predicting outcomes.

Isolated fractures can usually be man-aged nonoperatively if they are non-displaced and involve the distal portion of the malleolus. Very small avulsion fractures represent ligament injuries and do not re-quire casting and do quite well with func-tional bracing for support and early mobilization combined with ankle rehabili-tation. Nondisplaced, distal fibular frac-tures are usually stable and should be treated with a short leg walking cast for 4 to 6 weeks. A more detailed description of the evaluation and management of ankle frac-tures can be found in a standard orthopedic textbook (30).

TRANSCHONDRAL TALAR DOME FRACTURES

Description

Prolonged pain following an inversion injury of the ankle should raise suspicion of a transchondral talar dome fracture. These fractures often go unrecognized because the initial radiographs are negative or difficult to interpret. Approximately 6.5% of all ankle sprains are associated with transchondral fractures of the talar dome (31).

Inversion injuries cause most talar dome fractures and they usually occur on the anterolateral or posteromedial aspect of the talus. Anterolateral fractures result from an inversion dorsiflexorion force and posteromedial fractures occur following inversion of the plantar flexed ankle. Transchondral fractures are classified according to their severity: stage I—com-pression; stage II—attached, nondisplaced fragment; stage III—detached, nondis-placed fragment; stage IV—displaced frag-ment (Figure 16.17).

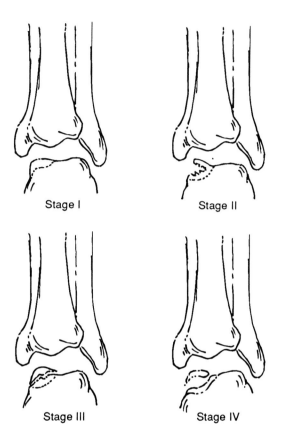

Figure 16.17. Four stages of transchondral talar dome fractures. Stage I—compression. Stage II—attached nondisplaced fragment. Stage III—detached nondisplaced fragment. Stage IV—detached displaced fragment.

History

The symptoms of a transchondral talar fracture can be nonspecific. The athlete may report stiffness, limitation of ankle joint motion, clicking, swelling, and pain with activity. The duration of symptoms before diagnosis may be several weeks to months. The severity of symptoms usually correlates with the severity (staging) of the lesion.

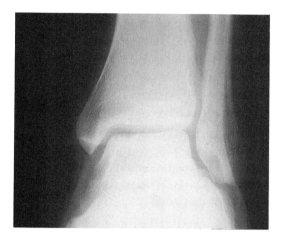

Figure 16.18. Transchondral talar dome fracture.

Physical Examination

There are no pathognomonic signs of a talar dome fracture. Findings consistent with the diagnosis include point tenderness in the area of the fracture, decreased range of motion, crepitus, and effusion.

Diagnostic Tests

Standard ankle radiographs should be obtained in any athlete who presents with persistent pain several weeks after an inversion ankle injury (Figure 16.18). If plain films are negative, a bone scan is highly sensitive in detecting talar dome lesions. If the bone scan is positive, a magnetic resonance imaging or computed tomography scan is often done to assist the orthopedic surgeon in determining the exact location, extent, and stage of the lesion (32).

Treatment

The symptoms and radiographic stage of the talar dome fracture determine treatment and prognosis. The vast majority of symptomatic stage I and II fractures respond well to conservative treatment of decreased activity, limited weight bearing, or immobilization. If symptoms persist or progress after 4 to 6 months of conservative therapy, surgical options such as excising the fragment or curettage or drilling of the subchondral bone should be considered. Best results are obtained by early operative treatment of stage III and IV talar lesions. Arthroscopy is becoming an increasingly helpful tool in the management of these fractures.

ANKLE REHABILITATION

The goals of ankle rehabilitation are to: 1) restore normal range of motion, strength, and proprioception; 2) decrease recovery time; 3) decrease morbidity such as functional instability, pain, and swelling; 4) prevent further injury or recurrent injury; and 5) maintain cardiovascular fitness level.

Ankle rehabilitation should include elements of flexibility, strength, coordination, and aerobic training.

Restoring normal ankle range of motion is the first step in a successful ankle rehabilitation program. As soon as pain permits, usually in the first 24 to 48 hours, the athlete should begin range of motion exercises. Partial weight-bearing ambulation with a heel-toe gait is begun immediately. The athlete should never be treated with non–weight bearing. Emphasis should be on regaining normal dorsiflexion and plantar flexion first. The "alphabet exercise," which is performed by tracing each letter of the alphabet in the air with the big toe, is a simple and useful way to improve range of motion in all directions. Performing this exercise in the supine position with the leg elevated helps mobilize local edema. During this initial rehabilitation phase, calf muscle stretching is also important to maintain muscle flexibility. Specific exercises to stretch the gastrocnemius and soleus muscles will assist in restoring ankle dorsiflexion (Figure 16.19).

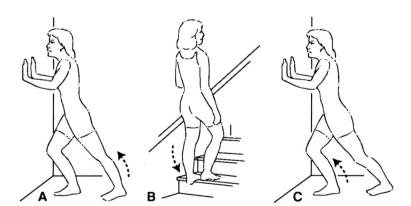

Figure 16.19. Calf muscle stretching exercises. *A.* Gastrocnemius muscle stretch performed with the rear knee straight. *B.* Another gastrocnemius stretch done with one or both heels overhanging a step. Body weight is supported on the front of the foot while steady downward pressure is applied. *C.* Soleus muscle stretch performed in the same manner as the gastrocnemius stretch except the rear knee is bent.

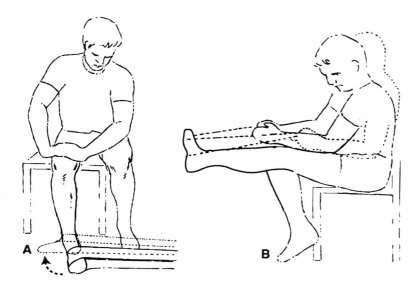

Figure 16.20. Use of an elastic band or surgical tubing to perform ankle strengthening exercises.

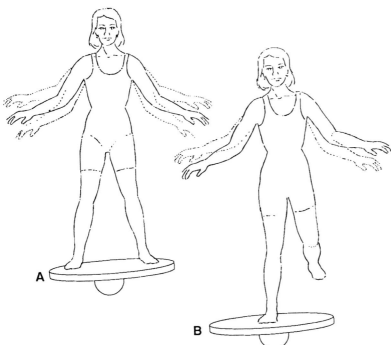

Figure 16.21. Balance board for proprioceptive training. The athlete should begin with two feet and progress to one foot centered over the half sphere.

Once the athlete has achieved near-normal range of motion, exercises to strengthen the muscles of the lower extremity should be started. Surgical tubing or some other elastic material can be used to provide resistance as the athlete performs range of motion exercises (Figure 16.20). Because the peroneal muscles are very important in overall ankle function and stability, emphasis should be on strengthening these muscles through resistance of ankle eversion. Heel and toe walking are additional ways to strengthen the calf muscles.

Following an ankle sprain, balance is often impaired even when range of motion and strength are normal. This can be assessed by comparing the athlete's ability to balance first on the uninjured foot alone, and then on the injured foot, with the eyes open and closed. A balance deficit results from disruption of the proprioceptive nerve receptors contained in the ligaments and joint capsule. Proprioception or balance training in athletes with chronic instability has been shown to decrease symptoms of functional instability and decrease the rate of reinjury (33,34). Proprioception training is usually performed with the use of a wobble board, a flat surface with a half sphere or perpendicular board attached (Figure 16.21). If this device is not available, the athlete can practice balancing on an uneven surface such as a folded-over pillow. The addition of a simple proprioceptive training program following lateral ankle sprains can reduce the incidence of functional instability from nearly 50% to less than 10%. Coordination drills such as rope skipping, running circles, zig-zags, and ahead and backward running should be started when balance is restored and the athlete has no feeling of instability. Progressive return to sport-specific agility drills will further prepare the athlete for return to competition.

Aerobic activities such as swimming or stationary biking or rowing will help the athlete maintain cardiovascular fitness during ankle rehabilitation.

References

1. Garrick JG, Requa RK. The epidemiology of foot and ankle injuries in sports. Clin Sports Med 1988;7:29–36.

2. Mack RP. Ankle injuries in athletics. Clin Sports Med 1982;1:71–84.

3. Maehlum S, Daljord OA. Acute sports injuries in Oslo—a one year study. Br J Sport Med 1984;18:181–185.

4. Jackson DW, Ashley RL, Powell JW. Ankle sprains in young athletes: relation of severity and disability. Clin Orthop 1974;101:201–215.

5. Sujitkumar P, Hadfield JM, Yates DW. Sprain or fracture? An analysis of 2000 ankle injuries. Arch Emerg Med 1986;3:101–106.

6. Stiell IG, Greenberg GH, McKnight RD, et al. Decision rules for the use of radiography in acute ankle injuries. JAMA 1993;269:1127–1132.

7. Dunlop MG, Beattie TF, White GK, Raab GM, Doull RI. Guidelines for selective radiological assessment of inversion ankle injuries. Br Med J 1986;293:603–605.

8. Taylor DC, Englehardt DL, Bassett FH. Syndesmosis sprains of the ankle: the influence of heterotopic ossification. Am J Sports Med 1992;20:146–150.

9. Konradsen L, Holmer P, Sondergaard L. Early mobilizing treatment for grade III ankle ligament injuries. Foot Ankle 1991;2:69–73.

10. Korkala O, Rusanen M, Jokipii P, Kytomaa J, Avikainen V. A prospective study of the treatment of severe tears of the lateral ligament of the ankle. Int Orthop 1987;11:13–17.

11. Brakenbury PH, Kotowski J. A comparative study of the management of ankle sprains. Br J Clin Pract 1983;37:181–185

12. Brooks SC, Potter BT, Rainey JB. Treatment for partial tears of the lateral ligament of

the ankle: a prospective trial. Br Med J 1981;282:606–607.

13. Caro D, Craft IL, Howells JB, Shaw PC. Diagnosis and treatment of injury of lateral ligament of the ankle joint. Lancet 1964;2:720–723.

14. van den Hoogenband CR, van Moppes FI, Coumans PF, Stapert JW, Greep JM. Study on clinical diagnosis and treatment of lateral ligament lesions of the ankle joint. Int J Sports Med 1984;5(suppl):159–161.

15. Linde F, Hvass I, Jurgensen U, Madsen F. Early mobilizing treatment in lateral ankle sprains. Scand J Rehab Med 1986;18:17–21.

16. Wilkerson GB. Treatment of the inversion ankle sprain through synchronous application of focal compression and cold. JNATA 1991;26:220–237.

17. Gross MT, Bradshaw MK, Ventry LC, Weller KH. Comparison of support provided by ankle taping and semirigid orthosis. J Orthop Sports Phys Ther 1987;9:33–39.

18. Fumich RM, Ellison AE, Guerin GJ, Grace PD. The measured effect of taping on combined foot and ankle motion before and after exercise. Am J Sports Med 1981;9:165–170.

19. Myburgh KH, Vaughan CL, Isaacs SK. The effects of ankle guards and taping on joint motion before, during and after a squash match. Am J Sports Med 1984;12:441–446.

20. Greene TA, Hillman SK. Comparison of support provided by a semirigid orthosis and adhesive ankle taping before, during and after exercise. Am J Sports Med 1990;18:498–506.

21. Rarick GL, Bigley G, Karst R, Malina RM. The measurable support of the ankle joint by conventional methods of taping. J Bone Joint Surg 1962;44A:1183–1190.

22. Garrick JG, Requa RK. Role of external support in the prevention of ankle sprains. Med Sci Sports 1973;5:200–203.

23. Firer P. Effectiveness of taping for the pre-vention of ankle ligament sprains. Br J Sports Med 1990;24:47–50.

24. Rovere GD, Clarke TJ, Yates CS, Burley K. Retrospective comparison of taping and ankle stabilizers in preventing ankle injuries. Am J Sports Med 1988;16:228–233.

25. Sitler MR. The efficacy of a semi-rigid ankle brace to reduce acute ankle injuries in basketball: a randomized clinical study at West Point. American Orthopedic Society for Sports Medicine, 18th Annual Meeting, San Diego, 1992. Abstract.

26. Staples OS. Result study of ruptures of lateral ligaments of the ankle. Clin Orthop 1972;85:50–58.

27. Cetti R. Conservative treatment of injury to the fibular ligament of the ankle. Br J Sports Med 1982;16:47–52.

28. Freeman MAR. Instability of the foot after injuries to the lateral ligament of the ankle. J Bone Joint Surg 1965;47B:669–677.

29. Trevino S, Baumhauer JF. Tendon injuries of the foot and ankle. Clin Sports Med 1992;11:727–739.

30. Rockwood CA, Green DP, Bucholz RW, eds. Rockwood and Green's fractures in adults, 3rd ed. Philadelphia: JB Lippincott, 1991.

31. Flick AB, Gould N. Osteochondritis dissecans and the talus (transchondral fractures of the talus): review of literature and new surgical approach for medial dome lesions. Foot Ankle 1985;5:165–185.

32. Shea MP, Manoli A. Recognizing talar dome lesions. Physician Sports Med 1993;21:109–121.

33. Freeman MR, Dean ME, Hanham IF. The etiology and prevention of functional instability of the foot. J Bone Joint Surg [Br] 1965;47:678–685.

34. Tropp H, Askling C, Gillquist J. Prevention of ankle sprains. Am J Sports Med 1985;13:259–262.

INJURIES OF THE LOWER LEG, BETWEEN THE KNEE AND ANKLE

17

RICHARD M. WILK

Anatomy
History
Risk Factors
Physical Examination
Diagnostic Studies
Treatment
Medial Tibial Stress Syndrome
Stress Fractures
Compartment Syndrome
Gastrocnemius Muscle Tears
Exercise

When dealing with sports injuries, clinicians have to understand the concept of overuse injuries—that is, injuries that result from repetitive stress to an anatomic region. With overuse injuries, the body is unable to adapt to the stresses of a particular activity, and as a result, symptoms of pain develop that interfere with the athlete's performance.

Most problems involving the lower leg are secondary to overuse. These injuries are the sequelae of the forces acting on the bony and soft-tissue structures during walking, running, and jumping activities. Athletes of all ages can experience overuse injuries because they often result from improper training methods, improper equipment, or an underlying biomechanical abnormality.

Acute injuries of the lower leg are usually of a more severe nature and include fractures of the tibial or fibular shafts, bone or muscle contusions, muscle tears, and traumatic acute compartment syndrome. Chronic or overuse injuries are represented by medial tibial stress syndrome ("shin splints"), stress fractures, and exercise-induced (chronic) compartment syndromes. This chapter focuses on the more common overuse injuries of the lower leg.

ANATOMY

The lower leg refers to the area of the lower extremity between the knee and ankle (1). The two long bones in the lower leg are the tibia (larger) and the fibula (smaller). Injuries involving the proximal tibia and fibula are covered in Chapter 15 on knee injuries, and injuries involving the distal tibia and fibula are discussed in Chapter 16 on ankle injuries.

The tibia is the primary weight-bearing bone of the lower leg, and it is subjected to considerable forces of impact, twisting, and bending throughout an athletic activity. The fibula, which is lateral to the tibia, is essentially a non–weight-beating bone, its primary functions being the lateral stabilizing bony structure of the ankle and a site of muscle attachment. The fibula is subjected to rotational and bending forces transmitted through the complex motions of the ankle. The two bones form the tibia/fibular joint proximally, and they form the ankle mortise distally (Figure 17.1). They are attached to each other along their shafts by the thick interosseous membrane. The tibia is subcutaneous over its anterior border, lacking a significant protective soft-tissue envelope, and as a result, it is vulnerable to direct trauma during many contact sports. The fibula is surrounded by muscle throughout most of its length and is therefore less likely to be injured by direct trauma.

The muscles of the lower leg are organized into four compartments, each surrounded by a fascial tissue layer (Figures 17.2 and 17.3). The anterior compartment muscles arise from the lateral border of the tibial shaft, anterior aspect of the interosseous membrane, and the anteromedial aspect of the fibula. The tibialis anterior is the largest muscle of the group, and it courses distally and medially to insert on the medial aspect of the tarsal navicular bone, serving as a dorsiflexor and supinator of the ankle. The extensor hallucis longus inserts on the proximal phalanx of the great toe and acts to dorsiflex the great toe and supinate the foot. The extensor digitorum longus inserts on the proximal phalanges of each of the lesser toes and facilitates dorsiflexion of the lesser toes. The deep branch of the peroneal nerve is the motor nerve to the anterior compartment muscles and the sensory nerve to the dorsal aspect of the first web space of the foot. The nerve runs through the anterior compartment af-

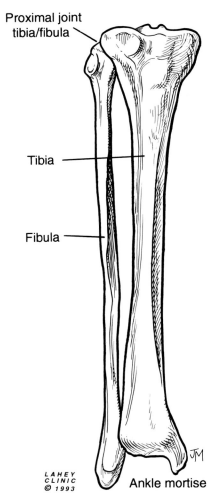

Proximal joint
tibia/fibula

Tibia

Fibula

Ankle mortise

LAHEY
CLINIC
© 1993

Figure 17.1. Bony anatomy of tibia and fibula.
(Reproduced by permission of the Lahey Clinic.)

ter it splits from the common peroneal
nerve around the neck of the fibula. The
deep peroneal nerve runs adjacent to the
anterior tibial artery.

The lateral compartment consists of the
peroneus brevis and longus muscles. These
muscles originate from the lateral aspect of
the fibula and descend into the foot behind
the lateral malleolus where they insert

distally on the base of the fifth metatarsal
and the plantar aspect of the base of the first
metatarsal, respectively. They function as
plantar flexors and pronators of the foot.
These muscles are innervated by the superficial peroneal nerve, the other terminal
branch of the common peroneal nerve. The
superficial peroneal nerve also supplies
sensation to the dorsum of the foot.

The gastrocnemius, soleus, and plantaris
muscles lie within the superficial posterior
compartment. The gastrocnemius muscle
originates from the posterior aspect of the
distal femur along with the plantaris,
whereas the soleus muscle arises from the
posterior aspect of the proximal tibia. All
three muscles insert into the calcaneus and
act as plantar flexors of the foot. The
gastrocnemius and the soleus muscles unite
to form the Achilles tendon distally.

The deep posterior compartment contains the tibialis posterior, flexor digitorum
longus, flexor hallucis longus, and popliteus muscles. They arise from the interosseous membrane, posterior border of the
tibia, posterior border of the fibula, and
proximal posterior tibia, respectively. The
tibialis posterior, flexor digitorum longus,
and flexor hallucis longus run distally
behind the medial malleolus. The tibialis
posterior inserts into the medial aspect of
the tarsal navicular and acts as a plantar
flexor and supinator of the foot. The flexor
digitorum longus inserts into the plantar
aspect of the proximal phalanges of the
lesser toes and helps to plantar flex the foot
and toes. The flexor hallucis longus inserts
into the plantar aspect of the proximal phalanx of the great toe and functions as a
plantar flexor of the foot and great toe. The
popliteus muscle runs proximally across
the knee joint to insert on the lateral femoral
condyle. Part of its course is intra-articular.
It functions to "unscrew" the knee from full
extension and initiates flexion. The muscles

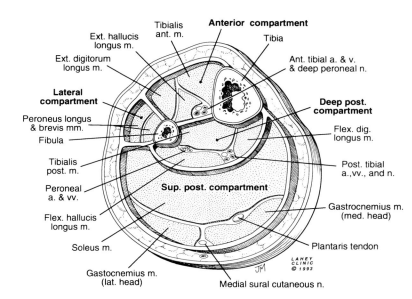

Ext. hallucis longus m.
Ext. digitorum longus m.
Lateral compartment
Peroneus longus & brevis mm.
Fibula
Tibialis post. m.
Peroneal a. & vv.
Flex. hallucis longus m.
Soleus m.
Gastocnemius m. (lat. head)

Tibialis ant. m.
Anterior compartment
Tibia
Ant. tibial a. & v. & deep peroneal n.
Deep post. compartment
Flex. dig. longus m.
Post. tibial a.,vv., and n.
Sup. post. compartment
Gastrocnemius m. (med. head)
Plantaris tendon
Medial sural cutaneous n.

LAHEY CLINIC © 1993

Figure 17.2. Cross-sectional anatomy of lower leg at the midcalf level. (Reproduced by permission of the Lahey Clinic.)

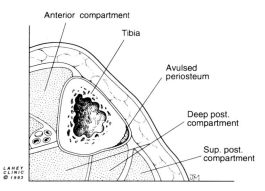

Anterior compartment
Tibia
Avulsed periosteum
Deep post. compartment
Sup. post. compartment

LAHEY CLINIC © 1993

Figure 17.3. Cross section of lower leg illustrates medial tibial stress syndrome of periosteum at the insertion into the posteromedial border of the tibia. (Reproduced by permission of the Lahey Clinic.)

of the deep and superficial compartment are innervated by the tibial nerve, which runs between the deep and superficial compartments with the posterior tibial artery. The posterior tibial artery and tibial nerve continue distally and run behind the medial malleolus into the foot. There, the tibial

nerve supplies motor function to the plantar musculature and sensation to the plantar aspect of the foot. Remember the mnemonic for the order of the structures from anterior to posterior as they course behind the medial malleolus: Tom, Dick, And Not Harry (Tibialis posterior, flexor Digitorum longus, posterior tibial Artery, tibial Nerve, and flexor digitorum Hallucis).

The motor nerves to the lower leg arise from the sciatic nerve as it branches into the common peroneal and tibial nerves above the popliteal fossa. As the common peroneal nerve runs distally, it wraps around the fibular neck where it divides into the superficial and deep branches. Their functions were discussed earlier. The saphenous nerve is the terminal branch of the femoral nerve and provides sensory branches to the medial aspect of the lower leg.

The blood supply to the lower leg is derived from the popliteal artery, which bifurcates distal to the popliteal fossa into the anterior and posterior tibial arteries. The anterior tibial artery runs through the anterior compartment adjacent to the deep peroneal nerve, whereas the posterior tibial artery lies next to the tibial nerve as the two run between the superficial and deep posterior compartments. The peroneal artery branches off from the posterior tibial artery and courses through the deep posterior compartment.

HISTORY

Most sports injuries of the lower leg can be diagnosed with a thorough history and physical examination. It is important to try and differentiate between acute, traumatic injuries and the more chronic, overuse injuries that can affect the lower leg. Most patients with severe traumatic injuries will be referred to an emergency department for initial evaluation; however, primary care physicians are increasingly being called on to assess less severe injuries. In general, if an athlete is able to get up and walk after an injury, it is unlikely that the injury is severe.

Knowledge of the sport an athlete pursues, and with what frequency, provides a clue to the potential mechanisms of injury. Does the athlete recall a specific injury or did the problem develop insidiously? How long have the symptoms been present? Frequently, the athlete may have changed the exercise routine several days or weeks before the onset of symptoms. When athletes with pain in the lower leg are evaluated, it is helpful to localize the symptoms to a particular region. Different pathologic processes will affect different areas of the leg. Additionally, the relationship of the sports activity to the symptoms is important. Does the pain start at the beginning of exercise or does it develop after the athlete has been exercising for a few minutes or longer? Is the athlete able to play through the pain or is he or she forced to stop exercising because of the discomfort? Do the symptoms disappear with rest or do they persist for a period of time? How do the symptoms affect the athlete's ability to walk? Does anything make the pain better? Is associated swelling, numbness, or weakness of the leg present? What has the athlete done to try and relieve the problem?

In general, these athletes will be seen in your office when the symptoms have greatly interfered with their ability to perform their regular exercise routine. The patients are often frustrated with their disability, and they are anxious to return to their previous level of function. In some patients, the inability to exercise can result in a mild or moderate depression. Our goal as physicians is to return the athlete to his or her sport as soon as the injuries have been permitted to heal and the affected area has been rehabilitated. As part of the treatment of these patients, we must try to provide a means of exercise through *cross training*, that is, permitting a form of exercise that does not stress the injured body part but will still provide the athlete with the physiologic and psychologic benefits of exercise.

RISK FACTORS

Overuse injuries of the lower leg can often be attributed to several underlying causes: training errors, improper equipment, biomechanical abnormalities, and metabolic abnormalities (2,3). Recognizing these factors will enable the physician to make specific recommendations to facilitate an athlete's proper conditioning and rehabilitation from an injury.

Training Errors

Training errors are responsible for most overuse injuries and include inadequate warm-up and stretching, inadequate conditioning, excessive mileage or abrupt increase in distances for runners, excessive running or jumping for aerobic dancers and running sports participants, frequent running on hills or uneven surfaces, and lack of cross training (2,4–6). Training errors are commonly seen in patients who suddenly decide to "get in shape" and in athletes who have been exercising regularly for months or years. What often causes a problem is any significant change from the normal exercise routine, such as increased frequency, increased intensity, or increased duration of participation in a particular sport (7–11). Cross training is a new concept that involves exercising through a variety of activities that stress different anatomic structures in different ways, avoiding the repetitive forces associated with a single sport that can lead to an overuse injury. This concept is especially important in prescribing an exercise regimen that an athlete can follow during recovery from an injury.

Improper Equipment

Improper equipment generally implies inappropriate footwear for a particular sport. Tennis shoes are designed for tennis, not for jogging, and vice versa. Athletic shoes have become sophisticated, and shoes are available for almost any sport activity. The cost of athletic shoes has risen considerably, so it may not be feasible for an athlete to purchase different shoes for each different sport. The athletic shoe companies have recently developed shoes for cross training, that is, shoes that can be used safely in a variety of different sport activities. Generally, this concept works well; however, with joggers, it is still preferable for those athletes to invest in a good pair of running shoes.

When these patients are evaluated, it is helpful to examine the athletic shoes they are wearing. Shoes that are poorly made or worn out do not provide adequate cushioning or stability and may be more likely to cause problems. Look for signs of abnormal wear that may point to a biomechanical abnormality of the lower leg. For example, an athlete with hyperpronation of the foot will often wear the inside of the sole, emphasizing the need for a shoe that has a sturdy heel counter. An excellent guide to selecting the proper running shoe is published at least once a year in *Runner's World* magazine (Emmaus, PA). The article discusses the shapes of feet, types of runners, and the types of running shoes that are available, depending on a patient's body habitus, running style, and anatomic abnormalities. A person committed to jogging or running on a regular basis needs to make a financial commitment to purchase quality running shoes as well. When athletes ask for specific recommendations, they can be referred to an athletic shoe store or they can review the yearly running shoe guide in *Runner's World*.

Biomechanical Abnormalities

Abnormal biomechanics can lead to abnormal distribution of forces throughout the entire lower extremity from the foot to the hip. During running activities, the athlete usually takes between 800 and 2000 steps per mile, each leg absorbing a force of between two and four times body weight. For a 150-lb jogger, that adds up to about 500 tons of force per mile (2)! That is a tre-

**Phases of
running gait**

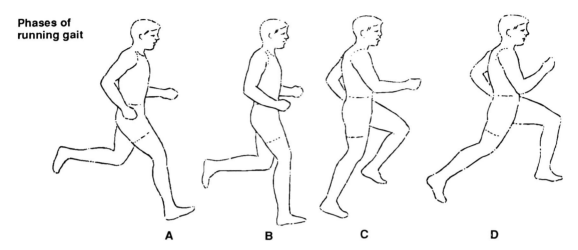

A   B   C   D

Figure 17.4. The components of the running gait. *A.* Footstrike. *B.* Midstance. *C.* Toe-off. *D.* Swing-through.

mendous amount of stress to the lower extremity, and when the forces are not distributed properly, an injury can occur.

To understand better the biomechanics, it is helpful to look at the different phases of running. The running gait can be broken down into four major components: footstrike, midstance, toe-off, and swing-through (Figure 17.4) (2). When the foot is in the swing-through phase, it assumes a position of supination. This means the foot is inverted and the arch is accentuated. When foot-strike occurs, the foot is still supinated, but the force of impact causes the foot to pronate during the midstance phase. This causes the foot to evert, with some flattening of the arch. When toe-off occurs, the foot will begin to supinate as it comes into the swing-through phase. A common biomechanical abnormality responsible for overuse injuries of the lower extremity is hyperpronation (Figure 17.5) (4,6,12–14). When the foot is in midstance, the arch collapses, resulting in excessive internal rotation of the tibia, putting abnor-

mal stresses on the knee and muscle-tendon units of the lower leg. These abnormal stresses can lead to the development of problems.

Metabolic Abnormalities

Metabolic abnormalities can predispose athletes to overuse injuries of the lower leg

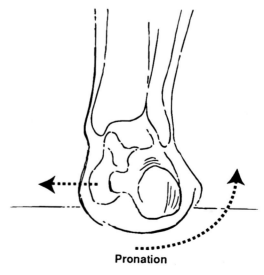

Pronation

Figure 17.5. Pronation of the foot during weight bearing.

(3,15). Usually, these metabolic deficiencies interfere with normal bone metabolism, and athletes may be at increased risk for stress fractures of the lower extremity. Patients must be evaluated for any underlying metabolic problems that may alter bone metabolism. Amenorrhea, osteomalacia, osteoporosis, rickets, and Paget's disease are a few of the potential causes.

PHYSICAL EXAMINATION

Examination of these patients should begin with visual assessment of the alignment of the lower extremity, looking for any obvious bony deformity that may occur with a fracture or dislocation or for a more subtle malalignment that may result in abnormal biomechanics. It is important to examine the hips, knees, feet, and ankles of any patient with lower leg problems. The reader is referred to the chapters on hip, knee, foot, and ankle problems for a discussion of the physical examination of those structures.

When an athlete is unable to stand, he or she should be referred for radiography to rule out a fracture before a thorough examination. When a severe injury has been ruled out, the examination begins with the patient standing in bare feet. Look for the presence of any malalignment of the lower extremity (Figures 17.6 and 17.7): genu valgus or genu varus (knock-knee or bowleg deformity), hyperpronation (pes planus), or cavus deformity of the foot. Watch the patient walk, looking for signs of a limp and try to evaluate whether the longitudinal plantar arch of the foot is present or whether it disappears with weight bearing. If the arch disappears during weight bearing, this may represent hyperpronation from a pes planus (flat foot) deformity. A high plantar arch may be seen with a

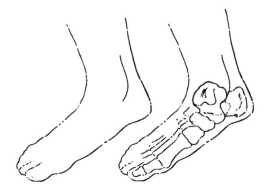

Figure 17.6. Hyperpronation or pes planus.

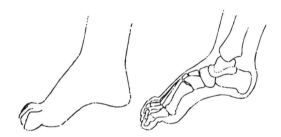

Figure 17.7. Abnormally high arch or pes cavus.

cavus foot deformity. Detailed descriptions of examination of the ankle and foot are presented in Chapters 16 and 18, respectively.

Most of the examination of the lower leg between the knee and ankle consists of palpating for areas of diffuse or local tenderness as well as palpating for fascial defects and muscle herniations. As mentioned previously, the location of tenderness can help elucidate the underlying cause of the patient's symptoms. It is also important to assess muscle strength and sensation because these can be affected by various pathologic processes. The physical findings associated with a specific overuse injury of the lower leg are discussed separately.

DIAGNOSTIC STUDIES

As clinicians, we must decide whether a diagnostic test is going to alter our treatment of a patient or just confirm what our clinical history and physical examinations have determined. Certainly, in the setting of an acute traumatic injury when a fracture is suspected, radiography is indicated because it will help in planning the appropriate treatment of the fracture. However, in overuse injuries of the lower leg, results of routine radiography are unlikely to change the initial management of those problems.

In general, radiography is indicated to rule out a fracture, neoplasm, or infectious process involving the tibia or fibula. In children, overuse injuries are uncommon, and radiography is appropriate to evaluate almost any bony tenderness, looking for any of the pathologic processes mentioned earlier. In the initial evaluation of an adult, however, radiography is not mandatory and should be obtained only when a high index of suspicion exists for the possibility of a bony abnormality.

Bone scans are useful for identifying the presence of stress fractures (16,17). That is their primary role in evaluating lower leg injuries. They are also helpful in diagnosing medial tibial stress syndrome (MTSS), as will be discussed shortly. Additionally, bone scans can be used to detect the presence of osteomyelitis or a neoplastic process.

The role of magnetic resonance imaging (MRI) in evaluating lower leg injuries is limited. It is an expensive diagnostic tool, and, generally, other less expensive modalities are available to provide diagnostic confirmation when necessary. The importance of the clinical history and physical examination cannot be overestimated (18).

In patients with a suspected exercise-induced compartment syndrome, definitive diagnosis requires measurement of the actual compartment pressures of the symptomatic compartment before and after exercise. This invasive study requires special equipment and should only be performed by clinicians with appropriate training. This procedure is discussed further in the section on Compartment Syndrome.

TREATMENT

The treatment of patients with lower leg injuries begins with an analysis of what factors may have caused the symptoms and an effort to correct errors of training, equipment, or biomechanical abnormalities. The athlete must recognize the need for a period of rest, ranging from a few days to 6 weeks, depending on the chronicity and severity of the symptoms. Most athletes will benefit from at least 2 to 3 weeks of activity modification, that is, avoiding activities that produce the symptoms of pain. Low-impact or no-impact sports, such as bicycling, water running, stair machines, in-line skating, rowing, or swimming offer the athlete the ability to exercise while avoiding the stresses of running or other high-impact activities. If these athletes still have symptoms while trying these other sports, they should be advised "if it hurts, don't do it."

Physical therapy exercises, consisting of stretching the calf muscles and heel cord as well as lower leg stretching in general, will help to improve flexibility and restore normal range of motion. Strength training is important to rehabilitate injured muscle tissue and to prevent or correct muscle atrophy that may develop as a result of an injury. Isometric and isotonic strengthening with weights or resistive rubber straps (Thera-band [The Hygenic Corp, Akron, OH]) are easily performed by the athlete without supervision. For most patients, a single consultation with a physical therapist can facilitate the development of a home exercise program the athlete can follow independently. When the injury is severe, modalities such as ice massage or ultrasound to the posteromedial border of the tibia will help to diminish local tenderness (19,20). Additionally, anti-inflammatory medication can help to relieve some of the local symptoms of pain caused by soft-tissue inflammation. Little if any role exists for corticosteroid injections in the treatment of patients with lower leg injuries.

Athletes with hyperpronation should be fitted with an antipronation orthotic to correct the abnormal position of the foot during sports that may have precipitated the symptoms. In general, most athletes with a mild deformity can be managed with off-the-shelf orthotics to control pronation. They are affordable and will usually be sufficient for most athletes. The orthotic should be a full-length device because it will replace the insole that will be removed from the athletic shoe. Occasionally, patients with more severe deformity or patients who did not improve with an off-the-shelf orthotic can be fitted for a custom orthotic. These custom orthotics are molded to the athlete's foot or fabricated from a cast of the athlete's foot, and they can cost several hundred dollars. For most athletes, a soft or a semirigid full-length "sport orthotic" covered with a neoprene liner is preferred.

When the athlete's symptoms have abated, a gradual return to activity is critical (2,5,20,21). Runners need to start off at no more than a half a mile a day, 2 to 3 days a week, with a gradual progression as they increase their distance and frequency of running. It is often appropriate for an athlete to resume running with a "walk-jog" program, where he or she begins by walking and gradually intersperses jogging into the program. The athlete should be advised that it will take at least 4 to 8 weeks to get back to the preinjury status, encouraging walking and other low-impact activities to supplement the workout. Using small incremental increases, such as 2 minutes a week, helps to avoid reinjury. The most important aspect of the treatment involves a gradual return to activity to avoid overstressing the injured body part after it has had a chance to heal. Often, these athletes require extra attention to their emotional needs because they are forced to modify their exercise regimen at a significant psychological cost. The change in activity can precipitate a depressive episode, and it is important to emphasize cross training as a means of permitting the athlete to continue exercise while the injury is healing. Proper training is the key to avoiding these problems in the future.

MEDIAL TIBIAL STRESS SYNDROME

Clinical Case #1

An 18-year-old woman comes to your office complaining of pain in her right shin. The pain started 4 months ago and is now increasing in severity. She is a runner. The pain is mild when she walks and becomes severe about 10 minutes after she runs. She had stopped running for 3 weeks and the pain disappeared, but when she starts running again the pain reappears. Examination reveals that she is a pronator and has tenderness over the posterior medial border of the tibia from 2 cm above the medial malleolus for 6 cm.

The term "shin splints" has been exploited in the medical literature to describe pain that develops in the lower leg between the knee and the ankle. According to the American Medical Association (22) in 1966, *shin splints* is defined as "pain and discomfort in the leg from repetitive running on a hard surface or forcible, excessive use of foot flexors: diagnosis should be limited to musculotendinous inflammation, excluding fracture or ischemic disorder." This definition is generally thought to be outdated and too restricting in its categorization of pain in the lower leg. According to Slocum (23), shin splint syndrome represents a symptom complex characterized by pain and discomfort in the lower part of the leg after repetitive overuse in walking or running.

Differential Diagnosis

In common practice, shin splints have referred to pain in the medial, lateral, or anterior aspect of the lower leg, including the diagnoses of periostitis, stress fracture, exertional or exercise-induced compartment syndrome, and posterior tibial tendinitis (12,13,21,24–26). These diagnoses represent a spectrum of injuries that can produce symptoms of pain in the same anatomic region, usually the posteromedial border of the tibia. Recently, several authors (21,25,27,28) classified the symptoms of pain along the posteromedial border of the tibia separately from anterior and lateral symptoms (Figure 17.8). MTSS has gained popularity as the cause of pain along the posteromedial border of the tibia (28).

Some overlap exists in the clinical presentation of MTSS, stress fractures, and exercise-induced compartment syndrome that

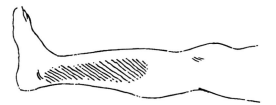

Figure 17.8. Area of pain in medial tibial stress syndrome (MTSS).

can only be differentiated through diagnostic studies and a carefully performed physical examination.

Etiology

It has been estimated (5) that this problem represents 12% to 18% of running injuries; women experience this injury more often than men. Several etiologic factors have been identified, including running on hard surfaces, running on uneven terrain, overtraining without proper conditioning, improper footwear, and abnormal biomechanics, especially hyperpronation of the foot. According to Clement (21), cyclic training stress induces a local muscle fatigue in the lower leg. This causes a loss of shock-absorbing function, and structural stress to bone increases, creating a painful periostitis. Resultant disuse muscular atrophy furthers the loss of shock absorption, and the cycle is reinforced (21).

The symptoms of MTSS seem to be caused by a painful periostitis or periostalgia of the posteromedial border of the tibia (25). This develops as a result of the repetitive stresses on the tibia that occur with prolonged running exercises. The stress can induce partial tearing of the periosteum resulting from traction from muscle strain or partial detachment of the periosteum from subperiosteal hemorrhage from micromuscle tearing (see Figure 17.3).

History

The specific complaints a patient may have depend on chronicity of the symptoms. In the earlier stages of MTSS, a patient will report discomfort that is usually of an aching nature over a diffuse area of the posteromedial aspect of the tibia between the middle and distal third of the lower leg. The pain may be present at the beginning of the workout and disappear after a period of warm-up, only to recur at the latter part of the exercise period and for a varying length of time thereafter (24). As the symptoms become more chronic, they may persist during the workout and even when the athlete is not exercising at all. When symptoms are severe, the athlete may have pain with routine walking activities. The pain is often relieved by over-the-counter analgesics. Occasionally, the athlete may note some swelling of the involved extremity. Often, the symptoms are bilateral.

Physical Examination

On physical examination, these patients will usually have an area of tenderness over the posteromedial border of the tibia that *begins a few centimeters above the medial malleolus and extends proximally for a distance of 4 to 10 cm* (see Figure 17.8). Some associated soft-tissue swelling may also be present. It is important to quantify the extent of the tenderness because patients with tibial stress fractures may also have tenderness in this region, although the area of tenderness seen with a stress fracture is much more localized (usually <2 cm). These patients will usually have normal strength and normal sensation throughout the lower leg.

Diagnostic Studies

Routine radiography is not necessary in the initial evaluation of these patients unless a neoplasm or osteomyelitis is clinically suspected, both of which are rare. Athletes who have prolonged symptoms of MTSS are at risk for the development of a stress fracture if they continue to participate in the sport causing their symptoms (21). In the patient in whom a stress fracture is suspected, a bone scan may be helpful in differentiating between MTSS and a stress fracture. This would rarely be indicated because early treatment is the same. Typically, in a three-phase bone scan, patients with MTSS will have normal results on radionuclide angiography and blood pool phases of the scan and abnormal diffuse increased uptake along the posteromedial border of the middle and distal third of the tibia during the delayed imaging phase (Figure 17.9). Patients with a stress fracture will have abnormal results on radionuclide angiography and blood pool phase of the scan, along with an area of focal increased uptake in the region of the stress fracture (16).

Treatment

The treatment of patients with MTSS includes all of the points discussed in the previous section of general injuries of the lower leg. Rest, proper stretching and strengthening of the lower leg muscles, nonsteroidal anti-inflammatory drugs (NSAIDs), orthotics, and a gradual return to activity are the core of the rehabilitation program. The most important aspect of the treatment of this problem is a gradual return to exercise

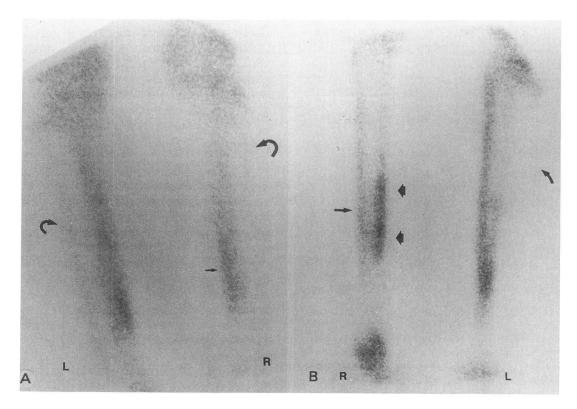

Figure 17.9. Bone scan demonstrates abnormal uptake along the postermedial border of the tibia seen in medial tibial stress syndrome. (Reproduced by permission from Michael RH, Holder LE. The soleus syndrome: a cause of medial tibial stress [shin splints]. Am J Sports Med 1985;13:88.)

after the symptoms have resolved. Proper training techniques, including cross training, and proper athletic shoes are essential to prevent recurrence of the symptoms.

Despite a proper treatment program, some athletes may continue to have symptoms that can preclude participation in their desired activity. It is important to establish an accurate diagnosis. In some patients with long-standing symptoms, the condition can progress to a stress fracture of the tibia, which may require a bone scan for definitive diagnosis. Other patients may have a deep posterior compartment syndrome that may require compartment pres-

sure measurements for diagnosis. When other conditions have been ruled out and the patient continues to have tenderness along the posteromedial border of the tibia, he or she may possibly be a candidate for surgical intervention. Several authors (13,25) have recommended release of the fascia and periosteum along the posteromedial border of the tibia along with cauterization of the periosteum to relieve the symptoms of pain. In general, though, most patients respond to nonoperative treatment and failure to adhere to your suggestions is a common cause of continued pain.

STRESS FRACTURES

The concept of a stress fracture of the bone was first discussed in 1855 by Briethaupt, a military physician who described a "march fracture" of the metatarsal in military recruits (8). In simple terms, a stress fracture represents mechanical failure of the bone from repetitive loading (15). Bone is constantly being remodeled in response to stress. In normal bone metabolism, resorption of bone occurs as osteoclast activity increases as a result of the forces acting on a bone. At the same time, osteoblasts are stimulated to lay down new bone to reinforce the remodeled bone. A stress fracture occurs when the rate of bone resorption exceeds the rate of bone reformation. Stress fractures have also been referred to as fatigue fracture, spontaneous fracture, pseudofracture, exhaustion fracture, and insufficiency fracture (10).

In athletes, stress fractures of the lower extremity can occur as a result of the repetitive loading seen with sports that involve running, jumping, and dancing. These activities can produce fatigue of the muscles of the lower leg, and according to some authors (8,9), this leads to diminished impact absorption of the soft tissues with consequent increased impact transmitted to the bony structures. The sequela of the increased forces on the bone can be a stress fracture.

Etiology

As with other overuse injuries of the lower extremity, the cause of stress fractures is multifactorial. Training errors, such as a sudden increase in the amount, frequency, or intensity of a workout, can cause a stress fracture. Athletes who run more than 20 miles a week may be at risk for stress fractures (29). The surface or terrain an athlete runs on, for example, running downhill or changing the terrain, can contribute to the development of a stress fracture. Biomechanical abnormalities, including hyperpronation, cavus feet, tibia vara, and limb length discrepancies, have been implicated as well. Improper or worn out footwear can also be a factor in the development of a stress fracture (11). The mediolateral width of the tibial shaft has been correlated with stress fractures, that is, a smaller width may be associated with a higher likelihood of stress fracture (30). Tibial stress fractures have also been correlated with amenorrhea, smoking, anorexia, low bone density, and low dietary calcium (3).

The tibia and the femur are most commonly involved, followed by the fibula and the metatarsals (9,29). Most stress fractures of the lower leg occur in the middle and distal third of the leg. Occasionally, stress fractures can develop in the tibial plateau (15).

History

Clinical Case #2

A 27-year-old female runner is seen for medial leg pain of several weeks duration. Onset was sudden several weeks after she began training for a recreational race. She notes the pain is distal and medial; she has been forced to markedly reduce her running because of this.

The athlete will usually be seen because of the relatively sudden onset of localized pain in the affected bone, and usually a change in the training routine precedes the onset of symptoms. Sometimes the patient may have some localizing symptoms in the weeks before being seen in the office. Symptoms of pain may initially develop after a run, only to progress to pain at the beginning of a run, which improves initially but recurs at the end of the run. In more severe injuries, the pain is constant, and the athlete is unable to run at all. Neglected stress fractures may even cause pain with routine walking (11).

Physical Examination

On physical examination, the athlete with a stress fracture will have localized tenderness to palpation, usually over an area of less than 2 cm, occasionally with associated soft-tissue swelling. In the tibia, stress fractures are found most commonly in the middle and distal third of the tibial shaft in runners, whereas in athletes involved in jumping sports, they are often seen in the proximal third of the tibia (3). Middle one third stress fractures are usually anterior, whereas proximal or distal lesions are medial. In the fibula, stress fractures are found primarily in the distal third (31).

Diagnostic Studies

A high index of suspicion should minimize the need for diagnostic studies. In the initial evaluation of a patient with a suspected stress fracture, results of routine radiography of the lower leg will usually be normal, and are not indicated unless the symptoms have been present for more than several weeks. Early radiographic changes may include periosteal or endosteal new bone formation or both, cortical hypertrophy, and medullary sclerosis (3,29) (Figure 17.10A and B). In more chronic injuries, late radiographic changes can reveal evidence of a healing fracture line or a break in cortical bone (Figure 17.10C and D). In children and adults, these changes can be seen with osteomyelitis or a bone neoplasm; therefore, clinical correlation is vital to arrive at the proper diagnosis.

If routine radiography is negative then the diagnostic study of choice for stress fractures is a bone scan. As early as 3 days after symptoms develop, results of a bone scan may be positive, revealing a focal area of increased uptake associated with the stress fracture (8) (Figure 17.11). Several classification systems have been devised to assess stress fractures. In general, the quantitative uptake on bone scan correlates with the severity of the stress fracture. Zwas and colleagues (17) created a system with four grades ranging from a small area of increased activity in the cortex (grade I) to intense diffuse uptake involving the width of the tibia (grade IV) (Figure 17.12). Matin (16) developed a system that included five stages of bone involvement, based on the percent of the width of the tibia involved in the stress fracture. Matin (16) also emphasized the importance of looking at both anteroposterior and lateral images of the bone scan to evaluate better the extent of involvement. These systems are helpful in determining the treatment plan for a particular patient. The higher the grade or stage of involvement, the longer the period of relative rest to permit healing of the stress fracture.

The role of MRI in the evaluation of stress fractures remains to be elucidated. MRI is sensitive at detecting abnormalities of bone, which usually appear as changes in the signal of the bone marrow. However, MRI is not specific, and it can be difficult to differentiate among a stress fracture, osteomyelitis, or a neoplasm. At this time, no role exists for MRI in the evaluation of stress fractures.

Treatment

The treatment of stress fractures of the lower leg is fairly straightforward: relative rest and temporary avoidance of the activ-

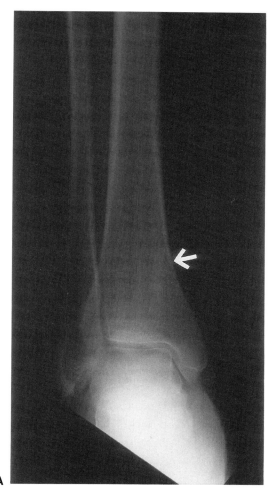

A

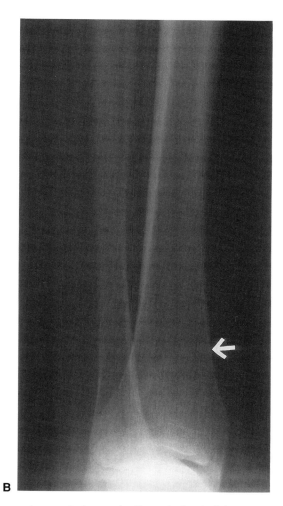

B

Figure 17.10. *A.* Early radiograph in antero-posterior projection of distal tibia stress fracture. Note metaphyseal sclerosis along medial distal metaphysis (*arrow*). *B.* Early radiograph in lateral projection of distal tibia stress fracture. Note linear sclerosis of distal metaphysis (*arrow*). *C.* Late (3 months) radiograph in anteroposterior projection of distal tibia stress fracture. Note cortical hypertrophy and periosteal reaction with medullary sclerosis (*arrow*). *D.* Late (3 months) radiograph in lateral projection of distal tibia stress fracture. Note linear sclerosis of distal metaphysis (*arrow*).

ity that precipitated the symptoms. The treatment of the *patient* with a stress fracture of the lower extremity is more complex. Typically, these patients are involved in a regular exercise routine, and to permit the stress fracture to heal, they will have to alter their activities. For many patients, this can create a significant amount of emotional stress because they are forced to alter their workout schedule. As physicians, we must address the anatomic problem, that is, the stress fracture, as well as the psycho-

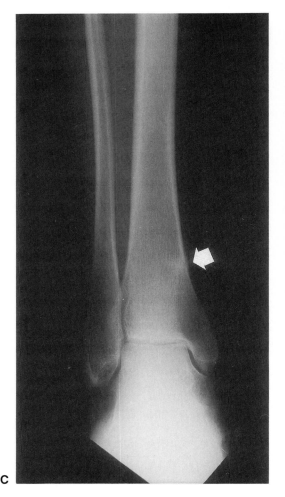

C

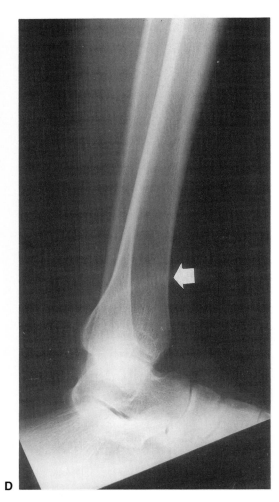

D

Figure 17.10. *Continued*

logical problem that can result as a consequence. It is important to emphasize to the
patient that the injury will heal if the athlete
will modify activity during the healing
phase. As with all overuse injuries, cross
training enables the athlete to continue to
exercise while permitting an injured body
part to heal. For stress fractures of the lower
leg, swimming, bicycling, water running,
rowing, and stair machines may permit the
athlete to exercise while healing takes place.

The athlete again has to be cautioned "if it
hurts, don't do it."

The exact period of rest depends on the
severity of the symptoms and the stage of
involvement demonstrated by diagnostic
studies. According to Zwas and coworkers
(17) grades I and II stress fractures need
between 3 and 4 weeks of rest, whereas
grades III and IV need 4 to 6 weeks to heal.
In general, the more severe the symptoms,
the longer the period of rest or activity

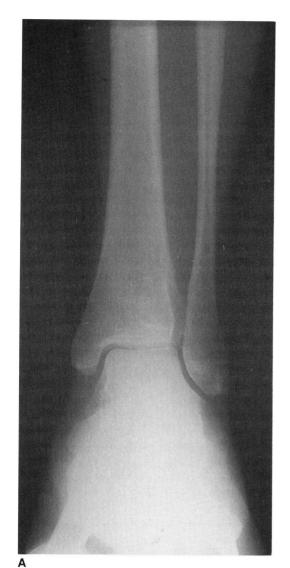

A

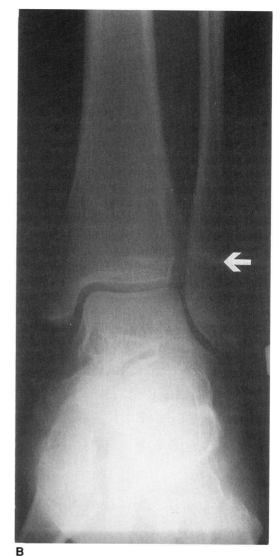

B

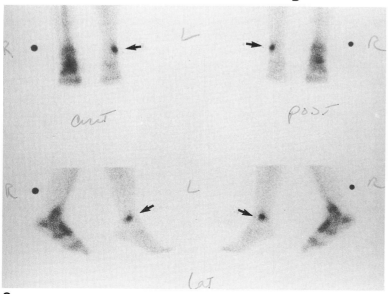

C

Figure 17.11. *A.* Early radiograph of distal fibula stress fracture. No abnormalities noted. *B.* Bone scan of distal fibula stress fracture 3 weeks after symptoms developed. Note focal area of uptake (*arrow*). *C.* Late (6 weeks) radiograph of distal fibula stress fracture. Note linear sclerosis of metaphysis of distal fibula.

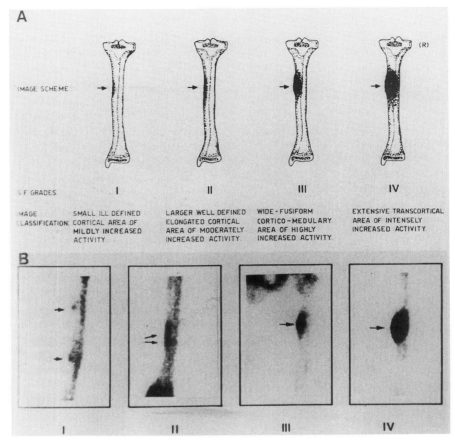

Figure 17.12. Bone scans demonstrating the four grades of stress fractures. (Reproduced by permission from Zwas ST, Elkanovitch R, Frank G. Interpretation and classification of bone scintigraphic findings in stress fractures. J Nucl Med 1987;28:453.)

modification to permit healing of the stress fracture.

When a patient is limping with routine walking activities, he or she should be instructed on partial weight-bearing ambulation with crutches or a cane. This should continue until the athlete can ambulate with no pain. With stress fractures of the tibia and fibula, the patient may be more comfortable in a splint during walking activities and ultimately during sports. Several studies (32,33) have evaluated the use of a pneumatic leg brace for stress fractures of the lower leg. Although the studies can be criticized for lacking a control group for comparison, the evidence suggests that patients can ambulate more comfortably and resume their exercise regimen earlier than might otherwise have been possible without the leg brace. It is even possible for an athlete with a fibular stress fracture to compete in a long pneumatic leg brace (32). Rarely do stress fractures of the lower leg require immobilization in a cast. These fractures will heal without immobilization, and it is possible to avoid "cast disease" that results in muscle atrophy and stiffness of the joints from immobilization.

In addition to rest, NSAIDs can provide relief of pain symptoms. In women who are amenorrheic, hormone therapy can be considered to regulate the menstrual cycle and help normalize bone metabolism, which can be affected adversely by abnormal estrogen levels seen with amenorrhea (see Chapter 23). There is a high frequency of eating disorders in women athletes with stress fractures. This possibility should be investigated.

The use of physical therapy modalities, such as ice massage and ice whirlpools, can help relieve pain symptoms. Ultrasound is contraindicated, however, because it can often cause increased pain. The athlete can be instructed on lower leg strengthening exercises that do not involve weight bearing, such as leg extension and leg curls and strengthening of the lower leg muscles using the Thera-band. Leg press and squat machines should be avoided.

It is possible to treat these patients based on results of their clinical history and physical examination without obtaining any diagnostic studies. An athlete with classic signs and symptoms of a stress fracture can start a treatment program of rest and modified activity and be seen for follow-up examination within 3 to 4 weeks to assess improvement of his or her discomfort. If there is less pain, the presumptive diagnosis of a stress fracture would appear to have been correct. If the pain symptoms are still fairly bothersome, diagnostic studies should be obtained to rule out any other abnormality. At that time, routine radiography can be carried out. When results of radiography are inconclusive, a bone scan may be ordered to rule out a stress fracture or other abnormality.

An athlete can return to participation in sports when the symptoms of pain have completely resolved. The athlete should be cautioned to resume activities on a gradual basis and to avoid the training errors that may have contributed to the development of the stress fracture. Obviously, biomechanical abnormalities and equipment problems should be corrected before the sport is resumed.

COMPARTMENT SYNDROME

The term *compartment syndrome* describes a pathologic state in which elevated tissue pressure within a closed muscle compartment leads to ischemia as a result of diminished perfusion through the microcirculation (22). Compartment syndromes can occur acutely as a result of trauma to an extremity or as a result of intense exercise. An acute compartment syndrome can also occur with bleeding disorders, burns, swelling after an arterial injury or thrombosis, drug or alcohol overdose, or venous obstruction (22). Compartment syndromes of the lower leg can also occur on an intermittent or chronic basis as a result of regular exercise. An acute compartment syndrome is a medical emergency and requires immediate surgery to decompress the involved compartments and prevent tissue necrosis that can occur as a result of the altered perfusion. A chronic compartment syndrome of the lower leg is not a medical emergency and can be managed initially with modifications of the exercise regimen and shoe wear. Operation is reserved for patients with recalcitrant symptoms.

Acute Compartment Syndrome

The muscles of the lower leg are divided into four distinct fascial compartments as discussed earlier in the anatomy review (see Figure 17.2). The individual compartments are surrounded by a layer of tissue that is relatively inelastic and effectively creates a closed space. Little room is available to accommodate bleeding or soft-tissue swelling that can occur with trauma, such as a fracture of the tibia, or severe contusion of the soft tissues. The bleeding and swelling within a closed tissue space will raise the pressure within that compartment. As the pressure rises, perfusion of the muscles and nerves within the compartment can be compromised, and ischemia can occur. If the diminished perfusion persists for longer than several hours, irreversible necrosis of the soft tissues can occur, leading to muscle contractures and loss of function (22). Prompt recognition of this injury is imperative to avoid the potential complications associated with this problem. Acute compartment syndrome is an emergency requiring urgent surgical decompression. Any patient with a suspected compartment syndrome should be evaluated emergently.

History

Clinical Case #3

A high school soccer player was kicked in the leg at a game 3 hours before coming to your office. She is complaining of pain that has gone from mild to severe. She notes numbness and decreased ability to dorsiflex her foot because it aggravates the pain.

The patient with an acute compartment syndrome will usually report a history of trauma to the lower leg before the onset of symptoms. Direct trauma to the lower leg can cause a fracture or severe muscle contusion leading to swelling as a result of bleeding in the injured extremity. A patient with an acute compartment syndrome will present initially with complaints of severe pain in the affected area. The pain may seem out of proportion with the degree of injury suspected. The patient may also complain of numbness of the area supplied by the sensory nerve within the affected compartment; for example, the dorsum of the foot may be numb as a result of a compartment syndrome of the lateral compartment. The symptoms of pain are not relieved by ice, elevation, or NSAIDs. With time, the pain symptoms can become excruciating. It is imperative to make the diagnosis of acute compartment syndrome to avoid the potential complications mentioned.

When these patients are evaluated, it is important to consider the possibility that an arterial or nerve injury may be the primary problem or that an associated injury may be present.

Physical Examination

A patient with an acute compartment syndrome of the lower extremity may present with an obvious bony deformity resulting from a fracture or soft-tissue swelling and ecchymosis from a severe contusion or both. The reliability of the examination is predicated on the alertness and cooperation of the patient.

The anterior compartment is most commonly involved in acute compartment syndrome; the lateral compartment and posterior compartments are less commonly involved (22). Palpation of the lower leg may reveal fullness and tightness of the muscle compartments, with some tenderness on palpation. Comparison to the uninjured leg is helpful to appreciate the extent of the swelling.

One of the most sensitive findings on physical examination is the severe pain that is caused by passive motion of the muscles within the affected compartment. By passive plantar flexing of the ankle and toes, the muscles of the anterior compartment are stretched, and the patient will almost invariably have severe pain if a compartment syndrome is present. Conversely, with passive dorsiflexion of the ankle and toes, a patient with a compartment syndrome of the deep posterior compartment will have severe pain. With passive inversion of the ankle, pain will be produced if the lateral compartment is involved. Patients with a compartment syndrome will often have weakness of the affected muscles because of the pain associated with muscle contraction.

If a compartment syndrome has been present for a few hours, the patient may have paresthesias over the area supplied by the sensory nerve within the affected compartment (22). For the anterior compartment, the first web space of the foot, which is supplied by the deep peroneal nerve, should be checked. The superficial peroneal nerve runs through the lateral compartment and supplies the dorsum of the foot. The plantar surface of the foot is innervated by the tibial nerve that courses through the deep posterior compartment. If paresthesias are present, immediate decompression is vital to prevent long-term deficits.

In most patients with acute compartment syndrome, the pedal pulses are palpable. When pulses are not detected, an arterial injury must be considered (22). It is imperative that the proper diagnosis be made and treatment instituted immediately.

Diagnostic Tests

A patient with a suspected compartment syndrome of the lower leg as a result of trauma should have routine radiographs to look for a fracture of the tibia or fibula. The definitive diagnosis of a compartment syndrome is made by direct measurement of the pressure within the compartment. This is an invasive test requiring the insertion of a special needle or catheter into the muscle compartments, and it should be performed by properly trained individuals.

Treatment

The treatment for acute compartment syndrome is emergency surgical decompression of the affected compartments.

Chronic Exertional Compartment Syndrome

In response to exercise, blood flow increases to the muscles that are performing work. The increase in blood flow leads to swelling of the muscle tissue as the metabolic activities within the muscle demand more oxygen and nutrients and results in evacuation of metabolic waste products. It is evident that muscle volume can increase by 20% in response to exercise (34). Normally, space in a muscle compartment is sufficient to permit the transient increase in muscle volume as a result of exercise; in certain individuals, however, the space in a particular compartment is limited because of anatomic constraints. As the muscles swell, tissue pressure increases within the compartment (35). As the muscles forcefully contract during exercise, the pressure within the compartment rises further (36). When the pressure reaches a certain point, the smaller capillaries can become compressed as a result of an altered arteriovenous gradient, and thus perfusion of the muscle can be diminished (36,37). With continued exercise, ischemia worsens as the tissue perfusion is compromised by the increased pressure within the compartment. Ischemia of the muscle causes pain, and the athlete finds it difficult to perform the exercise that started the whole process (34–36).

This is known as a chronic exertional or recurrent compartment syndrome (CECS) (22,36).

History

Clinical Case #4

A 23-year-old recreational runner presents with running-related pain in the leg. The athlete first noted the pain when he began to increase his speed a few months ago. The pain occurs after 3 miles and he must stop or slow down dramatically to be able to continue. He is absolutely pain free at rest.

In 1956, Mavor described what he termed anterior tibial syndrome of the lower leg that resulted from exercise (38). He was referring to pain in the lower leg that developed in a football player during running activities. The symptoms were only present during exercise, and the pain disappeared with rest. Mavor attributed the patient's symptoms to exercise ischemia of the anterior tibial muscles (38).

Patients in whom CECS of the lower leg develops report symptoms that develop after they start their exercise workout. The onset of pain usually occurs after a fixed amount of exercise. As they continue to exercise, the pain can often become so severe that they are forced to stop exercising, at which point the symptoms improve over a short period of time (39). In a rare situation, acute compartment syndrome can develop as a result of sudden vigorous exercise. An athlete with an acute compartment syndrome will not get relief of pain even with rest. This is an emergency situation and should be treated as discussed previously.

In addition to symptoms of pain, athletes may complain of cramping, tightness, and weakness of the involved muscles, and, occasionally, paresthesias of the sensory nerve in the affected compartment (34,40). The deep posterior and anterior compartments are most commonly involved. The symptoms are often bilateral. Figure 17.13 shows areas of pain for the different compartments.

Physical Examination

When a patient is seen in the office with symptoms suggestive of CECS, the findings on physical examination at that time are usually limited. Some patients may have palpable defects in the fascia, generally overlying the anterior compartment (34,36,40). These fascial defects are sequelae of increased pressure within the muscle

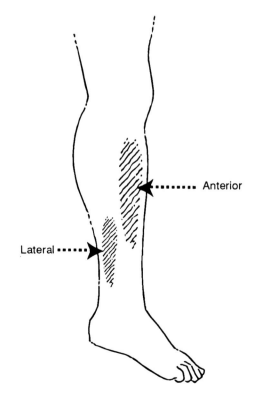

Figure 17.13. Typical areas of pain in anterior and lateral compartment syndromes.

compartment. With exercise, the muscle can herniate through the fascial defect, resulting in ischemia and pain.

To evaluate the patient better, it may be necessary to have the patient exercise to produce symptoms. This may be difficult in an office setting and may require having the athlete exercise outside the office or on a treadmill if one is available and then return for an examination as soon as symptoms develop. At that time, the lower leg can be palpated for fullness of the muscle compartments, fascial defects, weakness, and areas of tenderness (39). It is important to distinguish tenderness of the muscle compartments from localized tenderness of the tibia seen with MTSS and stress fractures. Additionally, the athlete may experience pain with passive stretching of the muscles of the involved compartment (34). Specifically, when the patient has CECS of the anterior compartment, pain symptoms may be exacerbated by passive plantar flexion of the ankle and toes. In similar fashion, when the deep posterior compartment is involved, the pain symptoms may be worse with passive dorsiflexion of the ankle and toes.

Diagnostic Tests

Radiography or a bone scan is not needed unless the examiner believes the symptoms may represent MTSS or a stress fracture. In general, however, the clinical history is enough to make a tentative diagnosis. The only way to arrive at a definitive diagnosis of CECS is to perform compartment pressure measurements before and after exercise. This is an invasive test that requires inserting a pressure measurement device into the affected muscle compartments for direct measurement of the pressures.

Numerous studies (34,37,40–42) have addressed the criteria for CECS. Although no consensus exists, it is believed that any of the following represent reasonable criteria for a diagnosis of exercise-induced compartment syndrome:

1. A resting compartment pressure of more than 15 mmHg.
2. A delayed normalization of the pressure after exercise stops (>6 minutes).
3. A postexercise measurement of more than 15 mmHg measured 15 minutes after the completion of the exercise.

Compartment pressure measurements are necessary to verify the need for surgery if a patient does not improve with nonoperative treatment.

Treatment

The options for treating patients with CECS are limited because the condition develops as a result of the patient's anatomy. Stretching exercises for the muscles of the involved compartment and the entire lower leg may help to increase flexibility and possibly increase compliance of the fascial layer surrounding the muscle tissue. Proper warm-up before beginning the exercise that precipitates symptoms may help to precondition the muscle and lessen the rapid change in blood flow through the muscle and subsequent swelling that occurs with vigorous exercise. It is also important to correct any biomechanical abnormalities with orthotics when indicated.

Athletes who continue to have symptoms despite these measures can either limit the activity that caused the symptoms while pursuing other forms of exercise or consider surgery. Before surgical intervention is considered, it is imperative that an accurate diagnosis be obtained by performing compartment measurements. The surgical procedure involves incising the fascia to decompress the muscles within that compartment. Recovery from the operation takes about 3 weeks, and the procedure is associated with a high success rate in properly selected patients (34).

GASTROCNEMIUS MUSCLE TEARS

Clinical Case #5

A 38-year-old male tennis player comes to the office the day after injuring his leg playing doubles tennis. He felt a sudden pain in the calf while moving to the net, almost as if his partner hit him with his racket. He looked around and his partner was back at the baseline.

Athletes who participate in sports that involve sudden bursts of running or change in direction are at risk for traumatic tearing of the muscles of the lower leg. The term "tennis leg" was used by Powell (43) in 1883, referring to a presumed rupture of the plantaris tendon that occurred in a tennis player. Subsequent investigators (44,45) have determined that the injury is actually a tearing of the medial head of the gastrocnemius muscle. Several case reports have appeared (46,47) of an acute compartment syndrome of the lower leg resulting from a tear of the medial head of the gastrocnemius muscle.

Etiology

This injury is seen most commonly in middle-aged athletes and is thought to be caused by slight degeneration of the muscle-tendon unit, often seen with aging (47). Other factors associated with this injury include an excessively tight gastrocnemius-soleus-Achilles tendon complex and lack of adequate stretching and warm-up before an athletic activity. The injury results from sudden dorsiflexion of the ankle with the knee in extension (45). In many patients, the injury occurs with vigorous push-off during a running sprint.

History

The athlete will be seen because of a complaint of sudden onset of pain in the middle to upper calf region and often may report hearing or feeling a "pop" at the time of the injury (46,48). Athletes may state that it felt like the back of the calf was being hit with a hard object. They will often have difficulty walking because of the pain. Some patients may recall general symptoms of discomfort in the region for a day or so before the injury (49).

Physical Examination

Most athletes will present with a varying degree of swelling and tenderness of the calf region (Figure 17.14). If the athlete is examined soon after the injury, a defect may be palpable in the region of the midcalf (47). Within a few days, ecchymosis of the midcalf may extend down toward the ankle (50). Initially, pain may be produced by dorsiflexion of the ankle, and the athlete may be unable to perform a single leg-toe raise on the affected side (19).

Diagnostic Tests

As with many of the problems affecting the lower leg, a thorough history and physical examination should be sufficient to diagnose a tear of the medial head of the gastrocnemius muscle. Routine radiography is not necessary. If a compartment syndrome is clinically suspected, it may be necessary to refer the patient for further evaluation and compartment pressure measurements.

Treatment

The treatment of patients with this injury involves the typical approach to sports injuries: rest, ice, elevation, compression, and

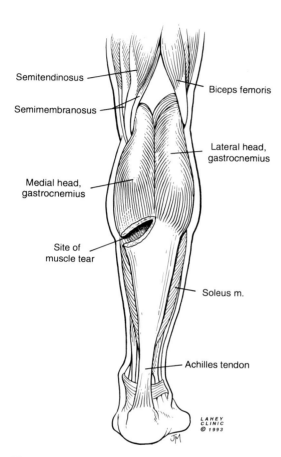

Figure 17.14. Anatomy of calf demonstrates a tear of the medial head of the gastrocnemius at the musculotendinous junction. (Reproduced by permission of the Lahey Clinic.)

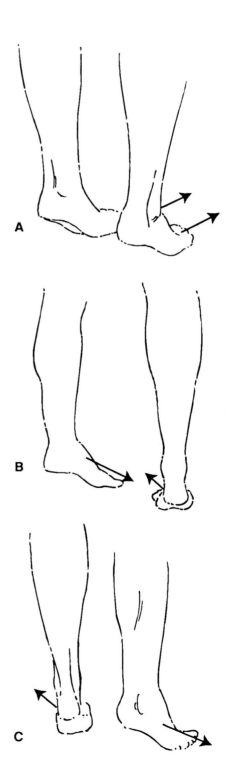

Figure 17.15. Toe raising for muscle strengthening of the calf. *A.* Legs straight for gastrocnemius-soleus. *B.* Toes in for posterior tibialis. *C.* Toes out for peroneals.

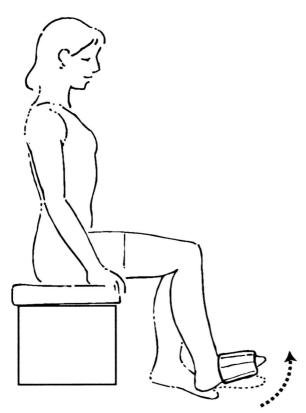

Figure 17.16. Strengthening dorsiflexors of foot with small weight on foot.

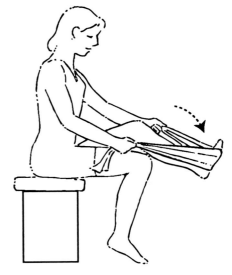

Figure 17.17. Strengthening plantar flexors (less strenuous than Figure 17.15) with elastic sheeting.

NSAIDs. The patient can be fitted with a heel lift to take some of the strain off the injured muscle. Several authors (19,20) advocate a neoprene calf sleeve to help control swelling. The patient should be given instructions in partial weight-bearing ambulation, advancing to full weight bearing as tolerated. A referral to a physical therapist may be helpful. Additionally, the patient can start passive stretching of the calf muscles, using modalities to relieve some of the discomfort. As the pain symptoms resolve,

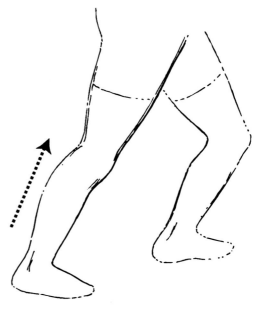

Figure 17.18. Stretching for gastrocnemius and soleus muscles and Achilles tendon.

the athlete can begin strengthening of the muscles, starting with Thera-band, routine walking, cycling, and progressing to toe raises as tolerated. Most athletes can expect a full return to sports within 6 to 7 weeks (19). Shields and colleagues (19) have shown that no strength deficit results when the patient goes through a structured physical therapy program.

EXERCISE

Some basic exercises that can be used with lower leg injuries can be seen in Figures 17.15 through 17.18.

References

1. Clemente CD. Anatomy: a regional atlas of the human body, 2nd ed. Baltimore: Urban & Schwarzenberg, 1981.

2. Brody DM. Running injuries: prevention and management. Clin Symp 1987;39:1–36.

3. Taube RR, Wadsworth LT. Managing tibial stress fractures. Physician Sports Med 1993;21:123–130.

4. Rasmussen W. Shin splints: definition and treatment. Sports Med 1974;2:111–117.

5. Briner WW Jr. Shinsplints. Am Fam Phys 1988;37:155–160.

6. Jones DC, James SL. Overuse injuries of the lower extremity: shin splints, iliotibial band friction syndrome, and exertional compartment syndromes. Clin Sports Med 1987;6:273–290.

7. Holder LE, Michael RH. The specific scintigraphic pattern of "shin splints in the lower leg": Concise communication. J Nucl Med 1984;25:865–869.

8. Markey KL. Stress fractures. Clin Sports Med 1987;6:405–425.

9. Ha KI, Hahn SH, Chung M, Yang BK, Yi SR. A clinical study of stress fractures in sports activities. Orthopaedics 1991;14:1089–1095.

10. Belkin SC. Stress fractures in athletes. Orthop Clin North Am 1980;11:735–742.

11. Fitch KD. Stress fractures of the lower limbs in runners. Aust Fam Phys 1984;13:511–515.

12. Bryk E, Grantham SA. Shin splints: a chronic deep posterior ischemic compartmental syndrome of the leg? Orthop Rev 1983;12:29–40.

13. Michael RH, Holder LE. The soleus syndrome: a cause of medial tibial stress (shin splints). Am J Sports Med 1985;13:87–94.

14. Viitasalo JT, Kvist M. Some biomechanical aspects of the foot and ankle in athletes with and without shin splints. Am J Sports Med 1983;11:125–130.

15. Nix RA. Stress fractures in the lower extremity. J Arkansas Med Soc 1983;80:10–13.

16. Matin P. Basic principles of nuclear medicine techniques for detection and evaluation of trauma and sports medicine injuries. Semin Nucl Med 1988;18:90–112.

17. Zwas ST, Elkanovitch R, Frank G. Interpretation and classification of bone scintigraphic findings in stress fractures. J Nucl Med 1987;28:452–457.

18. Martin SD, Healey JD, Horowitz S. Stress fracture MRI. Orthopaedics 1993;16:75–78.

19. Shields CL Jr, Redix L, Brewster CE. Acute tears of the medial head of the gastrocnemius. Foot Ankle 1985;5:186–190.

20. Mulligan E. Lower leg, ankle and foot rehabilitation. In: Andrews JR, Harrelson GL, eds. Physical rehabilitation of the injured athlete. Philadelphia: WB Saunders, 1991:197–266.

21. Clement DB. Tibial stress syndrome in athletes. J Sports Med 1974;2:81–85.

22. American Medical Association. Subcommittee on Classification of Sports Injuries. Standard Nomenclature of Athletic Injuries. Chicago: American Medical Association, 1966:122–126.

23. Slocum DB. The shin splint syndrome: medical aspects and differential diagnosis. Am J Surg 1967;114:875–881.

24. Jackson DW. Shinsplints: an update. Physician Sports Med 1978;6:51–68.

25. Detmer DE. Chronic shin splints: classification and management of medial tibial stress syndrome. Sports Med 1986;3:436–446.

26. Devas MB. Stress fractures of the tibia in athletes or "shin soreness." J Bone Joint Surg 1958;40B:227–239.

27. Puranen J. The medial tibial syndrome: exercise ischaemia in the medial fascial compartment of the leg. J Bone Joint Surg 1974;56B: 712–715.

28. Mubarak SJ, Gould RN, Lee YF, Schmidt DA, Hargens AR. The medial tibial stress syndrome: a cause of shin splints. Am J Sports Med 1982;10:201–205.

29. Sullivan D, Warren RF, Pavlov H, Kelman G. Stress fractures in 51 runners. Clin Orthop 1984;187:188–192.

30. Giladi M, Milgrom C, Simkin A, et al. Stress fractures and tibial bone width: a risk factor. J Bone Joint Surg 1987;69B:326–329.

31. Dugan RC, D'Ambrosia RD. Fibular stress fractures in runners. J Fam Pract 1983;17: 415–418.

32. Dickson TB Jr, Kichline PD. Functional management of stress fractures in female athletes using a pneumatic leg brace. Am J Sports Med 1987;15:86–89.

33. Whitelaw GP, Wetzler MJ, Levy AS, Segal D, Bissonnette K. A pneumatic leg brace for the treatment of tibial stress fractures. Clin Orthop 1991;270:301–305.

34. Eisele SA, Sammarco GJ. Chronic exertional compartment syndrome. Instr Course Lect 1993;42:213–217.

35. Styf JR, Körner LM. Chronic anterior-compartment syndrome of the leg. J Bone Joint Surg 1986;68A:1338–1347.

36. Fronek J, Mubarak SJ, Hargens AR, et al. Management of chronic exertional anterior compartment syndrome of the lower extremity. Clin Orthop 1987;220:217–227.

37. Styf J, Körner L, Suurkula M. Intramuscular pressure and muscle blood flow during exercise in chronic compartment syndrome. J Bone Joint Surg 1987;69B:301–305.

38. Mavor GE. The anterior tibial syndrome. J Bone Joint Surg 1956; 38B:513–517.

39. Veith RG, Matsen FA III, Newell SG. Recurrent anterior compartmental syndromes. Physician Sports Med 1980;8:80–88.

40. Rorabeck CH, Fowler PJ, Nott L. The results of fasciotomy in the management of chronic exertional compartment syndrome. Am J Sports Med 1988;16:224–227.

41. Rorabeck CH, Bourne RB, Fowler PJ, Finlay JB, Nott L. The role of tissue pressure measurement in diagnosing chronic anterior compartment syndrome. Am J Sports Med 1988;16:143–146.

42. Pedowitz RA, Hargens AR, Mubarak SJ, Gershuni DH. Modified criteria for the objective diagnosis of chronic compartment syndrome of the leg. Am J Sports Med 1990;18:35–40.

43. Powell RW. Lawn tennis leg. Lancet 1883; 2:44.

44. Arner O, Lindholm Å. What is tennis leg? Acta Chir Scand 1958;116:73–77.

45. Miller WA. Rupture of the musculotendinous juncture of the medial head of the gastrocnemius muscle. Am J Sports Med 1977;5:191–193.

46. Straehley D, Jones WW. Acute compartment syndrome (anterior, lateral, and superficial posterior) following tear of the medial head of the gastrocnemius muscle: a case report. Am J Sports Med 1986;14:96–99.

47. Anouchi YS, Parker RD, Seitz WH Jr. Posterior compartment syndrome of the calf resulting from misdiagnosis of a rupture of the medial head of the gastrocnemius. J Trauma 1987;27:678–680.

48. Millar AP. Strains of the posterior calf musculature. Am J Sports Med 1979;7:172–174.

49. Froimson AI. Tennis leg. JAMA 1969; 209:415–416.

50. McClure JG. Gastrocnemius musculotendinous rupture: a condition confused with thrombophlebitis. South Med J 1984;77:1143–1145.

THE FOOT

MICHAEL PETRIZZI

18

Anatomy
Biomechanics
Athletic Footwear
History and Physical Examination
Hindfoot Injuries
Midfoot Injuries
Forefoot Injuries

Foot injuries represent a significant threat to both the competitive and the recreational athlete (1). The foot is an amazing combination of bones (tarsals, metatarsals, phalanges, sesamoids), ligaments, muscles, and their tendons. The foot must serve two functions. It routinely supports the weight of an individual's body with the minimum use of muscular action, therefore, conserving energy. However, in a moment's notice it launches a person forward or provides the support needed when landing. With each running step, the foot is exposed to forces equal to three to four times the body weight of the athlete. This makes the foot the site of many injuries in the running athlete.

ANATOMY

The foot is a complex organ assembled from 26 bones with numerous ligamentous interconnections. The myriad intrinsic muscles as well as the extrinsic muscle-tendon units add to this complexity (2). A thorough knowledge of the anatomy and the biomechanics of the foot is necessary for the diagnosis and treatment of athletic injuries to the foot and remaining lower extremity.

The foot is divided into three different segments (Figure 18.1): the hindfoot, which is made up of the talus and calcaneus; the midfoot, which consists of the navicular, cuboid, and three cuneiforms; and the forefoot, containing the metatarsals, phalanges, and sesamoid bones. The main joints of the foot are the talocrural or ankle joint, the talocalcaneal or subtalar joint, the midtarsal joints, the tarsometatarsal joints, and the metatarsophalangeal joints. The many joints and their ligamentous interconnections contribute to the shape and function of the foot. This is dependent on the two arches which they form: the longitudinal arch and the transverse arch (Figure 18.2).

The longitudinal arch runs from the calcaneus to the metatarsal heads on the medial side of the foot. Its structure is maintained both statically and dynamically (Figure 18.3). The prime static stabilizer is the calcaneonavicular (spring) ligament. The secondary static stabilizers are the multiple capsular ligaments and plantar aponeurosis. The prime dynamic stabilizer of the longitudinal arch is the posterior tibial muscle, secondarily supported by the anterior tibial and peroneus longus muscles.

The transverse (metatarsal) arch is located in the frontal plane in the forefoot. It is apparent only when the foot is non–weight bearing. The transverse arch is supported by the intermetatarsal ligaments and collapses with weight bearing to allow weight to be distributed to all metatarsal heads.

BIOMECHANICS

It is important to understand the biomechanics of the foot in the running gait cycle to appreciate the cause and treatment of many foot and leg injuries. The gait cycle (Figure 18.4) begins with the heel-strike and ends with heel-strike of the same foot. It is divided into stance and swing phase. The running gait differs from the walking gait in that there is a segment of double limb support (both feet on the ground) in walking, and there is only single limb support during the stance phase while running. There is also a float phase in running, with both feet off the ground. This increases the forces on the foot and leg with running. As the athlete runs faster, the duration of

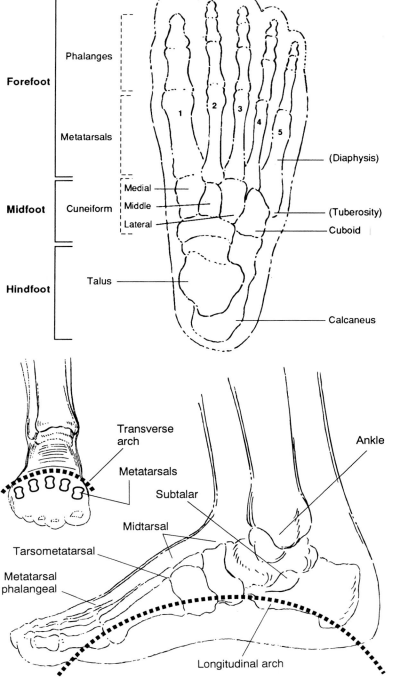

Figure 18.1. Bony anatomy expanded to show forefoot, midfoot, and hindfoot.

Forefoot

Phalanges

Metatarsals

(Diaphysis)

Midfoot

Cuneiform

Medial
Middle
Lateral

(Tuberosity)

Cuboid

Hindfoot

Talus

Calcaneus

Figure 18.2. Longitudinal and transverse arches of the foot.

Transverse arch

Metatarsals

Subtalar

Midtarsal

Tarsometatarsal

Metatarsal phalangeal

Ankle

Longitudinal arch

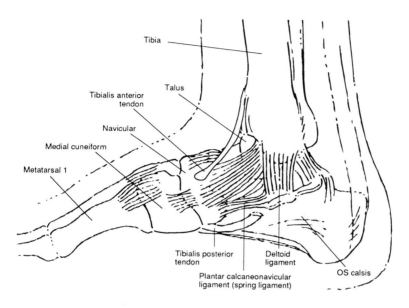

Figure 18.3. Static and dynamic stabilizers of the longitudinal arch.

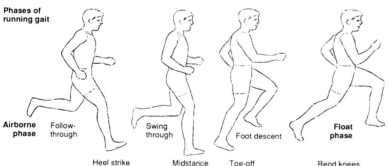

Figure 18.4. Running gait.

the stance phase decreases and the forces increase further.

The foot goes through a complex series of motions with gait, termed supination and pronation (Figure 18.5). These motions are part of the normal biomechanics of the foot, which is typically supinated during the swing phase to heel-strike. The foot then pronates rapidly in early stance, only to supinate again just before toe-off.

Many of the important motions of the foot occur at the subtalar joint, which is ac-

tually the talocalcaneal joint. This joint has significant ligamentous support and yet can have motions in three different planes. Because most of the injuries of the foot occur where there is contact with the ground, a closed kinetic chain must be considered. Therefore, the remaining joints of the foot do play a part. Included in these are the midtarsal joints, the tarsometatarsal joints, and the metatarsophalangeal joints.

The posterior tibial and anterior tibial muscles maintain the foot in the supinated

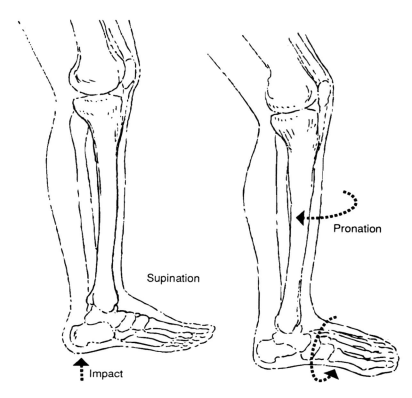

Figure 18.5. *Supination*:
foot is supinated during
swing phase from toe-off to
heel-strike. At heel strike
there is rapid *pronation* to
dissipate energy.

Supination

Pronation

Impact

position during the swing phase of gait. The calcaneus is under the talus and the foot is relatively stiff. With heel-strike, the calcaneus moves into a more pronated position and the foot "rolls in" (see Figure 18.5). The posterior and anterior tibial muscles contract eccentrically (maximally lengthened while they are contracting) as this occurs. This dissipates some of the energy (three to four times body weight) that must be absorbed with each step. In the stiffer high-arched (cavus) foot, very little energy is dissipated in the foot, and excessive forces are transmitted up the leg, which may lead to injuries in the leg, knee, or thigh. At the anatomic level, in pronation the calcaneus moves laterally and the head of the talus adducts and plantar flexes. There is medial rotation of the tibia and the medial arch flattens out. The joints of the

foot become looser, allowing better adaptation of the varied surfaces that the foot contacts. In the foot with excessive pronation, there is both increased medial rotation of the tibia and eversion of the calcaneus. There is increased stress on the anterior and posterior tibial muscles. These predispose to injuries of the leg.

At toe-off, the foot moves back into supination, both through anterior and posterior tibial muscular activity, and the tightening of the plantar fascia as the toes are dorsiflexed. As mentioned earlier, it is excessive degrees of these two normal motions, pronation and supination, that are responsible for many common foot and leg overuse injuries in athletics. Even though the foot needs to pronate both to dissipate energy and to adapt to uneven surfaces, there is the tradeoff because excessive pronation leads to an increase in torsional forces on the connective tissues. On the other hand, although the supinated foot may be great for pushing off, the supinated foot is a rigid structure that may not be able to dissipated the shock of the forces transmitted to it. This, too, can lead to problems in the foot and leg.

ATHLETIC FOOTWEAR

There has been an explosion in the types of athletic footwear over the past 25 years. Beginning with running shoes in the late 1960s, the number and complexity of shoe types has markedly increased. It is important to understand basic terminology and construction of these athletic shoes (Figure 18.6).

The *last* is the basic shape of the shoe—it can be a board last (stiffer = more support) or a slip last (more flexible = more cushion). Therefore, in addition to a comfortable fit, "functional fit" is important.

The *counter* is the heel cup configuration

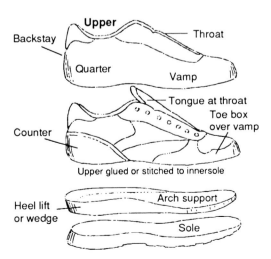

Figure 18.6. Athletic footwear.

of the shoe. It should be firm, well padded, and rigidly attached to the last. With alignment abnormalities of the foot, the counter and its attachment to the last are often the first part of the shoe to break down.

The *toebox* is the portion of the shoe that accommodates the forefoot. It should have enough room to allow for easy motion of the toes. There should be $\frac{1}{4}''$ to $\frac{3}{8}''$ in front of the long toe. Excessive space, however, can cause trouble if the foot slides in the shoe.

The shoe should have an adequate *longitudinal arch support*. This is most often supplied as a separate insert in running or walking shoes and as a glued in support in other athletic footwear. Typically, the arch support supplied will accommodate a foot with a normal arch. Athletes with either a flat foot or high-arched foot will usually require a more substantial, often custom made, orthotic for comfort and to reduce the risk of injury.

The *sole* of athletic shoes these days is usually a composite of several layers. The outersole typically is designed for either traction or abrasion resistance, while the main sole structure is for cushioning and flexibility. Shoes for distance running should be flexible in the forefoot; shoes for walking or racquet sports should have a stiffer forefoot. More expensive running shoes often have a gel or airbag system in the heel to help absorb energy. Most running shoe companies have a shoe designed for the pronated foot, which uses a stiffer material for the sole on the medial heel and arch.

Because the average foot strike is on the lateral heel and push-off is from the great toe, these are the areas that typically show wear (Figure 18.7). A runner's shoes should be inspected for the wear pattern. Some extension of the life of a running shoe can be gained by using a liquid rubber solution (usually obtainable at sporting goods

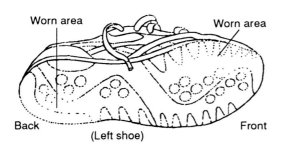

Worn area

Worn area

Back

Front

(Left shoe)

Figure 18.7. Typical wear pattern in the running shoe.

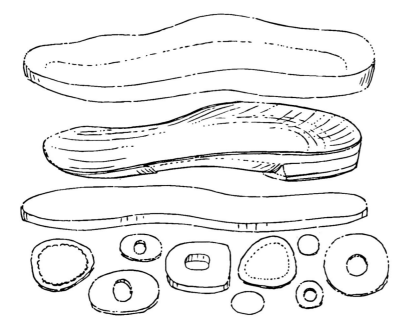

Figure 18.8. Orthotic: *posting* can compensate for hindfoot malalignment, which can also help with reducing pronation, the arch provides additional support, *relief points* can take pressure off bony prominences.

stores) to build up the areas of early sole wear. Excessive sole wear can accentuate any biomechanical variant in the runner and predispose to injury. The longevity of a running shoe is usually determined by how long the sole maintains its cushioning. This is between 350 and 500 miles, depending on the weight of the runner and the quality of the shoe. Runners should be counseled to change shoes regularly before 500 miles or even sooner for heavier athletes. It is often best in the aggressive distance runner to use

several pairs of shoes simultaneously so that break in can occur gradually.

Orthotics are inserts for the shoe designed to correct for an alignment or biomechanical abnormality of the runner's foot (Figure 18.8). Most commonly they are used to correct pronation or to relieve pressure from an area of the foot. Orthotics come in three basic groups: soft, semirigid, and rigid. Soft orthotics are made of felt or soft foam and are available over-the-counter at running and sporting goods stores.

Semirigid orthotics are custom made from a moldable plastic, such as plastazote. Rigid orthotics are made from hard plastic and usually require a casting of the athlete's foot. Semirigid orthotics are cheaper and somewhat easier to fabricate. They are more forgiving, so that the mold does not have to be perfect. They are used most commonly to relieve pressure or in mild to moderate pronators. Rigid orthotics are more expensive and harder to fit. They often cause problems if used on a high-arched foot. Rigid orthotics are best suited for moderate to severe pronators, when semirigid orthotics fail to alleviate the runner's symptoms.

HISTORY AND PHYSICAL EXAMINATION

In evaluating the athlete who presents with a complaint of foot pain, history is important. Location of the pain and an understanding of the anatomy are the bases of the diagnosis. Determining whether there are factors relating more likely to overuse versus traumatic injury may be the key point in your decision tree. Some factors that may lead to overuse injuries are a change in shoes, a change of surface, an increase in mileage, or an increase in the intensity of training. There may have been no change whatsoever, with the injury arising from chronic overuse related to anatomic or biomechanical abnormalities.

The physical examination of the foot consists of three different components: static observation, dynamic examination, and shoewear.

In static observation, observe the athlete both in the weight-bearing and non–weight-bearing phases. Are there any obvious deformities? Is there significant bow-ing of the Achilles tendon or significant flattening out of the arch with or without weight bearing. While looking at the skin, check to see if there is any callous formation indicating areas of excessive pressure.

The dynamic examination includes gait, range of motion, and strength examinations. Analyze gait with the athlete barefoot, walking in the hallway. Stand or squat while the athlete walks both toward you and away from you, several times. Concentrate on only one part of the foot on each cycle. With continued observation and practice, it is often possible to be able to determine excessive degrees of supination or pronation as well as other gait abnormalities. A video camera can be used to analyze gait while the athlete is running on a treadmill.

Assessing the range of motion of the various joints of the foot is demonstrated in Figure 18.9. Motion of the hindfoot, or subtalar joint, is assessed by cupping the heel in one hand and alternately inverting and everting it (Figure 18.9A). Midfoot motion and motion at the midtarsal and tarsometatarsal joints is assessed by maintaining the hindfoot in neutral while inverting (Figure 18.9B) and then everting (Figure 18.9C) the forefoot. Motion in the forefoot is dorsiflexion (Figure 18.9D) and plantar flexion (Figure 18.9E) at the metatarsophalangeal joints. Although a major function of the leg muscles is stabilization of the foot, they can be tested by isolating their functions as shown in Figure 18.9B.

The third part of the examination is footwear. Athletes should bring in not only the shoes that they compete in, which for some sports may be less than an hour a day, three to four times a week, but also the footwear they are in for the rest of the day. This can be a valuable part of your evaluation. Look for patterns of excessive wear (e.g., medial

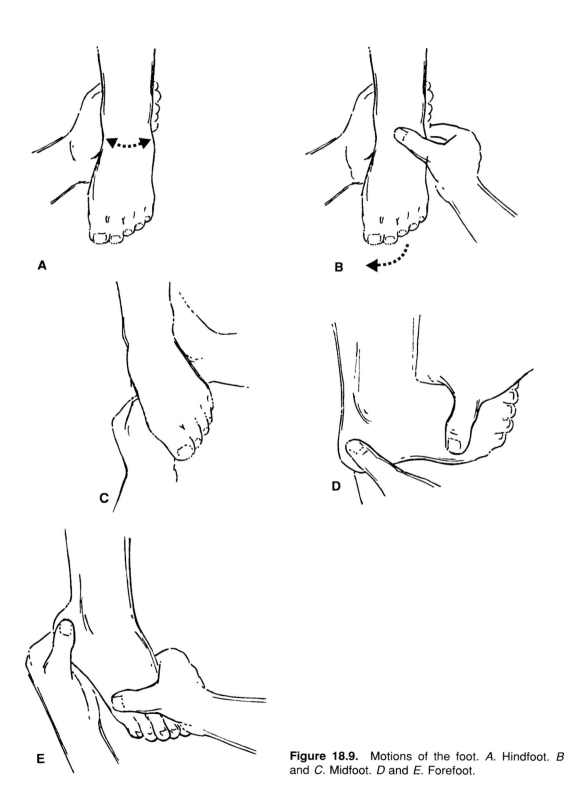

Figure 18.9. Motions of the foot. *A.* Hindfoot. *B* and *C.* Midfoot. *D* and *E.* Forefoot.

heel collapse with hyperpronation; see Figure 18.7).

In terms of diagnostic tests, x-rays are frequently needed. Dr. D. J. Morton was quoted in the 1930s as saying, ". . . the x-ray was absolutely invaluable . . ." (3). However, in this era of cost-effective medicine, one should consider whether the history and physical examination clearly point to a soft-tissue injury, and whether or not the x-ray has a reasonable likelihood of adding anything to the diagnosis. The x-rays may not initially show any findings in the case of stress fractures in the foot. In this instance, a bone scan may be indicated. It may be helpful to use the tuning fork test. This is done by vibrating the tuning fork and locating its hub over the tender areas. Although this test cannot separate periostitis from a stress fracture, the presence of excruciating discomfort often indicates true bony pain as opposed to soft-tissue disease. This can be helpful in further clarifying the decision to request a bone scan.

Because injuries can result from either abnormal stresses (such as a rapid increase in mileage) on a normal structure, or normal stresses placed on an abnormal structure (such as the excessively pronated flat foot), it is important to keep this principle in mind to guide treatment. This may also lead to the prevention of further injuries. When the abnormal structure can be identified, the use of orthotics or better constructed athletic footwear can help resist the abnormal motion and can be an important part of the treatment.

HINDFOOT INJURIES

This area includes the talus and calcaneus, as well as the Achilles tendon, origin of the plantar fascia, heel pad, and the tarsal tunnel. The peroneal, as well as anterior and posterior tibial tendons, traverse this area going to their more distal insertions, but the hindfoot is their most common site of injury.

Achilles Tendinitis

Epidemiology

Tendinitis typically occurs in somewhat older athletes in running or jumping sports.

Clinical Case #1

Mr. S. and Mr. L. are 33-year-old white collar workers who have been friends since high school. They have been recreational runners for years and decided to train for an upcoming marathon. Their weekly mileage as they begin to train up for the marathon was about 20 miles. Several weeks into their program, they have both developed heel pain. They have been running many hills and have doubled their weekly mileage over 3 weeks. Mr. S. has flat feet and has frequently had "shin splints" during his athletic career. Mr. L. has a very high instep and arch. He has a history of frequent sore calves and frequent leg cramps when he was a high school running back. He follows the same training as Mr. S. and complains of the same kind of pain.

At times the issues associated with either static or functional hyperpronation, as in Mr. S., are an issue, whereas Mr. L. is an individual with cavus foot by history. Both individuals suffer from the problem of the training error of the sudden increase in mileage and course conditions. Mr. S. does have a functional problem with hyperpronation. His Achilles tendon showed some bowing medially and was warm and tender to the touch. He had no pain in front of the tendon nor did he have any bony tenderness. The only difference on examination of Mr. L. was the cavus foot deformity.

Mr. S. was suffering from a problem of Achilles tendinitis, probably due to increased torsional forces on the tendon from excessive pronation. His training error of suddenly increasing his distance, as well as the hill work, contributed to bringing out this problem. Mr. L. suffered from the problem of not having very good shock absorption. So, every time he took a step, a force two to three times his body weight was transmitted to his Achilles tendon. The differential for posterior heel pain in this age group would also include retrocalcaneal bursitis. In this case, there would be tenderness found anterior to the tendon, overlying the bony tuberosity of the calcaneus (Figure 18.10). Sometimes swelling of the tendon can be appreciated in the case of Achilles tendinitis. This is more typical of chronic injuries. If there is swelling, it is usually a fusiform type and it is felt within the body of the tendon itself. Patients who are suffering from a case of retrocalcaneal bursitis may also have a Haglund's deformity, which is a bony prominence on the posterior aspect of the calcaneus, or they have had a shoe with poor padding in the counter, which causes irritation. If the complaint of pain is brought to you by a 7- to 13-year-old, one must keep the diagnosis of Sever's disease in mind. This is a case of calcaneal apophysitis, a self-limiting condition that would have no effect on linear growth (Figure 18.11). Treatment for Sever's disease can be as simple as a heel lift. It may be disabling enough to require rest from all athletic participation. In the case of a 12-year-old, x-rays may be necessary, and one should see that the calcaneal apophysis is present and more dense than usual.

Both Mr. S. and Mr. L. would benefit from the use of ice and judicious use

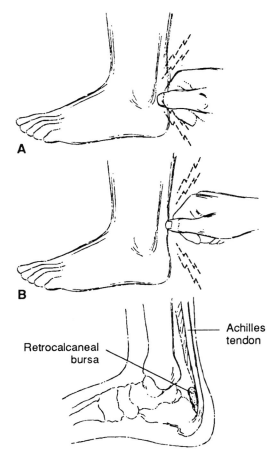

Figure 18.10. *A.* Tenderness anterior to Achilles tendon—retrocalcaneal bursitis. *B.* Tenderness in tendon itself—Achilles tendinitis.

of a nonsteroidal anti-inflammatory drug (NSAID). If seen early enough in the course of the disease, total rest may not be required but simply a reduction in training intensity. For Mr. S., correction of his tendency toward hyperpronation with a shoewear change or orthotic would be a key to future successful participation in any athletic endeavor. Mr. L., on the other hand, would derive the most benefit from the same ini-

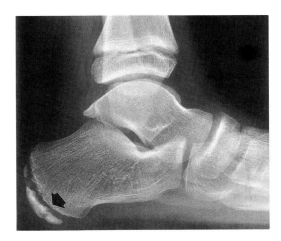

Figure 18.11. Sever's disease: sclerosis and fragmentation of the calcaneal apophysis (*arrow*).

tial treatments but a rehabilitation program that included calf stretching exercises would also be beneficial (Figure 18.12). One starts to stretch by placing the affected leg about an arm's length away from the wall, keeping the heel in contact with the ground as one stretches forward. The knee is kept straight to stretch the gastrocnemius muscle. Then, to get more stretch to the soleus muscle, allow the knee to bend. The use of well-cushioned running shoes would be advisable. A $\frac{1}{4}''$ commercial heel lift will slightly decrease the forces in both men. Injection of corticosteroids into the area is *not* recommended because of the fear of Achilles tendon rupture. The athlete can safely return to complete participation when there is little or no pain.

Retrocalcaneal bursitis can be injected with corticosteroids, if necessary. The bursa is between the tendon and bone. One must be careful not to have any steroid go into the body of the Achilles tendon. However, improved footwear, icing, and NSAIDs may be adequate treatment.

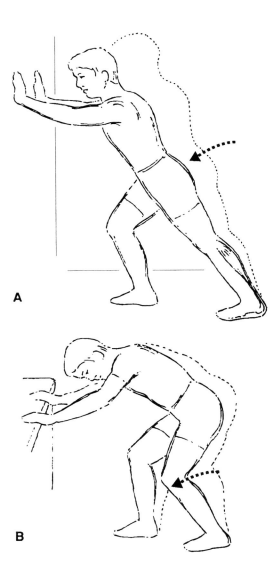

Figure 18.12. Stretching of tendoachilles: straight knee for gastrocnemius muscle (*A*), bent knee for soleus muscle (*B*).

Achilles Tendon Rupture

Epidemiology

Achilles rupture most often occurs in male athletes in their thirties and forties. It commonly occurs in sports with starting-stopping running activities. Many, but certainly not all, athletes with Achilles tendon rupture have had prior tendinitis.

Clinical Case #2

A 35-year-old avid tennis player plays two to three times per week. Midway through the third set one weekend he rushes the net. He feels a sharp tear in his anke and falls. He has quite a bit of pain, but he is able to bear weight. The next day he comes to your office. Although feeling something tear, there was no twisting of the ankle. (The injury usually occurs when the athlete is tired or has not fully warmed up.) The ankle is swollen and ecchymotic. There is no tenderness over the malleoli or the ligaments. The Achilles tendon is swollen and painful. He has very little strength of plantar flexion. With the patient prone, squeezing his calf muscle results in no plantar flexion of the foot (Figure 18.13). This is the Thompson test and indicates a complete rupture of the Achilles tendon.

Rupture of the Achilles tendon may be confused with ankle sprains. The lack of twisting in the injury and no tenderness over the ligaments should focus the examiner on other injuries.

The options for treatment are surgical repair or casting. For casting to be successful, the ends of the tendon must be approximated when the foot is allowed to rest in plantar flexion. If this does not happen, then surgical repair is necessary. If the ends of the tendon come together with plantar flexion, then nonoperative treatment can be considered. The advantages of surgery are better long-term strength and endurance, with a decreased risk of rerupture. Nonoperative treatment avoids the risks of surgery and anesthesia, but recovery is slower, rerupture is higher, and long-term function is not quite as good.

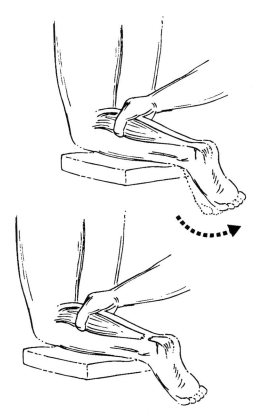

Figure 18.13. Thompson test. Absence of plantar flexion of foot when squeezing the calf muscle is a positive test, indicating rupture of the Achilles tendon. (Modified from S Hoppenfeld. Physical Examination of the Spine Extremities. Norwalk, CT: Appleton & Lange, 1976: 218.)

Heel Pain—Plantar Surface

Epidemiology

Pain in this area is often seen in runners and aerobics participants. The most common diagnosis is plantar fasciitis.

Clinical Case #3

Mrs. W. is a 28-year-old bank executive who realized the need to get back into shape after she saw her family physician for her yearly checkup.

She joined a local fitness club and began doing aerobics. After 2 weeks of class, she came back to her family physician disheartened, complaining of sharp pains in the bottom of her foot. The pain is most severe on first arising in the morning.

Clinical Case #4

Mrs. J. is a 47-year-old university official who presents complaining of heel pain when she first gets up in the morning and whenever she gets out of a chair after a long meeting. She has gained 25 lb over the last 2 years and has trouble finding shoes that fit because of her high arch. She recently began a walking/running program to help lose weight.

Both patients complain of pain at the bottom of their heel and describe it as occurring at its worst when the foot is first put down on the ground. Mrs. W. is found to have a problem with hyperpronation. In addition, the shoes that she used for aerobics were quite old and had a very poor heel counter. The physical findings in Mrs. J. confirm pain at the base of the heel (Figure 18.14). It is made worse when her toes are dorsiflexed passively and the examiner would note the cavus foot deformity. If x-rays are ordered, and it could be argued that most cases of plantar fasciitis do not need an x-ray, one may find a heel spur (Figure 18.15), which is simply calcification of the attachment of the plantar fascia. This finding is also often seen in many asymptomatic individuals.

The plantar fascia is a thick band of connective tissue that originates at the bottom of the heel and progresses forward toward the ball of the foot. It helps maintain the arch of the foot. The stiff "high-arch foot" can be plagued with painful swelling of this tissue because the force is concentrated at the origin of the plantar fascia, as was noted

in Mrs. J.'s case. Mrs. W. had the problem of excessive pronation, which caused her problems because of the increased torsional forces as mentioned. Once again the combination of the tendency toward hyperpronation challenged by the training error of sudden increase in activity was a significant factor in her problem. For Mrs. J., not only did the cavus foot contribute to the problem, but at age 47 with a 25-lb increase in weight, there is even more force concentrated there.

In the differential diagnosis of heel pain on the sole of the foot, one should also consider fat pad syndrome, fat pad contusion, and tarsal tunnel syndrome. The fat pad of the heel is a specialized cushioning area, where there are thick fibrous septae dividing the pad into numerous compartments (see Figure 18.14B). This specialized area cushions heel-strike by functioning like a waterbed. With aging, atrophy of the fat within these compartments may decrease the cushioning effect and lead to heel pain in the fat pad itself. Direct trauma may lead to bleeding into the fat pad, which also causes pain here in athletes. Tarsal tunnel syndrome is caused by pressure on the posterior tibial nerve, or one of its terminal branches (medial or lateral plantar nerves and calcaneal branch), at the level of the flexor retinaculum or more distally. This often leads to activity-related pain in the heel or sole of the foot. This is analogous to carpal tunnel syndrome in the hand. The pain is usually poorly localizable, and reproduced by a positive Tinel's sign at the site of entrapment. An electromyogram and nerve conduction studies are necessary to confirm this diagnosis.

It is important to counsel the athlete that the problem of plantar fasciitis can often be a slow healing process. The tissue is not very well vascularized and constantly being stressed, even in sedentary activities.

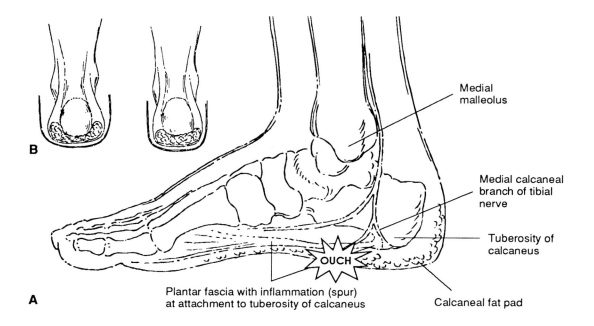

B

Medial
malleolus

Medial calcaneal
branch of tibial
nerve

Tuberosity of
calcaneus

OUCH

A

Plantar fascia with inflammation (spur)
at attachment to tuberosity of calcaneus

Calcaneal fat pad

Figure 18.14. *A*. Tenderness at base of heel in plantar fasciitis. *B*. Heel fat pad, note multi-septate anatomy for cushioning.

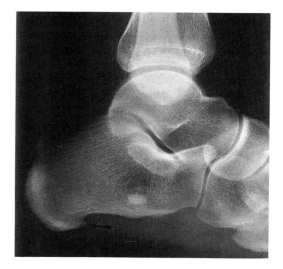

Figure 18.15. Heel spur (*arrow*) calcification of origin of plantar fascia.

Mechanical problems should be addressed. The use of orthotics is appropriate for excessive pronation. A heel cup, particularly one that is soft and well padded, can help plantar fasciitis in the high-arched foot. Heel cups are often of benefit in pain from the heel pad. Ice is helpful along with use of NSAIDs. With plantar fasciitis, the judicious injection of a corticosteroid and local anesthesia, taking care to avoid the calcaneal fat pad, may be of benefit. Corticosteroids may cause fat atrophy, and repetitive injections should be avoided. Once again the fear of rupture of the fascia needs to be considered.

Both athletes will benefit from the use of a good running shoe with an excellent heel counter. This shoe should be worn as often as possible (e.g., including a walk to the bathroom in the middle of the night). The decrease of any strain on the fascia can help the healing process. Mrs. J. would particularly benefit from stretching exercises for both her calves as well as the plantar fascia.

We often put athletes on relative rest for this problem. One should also consider re-developing the strength of the intrinsic muscles of the foot with exercises such as towel curls (pulling a towel toward the back of the foot through the use of the toes). Also, when there is significant decrease in the pain of the heel itself, walking on soft surfaces such as the sand or grass can strengthen intrinsic muscles. Rarely, for the patients with extremely tight calf muscles and plantar fascia, use of a nighttime splint putting the foot into as much dorsiflexion as can be tolerated may be of benefit.

Posterior Tibial Tendinitis and Rupture

Epidemiology

These occur in middle-aged athletes in running sports. The degeneration of the tendon from chronic tendinitis is felt to lead to most of the cases of tendon rupture. Rupture may occur insidiously or following a trauma.

Clinical Case #5

Mr. V. is a 48-year-old recreational runner who has developed pain in both feet, on the medial foot and ankle. He is aware of swelling, has self-treated with over-the-counter ibuprofen, but is not really improving. He has already decreased his mileage.

Clinical Case #6

Mrs. Q. is a 52-year-old tennis player who injured her right ankle during a match several days ago. She comes to the office with significant pain and swelling medially below the ankle.

Posterior tibial tendinitis usually presents with pain and swelling, just distal to the medial malleolus. About 50% of the pa-tients who rupture the tendon will have a traumatic injury. This may be confused with ankle sprain. The swelling and tenderness from posterior tibial tendinitis or rupture is distal to the ankle. It can be traced to the insertion of the tendon onto the navicular. With chronic cases of tendinitis, there is degeneration of the tendon and a loss of normal arch. With rupture of the tendon, the arch collapses even further. Acute tendon rupture, when mistaken as a sprain, will not improve as expected and a progressive flat foot will ensue.

With rupture of the tendon, the athlete will have the "too many toes sign" when observed from behind (Figure 18.16). The athlete will also have a unilateral flat foot and the inability to invert the foot when going up on the toes.

The posterior tibial tendon may undergo degeneration and intersubstance rupture. When sudden rupture occurs, it may be mistaken for an ankle sprain. Remember that medial ankle sprains are unusual.

Molded, rigid, or semirigid orthoses are indicated in treatment of posterior tibial tendinitis. NSAIDs and activity reduction are appropriate. For athletes with a traumatic rupture, consideration for early surgical repair is appropriate. Treatment for chronic rupture is the same as in tendinitis. Surgical treatment may be considered for resistant tendinitis or ruptures that remain symptomatic.

Other Tendons

Tendinitis of peroneal tendons or the anterior tibial tendon is usually caused by training errors, either a sudden increase in duration or intensity of activity. Focal pain, swelling, and tenderness are typical. Not infrequently there will be a fine crepitance (almost "squeaky") with motion. Treatment

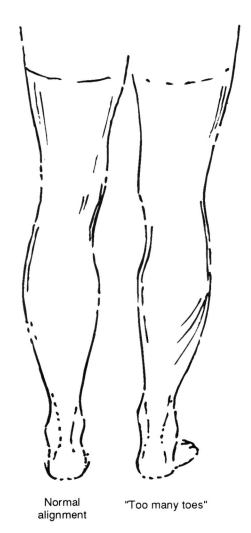

Normal   "Too many toes"
alignment

Figure 18.16. "Too many toes" sign indicative
of unilateral posterior tibial tendon rupture.

is with NSAIDs, icing, and temporary activity modification.

MIDFOOT INJURIES

A number of conditions that may present with symptoms in the midfoot have already been discussed. These include plantar fasciitis and the various tendons. The tarsal navicular is a common site of athletic injury. It is the keystone of the longitudinal arch, and, therefore, under considerable stress with running and jumping.

Clinical Case #7

A 17-year-old high school basketball player has pain in his foot about halfway through the season. The pain developed insidiously. He is a jumping athlete putting significant stress on his foot. There is tenderness in the midfoot, over the navicular bone. There is no particular bony prominence.

A bony prominence might indicate an accessory navicular (Figure 18.17). This is a portion of the bone, formed from a secondary ossification center, which did not unite with the body of the navicular. These are often painful due to rubbing on the shoe or the posterior tibial tendon.

Radiographs are necessary to diagnose an accessory navicular. If the films are nor-

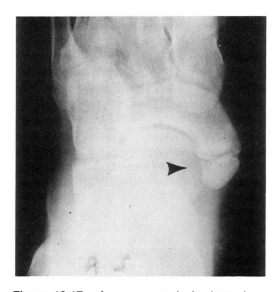

Figure 18.17. Accessory navicular (*arrow*).

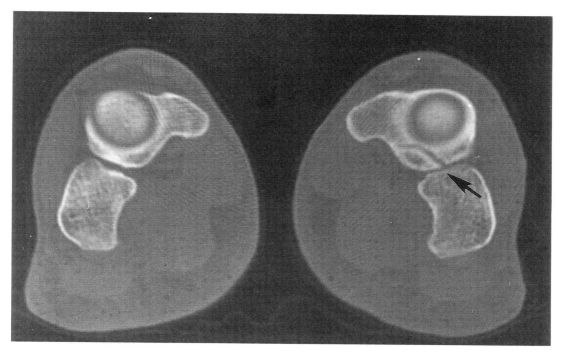

Figure 18.18. Stress fracture of the navicular (*arrow*) seen only on computed tomography scan.

mal, the physician must have a high suspicion of a stress fracture of the navicular. Failure to treat a stress fracture of this bone appropriately may result in a true fracture, requiring surgery. A technetium bone scan or computed tomography scan is indicated to make the diagnosis (Figure 18.18). If identified early, treatment is usually casting and non–weight bearing. If there is a delay in diagnosis, treatment may be more complex and even require surgery.

Kohler's disease, or avascular necrosis of the navicular, might present with similar symptoms. X-rays would demonstrate the sclerotic, collapsed bone of osteonecrosis (Figure 18.19). Treatment is usually symptomatic with arch support.

FOREFOOT INJURIES

The forefoot is subjected to substantial stress in the push-off phase of running. Jumping sports accentuate the risk of injury to the forefoot. The structures at risk are diverse. The subcutaneous location of the structures makes physical examination the key to accurate diagnosis.

Metatarsalgia

Epidemiology

Running, aerobics, and court sports are frequent causes.

Clinical Case #8

A 17-year-old high school senior is actively being recruited by many university basketball programs. Just about every year, in the late season, he complains about a dull achy foot. He

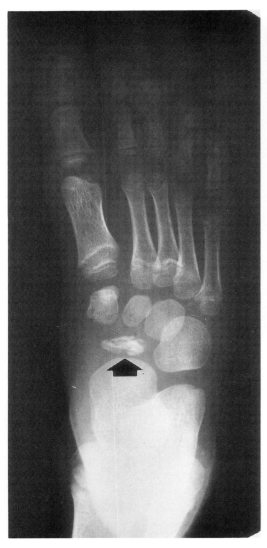

Figure 18.19. Sclerosis and collapse of the navicular (*arrow*) indicative of Kohler's disease.

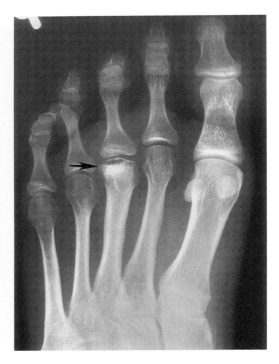

Figure 18.20. Freiberg's infraction of third metatarsal (*arrow*).

subjects the foot to constant pounding and complains of a dull ache. On static examination, he seemed to have an adequate arch. Dynamic evaluation revealed significant splaying out of the foot. Tenderness was found in the region of the metatarsals but there was no one specific area of bony tenderness.

Metatarsalgia is a term used to describe pain under the metatarsal heads, typically concentrated under the second and third. This specific example describes one of overuse. However, there are clinically important differences based on the location of pain, which will be discussed in further examples. Radiographs are indicated if the tenderness is limited to a single metatarsal head. This may demonstrate collapse of the metatarsal head (typically the second or third). This is termed Freiberg's infraction (Figure 18.20). Metatarsalgia is often encountered in older athletes who have lost some of the fat that cushions the metatarsal heads.

In the treatment of metatarsalgia, NSAIDs can be helpful, and correction of the tendency toward hyperpronation with

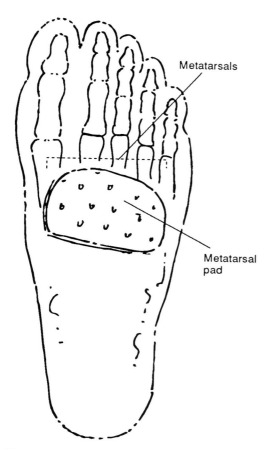

Metatarsals

Metatarsal pad

Figure 18.21. Metatarsal pad to relieve pressure on metatarsal heads.

improved footwear or orthotics is indicated. Often the use of a metatarsal pad, placed in the shoes proximal to the metatarsal heads, will distribute the forces to a wider area and relieve the symptoms (Figure 18.21).

Metatarsal Stress Fractures

Clinical Case #9

Mr. J. another high school athlete, a soccer player, presents with severe pain right in the middle of his foot. He presents with localized pain. The pain has been present for 10 days.

Clinical Case #10

Mr. W. is a 37-year-old 6'6" weekend basketball player who during the week "pounds the pavement" as a car salesman. One particular Sunday, while coming down with a rebound, he hears a crack (he presents to you at Monday night office hours complaining of pain and swelling over the fifth metatarsal). Mr. W. is hinting toward chronic overuse issues and repetitive microtrauma with an acute event.

Mr. J. was found to have problems toward hyperpronation, but also a detectable, small amount of swelling was located over the third metatarsal. Mr. W. was complaining of pain over the fifth metatarsal. You note his tendency toward oversupination as he walks, which at this point is difficult because of the pain. Both individuals complain of significant pain when a vibrating tuning fork is applied to the area of their discomfort. Since both individuals complained of bony pain, x-rays were obtained. Mr. J.'s initial films were negative. When Mr. J. returned with the pain improving 2 weeks later, a repeat x-ray was taken (Figure 18.22) and the callous formation of a healing stress fracture was noted. Mr. W.'s x-ray demonstrated a fracture in the fifth metatarsal in the diaphyseal region.

Both individuals are suffering from a problem with stress fractures of the metatarsals (4). However, stress fractures of the second through fourth metatarsals are different from fractures to the diaphysis of the fifth metatarsal because of a higher rate of nonunion in the latter (5). This is an appropriate time to discuss the difference between a Jones' fracture (a fracture of the fifth metatarsal through the diaphysis) ver-

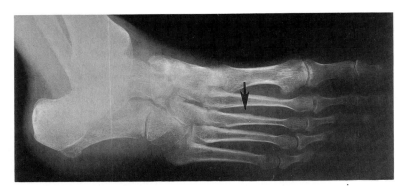

Figure 18.22. Stress fracture of third metatarsal shows early callous formation (*arrow*).

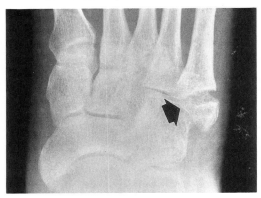

Figure 18.23. Avulsion of base of fifth metatarsal (*arrow*) from inversion injury.

sus an avulsion fracture of the base of the fifth metatarsal. The avulsion fracture occurs at the most proximal portion of the fifth metatarsal because of contraction by the peroneus brevis which causes the avulsion to occur with an inversion injury (Figure 18.23). Once again the management is very different because of the problems with nonunion with diaphyseal injuries. The avulsion fracture is in cancellous bone, and as long as the joint is not displaced, a stiff shoe or walking cast for comfort is adequate treatment.

A diaphyseal fracture may occur as a single traumatic event in otherwise normal bone, but in jumping athletes there is often an underlying stress fracture that goes on to true fracture. Radiographs will show this, with sclerotic margins, if there was a preexisting stress reaction.

Mr. J. was able to improve with a supportive taping technique to allow him to participate in the final week of the season. If this does not improve the pain, then the use of a stiff-soled shoe or wooden shoe is necessary. As you can see, not every individual would need to be casted but a short leg cast can certainly be used. In the case of Mr. W. with his stress-related Jones' fracture, high rates of nonunion have been discussed in the literature (5). In this instance, a conservative approach may include 4 to 6 weeks in a non–weight-bearing short leg cast followed by 4 to 6 weeks in a weight-bearing cast, with gradual rehabilitation after the casting period is over. The presence of a periosteal reaction at the time of the fracture indicates the preexisting stress fracture and increases the risk of nonunion. In the athlete who wishes to place high demands on the foot following treatment, consideration for early operative repair with bone graft or internal fixation by a screw needs to be considered. Mr. W. is a relatively classic example of a person with the Jones' fracture who has repetitive microtrauma to the area because of his tendency toward supination and "constant pounding" with an inversion mechanism that was "the straw that broke the camel's back."

Another syndrome as a cause of metatarsalgia is called the D. J. Morton's syndrome (3). Here the athlete will complain of pain at the base of the second or third metatarsal. Physical findings would include large callous formation of the second or third metatarsal head, palpation tenderness at the second metatarsal, and the second toe would be longer than the great toe. This syndrome is a combination of a short, hypermobile first metatarsal with sesamoids that are posteriorly displaced, and a thickened second metatarsal shaft that can be seen on x-ray. This can cause abnormal stresses placed on the hyperpronated foot.

If a diagnosis of D. J. Morton's syndrome can be made, then a Morton's extension pad, which is an insert that extends beyond the great toe to alter the biomechanics, can be used.

Morton's Neuroma (Not D. J. Morton)

Epidemiology

These injuries are seen in running, dancing, and aerobics. Women have a higher prevalence rate than men.

Clinical Case #11

A 23-year-old school teacher has always kept herself in great shape. When she began her career teaching second grade at the local school, she began wearing more fashionable shoes to class with approximately a 2-inch heel and needed to go to the local health club to use the stair stepper rather than getting a run in because of her schedule. She complains of discomfort and a tingling sensation in all of her foot, which radiates toward her toes.

The patient has both started to use a different form of aerobic exercise and is now wearing a shoe that puts more force on the metatarsals as well as narrows the foot (6). The patient may not have any functional abnormalities. Sometimes one can feel a "mass" between the metatarsal heads. Lateral compression of the metatarsal heads can accentuate the symptoms and cause the mass to "pop" out from between the metatarsal heads. Long-standing cases will have decreased sensation in the web space and the adjoining sides of the toes.

Morton's neuroma does not represent a true neuroma, but rather perineural fibrosis where the digital nerves are traumatized between the metatarsal heads (7). The most common location is between the third and fourth metatarsal heads, although the neuroma may be between the second and third or fourth and fifth metatarsal heads.

Often just having adequate space in the toe box to accommodate the metatarsal heads will be helpful. The use of a metatarsal pad will also help (see Figure 18.21). NSAIDs may be of additional benefit. If a neuroma has developed significant enough fibrosis, injection with a mixture of lidocaine and corticosteroids can be both diagnostic and therapeutic. The injection should be given dorsally, so that it is less painful. Cases of intractable pain can be referred for consideration of surgical removal. Because surgery leads to a permanent sensory deficit between the involved toes, a long trial of a conservative approach is well worth it.

Sesamoiditis Versus Sesamoid Stress Fractures

Epidemiology

Floor sports, dancing, basketball, and also running are the primary causes.

Clinical Case #12

A local dance school instructor has had formal training in ballet. She has just completed preparing all of her classes for the annual exhibition. This involved many additional hours of instruction on her part and she presents complaining of pain under her great toe, particularly when she pushes off.

Chronic overuse and the location of the pain are diagnostic in this patient. She has a cavus foot deformity and also is found to have some hallux valgus. The examiner will note palpable tenderness either medial or lateral to the first metatarsal head, which is made worse with passive dorsiflexion of the great toe. Palpation of the first metatarsophalangeal joint from the dorsal aspect does not reproduce pain. Interpretation of x-rays can be difficult because a bipartite sesamoid can be found in 10% to 30% of patients (Figure 18.24). There is

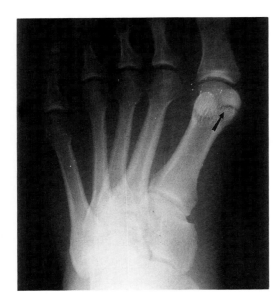

Figure 18.24. Bipartite medial sesamoid (*arrow*).

sclerosis at the separation of a bipartite sesamoid. Because bipartite sesamoids are bilateral (both feet) in 85% of cases, an x-ray of the other side can be helpful in the differentiation. In the case of a suspected stress fracture, a bone scan can be of help to identify this.

There are many locations for sesamoid bones in the foot. The sesamoids located in the medial or lateral location on the plantar surface of the first metatarsophalangeal joint are constant. They are located in the tendons of the flexor hallucis brevis. Repetitive microtrauma is what sets up the problem of sesamoiditis. A stress fracture can occcur because of an additional overload. The absence of pain on the metatarsophalangeal joint itself makes a diagnosis of arthritis less likely (including gout).

Use of ice and NSAIDs is helpful initially. In the long term, orthotics may be necessary. The use of a metatarsal pad to help relieve the pressure on the sesamoids can help. Sometimes a pad, with a "doughnut" cut out to avoid pressure on the sesamoid, is used. If a stress fracture is suspected, then a bone scan or repeat x-rays in 3 weeks are indicated. If a stress fracture is diagnosed, a short leg weight-bearing cast for 4 to 6 weeks followed by protective padding for an additional 6 weeks may be necessary. There would be no benefit in injection therapy with corticosteroids. In the case of a stress fracture, there is always the possible complication of nonunion.

Turf Toe

Epidemiology

Football players (particularly linemen), especially those playing on artificial turf, are susceptible to turf toe.

Clinical Case #13

An 18-year-old college freshman football lineman suffered through the two-a-day practices as he tried out for his college team as a walk on. He felt that he hurt himself during spider drills because, while performing the drill on all fours, he forced his great toe into an extremely bent position.

The use of flexible shoes allowing extreme dorsiflexion to occur should be elicited in the history. The patient will complain of pain trying to push off of the great toe and may have a mild amount of inflammation. The disability is always greater than physical findings.

Turf toe can be considered a sprain injury to the joint capsule and surrounding ligaments of the first metatarsophalangeal joint, which is brought on by severe dorsiflexion. Differential diagnosis might include fracture and sesamoiditis. Ice and NSAIDs can help; a buddy-taping technique to prevent dorsiflexion has been shown to be helpful. Often a steel or tin insert in the toe box can provide additional support for the toe that would still need to be taped. Unfortunately, it is difficult to find more rigid football shoes.

Ingrown Toenails

Epidemiology

Any athlete is subject to this problem.

Clinical Case #14

A 33-year-old marathoner has been in training for the Marine Corps marathon but is now in your office because of pain and swelling of the great toe. It is red and swollen on the lateral aspect of the nail. You can see that the toenail has been trimmed short and the edge is hidden among the swelling. There is no sign of more proximal infection. You also note a very thickened nail in general, with some resolving bruising underneath the nailbed. He tells you that he had noted blackness there months ago and so, after reading an article in a popular running magazine, began to trim his nails very closely.

The previous problem with a subungual hematoma caused this athlete to trim his nails excessively short. The absence of systemic infection but the chronic thickened nail and the buried edge are important issues.

The athlete had probably suffered from a subungual hematoma, which is often known as blacknail or "runner's toe." It occurs due to trauma to the nailbed. This often happens due to a combination of shoe fit and nail length, which causes the trauma. The shoe may be too short or too long. Unless this occurred because an acute trauma such as a weight dropped on it in the weight room, there is less frequently a need to relieve the pressure with the hot sterile needle technique. Unfortunately, as so often happens, the correction of one problem led to the problem of an ingrown toenail, which probably could have been avoided. It is well worth time counseling all athletes, perhaps during any preparticipation examination, about proper care of nails. If the nail is trimmed straight across, but not below the depth of the soft tissue, ingrown toenails will rarely occur.

This athlete is just weeks away from running in the marathon. The typical minor surgery procedure of removal of a portion of the nail is a less attractive option (Figure 18.25) because immediately postoperatively there can be increased swelling and difficulty maintaining conditioning. Antibiotics

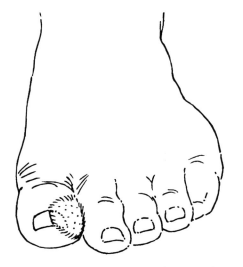

Figure 18.25. Removal of ingrown portion of
nail.

and frequent warm soaks can calm down
some of the inflammation as can the use of
an NSAID. Packing some cotton under the
edge of the nail to lift it out of the inflamed
soft tissue is usually of benefit. Another
temporizing technique that can be successful involves the use of intravenous tubing
in which a slit is placed so that it can cover
the edge of the nail, which can be reached
often with just local ice application or
anesthetic spray. By forming this barrier
between the jagged nail edge and inflamed
tissue, tissue can often heal until such time
as more definitive treatment may be necessary.

Foot injuries represent a significant
portion of complaints that the athletes will
bring to their primary care physicians. Despite its relatively small size in comparison
to the rest of the body, the foot is an amazingly complex structure. A better understanding of the kinesiology of the foot
enables the practitioner to more accurately
and effectively diagnose and treat these
injuries.

References

1. Blythe LS, Mueller FO. When and where
players get hurt. Physician Sports Med 1974;2:
45–52.
2. Norkin CC, Levangie PK. The ankle-foot
complex. In: Joint structure and function, a comprehensive analysis. Philadelphia: FA Davis,
1983:331–366.
3. Morton DJ. Foot disorders in general practice. JAMA October 2, 1937:112–119.
4. Alfred RH, Bergfeld JA. Diagnosis and
management of stress fractures of the foot.
Physician Sports Med 1987;15.
5. Lombardo JA, Micheli LJ, Bergfeld JA. Basketball player with pain over the fifth metatarsal,
a case conference. Physician Sports Med 1987;15.
6. Vereschagin KS, et al. Transient paresthesia
in stair-climber's feet. Physician Sports Med
1993;21:63–64.
7. Schon LC, Baxter DE. Neuropathies of the
foot and ankle in athletes. Clin Sports Med
1990;9:489–510.

Bibliography

Garfinkel D, Rothenberg MA, Lee A. Foot
problems in athletes. J Fam Pract 1984;19:239–
250.
Garrick JG, Requa RK. The epidemiology of
foot and ankle injuries in sports. Clin Sports Med
1988;7:29–36.
Jones DC. Tendon disorders of the foot and
ankle. J AAOS 1993;1:87–94.
Keene JS, Lange RH. Diagnostic dilemmas in
foot and ankle injuries. JAMA 1986;256:247–251.
Marshall P. The rehabilitation of overuse foot
injuries in athletes and dancers. Clin Sports Med
1988;7:175–192.
McBryde AM, Anderson RB. Sesamoid foot
problems in the athlete. Clin Sports Med
1988;7:51–60.
Torg JS, Pavlov H, Torg E. Overuse injuries in
sports: the foot. Clin Sports Med 1987;6:291–321.

HEAT ILLNESS

KARL WATTS
GERTJAN MULDER

19

Physiology
Pathophysiology
Heat Acclimation
Spectrum of Disease
Prevention

Heat stroke is the third leading cause of death among athletes during sporting events, behind head and neck injuries and cardiac abnormalities. The 1991–1992 National Collegiate Athletic Association (NCAA) Injury Surveillance System recorded 108 cases of heat exhaustion and one case of heat stroke in the NCAA during that year (1). Many other cases occur and go unrecognized. Even though heat illness is preventable, the risk of injury to the athlete persists. Education and prevention of heat illness has come a long way since the time when water was not allowed on the field during football practice. There is still much room for improvement. Illustrative of this point is that in the summer of 1993 a road cycling race was held in a southeastern city when the temperature was 100°F and the humidity 100%. Many cyclists dropped out secondary to the heat. This is an event that should have been postponed or canceled. With the mortality from heat stroke being as high as 80%, heat illness is an entity that cannot be taken lightly. In this chapter the spectrum of heat illness syndromes and their treatment are discussed. More importantly, prevention and recommendations for conducting athletic events are reviewed. Proper supervision, prevention, and education will ensure the safety of athletes during sporting events.

PHYSIOLOGY

Heat illness implies an overwhelmed thermoregulatory system that is unable to maintain body temperature within its required narrow physiologic range. Proper thermoregulation requires a balance between heat gain and heat dissipation. Heat gained comes from basal metabolic rate (BMR) (about 100 kcal/hr for a 70-kg person), exertion (300–600 kcal/hr for

moderate work), and from the environment (up to 300 kcal/hr from the sun) (2). Without concomitant heat loss, body temperature would rise 1.1°C/hr from BMR alone (3). During exertion an athlete's body temperature could reach up to 107.6°F (42°C). Given severe enough environmental conditions, heat illness can occur even without significant exertion, especially when combined with personal risk factors (Table 19.1).

Thermoregulation appears to be primarily mediated centrally by temperature sensitive neurons in the preoptic area of the anterior hypothalamus (4). This area presumably functions as a thermostat, attempting to maintain core temperature as near as possible to a thermal set point by affecting heat loss or heat gain mechanisms. Skin surface temperature probably affects heat loss mechanisms as well but is a less potent factor. Additional thermosensors are postulated elsewhere, such as in the spinal cord and extremity musculature.

The body's energy state can be expressed as follows:

$$\text{Heat storage} = M + W - (C + D + R + E)$$

where M = metabolic heat, W = work performed, C = convective heat gain/loss, D = conductive heat gain/loss, R = radiation heat gain/loss, and E = evaporative heat loss.

Cooling by sweat evaporation and radiant heat loss most significantly affects this equation, with conduction and convection being lesser factors. *Conduction* (heat transfer through direct contact) is of minimal importance because air is an effective insulator. *Convection* (heat transfer between the body and surrounding air or liquid) plays an important role. A cooling breeze offers significant relief in hot weather but can be disastrous in the cold (the wind chill factor). *Radiant* heat exchange through sun expo-

Table 19.1. Predisposing Factors for Heat Illness

Elderly athletes	Reduced cardiovascular reserve
	Tend to be more dehydrated
	Frequently have preexisting cardiovascular disease
Children	Lower sweat rates
	Higher sweat "set point"
	Relatively higher heat production
	Relatively lower cardiac output
	Slower to acclimate
	Faster dehydration
Obesity	Insulated with a lower surface-to-volume ratio
	Worse cardiac reserve
	Lower sweat gland density
	Lower specific heat results in greater rise in temperature for given heat load
Poor conditioning	
Nonacclimation	
Sickle cell trait	
Hyperthyroidism	Increased metabolic heat production
Pheochromocytoma	
Skin disorders	Interfere with sweating
	Miliaria
	Burns
	Scleroderma
	Cystic fibrosis
	Chronic idiopathic anhydrosis
	Anhydrosis from other causes
Febrile illness	
Dehydration	Gastroenteritis
Drugs	*β Blockers*—reduce cardiac reserve
	Stimulants—amphetamines, cocaine, PCP—increase heat production, may increase hypothalamic set point (amphetamines, LSD) and can induce seizures
	Anticholinergics—phenothiazines, antihistamines, tricyclic antidepressants, antispasmotics, lithium—inhibit sweating and disrupt hypothalamic function
	Diuretics, laxatives—dehydration
	Salicylates—uncouple oxidative phosphorylation
	Mind-altering drugs—alcohol, etc—impair judgment and awareness
Restrictive clothing and gear	

sure can result in a heat gain of 55 to 140 kcal/m² per hour, which is enough to raise the core temperature by 1°C/hr. On the other hand, radiation can account for as much as 65% of heat loss in a cool environment (2). Sweat evaporation provides the most significant contribution to minimizing the effects of heat stress, amounting to 0.58 kcal of heat loss for each milliliter of evaporated sweat.

Once heat stress is perceived, mechanisms spring into action to facilitate heat loss. Under influence of both central and local control, blood flow to skin increases dramatically (up to 8 L/min) while there is concommitant splanchnic vasoconstriction and increased cardiac output in order to maintain adequate blood pressure. Increased skin perfusion makes more body heat available for dissipation to the environment (2). Increased skin temperature causes local vasodilation of cutaneous vessels, a response which augments centrally and sympathetically mediated vasodilation (4). Cholinergic nerve fibers stimulate sweat production, up to 2 L/hr in marathon runners (4)

At rest, body temperature can be maintained at normal ranges by convection of heat to the skin surface and radiation heat loss to the atmosphere. With exercise or an increase in atmospheric temperature, blood is shunted to the skin for increased dissipation of heat. Evaporation of sweat becomes the major mechanism of heat loss when environmental temperature approaches or exceeds body temperature.

PATHOPHYSIOLOGY

Heat illness occurs when the athlete's ability to dissipate heat is overwhelmed by heat absorption and production. Eventually this results in system failure. Recent research has focused on the "energy depletion model" (5). Key events are probably occurring on a cellular level. In heat, ion diffusion across cell membranes is increased, resulting in dramatically increased metabolic demands to maintain cellular homeostasis. At the same time it appears that cellular, and in particular mitochondrial, metabolism becomes less efficient.

Muscular work combines with cellular demands to deplete cellular adenosine triphosphate (ATP). As ATP is depleted, intracellular hydrogen ions accumulate, and cellular function worsens. Glycolysis is impaired due to this acidosis and the system fatigues. Systemic lactic acidosis and dehydration further disturb transmembrane ion balance (4,5). Free radicals may be involved in the destruction of cell membranes as well. Grossly, a struggle occurs between compensatory and autoregulatory mechanisms. Significantly reduced cardiac filling pressure and reduced functional blood volume are caused by a combination of increased blood flow to exercising musculature, maximum dilation of peripheral vessels, and fluid losses from sweating. Negative inotropic effects from acidosis and energy depletion probably result in reduced stroke volumes, necessitating increased heart rate. Eventually, splanchnic vasoconstriction falters, reducing effective blood flow to the skin and further impairing heat exchange (4). Sweating itself becomes impaired due to volume losses, as well as from sweat gland dysfunction in severe cases. In the face of rising body temperature and overwhelmed thermoregulatory coping mechanisms, system failures occur and are manifest as heat illness.

HEAT ACCLIMATION

Clinical Case #1

It has been a particularly cold winter and early spring. Your patient, a 43-year-old man, has been training regularly for a half marathon to be held in a few weeks in south Florida. He is in the office for his annual checkup. What advice should you give him in preparation for running in the potentially warm, humid conditions?

Acclimation is the process of physiologic adjustment by an organism to environmental change. Heat acclimation allows human beings to increase their tolerance to heat stress. Once acclimated, athletes tend to have lower core temperatures with exertion, improve their exercise tolerance, and have a lower incidence of heat illness, although reduced incidence of heat stroke has not been proven. Preexisting cardiorespiratory fitness helps determine the speed of acclimation, but generally this takes 10 to 14 days. Passive acclimation in heat, that is, without exercise, results only in increased heat dispersal capability. Training in cool and dry environments only improves body system efficiency without adapting heat dispersal. Complete acclimation requires daily exercise in the heat, especially humid heat (6). The potential for heat tolerance appears to be equal between equally fit men and women.

Physiologically, heat acclimation is made possible by several adaptations. On a cellular level, metabolic efficiency is increased, probably related to enhanced mitochondrial function. Cardiovascular adaptation results in a reduction of peak heart rate and an increase in stroke volume. There is either no change or an increase in cardiac output, and an overall reduced cardiovascular strain for a given level of exercise in the heat. Heat dissipation becomes more effective. The athlete starts sweating at lower temperatures and sweat production may increase by a factor of two or more. For this reason it is critical for the athlete to increase fluid intake. Dehydration impairs the process of heat acclimation, causes cardiovascular impairment, and predisposes to heat exhaustion (4,6).

With heat acclimation, activation of the renin-angiotensin system causes an increase in aldosterone levels. This in turn causes reduced sodium concentration in sweat and urine at the expense of some potassium losses. This reduces the acclimated athlete's need for sodium replenishment during exercise. Sodium conservation results in a 10% to 25% plasma volume expansion. Furthermore, antidiuretic hormone initially increases, which results in reduced water and electrolyte losses in urine. Cortisol levels are initially increased as well, but fall as acclimation is accomplished and physiologic strain is reduced (7).

Prior to starting any acclimation it is recommended to first achieve cardiovascular fitness under cool conditions. Once fit, acclimation can be started with multiple but relatively brief intense aerobic workouts in the heat. An example would be to participate in 20-minute sessions of moderate intensity (up to a maximum oxygen consumption of 50%) with cooling off periods in between and a total workout time of up to 90 to 120 minutes. If these are tolerated, sessions are prolonged and possibly intensified after about 5 days. Unlimited fluids are made available throughout acclimation and intake is encouraged. Once achieved, maintenance of heat acclimation requires continued frequent exertion in heat, although this need not be as intense as in the acquisition period (4). In this phase, intense workouts are done during the cool hours, with lighter workouts during the heat of the day. During heat acclimation as well as during the maintenance phase, daily measurement of weight is advisable. If weight drops 2% to 3%, oral fluids are pushed. With a 4% to 5% drop, workouts are reduced. With a 7% or greater drop, workouts should be discontinued and medical attention is advisable. Unfortunately, acclimation decays within days on cessation of exercise in the heat. The cardiovascular benefits, which were the first to be acquired, are the first to be lost as well.

In summary, heat acclimation requires moderate exercise in hot conditions, requires caution to prevent the precipitation of heat illness, and should involve adequate and frequent hydration. It improves energy economy and increases exercise tolerance in hot humid weather. It probably benefits endurance athletes in cooler weather as well.

If your patient who is headed south for the half marathon has a few weeks prior to the trip, he can train in clothing that decreases evaporative heat loss. This will help with heat acclimation. He would have to head south 2 weeks before the race to be able to benefit from training in the local weather conditions. He should certainly be advised of his increased need for fluids and electrolytes (see section on Fluid and Electrolyte Replacement) in the unacclimated state.

SPECTRUM OF DISEASE

Heat Cramps

Clinical Case #2

It is particularly hot and humid for the first high school football game of the season. Despite the trainer's best efforts to have the players drink frequently and cool with wet towels, several players develop cramps in the calves.

Heat cramps occur in the large skeletal (voluntary) muscle at the time of or shortly after strenuous exertion in the heat. These cramps can be excruciating. Typically they are brief and have been described as involving subsections of large skeletal muscle, such that as one portion starts to relax, an adjacent one begins to spasm. The gastrocnemius and hamstring muscles, as well as abdominal wall muscles, are frequently involved. Most researchers feel they are related to reduced serum sodium and chloride levels, which may be a result of salt losses from sweating. Heat acclimation may reduce the incidence of cramps. The differential diagnosis for heat cramps includes exercise-induced muscle soreness, muscle spasm secondary to strain, hyperventilation-induced tetany (as in heat exhaustion or stroke), gastroenteritis, and cramps from other low-sodium states (cholera, dialysis). Treatment involves rest and fluid and electrolyte replacement. Salt tablets are not recommended because they are significant gastrointestinal irritants. Mild cramps can be treated orally with 0.1% to 0.2% sodium chloride solution (e.g., by mixing $\frac{1}{4}$ to $\frac{1}{2}$ teaspoon of table salt in one quart of water). Severe cramps may require intravenous normal saline. Prevention involves adequate rest and hydration during heat exertion as well as avoidance of low-sodium diets. Typical American diets include plenty of salt; supplemental salt is usually unnecessary and, in fact, may impair heat acclimation by preventing the associated rise in aldosterone and concomitant sodium conservation. On the field treatment of at gastrocnemius heat cramp includes forced dorsiflexion stretching of the foot for 1 or 2 minutes. Drinking of at least 0.5 L of an electrolyte-rich solution is encouraged (see section on Fluid and Electrolyte Replacement) as is continued drinking during the remainder of the game. Athletes can return to action but are susceptible to recurrence. Prevention is the best treatment.

Clinical Case #3

It is early July and a girls' softball tournament has been going on all day in the hot, humid conditions. You arrive for the championship game. Shortly thereafter one of the outfielders collapses. Immediate treatment necessitates moving her to the shade, rapid cooling, and an assessment of the severity of her heat illness.

Heat Syncope

Syncope can occur in heat after prolonged standing or after an intense workout. It is related to peripheral vasodilation and subsequent pooling of blood in the legs, frequently in the face of decreased cardiovascular reserve as well as inadequate hydration. It is most common in the elderly. Other causes of syncope must be considered, especially if syncope or near-syncope occurs during exertion. Treatment involves adequate hydration and preventive measures. Prevention includes avoidance of prolonged standing, frequent flexing of leg muscles if prolonged standing is necessary, and an adequate cool-down period after intense workouts.

Heat Exhaustion (Heat Prostation)

Heat exhaustion represents a more serious form of heat strain. It may develop over the course of several days and presents with weakness, fatigue, and thirst. Victims often complain of a frontal headache, vertigo, and nausea, and they may have emesis. Impaired judgment may be evident, but otherwise patients are neurologically intact. Tremulousness, muscle cramps, orthostatic symptoms, and even frank syncope can occur. Heat-induced hyperventilation may cause subjective dyspnea as well as paresthesias. Core temperature in heat exhaustion is frequently elevated, can be normal, and as opposed to heat stroke, never exceeds 104°F (40°C). Other characteristics that distinguish exhaustion from stroke are the intact neurologic examination and lack of hepatic damage.

Heat exhaustion results from heat strain in the face of varying degrees of water and salt depletion. Inadequate fluid replacement is common among athletes. Even when athletes are encouraged to take in plenty of readily available fluids, they tend to voluntarily replace only one half to two thirds of their losses. When this continues over the course of several days, hypernatremia and dehydration develop, predisposing the athlete to heat exhaustion or stroke. If the athlete ingests adequate but hypotonic fluids, heat exhaustion tends to be slower in onset and may be due primarily to salt deficiency. In the later form of heat exhaustion, temperature is commonly normal. As one might expect, heat cramps may be experienced concurrently. Heat exhaustion can also be present in an individual exposed to hot environments without adequate access to water. This type may be a forerunner to heat stroke.

Heat exhaustion treatment is based on clinical parameters. Orthostatic vital signs, temperature, level of dehydration, and clinical appearance help to guide therapy. The patient should be weighed, especially if a preevent measurement is available. Blood urea nitrogen (BUN), hematocrit, urine osmolality, and serum and urine sodium levels may add to the clinical impression. Following urine output during treatment is helpful. Mild exhaustion can be treated orally with the equivalent of 0.1% to 0.2% saline ($\frac{1}{4}$ to $\frac{1}{2}$ teaspoon table salt in one quart water). Again there is no role for salt tablets. On the field cooling by removing clothing, fanning, and keeping the skin wet should also be initiated. If the athlete can take fluids, is coherent, and not hypotensive, hospital care may not be needed.

Worse conditions can require intravenous fluid replacement with normal saline until the patient is hemodynamically stable. Following this, half of the free water deficit should be replaced over 24 hours, with the remainder given over the next 24 to 48 hours. Osmolality should be dropped at less than 2 mOsm/hr and sodium concentration less that 1 mEq/L per hour. More rapid correction can result in central nervous system (CNS) edema and seizures. Therefore, sodium concentration or serum osmolality should be followed approximately every 6 hours.

Calculate water deficit in liters as follows (8):

Water deficit (L) = CBW × ([Na]/140 − 1)

CBW = Current body weight (kg) × 0.4
for women (× 0.5 for men)

Calculate osmolality as follows:

Serum osmolality = 2(Na mEq/L)
+ (Glu mg/dl)/18
+ (BUN mg/dl)/2.8

Heat Stroke

Heat stroke is the most severe manifestation of heat illness, with high potential for permanent neurologic damage and death. This section focuses primarily on exertional heat stroke, since classic or epidemic heat stroke is not common in athletes.

In heat stroke core body temperature rises to above 105.8°F (41°C). About 20% of victims note prodromal symptoms similar to those in heat exhaustion, but in 80% delirium or coma occur suddenly and without much warning. The classic triad of extreme pyrexia, severe CNS dysfunction, and dry skin occurs in some, but sweating persists in more than half of exertional heat stroke victims. Dry skin is thought to be a late phenomenon. Heat stroke presents as collapse, with tachycardia, hypotension, and dehydration. Most if not all victims suffer coma, severe confusion, and neurologic irritability. Convulsions are common (72%) as is vomiting (71%) (9,10). Severe hypotension, dry skin, and diarrhea are less common (22% to 44%) (9,10). Many cases may be misdiagnosed, especially in milder climates when the index of suspicion is low. This is especially likely because some cooling off usually starts on collapse, so that on arrival to the emergency room core temperature may be significantly reduced.

The diagnosis of heat stroke is made by using observations of witnesses, knowledge of activities and weather conditions prior to the collapse, any obtainable past medical history, as well as the clinical presentation of the patient. Elevation of serum liver enzymes (aspartate aminotransferase, alanine aminotransferase and lactic dehydrogenase) is typical of heat stroke, often exceeding 1000 IU/L. This does not occur in most of the other conditions in the differential diagnosis (Table 19.2). Because this rise in liver enzymes as well as other complications of heat stroke may not occur until 1 to 2 days after presentation, it is recommended to observe patients for 48 hours.

Treatment

Heat stroke is an absolute medical emergency. Outcome directly relates to severity and duration of hyperthermia. Therefore, rapid cooling to a core temperature below 102.2°F (39°C) is critical.

Table 19.2. Differential Diagnosis of Heat Stroke

Heat syncope
Hysteria
Dehydration
Viral hepatitis
Febrile illness with CNS changes
    Malaria
    Typhus and typhoid
    Encephalitis
    Meningitis
Status epilepticus
Drugs
    Anticholinergics

Field Management

Management begins in the field with the usual ABCs (airway, breathing, circulation), with due consideration to the presence of unexpected conditions, including cervical spine injuries. Due to severe CNS depression, seizures, and vomiting, the airway is frequently compromised. Endotracheal intubation should therefore be considered, if feasible. Nasogastric suction reduces chance of aspiration as well. Both should ideally be in place prior to any significant transportation if aspiration risk appears to be high.

Cooling measures are critical and need to be started at once. Unless contraindicated, the victim should be moved to a shady, cool, and ventilated place, preferably near a source of cool water or ice. Clothing should be removed. Vital signs should be obtained if possible and should include a rectal temperature. Cooling is effectively accomplished by wetting the body and fanning. Ice packs can be placed wherever there are large superficial blood vessels (groin, axillae). Immersion in a stream, pond, or ice water bath is extremely effective; however, this may complicate necessary procedures and is contraindicated in the face of seizures and severe agitation. Cooling from an ambulance or helicopter ride (with the windows open), and even from helicopter rotor downdraft, have been effective. Athletes with heat stroke should be transported to the nearest hospital for further care.

PREVENTION

Education of the athlete, coach, athletic trainer, and parents is the most critical point in the prevention of heat illness. Many advances have been made in the field of sports medicine in the area of heat illness and fluid replacement. These advances are of little use if not related to the above individuals. The team physician is often looked on to provide new information and to squelch misconceptions.

1. Detailed medical histories should be available on all athletes. History of prior heat illness (especially heat exhaustion and heat stroke) and systemic disease should be noted. Athletes at higher risk require increased caution in situations of high heat stress.

2. Daily weights, before and after practice, should be documented. If loss of 2% to 3% of body weight occurs, oral fluids should be pushed. With loss of 4% to 5%, oral fluids should be pushed and workouts reduced. With loss of greater than 7%, workouts should be discontinued, intravenous fluids considered, and medical attention given.

3. Heat stress index measurements should be obtained on a daily basis using the WBGT, WBT, or DBT/humidity tables. Special precautions or restructuring of workouts should then be implemented as recommended in the tables.

4. Both water and glucose/electrolyte solutions should be readily accessible.

5. Identify athletes who may have problems secondary to being poorly conditioned and unacclimated.

6. Allow adequate time at the beginning of the season for conditioning and acclimation.

7. Schedule events and practices during the cooler parts of the day. Reschedule events or practices as needed depending on the heat stress. Remember that adequate acclimation for events in the heat of the day cannot be achieved with practice sessions during cooler parts of the day.

8. Proper clothing is important. Avoid excessive clothing or equipment. Loose, porous light-colored clothing is optimal. Avoid continued use of sweat saturated clothing or prolonged exposure of the skin to direct sunlight.

9. Discourage dehydration techniques as a method of weight loss.

10. Encourage athletes to become accustomed to the hydration methods used in events during practice. This is especially true for distance runners and cyclists.

Heat Stress Index

Understanding of heat stress and the heat stress index is necessary when considering prevention of heat illness. The stress that the body encounters in a hot environment depends on other factors besides the temperature. Humidity, radiation of heat from other objects, and wind velocity are also important. The wet bulb globe temperature (WBGT) index is a measure of the heat stress in the environment and takes into account the above factors. The WBGT index is calculated as follows:

$$WBGT = 0.7(WBT) + 0.2(DBT) + 0.1(BGT)$$

where WBT = wet bulb temperature, DBT = dry bulb temperature, and BGT = black globe temperature. The DBT is a conventional measure of the ambient temperature. The WBT is essentially the DBT depressed by the vaporization of water. As humidity increases the WBT approaches the DBT. When humidity is 100%, the DBT equals the WBT. The BGT takes into account radiant heat. Of note is the significant contribution the WBT plays in the heat stress index. This is due to the large role humidity plays in the heat stress the body perceives. In temperatures above 65°F (18.3°C), the main mechanism of heat dissipation from the body is via evaporation of sweat from the skin. As the humidity increases the ability of the body to dissipate heat by this mechanism decreases. One continues to sweat but there is less evaporation of the sweat from the body. In 100% humidity there is no evaporation at all.

The WBGT index can be measured with commercially available devices, which can be rather costly. Alternatively, one can use the following formula:

$$WBGT = 0.567(DBT) + 0.393(Pa) + 3.94$$

where Pa = environmental water vapor pressure. Because WBT makes such a significant contribution to the WBGT index, many have advocated using it alone as an estimate of the environmental heat stress. The WBT can be measured quite easily with a portable and inexpensive device called the sling psychrometer. With such a device one can determine the WBT, DBT, and humidity at the site of an athletic event. The heat stress can be determined using temperature/humidity tables or by using the WBT alone. Because temperature and humidity can vary locally one should not totally rely on reports from the weather service or media, but should have measurements from the site of competition if possible. Once the heat stress index is obtained one can use recommendations such as made available by the American College of Sports Medicine (ACSM) in their position stand on the prevention of thermal injuries to decide if special precautions need to be implemented, or whether the event should be postponed or canceled (Tables 19.3 and 19.4).

Fluid and Electrolyte Replacement

Fluid ingestion during exercise has the goals of supplying water and electrolytes to

Table 19.3. ACSM Guidelines on Risk of Thermal Stress by WBGT

Flag/WBGT	Risk	Recommendations*
Black: WBGT >28°C >82°F	Extreme	Cancel event
Red: WBGT 23–28°C 73–82°F	High	High risk for heat illness Heat sensitive athletes should be excluded Frequent breaks and unlimited fluids Light workout
Amber: WBGT 18–23°C 65–73°F	Moderate	Frequent breaks and unlimited fluids
Green: WBGT 10–18°C 50–65°F	Low	No special precautions necessary
White: WBGT <10°C <50°F	Very low	Hypothermia risk

*The black flag designation and the recommendations are not part of the
ACSM guidelines.
ACSM = American College of Sports Medicine; WBGT =wet bulb globe
temperature.

Table 19.4. Guidelines on Risk of Thermal Stress by Wet Bulb Temperature*

Wet Bulb Temperature	Risk	Recommendations
>25.5°C >78°F	Danger level	Alter practice schedule to provide a lighter practice routine, or conduct sessions in shorts Mandatory water breaks Exclude susceptible players and those with >3% weight loss
19–25°C 66–78°F	Caution	Unlimited fluids and frequent breaks
<19°C <66°F	Safe	No precautions are necessary Susceptible individuals should be watched

* If relative humidity is more than 95%, danger-level procedures should be observed, regardless of wet bulb
reading.

replace the losses incurred by sweating and
of providing a source of carbohydrate fuel
to supplement the body's limited stores.
Over the past several years there have been
several studies and reviews debating the
optimal fluid to ingest during exercise. Although there is not universal agreement the
majority of evidence thus far points to solutions supplemented with carbohydrate and
sodium.

When considering fluid replacement
there are four main factors to consider: the
ingested fluid, the individual, the activity,
and environmental conditions.

The majority of the research conducted in the area of fluid replacement has been focused on defining the optimal replacement solution. In the past water has been advocated as the best replacement. Current evidence seems to point away from this conclusion. Ingestion of water alone during exercise causes a fall in serum sodium concentrations and serum osmolality (11). In a study by Nose and colleagues, rehydration after exercise with plain water resulted in a rapid fall in the plasma sodium concentration and in plasma osmolality (12). These changes have the effect of reducing the stimulus to drink and of stimulating urine output, both of which will delay the rehydration process (13) and can lead to dehydration. There is evidence that the ingestion of sodium-containing solutions during exercise may prevent the fall in plasma volume more effectively than the ingestion of pure water (11).

Absorption of glucose occurs in the small intestine and is an active, energy-consuming process linked to the transport of sodium. There is no active transport mechanism for water, which will cross the intestinal mucosa in either direction depending on the local osmotic gradients (14). Basically, water will follow glucose and sodium. Coyle and Montain (15) demonstrated no significant difference in gastric emptying times and intestinal absorption for water and solutions containing up to 8% carbohydrate. High carbohydrate concentrations will delay gastric emptying, and very high concentrations will result in the secretion of water into the small intestine.

Numerous reports abound in the literature of hyponatremia in endurance athletes. The cause in many cases is multifactorial, being mainly a combination of sodium loss in sweat and ingestion of hypotonic fluids. Sodium is adequately supplied in the diet. The role sodium plays in preventing the

exercise-related fall in plasma volume and in the active transport of glucose are significant reasons for its inclusion in sport drinks. High sodium concentrations tend to lead to gastrointestinal upset and can make drinks unpalatable.

Gastric emptying time can vary from individual to individual and is a major factor in rehydration during exercise. The volume of gastric contents is important in regulating the rate of gastric emptying; emptying follows an exponential time course and rapidly falls as the volume remaining in the stomach decreases (13). A high rate of emptying is promoted by keeping the gastric volume high (500–600 mL) by repeated drinking. The most recent evidence suggests that the gastric emptying of hot and cold drinks is not different (14).

Rate of sweating can differ depending on the individual, intensity of exercise, environmental conditions, and state of hydration. Sweat rates can average 1–2 L/h in runners. When one considers that most runners drink only about 500 mL/h, it is apparent that they can dehydrate 500–1500 mL/h. Athletes should try to estimate the magnitude of dehydration after workouts by obtaining body weight before and after. Every pound lost represents approximately 500 mL (16 oz) dehydration.

The volume of fluid to ingest during an event should be considered individually on the basis of ongoing losses. It has been assumed that the optimum rate of fluid ingestion is equal to the rate of fluid loss. However, this has not been proven. The majority of athletes would not tolerate replacing the 1–2 L/h that they lose via sweat. The ACSM recommends drinking 400–600 mL, 15 to 20 minutes prior to exercise, then 100–200 mL every 2–3 km. Depending on the individual, this amount may not be tolerated by the elite athlete and may be insufficient for slower athletes. It is rational to use precompetition hydration to increase the gastric volume, thus enhancing gastric emptying time during the event. Individuals need to realize they need to drink prior to thirst. Slowing or cessation of sweating is a sign of inadequate intake.

The length and intensity of the event or activity play important roles in sweat rate, fluid loss, and depletion of carbohydrate stores. Endurance events lasting longer than 60 to 90 minutes (distance running, cycling), as well as sports that require bursts of high-intensity activity over a prolonged period of time (soccer, football, tennis, hockey), are likely to significantly deplete carbohydrate stores. Carbohydrate replacement during such events probably benefit performance. Activities which are shorter than 30 minutes in duration usually do not require supplementation during the event.

Environmental conditions obviously play a critical role in fluid loss and the need for fluid supplementation.

In summary, there is no consensus among investigators concerning fluid replacement. Current evidence suggests the optimal solution contains 4% to 8% carbohydrate and a low sodium concentration. Most sport drinks contain 6% to 7% carbohydrate and 10–25 mmol/L of sodium, which is sufficient and palatable. Pre-event hydration and forced fluid ingestion as tolerated during the event are recommended for enhanced performance and reduced incidence of heat illness.

References

1. NCAA Injury Surveillance System, 1991–1992.

2. Auerbach PS, Geehr EC. Management of wilderness and environmental emergencies. St. Louis: CV Mosby, 1989.

3. Knochel J. Environmental heat illness. Arch Intern Med 1974;133:841–864.

4. Pandolf K, Sawka M, Gonsalez R. Human performance physiology and environmental medicine at terrestrial extremes. Indianapolis: Benchmark Press, 1988.

5. Hubbard R. Heatstroke pathophysiology: the energy depletion model. Med Sci Sports Exerc 1990;22:19–28.

6. Armstrong LE, Maresh CM. The induction and decay of heat acclimatisation in trained athletes. Sports Med 1991;12:302–312.

7. Bouchama A, et al. Ineffectiveness of dantrolene sodium in the treatment of heatstroke. Crit Care Med 1991;19:176–180.

8. Rubenstein E, Sederman DD. Scientific American Medicine. New York: Scientific American, 1993.

9. Shibolet S, Lancaster M, Danon Y. Heat stroke: a review. Aviation Space Environ Med 1976;47(3):280–301.

10. Simon HB. Extreme pyrexia. Hosp Pract 1986;21(54):123–129.

11. Noakes T. Fluid replacement during exercise. Exerc Sport Sci Rev 1993;21:297–330.

12. Nose H, et al. Water and electrolyte balance in the vascular space during graded exercise in humans. J Appl Physiol 1991;70(6):2757.

13. Maughan RJ. Fluid and electrolyte loss and replacement in exercise. J Sports Med 1991; 9:117–142.

14. Maughan RJ, Noakes TD. Fluid replacement and exercise stress: a brief review of studies on fluid replacement and some guidelines for the athlete. Sports Med 1991;12:16–31.

15. Coyle E, Montain S. Benefits of fluid replacement with carbohydrate during exercise. Med Sci Sports Exerc 1990;23:811–817.

Bibliography

American Academy of Pediatrics. Committee on Sports Medicine. Climatic heat stress and the exercising child. 1982;69:808–809.

American College of Sports Medicine. Prevention of thermal injuries during distance running, 1984.

American Red Cross, Emergency Response. Mosby Lifeline. Heat and cold emergencies 1993;18:353–363.

Ash C, et al. The use of rectal temperature to

monitor heat stroke. Missouri Med 1992;89: 283–288.

Barr S, Costill D, Fink W. Fluid replacement during prolonged exercise: effects of water, saline, or no fluid. Med Sci Sports Exerc 1990;23:811–817.

Bock H, et al. Demographics of emergency medical care at the Indianapolis 500 Mile Race (1983–1990). Ann Emerg Med 1992;21:1207.

Bracker M. Environmental and thermal injury. Clin in Sports Med 1992;11:419–437.

Brown DW. Heat and cold in farm workers. Occup Med 1991;6:371–389.

Bruss D, et al. Heat illness. Minnesota Med 1990;73:33–35.

Callaham M. Heat illness. Emerg Med 1983;1:498–522.

Clowes HA, O'Donnell T. Heat stroke. N Engl J Med 1974;291:564–566.

Costrini A. Emergency treatment of exertional heatstroke and comparison of whole body cooling techniques. Med Sci Sports Exerc 1989;22: 15–18.

Costrini A, et al. Cardiovascular and metabolic manifestations of heat stroke and severe heat exhaustion. Am J Med 1979;66:296–301.

Cuidotti T. Human factors in firefighting: ergonomic-, cardiopulmonary-, and psychogenic stress-related issues. Int Arch Occup Environ Health 1992;64:1–12.

Dann E, Berkman N. Chronic idiopathic anhydrosis—a rare cause of heat stroke. Postgrad Med J 1992;68:750–752.

Davidson M. Heat illness in athletics. Athl Train 1985;96–101.

Epstein Y. Heat intolerance: predisposing factor or residual injury? Med Sci Sports Med 1989; 22:29–35.

Favata E, Buckler G, Gochfeld M. Heat stress in hazardous waste workers: evaluation and prevention. Occup Med 1990;5:79–91.

Fortney S, et al. Circulatory and temperature regulatory responses to exercise in a warm environment in insulin-dependent diabetes. Yale J Bio Med 1981;54:101–109.

Gordon N. Effect of selective and nonselective beta-adrenoceptor blockade on thermoregulation during prolonged exercise in heat. Am J Cardiol 1985;55:74D–78D.

Gottschalk P, Thomas J. Heat stroke: recognition and principles of management. Clin Pediatr 1967;6:576–578.

Hamilton M. Fluid replacement and glucose infusion during exercise prevent cardiovascular drift. Am Physiol Soc 1991;71:871–877.

Harrison MH. Heat, exercise and blood volume. Sports Med 1986;3:214–233.

Hassanein T, et al. Liver failure occurring as a component of exertional heatstroke. Gastroenterology 1991;100:1442–1447.

Hassanein T, et al. Heatstroke: its clinical and pathological presentation, with particular attention to the liver. Am J Gastroenterol 1992; 87:1382–1389.

Hubbard RW. An introduction: the role of exercise in the etiology of exertional heatstroke. Med Sci Sports Exerc 1990;22:2–5.

Kenny L. Physiological correlates of heat intolerance. Sports Med 1985;2:279–286.

Knochel J. Catastrophic medical events with exhaustive exercise: "white collar rhabdomyolysis". Kid Int 1990;38:709–719.

Knochel J. Dog days and siriasis. JAMA 1975;233:513–515.

Knochel J, Caskey J. The mechanism of hypophosphatemia in acute heat stroke. JAMA 1977;238:425–426.

Knochel J, Dotin L, Hamburger R. Pathophysiology of intense physical conditioning in a hot climate. J Clin Invest 1972;51:242–255.

Kobayashi Y, et al. Effects of heat acclimation of distance runners in a moderately hot environment. Eur J Appl Physiol 1980;45:189–198.

Maughan RJ. Fluid replacement in sport and exercise—a consensus statement. Br J Sport Med 1993;27:34–35.

McDiarmid M, Agnew J, Lees P. Pregnant firefighter performance. J Occup Med 1991; 33:446–448.

McKeag DG, Hough DO. Management of onsite emergencies. Prim Care Sports Med 1993; 9:203–222.

McKeag DG, Hough DO. Common sports-related injuries and illnesses—hematology, endocrine and environment. Prim Care Sports Med 1993;16:483–508.

McLeod R. Heat illness in early season football practice. J Ky Med Assoc 1972;70:613–614.

Millard-Stafford M. Fluid replacement during exercise in the heat. Sports Med 1992;13:223–233.

Milunsky A, et al. Maternal heat exposure and neural tube defects. JAMA 1992;268:882–885.

Mitchell GW. Rapid onset of severe heat illness: a case report. Aviation, Space, Environ Med 1991;62:779–782.

Murphy R. Heat illness. J Sports Med 1973; 1:26–29.

Nadel ER. Recent advances in temperature regulation during exercise in humans. Fed Proc 1985;44:2286–2292.

Noakes T. Hyponatremia during endurance running: a physiological and clinical interpretation. Med Sci Sports Med 1991;24:403–405.

O'Donnell T. Acute heat stroke. JAMA 1975; 234:824–828.

O'Donnell T Jr. The circulatory abnormalities of heat stroke. N Engl J Med 1972;287:734–737.

Pugh LGCE, Corbett JL, Johnson RH. Rectal temperatures, weight loss, and sweat rates in marathon running. J Appl Physiol 1967;23:347–352.

Savdie E, et al. Heat stroke following rugby league football. Med J Aust 1991;155:636–639.

Sawka M. Current concepts concerning thirst, dehydration, and fluid replacement. Med Sci Sports Med 1991;24:643–644.

Sawka M, et al. Human tolerance to heat strain during exercise: influence of hydration. J Appl Physiol 1992;73:368–374.

Schrier R, et al. Studies in military recruits during summer training, with implications for acute renal failure. Ann Intern Med 1970;73:213–223.

Shapiro Y, Seidman DS. Field and clinical observations of exertional heat stroke patients. Med Sci Sports Exerc 1989;22:6–13.

Shapiro Y, et al. Heat intolerance in former heatstroke patients. Ann Intern Med 1979;90: 913–916.

Shibolet S, et al. Heatstroke: its clinical picture and mechanism in 36 cases. Q J Med 1967; 144:525–548.

Sinclair RE. Be serious about siriasis. Postgrad Med 1985;77:261–276.

Squire D. Heat illness. Pediatr Clin North Am 1990;37:1085–1109.

Tek D, Olshaker J. Heat illness. Emerg Med Clin North Am 1992;10:299–310.

Vassallo S, Delaney K. Pharmacologic effects on thermoregulation: mechanisms of drug-related heatstroke. Clin Toxicol 1989;27:199–224.

THREE COMMON MEDICAL PROBLEMS IN SPORTS

20

KARL B. FIELDS

Upper Respiratory Infections
Infectious Mononucleosis
Exercise-induced Asthma

Medical illness causes more loss of time from training and competition than does injury. This fact often is unappreciated because dramatic injuries capture the attention of both the public and of the sports medicine community. In general, athletes are in better health than their peers throughout society. However, the demands of competition and training place special stresses on athletes, which the average individual does not face. In certain situations these stresses precipitate illness. In addition, frequent respiratory infections may be a marker for the athlete who has trained too vigorously or has some other high-risk health habits. Lack of sleep, improper eating, and the use of illegal drugs could all affect an athlete's resistance to common illness.

This chapter offers an overview of three common medical conditions seen in sports competition. The information is intended to guide team physicians so that they can help athletes safely return to training. Special risks and complications related to sports participation are also emphasized. The three problems discussed are upper respiratory infections, mononucleosis, and exercise-induced asthma.

UPPER RESPIRATORY INFECTIONS

Viral upper respiratory infections (URIs) are the most common infectious disease in athletes, accounting for over 90% of the infections that occur. A number of studies have compared the frequency of URIs in athletes versus the general population and show no difference with both groups averaging 1.5 to 2.0 infections per year. This remains true for all age spectrums from pediatric to master's level athletes. Aggravating factors for URIs include crowding, poor air quality, and exposure to many

people. These play a greater role than does athletic activity.

Upper respiratory infections cause significant time loss in team sports, over 75% of athletes miss training due to this type of illness. The average athlete loses 5 to 7 days. Secondary infections that complicate URIs include sinusitis, bronchitis, pneumonia, and otitis media. Worsening flares of asthma also add to the overall morbidity created by URIs.

Effects of Training and Other Factors

Because exercise has many positive benefits, the finding that exercise does not reduce the frequency of URIs is somewhat surprising. Even though the number of illnesses remained unchanged, some clinical studies have pointed to a potential beneficial effect of training. For example, several studies of moderate exercises show that specific cells within the immunologic defense systems are stimulated by consistent, moderate activity. One epidemiologic study of runners showed a lower than expected rate of upper respiratory problems of 1.2 infections per year. Additional studies showed that runners and other conditioned athletes seemed to recover faster from illness when compared to sedentary colleagues. Perhaps the key to the positive results in these studies was that the athletes engaged in moderate activity and not in stressful training or competition.

Peak training appears to increase the risk for infectious problems. One study demonstrated that Nordic skiers have decreased secretory IgA levels following races. Similarly, studies of cells in the immunologic defense barriers showed a depression of function for 24 to 48 hours after very stressful training sessions and long competitions like marathon races. Furthermore, epidemiologic studies document that vigorous training or competitions increases the risk of respiratory illness for the following 2 to 4 weeks.

Studies of athletes with respiratory infection have often found two groups: one of athletes who rarely have infections and another who have multiple infections. This led researchers to look at specific factors that might have changed the benefit-versus-risk ratio of training in the frequently infected individuals. One key factor is the consistent use of alcohol. Athletes tend to use alcohol at the same rate as nonathletes, but some sports traditionally have a postcompetition social norm of drinking beer or other alcoholic beverages. Athletes who tend to do this too frequently are often found among the frequently infected groups. Another factor was the presence of family support while the athlete was training. One supposition is that athletes who have family support probably have more regular meals and eat a better balanced diet. Another factor may be that family influences lead to more regular sleeping hours and less external stresses with activities of daily living. In any regard, once an athlete gets sick having help at home may maximize the ability to rest and recover.

Air pollution may be another factor for the athlete with frequent colds. This may play the largest role in runners who, during a vigorous 1 hour run, inhale an equal amount of oxygen as they would in 23 other hours of the day. The ability to increase ventilatory turnover to 20 to 25 times normal is one of the adaptations that allows the conditioned distance runner to perform at high levels. Nevertheless this physiologic adaptation also leads to inhalation of airborne particulates in direct proportion to the amount of air passed through the system. Perhaps, because of this, statistical studies show higher rates of respiratory infections in cities with high air pollution and

paralleling this are other studies that find higher respiratory rates after urban marathons than after rural marathons. So the possibility exists that air pollution triggers URIs particularly in runners.

Illness Severity in Athletes

Assuming that some athletes train too vigorously, do these athletes have a more severe illness? This question comes to mind when team physicians struggle to get a performer back to activity with what seems to have been a minor infection. No studies to date indicate that athletes experience a different illness severity. However, some studies suggest that athletes may delay seeing physicians unless they have a team physician readily available. This means that athletes who delay visiting a physician's office are more likely to have a secondary infection. In this regard, if one compares the athletes who see a physician for URIs with those who manage self-care, there does appear to be a difference in illness severity. The athletes who go to the physician often are treated with antibiotics and on average lose about twice as many days to training as would be expected. So despite the fact that athletes do not seem to have more severe illnesses than other individuals perhaps the physician should keep a high index of suspicion of secondary infection or a complicated illness by the time an athlete chooses to come for care.

Special Concerns and Complications in Athletes

The question then arises whether URIs lead to special risks or complications in athletes. Every team physician fears a viral infection that leads to a persistent low-grade fever and tachycardia. This infection cannot be excluded from an early myocarditis on the basis of clinical symptoms alone. Although myocarditis obviously is a rare process, fatalities have occurred in a number of athletes. Particular concern occurs when there are known coxsackie or influenza epidemics. One study demonstrated that 2 of 12 athletes who had poorer performance and no symptoms of viral infection had had the evidence of a recent coxsackie B infection (Roberts JA, 1986). Similarly, a British study of elite athletes with symptoms suggestive of overtraining and excessive fatigue showed that 2 of 14 had evidence of a recent persistent infection one of which was a subacute coxsackie myocarditis.

No clear clinical guidelines aide the physician's judgment to know exactly how to handle athletes with a common viral URI. Published case reports lead physicians to be cautious, particularly when athletes have temperature elevation or a resting tachycardia. One case report detailed death from progressive heart failure in an athlete who tried to train through a URI and then developed a coxsackie myocarditis. Similarly, athletes who try to train through influenza have been known to develop myocarditis and in 2 cases developed a bacterial meningitis after training through an episode of influenza B. Thus, while athletes may have the drive to train through what seems like a minor viral infection, the amount of immune suppression that they are experiencing cannot be judged simply from their willingness to train. In this regard, whenever clinical symptoms seem to persist, including fever, tachycardia, continued muscle aches, persistent respiratory symptoms, and excessive fatigue, rest from activity seems to be the best approach rather than allowing the athlete to compete.

Another risk that may be overlooked is the excessive use of over-the-counter medications. For example, the use of antihistamines may increase the fluid needs and the risk for hyperthermia in a given athlete. Similarly, too much use of vasoconstrictor products with α-adrenergic properties could be a factor in triggering arrhythmias in an athlete with an unsuspected myocarditis. In any regard, careful review of prescription and over-the-counter medication use by athletes may identify special reasons for caution. Team physicians can expect that 50% to 75% of their athletes will develop URIs during the course of the season. Because these are so common, giving out guidelines before the start of the season about safe medication usage and appropriate medical care may help athletes avoid mistakes in the self-care of their illness.

Summary

In summary, URIs account for as much as 90% of the infectious diseases seen among athletes. Although these are usually minor setbacks, they do cause major losses of time from both training and competition. Unfortunately, common URIs can suppress the immune system sufficiently to lead to fatal complications like myocarditis. In addition, the athlete must be cautioned about playing while sick and specifically about not training through an illness while symptoms are persistent. Studies demonstrate muscle abnormalities both at the biochemical and structural level that persist for 4 to 6 weeks after a number of common viral infections. Allowing the athlete easy workouts during a minor URI not accompanied by fever, tachycardia, or systemic symptoms is a common practice and seems appropriate. However, when the team physician suspects that a URI is more complex than the common low-grade "cold," then rest is indicated rather than return to training.

INFECTIOUS MONONUCLEOSIS

Nearly every team physician has had athletes develop mononucleosis in the course of a competitive season. This is not surprising because mononucleosis ranks among the more common infectious problems of athletes, and over 90% of adults have positive Epstein-Barr virus (EBV) titers by age 30 years. In white students between the ages of 14 and 24 the attack rate averages 3% to 5% per year. The attack rate in black students of this age group is lower even though black adults have similar positive titers. Theories suggest that black children may develop mononucleosis infections at younger ages in the primary grades. In developing countries, socioeconomic factors are thought to contribute to high infection rates before the age of 3 (in parts of Africa 80% of children have positive titers). Whether genetic factors or other unknown reasons contribute to earlier onset of infection or tendency toward asymptomatic illness has not been proven.

Clinical Presentation

Infectious mononucleosis has a relatively long incubation, sometimes lasting from 30 to 50 days. In adolescents the dominant mode of spread is salivary transmission. This led to nicknames including the "kissing disease." Regardless of social behavior, the level of contagious spread remains low despite the ubiquitous nature of the virus. For example, roommates of contact cases are at no greater risk of infection than are other students in college. In addition, epidemics of mononucleosis remain rare whether looking at high school or college age students.

Symptoms for mononucleosis include a nonspecific type of prodrome. This prodrome usually lasts from 5 to 7 days and the most prominent feature often is fatigue. Specifically, athletes who underperform or complain of chronic tiredness deserve evaluation for mononucleosis. Other symptoms that can be variable and nonspecific include headaches, anorexia, and myalgias. When the active infection phase begins it usually lasts 1 to 2 weeks and almost always resolves by 4 weeks. The acute phase includes fever, sore throat, often with tonsils having fairly extensive exudate, enlarged and tender lymph nodes that may occur in any location, sweats, and occasionally abdominal pain. Although these are the most common symptoms, the disease can present in a variety of ways. Examples of atypical presentations seen by the author include an athlete whose primary symptom was unilateral swollen eyelids accompanied by headache and low-grade fever. Another atypical presentation was an athlete with some myalgias and one tender inguinal lymph node. A third patient presented with right upper quadrant pain and nausea mimicking acute cholecystitis. Considering the variety of clinical manifestations, the physician must consider testing for mononucleosis in athletes who have an atypical infectious disease.

Diagnosis

Physical findings help support the history and commonly include an exudative pharyngitis and generalized lymphadenopathy. Rashes vary in appearance but often are nonspecific maculopapular type reactions. Petechiae of the soft palate and periorbital edema are seen in as many as 30% of patients. Less commonly, the abdominal examination may reveal hepatic or splenic enlargement and jaundice occurs in a few of these cases.

Fortunately, laboratory confirmation can usually give a rapid diagnosis. One test that perhaps is underutilized is the peripheral blood smear for atypical lymphocytes. These atypical lymphocytes are actually T cells that attack the EBV-infected B cells. A peripheral smear in a patient with vague infectious symptoms that shows 20% atypical lymphocytes suggests mononucleosis and should be treated as such unless other diagnoses become apparent. Mononucleosis spot tests have improved and are now greater than 90% sensitive and specific. Occasionally a negative test will require a titer for confirmation but this usually indicates that there is another viral infection that is mimicking mononucleosis. Mimicking infections include cytomegalovirus, coxsackie, other common respiratory viruses, and toxoplasmosis.

Special Concerns in Athletes

For years coaches have suggested that mononucleosis must be more common in athletes, but this has not been confirmed by studies that show athletes have the same rate as seen in other students of similar age. At least one study suggested that athletes recovered more rapidly from mononucleosis, but this has not been confirmed. One specific consideration in athletes is that a premature return to training may prolong the recovery, although moderate activity is clearly better than bed rest. For athletes this means that during the first 2 weeks after the diagnosis they can continue attending class and doing normal daily activities but should avoid training or any vigorous recreational activities. Athletes who develop complications or get into a prolonged course of mononucleosis require 3 months or longer to regain peak form.

There are a few special concerns in athletes, particularly in contact sports. Splenic rupture has been reported in

mononucleosis but is a rare condition. A survey of 45 student health physicians with an average of 13 years of experience recalled only 22 splenic ruptures. Football posed the highest risk with 17 of these injuries occurring in football. Only 8 of the 17 students, however, had diagnosed mononucleosis. Death from splenic rupture with mononucleosis remains quite rare and only two deaths have been recorded in the last 20 years.

The risk of splenic rupture from contact while rare is real and participation in football is not safe until any splenic swelling resolves. Therefore, most team physicians prefer to do an ultrasound evaluation of splenic size before allowing a player to return to football competition. Perhaps this is an overly cautious route but if the physician chooses not to do radiologic evaluation, he or she should at minimum hold the athlete from contact activities for 30 days. No ruptures of the spleen have occurred past 30 days from diagnosis. Physical examination is not a reliable way to assess splenic size. A number of studies looking at ultrasound comparison with examiners' estimates of splenic size reveal that two thirds of the enlarged spleens are not detectable on routine abdominal palpation.

A possible concern associated with mononucleosis is a greater risk of intracranial bleeds. This type of data comes from information in the Head and Neck Catastrophic Injury Registry, which shows that more athletes than statistically predicted who experienced catastrophic head injury test positive for mononucleosis. One speculation is that mononucleosis creates a vasculitis in central nervous system (CNS) vessels. But do these statistical data indicate a true complication that makes bleeding more common with head contact? No studies have confirmed this. Nevertheless the association of mononucleosis and fatal head injuries adds one more reason not to return the athlete with mononucleosis too quickly to contact or collision sports.

Treatment

Treatment of mononucleosis primarily is symptomatic and supportive. Special attention should be paid to the possibility of co-existent group A streptococcal pharyngitis. The exudate pharyngitis looks no different than what would be seen in streptococcal infections so that appearance and a positive mononucleosis diagnosis do not rule out the presence of two separate infectious disease processes.

Over the years there has been a debate on the appropriate use of corticosteroids for treatment of mononucleosis. Specific indications include complications such as life-threatening swelling of the tonsils, thrombocytopenia, hemolytic anemias, or rather extensive hepatosplenomegaly. Many team physicians, including the author, tend to use a 1-week course of oral prednisone, believing that this treatment speeds the symptomatic recovery of the athlete. Anorexia is a common symptom in mononucleosis and most athletes cannot afford extensive weight loss. Corticosteroid preparations seem to stimulate appetite. Still, no medical studies clearly indicate when steroid medications should be used or whether they make a difference in the disease process. On the positive side, one college health study showed an improvement in symptoms and a slightly quicker return to class in students who were treated with steroids versus those given only symptomatic care.

Part of the treatment process should be careful advice about the return to activity. Light activity may begin as soon as symptoms allow and can include the typical walking back and forth to class and routine activities of daily living. Training should not start before 3 weeks and the physician may wish to adjust the intensity of training to reflect the degree of illness that the individual athlete experienced. As noted above, contact sports should not start for a minimum of 30 days and after documentation that there is no splenic enlargement. In more prolonged bouts of mononucleosis judgment should come into play and specific strength testing may guide the return to contact sports. Most team physicians have treated some athletes with prolonged disability and chronic symptoms. Studies of this condition suggest that premorbid psychological traits may be a predictor of the athlete who does not recover after a mononucleosis infection. Chronic mononucleosis has not been proven to be a distinct clinical entity. True reactivation of EBV infection occurs rarely and in these cases generally the host has immunosuppression.

Summary

In summary, infectious mononucleosis occurs often enough that all team physicians treat adolescents with this condition. The athlete represents a special situation only in that return to training should be cautious and contact sports should be delayed for a full 30 days after the diagnosis of the illness. Treatment remains primarily symptomatic, but a number of physicians feel that 1 week of corticosteroid therapy helps athletes return more quickly to their normal functional status.

EXERCISE-INDUCED ASTHMA

Exercise-induced asthma (EIA) occurs frequently in all sports. Effective treatments exist, which usually enable the athlete to pursue a productive sports career without interference from the illness. Involvement in sports provides benefits to patients in that an active life-style helps individuals better control their asthma in all aspects of their life.

Asthmatics face problems from those who do not understand their disease. Often coaches label athletes with EIA as lazy or lacking in motivation. This can damage the self-esteem of young competitors. Successful treatment may alleviate clinical symptoms and completely turn around their sports performance. This improvement in competitive abilities builds confidence and may also have long-term psychological benefits.

Studies of U.S. Olympic teams revealed that 10% of these elite athletes were found to have EIA but only half of them had previously been diagnosed. The author has conducted studies of middle school, high school, and college athletes. Approximately 17% of these students tested positive for EIA on a simple screen using peak flow meters. Other studies using standard pulmonary function tests detected as high as 20% to 25% of participants. In all of these studies a large number of the athletes were unaware that they had EIA. In addition, even the athletes who had previously been diagnosed with asthma rarely had sufficient control of their condition.

Studies in the 1930s and 1940s identified factors that triggered symptoms of EIA in the laboratory setting. Specifically, trigger factors like dry air, cold air, or air containing certain chemicals or allergens all produced bronchospasm in the laboratory setting. The triggers alone would not provoke bronchospasm unless the athletes also had a high minute ventilation. These observations explain the association of EIA with exercise because the respiratory exchange is much greater than during normal activity. For this reason the provocative agents that trigger bronchospasm are entering the lungs in much higher quantities than in the nonexercising state. Clinicians recognized that a complex process occurs. Specific trigger factors in the appropriate setting, coupled with a high minute ventilation in susceptible individuals can induce a clinical syndrome indistinguishable from classic asthma.

Clinical Presentations

Persistent cough is a key symptom of EIA. This symptom occurs commonly enough to be described by sport specific names like the "1500 meter runner's hack" or "figure skater's cough." Athletic trainers frequently see this phenomenon during practices and may be the first to identify these patients.

Allergic Athletes

Allergic athletes develop cough that is typically associated with seasonal variation rather than temperature or humidity. For example, these athletes may be particularly sensitive when a particular tree pollinates. On these occasions the athlete coughs and may have watery eyes, runny nose, sneezing, or other clinical symptoms. Seasonal allergic rhinitis is an important part of the history because the athlete with "hay fever" has a 40% to 50% chance of developing EIA. Exercise occasionally leads to hives and on rare occasions a syndrome called exercise-induced anaphylaxis; both of these conditions possibly relate to allergy.

A careful history of atopic individuals who cough with exercise often reveals that they wheeze or cough extensively at times when they are not exercising. One of these times is after URIs when the individual requires a prolonged time to recover. In fact, their pulmonary function test pattern looks like an asthmatic 4 to 6 weeks after a lower respiratory infection. Other occasions that worsen the cough for atopic athletes include recent changes in environment such as new carpet or a move to a new house. Secondary infections such as chronic sinusitis with symptoms of postnasal drip, sore throat, nasal obstructions, or fatigue (from resting poorly at night) can complicate the athlete's ability to continue sports. In any regard, the individual with a strong allergic history who performs poorly during sports activities merits a careful screening for exercise-induced asthma.

Patients with Asthma

Virtually all true asthmatics will show a drop in peak flow levels with sustained aerobic exercise unless they are on an adequate dose of medication and consistently pretreat before exercise. This is of key importance because asthmatics have a continuous low-grade inflammatory process that plays a significant role in their symptoms. During exercise the cells that respond to the inflammatory response release chemicals that may trigger more severe bronchospasm.

Patients with Classic EIA

Patients with classic EIA frequently relate that their performance was fine until they exercised on a cold day. Cold temperatures also trigger true asthmatics to have respiratory difficulties but are a consistent trigger for EIA symptoms in classic patients. Dry air worsens bronchospasm nearly as much as cold temperatures and when both cold and dry air are present, the effects are additive. During the most severe environmental conditions the athlete should consider exercising indoors. Because these triggers vary for certain sports some have a higher likelihood of precipitating EIA. For example,

cross-country running and skiing have a much higher association with cold, dry air than a sport like swimming. All winter sports pose environmental problems. Other sports with high aerobic demand such as soccer or wrestling are difficult on the asthmatic. These sports trigger symptoms more commonly than those with stop and go action like football, regardless of environmental conditions.

Diagnosis

The most common way to diagnose EIA is a classic history followed by a successful trial of inhaled bronchodilators. When the history is not clear many physicians like to use a standard exercise challenge test which measures pre- and postexercise peak expiratory flow rates (PEFR). The most asthmogenic challenge uses free running in an outdoor environment. Treadmill testing is an option but precipitates fewer symptoms because the procedure is done in controlled humidified environment. Cycling, step tests, or other forms of exercise trigger symptoms less consistently than free running. The standard exercise challenge requires running for 6 to 12 minutes adjusted for the age of the athlete. Heart rates should read 80% of a predicted maximum. The PEFR should be measured before exercise and then at regular intervals for 15 to 20 minutes after exercise. The classic positive response occurs at 6 to 8 minutes after completion of exercise when the individual experiences a PEFR drop of 15% or greater. Although a 10% drop is suggestive of EIA, most researchers consider 15% the positive diagnostic point for mild EIA. When drops are 25% or greater the individual has moderate EIA. Drops greater than 50% suggest a severe EIA. Other screening tests that confirm the suspicion of EIA include a postexercise sputum that reveals eosino-phils. Similarly, a nasal smear for eosino-phils establishes the diagnosis of allergic rhinitis, which in turn, suggests a strong likelihood that the individual will at some point have EIA symptoms. A positive smear in an individual with a suggestive history gives enough information to begin a trial of treatment.

For difficult cases, an exercise challenge preceded and followed with standard pulmonary function tests is a more accurate indicator than a measure of PEFRs. Today a number of miniaturized pulmonary function tests can be used at track side and still give accurate screens.

Treatment

Once a diagnosis has been established, clinicians should treat aggressively. National Institutes of Health guidelines published in the 1990s have changed the focus of asthma treatment. In the past, physicians emphasized the treatment of bronchospasm, relying heavily on the use of theophylline products. Newer treatments target the inflammatory component of asthma which, when adequately controlled, may suppress the development of bronchospasm. In this sense, treatment has been directed to an earlier manifestation of the pathophysiologic process rather than treating the end result of the asthma sequence.

Physicians should adjust treatment individually according to the factors that trigger EIA in a given patient. For example, the patient with a strong history of atopic problems needs suppression of the allergy response. Treatment should begin prior to symptoms and at the earliest date of the individual's high-risk season. For example, the athlete with spring allergies would begin preventive medications 2 weeks before pollen appears. Inhaled steroid products,

both pulmonary and nasal, work extremely well and may be considered first-line treatment. Typically patients tolerate and respond to these drugs well. A lower percentage of patients respond to cromolyn sodium, but most physicians prefer starting the pediatric patient on this or a newer mast cell inhibitor. Clinical experience with these products in pediatric patients is more extensive than with inhaled corticosteroids.

Some clinicians favor using antihistamines in athletes, particularly newer formulations like loratadine, terfenadine and astemizole because these products have fewer side effects. These products, along with ketotifen (used in Europe), are the only antihistamines that seem to improve bronchodilation in asthma patients. Nevertheless antihistamines do pose specific risks in athletes. Even the best of these products may cause airway drying and hamper the ability of the athlete to tolerate heat stress. Athletes on chronic antihistamines also report a lack of energy and alertness referred to as "antihistamine fog." In addition, many athletes do not like the idea of taking a pill regularly. Due to these factors antihistamines remain a second choice to the inhaled products. Whether inhaled antihistamine will penetrate the U.S. market remains unknown at this time.

The atopic patient also needs bronchodilators but can usually limit their use to pretreatment before training and competition. Albuterol remains the drug of choice and numerous studies have documented its effectiveness. Other products including terbutaline, penbutolol, metaproterenol, and bitolterol also provide good bronchodilation and presumably should provide similar benefit. One new development in bronchodilation is the U.S. approval of a longer acting β-agonist product. Salbutamol appears to give 12 hours of bronchodilation and potentially could provide adequate coverage for athletes when used once or twice a day. If clinical trials prove promising this could become an attractive alternative.

Treatment of true asthmatic patients use the same protocols but the assumption must be that these individuals have chronic inflammatory change at all times of the year. To prevent significant bronchospasm, these patients need more aggressive suppression of their inflammation. True asthmatics do best on regularly scheduled maintenance doses of inhaled steroids or cromolyn plus β-agonists. The β-agonist dose also requires supplementation before and during exercise. Products such as ipratropium and theophylline may play a supplemental role but often can be avoided if good control of the inflammation is maintained.

At the earliest sign of complicating problems an asthmatic patient deserves re-evaluation. For example, the asthmatic patient with significant allergic rhinitis needs the addition of nasal steroids because of the increased risk for significant sinusitis. When sinusitis occurs, appropriate antibiotic coverage should start. The key clinical symptoms of this may be a change in the appearance of mucous secretions, increase of postnasal drainage, discolored sputum, and a sore throat each morning. The worsening asthmatic patient with sinusitis may benefit from a short burst of prednisone for 3 to 7 days but should be switched back to inhaled steroids as quickly as possible to lessen risk of long-term side effects.

Patients with classic EIA usually do not require multiple medications. These individuals respond well to environmental manipulations. For example, runners can use a scarf or a mask to warm cold air before it enters their airways. Better humidification of indoor workout areas may also lessen some symptoms of EIA. One trick that a number of coaches use is to take athletes who have EIA difficulties and have them do their warm-up inside at a gradual pace and then move outside to train. After a high minute ventilation in warm air, soft tissue of the airway does not cool off and they may be able to avoid the bronchospasm they would otherwise experience. When such individuals do require medication, most have an excellent response to a β-agonist like albuterol. Timing of this medication should be individualized for the particular sport and the length of competition. For example, one individual may need to use the inhaled medication 30 minutes before beginning training or competition. This may not work for a second individual who needs to start 30 minutes before competition and take a booster dose 10 to 15 minutes before the competition or after the start of the warm-up phase. A rigid guideline is not the best approach, and each athlete can experiment with the timing of product use to determine when he or she will achieve the maximum response.

When the patient with classic EIA does not seem to be responding as well as expected, perhaps an airway inflammation is present. These patients probably have a component of intrinsic asthma or allergic problems. In this situation inhaled anti-inflammatory agents like corticosteroids can improve control of breathing.

Treatment Failure

There are specific reasons that EIA patients may not respond to treatment. In particular, some patients display poor inhaler techniques. In addition, patients frequently have empty canisters, are too nervous to actuate them well, or forget their canisters at a time of practice or competition. Some of these problems can be eliminated by spacer devices that increase the amount of drug that is delivered to the patient. The aerochamber is an example of one of the more popular spacer devices. Another approach is to use a capsule that can be inhaled in a powdered form (e.g., Ventolin Rotacaps). Athletes may prefer the capsule because they take up little space and the delivery device can be hidden easily by holding it in the palm of the hand. Other individuals may not see the athlete use the medication and this helps adolescents avoid embarrassment.

Other causes of treatment failure include subtherapeutic dosing, undiagnosed occult infection, or poor timing in the administration of medications. The physician should also consider the possibility of a misdiagnosis even when there is a history of wheezing. Additionally, there are occasional situations when the allergic patient will find pollen counts so excessive that no amount of medication will allow them to comfortably participate in their given environment. The same sorts of difficulties exist when air pollution is extreme.

One final cause for treatment failure that should not be overlooked is that certain athletes have a need to fail. Athletes who have been pushed into their sport or have a poor relationship with a coach may fall into this category. The athlete who is under pressure imposed either by self, parents, coaches, or others can use the medical condition as a reason to end this relationship. These individuals may need the guidance of a team physician to understand the choice they are actually making.

Peak Flow Monitors

A final key factor in successful treatment of the asthmatic athlete is to give this individual control over the disease process. In the 1990s diabetics are rarely treated without allowing them to monitor their blood sugars and adjust their treatment regimen accordingly. However, a similar approach to the treatment of the asthmatic athlete has not occurred. Good peak expiratory flow meters are not expensive. With a few minutes of instruction, asthmatic athletes can learn where their relative baseline breathing capacity is at any given time and how the peak flow meter can be used to adjust the dosage according to the severity of their breathing impairment. This approach can markedly reduce medication usage by eliminating the unnecessary doses that routine schedules can generate. The athletes can also use peak flow meters as a type of behavioral modification tool to reward themselves for doing a good job in controlling their breathing difficulties.

Summary

In summary, EIA is an overwhelmingly common condition in athletes. Newer approaches to treatment that focus on inflammation hold the promise for athletes that they can lead a normal competitive life by preventing their asthmatic problems rather than treating them after symptoms become significant. Classifying EIA patients by the primary cause of their condition helps direct treatment but when inflammation is suspected it should always be treated vigorously. Careful monitoring of the asthmatic patient and an awareness of the factors that influence responses to treatment are all part of a successful treatment program.

Bibliography

Upper Respiratory Infections

Berglund B, Hemmingsson P. Infectious disease in elite cross-country skiers: a one-year incidence study. Clin Sports Med 1990;2:19–23.

Budgett RG, Fuller GN. Illness and injury in international oarsmen. Clin Sports Med 1989; 1:57–61.

Roberts JA. Viral illnesses and sports performance. Sports Med 1986;3:296–303.

Shephard RJ, Shek PN. Athletic competition

and susceptibility to infection. Clin J Sports Med 1993;3:75–77.

Simon HB. The immunology of exercise: a brief review. JAMA 1984;252:2735–2738.

Mononucleosis

Eichner ER. Hematologic problems. In: Grana WA, Kalenak A, eds. Clinical Sports Medicine. Philadelphia: WB Saunders, 1991:209–216.

Simon HB. Immune mechanisms and infectious diseases in exercise and sports. In: Strauss RH, ed, Sports medicine, 2nd ed. Philadelphia: WB Saunders, 1991:95–116.

Torg JS, Beer C, Bruno LA, Vegso J. Head trauma in football players with infectious mononucleosis. Physician Sports Med 1980;8:107–110.

Watson AS. Children in sport. In: Bloomfield J, Fricker PA, Fitch KD, eds. Textbook of science and medicine in sport. Melbourne, Australia: Blackwell Scientific Publications, 1992:436–466.

Exercise-induced Asthma

Badier M, Beaumont D, Orehek J. Attenuation of hyperventilation-induced bronchospasm by terfenadine: a new antihistamine. J Allergy Clin Immunol 1988;81:437–440.

Casale TB, Keahey TM, Kaliner M. Exercise-induced anaphylactic syndromes: insights into diagnostic and pathophysiologic features. JAMA 1986;255:2049–2054.

Eisenstadt WS, Nicholas SS, Velick G, Enright T. Allergic reactions to exercise. Physician Sports Med 1984;12:95–102.

Huftel MA, Gaddy JN, Busse WW. Finding and managing asthma in competitive athletes. J Respir Dis 1991;12:1110–1119.

Katz RM. Coping with exercise-induced asthma in sports. Physician Sports Med 1987;15:101–108.

McFadden ER Jr, Ingram RH Jr. Exercise-induced asthma: observations on the initiating stimulus. N Engl, J Med 1979;301:763–768.

U.S. Department of Health and Human Services. Guidelines for the diagnosis and management of asthma: National Asthma Education Program/Expert Panel Report. Publication no. 91-3042, Bethesda, MD: 1991.

EXERCISE IN PERSONS WITH CARDIOVASCULAR DISEASE

21

RANDAL J. THOMAS
RICHARD WEI

Benefits and Risks of Exercise
Sudden Death with Exercise
Physiology of Cardiovascular Disease and
    Exercise
Preparticipation Cardiovascular
    Evaluation of Athletes
Exercise Prescription
Exercise in Persons with Specific Types of
    Cardiovascular Disease
Cardiac Rehabilitation

"In all cardiac cases that are fit to walk about, outdoor exercise is beneficial, for it encourages health of mind and body."
—Sir Thomas Lewis (*Diseases of the Heart*. New York: Macmillan, 1933)

There is growing evidence that physical activity promotes good health and prolongs life among people who are free from significant health problems (1–4). But what about physical activity for individuals who have cardiovascular disease (CVD)? Is it safe? If so, what can a primary care physician do to ensure that such individuals are adequately cleared for physical activity and are prescribed safe exercise programs? And for whom should medically supervised, group-based exercise programs (i.e., supervised cardiac rehabilitation programs) be recommended?

These and many other questions confront primary care physicians as they consider the prescription of safe physical activity programs for their individual patients who have CVD. These issues, in fact, will be increasingly more important for physicians as the pool of patients with various forms of CVD continues to grow. This growth is occurring for at least two reasons: 1) the "aging of America" and more effective treatments for myocardial infarction are resulting in greater numbers of people living with coronary artery disease (CAD) (5), and 2) treatments for congenital heart disorders are producing older adults with such disorders, many of whom desire to remain physically active (6).

Primary care physicians play a crucial role in the prescription of safe exercise programs for their patients, especially those with CVD. Although physicians may feel comfortable identifying cardiovascular conditions that would make exercise dangerous, many feel uncertain about the prescription of specific exercise activities for eligible patients with CVD. Part of this uncertainty is due to the lingering questions raised by the tragic, exercise-related deaths of apparently healthy athletes. Such deaths, heavily covered by the media, are very rare, yet they serve as powerful reminders to physicians, patients, and parents alike of the potential risks of exercise. In addition, many aspects of exercise prescription of people with CVD are unclear or understudied, or both, particularly for young people with congenital heart disease.

BENEFITS AND RISKS OF EXERCISE

Despite these uncertainties and tragic events, substantial evidence indicates that exercise is safe and beneficial for persons with CVD. Among participants in supervised cardiac rehabilitation programs, for example, most of whom have CVD, the risk of exercise-related cardiac events is quite low. Haskell studied the experience of 30 rehabilitation programs in 1978 and found that one cardiac arrest occurred every 33,000 person-hours of exercise and one fatality every 120,000 person-hours of exercise (7). More recently in 1986, Van Camp and Peterson reported on the 5-year experience of 167 randomly selected programs in the United States (8). They found that one cardiac arrest occurred every 111,996 person-hours of exercise and that one fatality occurred every 783,972. For the average cardiac rehabilitation program, then, such events are extremely rare. This safety record, remarkable given the fact that most participants have severe CAD, is partly due to the thorough preparticipation screening and risk assessment that all participants undergo. This allows the cardiac rehabilitation personnel to prescribe and monitor a safe exercise program, tailoring the intensity, duration, frequency, and type of exercise to the particular participant.

In people over the age of 35 without known CVD, the possibility of an exercise-related death is also very rare. Thompson and coworkers studied the incidence of sudden death during intermediate- to high-intensity exercise (running/jogging) in Rhode Island from 1975 to 1980 and found one death per 7620 runners for a rate of one death for every 396,000 person-hours of running (9). Similar studies in other populations have yielded similar risk estimates, ranging from 0 to 2.5 deaths per 100,000 patient-hours of exercise (10).

The incidence of exercise-related sudden death (ERSD) among young persons under 35 years of age is not well characterized, but the scarce data that are available suggest that it is likely to be quite small. Driscoll and Edwards found that only 2% of deaths in children and adolescents in Olmsted Country, Minnesota from 1950 to 1982 were sudden and unexpected, giving an incidence of 1.3 sudden deaths per 100,000 person-years (11). Exercise-related sudden cardiac deaths occurred in less than 20% of cases, giving an incidence of approximately 0.2 exercise-related sudden cardiac deaths per 100,000 person-years. Other reports tend to concur with an incidence of 0.2 to 1.0 sudden deaths per 100,000 person-years (12,13), much less than the rate of ERSD in adults (approximately 0 to 2.5 deaths per 100,000 person-*hours*, as noted above).

In contrast to older athletes, very few young athletes who suffer ERSD have had previous symptoms of CVD (i.e., syncope, chest pain, or severe dyspnea on exertion) nor has their CVD been previously diagnosed (14,15). The actual rates of ERSD in young adults with preexisting congenital heart disease, therefore, are unknown, but are likely to be higher than in young persons without CVD. Rates of nonfatal exercise-related cardiac events in young persons with CVD are unknown.

The benefits of habitual physical activity are numerous. Among healthy persons, for example, regular exercise has been shown to increase life expectancy and to prevent, delay, or reverse the onset of CVD, diabetes, hypertension, obesity, and some cancers (1–4). At least a partial explanation of these benefits can be found in improvements in lipoprotein levels, body weight, insulin sensitivity, blood pressure levels, and coagulation factors that have been associated with regular exercise (16–20).

Similar benefits occur also in people with known CAD. In fact, several meta-analyses have assessed the effectiveness of supervised exercise programs (cardiac rehabilitation) on survival following an MI and have shown that mortality rates are 20% to 25% lower among persons who participate in such programs than among those who do not (21–23). Such exercise programs have been shown to decrease the rates of fatal but not nonfatal recurrent MI. They have also been shown to increase physical fitness, promote improvements in life–style-related CAD risk factors (i.e., hypercholesterolemia, smoking, hypertension, and obesity), expedite a patient's safe and early return to work, and improve the psychological well-being (24–26).

SUDDEN DEATH WITH EXERCISE

Exercise-related Cardiac Death in Young Athletes

Although cardiovascular disease is the leading cause of death in the United States today, life-threatening cardiovascular disorders are relatively uncommon, especially in people less than 30 years of age. *Inherited forms of CVD are not only the most com-*

mon forms of CVD in young persons, but they are also the most common cardiac causes of ERSD (Table 21.1).

In 1974, Lambert and coworkers (27) reported on 254 sudden cardiac deaths in children, ages 1 to 21, from 10 countries in Western Europe, Central America, and North America. The leading causes of *sudden death* were congenital aortic stenosis (18%), Eisenmenger's syndrome (15%), cyanotic congenital heart disease with pulmonary stenosis or atresia (10%), and hypertrophic cardiomyopathy (9%). Only 10% of deaths were *exercise-related*, of which 25% were due to hypertrophic cardiomyopathy (HCM) and 25% to aortic stenosis.

Maron and coworkers (14,28) studied in detail a group of 29 competitive athletes, ages 13 to 30 years, who died suddenly either during or immediately following exercise. CVD was noted in all but one of the athletes and was the definite cause of death in 76% of cases. HCM was the most common disorder (48% of cases), followed by anomalous coronary arteries (14%), CAD (10%), and aortic rupture (7%). One athlete was considered to have a normal heart, and the remaining six were considered to have

Table 21.1. Leading Causes of Exercise-related Cardiac Death (ERCD) in Younger (<35 yr) and Older (≥35 yr) Persons

Causes of ERCD in Younger Persons	Causes of ERCD in Older Persons
Hypertrophic cardiomyopathy	Coronary artery disease
Anomalous coronary arteries	Valvular heart disease
Valvular heart disease	Congenital heart disease
Marfan's syndrome	
Coronary artery disease	

cardiac abnormalities that were possibly linked to their sudden death.

Other investigators have suggested that anomalous coronary arteries are the most common cause of ERSD in young athletes. In a report by Waller (29), anomalous coronary arteries were found in 35% of the 87 cases he studied. HCM was the second most common cause of ERSD (22% of cases). Other less common causes of ERSD in young athletes included mitral valve prolapse (MVP) and CAD. Of note, a full 27% of deaths in Waller's series of cases were due to uncertain causes.

Exercise-related Cardiac Death in Older Athletes

Acquired forms of CVD, particularly CAD, are the most common cause of ERSD in athletes older than the age of 35. In fact, studies of sudden deaths in older athletes have found that 80% to 97% of cases were due to CAD, usually severe CAD (14,28,29). Other cardiac causes of ERSD in older adults are rare and include HCM and valvular heart disease.

Exercise-related Cardiac Death in Female Athletes

Surprisingly few cases of ERSD in women have been reported in the literature. In the report by Waller (29), for example, only 10% of 87 ERSDs occurred in young girls, and none of the 60 deaths in older athletes occurred in women. Among the series by Maron and coworkers, in which 29 athletes who suffered ERSD were studied, only 3 (10%) occurred in girls (14). Information collected by one of the authors (RT) in 1991 on 40 ERSDs in young athletes concurs with these other reports. Of the 40 deaths investigated, 37 (92.5%) were in male athletes and only 3 (7.5%) were in female athletes (2 were participating in gymnastics and one was playing softball) (R. Thomas, unpublished data).

This discrepancy between ERSD in women and men could be due to several possible factors. First of all, the incidence of ERSD in women may truly be lower than in men. This could be true if the true prevalence of CVD is lower in younger and older women than in men or if there is a difference in participation between women and men in those sports most associated with ERSD. In addition, the scarcity of ERSD reports in women may be due to errors in reporting and classifying deaths in female athletes.

Due to the scarcity of information on ERSD in women, any guidelines for the prescription of exercise in women with CVD could be inaccurate. New information is emerging, however, suggesting that the benefits and risks of exercise are similar in women and men following a myocardial infarction (30). The relative benefits and risks of exercise in young women and young men with CVD are unknown. It is probable that young women with CVD are at no higher risk and may be at lower risk of ERSD than young men. Until further sex-specific information becomes available, activity guidelines for young women with CVD should be similar to those for young men with CVD.

PHYSIOLOGY OF CARDIOVASCULAR DISEASE AND EXERCISE

Several physiologic abnormalities of the cardiovascular system occur in patients with CVD that are particularly important when considering their exercise prescription. These abnormalities can occur together or separately, with varying degrees of severity and related functional limita-

tions. They can be classified into four general, interrelated groups (Table 21.2):

1. Insufficient myocardial oxygen supply
2. Excessive myocardial oxygen demand
3. Myocardial dysfunction
4. Heightened myocardial excitability

Underlying structural abnormalities of CVD can be the cause of any or all of these physiologic abnormalities. In some cases, however, their presence is compounded by the reversible effects of deconditioning (i.e., being "out of shape" from a sedentary lifestyle), a condition often seen in persons with chronic medical diseases like CVD. Examples of the types of CVD in younger and older adults that are associated with these physiologic abnormalities are shown in Table 21.2.

Habitual exercise has been shown in healthy people to affect these physiologic parameters by improving oxygen supply, decreasing myocardial work at rest, improving myocardial function, and decreasing myocardial excitability (31,32). Regular exercise probably provides similar benefits in persons with acquired forms of CVD (33–35). *In persons with congenital heart disease, however, regular exercise may actually worsen physiologic as well as symptomatic limitations* (36,37).

One of the main benefits of exercise, in people with and without chronic disease, is to enhance cardiopulmonary fitness or exercise capacity. Sedentary people who begin an exercise program, in fact, can improve their exercise capacity by as much as 15% to 20% even among those who have chronic diseases like CVD (24). A person's exercise capacity, usually measured in terms of oxygen consumption ($\dot{V}O_2$, usually measured in mL O_2/kg per minute, where 3.5 mL/kg per minute is equivalent to 1 metabolic equivalent or MET, the energy expended at rest) at a

Table 21.2. Examples of Cardiovascular Disease in Younger and Older Adults by Type of Physiologic Limitation

Characteristics	Examples in Persons Younger than 35 Years	Examples in Persons 35 Years and Older
Insufficient myocardial oxygen supply	Anomalous coronary arteries Right-to-left shunt	Coronary artery disease
Excessive myocardial work (oxygen demand)	Cardiomyopathy Left-to-right shunt	Hypertension Cardiomyopathy
Myocardial dysfunction	Cardiomyopathy Valvular heart disease	Cardiomyopathy Valvular heart disease
Heightened myocardial excitability	Prolonged QT syndrome Wolf-Parkinson-White syndrome	Ventricular tachycardia

Table 21.3. Determinants of Exercise Capacity

I. Central factors
  A. Pulmonary performance
    Ventilation
    Alveolar-capillary oxygen diffusion
  B. Cardiac performance
    Myocardial function (stroke volume, heart rate)
    Myocardial oxygen supply and demand
II. Peripheral factors
  A. Skeletal muscle blood flow
  B. Oxygen extraction/utilization

maximum workload, is determined by both central and peripheral factors, as shown in Table 12.3. The central determinants of exercise capacity include pulmonary and cardiac performance characteristics; the peripheral determinants include characteristics of skeletal muscle blood flow and oxygen extraction. In sedentary, but otherwise healthy people, regular aerobic exercise can improve exercise capacity by improving both central and peripheral factors (31,38). Persons with CVD, on the other hand, increase their exercise capacity largely through improvements in peripheral factors because central adaptations are restricted by underlying central cardiovascular limitations (39).

PREPARTICIPATION CARDIOVASCULAR EVALUATION OF ATHLETES

The aims of the preparticipation cardiovascular evaluation of both younger and older athletes are twofold: 1) to identify any significant, previously undiagnosed *type* of cardiovascular disorders and 2) to assess the *severity* of any cardiovascular disorders that may be present. The severity of CVD is particularly important because it correlates with a person's risk of ERSD. A preparticipation evaluation, then, should involve both the *screening* of athletes for CVD and the *risk stratification* of those persons found to have CVD.

Screening for Cardiovascular Disease

The predictive value of any screening effort depends on the accuracy of the screening measure as well as the prevalence of the disorder of interest. The more accurate the screening measure and the more common the disorder, the more likely it is that screening efforts will correctly identify those persons with and without the disorder (40). Screening for CAD in a 30-year-old, for example, will generally be less fruitful than screening for CAD in a 70-year-old since the prevalence of CAD is much greater in the older than in the younger person.

The history and physical examination are basic yet critical tools in screening athletes for CVD. Important historical findings that may help identify underlying CVD include a family history of sudden cardiac death before age 50, syncope, unusual shortness of breath or fatigue, palpitations, and exertional chest pain. Unfortunately, many athletes—particularly young athletes—do not have forewarning symptoms prior to an exercise-related cardiac arrest. Maron and coworkers, in fact, found in their series of 29 young athletes who died during exercise that only 8 (28%) had reported previous symptoms (14). However, forewarning symptoms of CVD, particularly exertional chest pain, are common in older athletes who die from an exercise-related sudden cardiac arrest (41).

The physical examination of the heart can be particularly helpful in detecting murmurs associated with congenital heart disease or acquired valvular disorders. Functional or so-called innocent murmurs are common in young adults and should be differentiated from significant murmurs (42). These murmurs include:

1. *Systolic ejection murmur*, which is generally soft (grade II or softer), is heard best early in systole at the third or fourth intercostal space along the left sternal border and usually lessens in intensity on standing.
2. *Venous hum*, which can be confused with the murmur of a patent ductus arteriosus, is characterized by a continuous murmur heard best above the right clavicle as a patient is sitting up or as the patient looks away from the side of the murmur. Unlike many continuous murmurs, the venous hum is not loudest near the end of systole, but rather during diastole.
3. *Mammary souffle*, typically noted only during pregnancy or during the postpartum period, is a high-pitched, systolic or continuous sound heard best along either sternal border. The sound can usually be muffled by pressure over the site where it is heard. Its origin is thought to be related to the increased flow of blood into the breasts during and soon after pregnancy.

Other screening measures for CVD include fairly simple, noninvasive tests such as chest x-ray, electrocardiography (ECG), echocardiography, and exercise ECG. In addition, more invasive tests, such as pharmacologic stress testing, nuclear medicine imaging, and coronary angiography, add additional diagnostic strength in screening for CVD. Unfortunately, most of these tests are not feasible to do in all preparticipatory evaluations of athletes because they are associated with significant costs (financial costs as well as potential health risk costs). The most cost-effective method for using these tests in unclear. Some forms of CVD, such as aortic stenosis and cyanotic heart disease, can often be diagnosed by findings from the patient's history and physical examination. Still other forms of CVD, however, such as anamolous coronary arteries and HCM, may only be detected after more elaborate and expensive testing. Echocardiography, in fact, would be a very accurate way to detect HCM but at current costs would not be cost effective for screening purposes. The use of ECG would be cheaper than echocardiography as a screening tool, but its ability to definitively diagnose CVD is relatively limited. Currently most research in the area suggests that more extensive and expensive screening efforts in potential athletes should be reserved for those with findings from their history or cardiac examination that are strongly suggestive of CVD (43). Despite its relatively low sensitivity and specificity for detecting CVD, exercise ECG should still be considered as an initial screening tool in adults prior to initiating an exercise program, particularly in men over the age of 40 and women over the age of 50 who have multiple risk factors for CVD (44).

Risk Stratification of Patients with Cardiovascular Disease

An individual's risk of ERSD is associated with the severity of CVD involved. In many cases of CVD, a considerable amount of information on disease severity can be ascertained from the patient's history and physical examination. Indeed, a patient with any form of CVD who is symptomatic by history (e.g., syncope, exertional chest pain, severe dyspnea) generally has a higher risk of ERSD than a person who is asymptomatic with the same type of CVD. In most athletes with CVD, however, certain tests (exercise ECG, echocardiography, cardiac catheterization, etc) are able to add important information regarding the patient's risk of sudden death. The appropriate tests for risk assessment vary from patient to patient and are covered later in this chapter.

EXERCISE PRESCRIPTION

Exercise prescriptions can be individualized to specific patients by considering the intensity, frequency, duration, and type of exercise appropriate for a given patient. For patients with CVD who are cleared for participation in sports activities (see below), *exercise intensity* is of particular importance. Intensity of exercise can be determined and monitored by three general methods (45). First, a person's heart rate response to an activity can be a useful guide to exercise intensity, but it is difficult for some people to consistently check while exercising. Low-intensity exercise would be of sufficient intensity to increase the heart rate to approximately 50% or less of a person's maximum heart rate (preferably measured during exercise testing, in some cases not requiring preparticipation exercise testing; maximum heart rate can be estimated by the formula: 220 − age). Intermediate-intensity exercise would increase the heart rate to approximately 50% to 70% of maximum heart rate, and high-intensity exercise would increase the heart rate to greater than 70% of maximum heart rate. For example, if a person attained a maximum heart rate of 170 beats per minute during exercise testing and was cleared for participation in low-intensity activities, the target heart rate should be no higher than 85 beats per minute (50% of 170). If cleared for intermediate-intensity exercise (50% to 70% of maximum heart rate), a person's target heart rate would be between 85 and 119 beats per minute. For those cleared to participate in high-intensity exercise (>70% of maximum heart rate), their target heart rate would be greater than 119 beats per minute. Other methods for estimating target heart rates have been devised, but the method described above is the simplest and most practical for use in patients with CVD.

Exercise intensity can also be estimated by the *rate of perceived exertion* (RPE) during a given activity, but this method is somewhat more difficult to accurately quantify and monitor than heart rate. Similar to the heart rate method, the RPE during a specific activity can be compared to that experienced during maximum exercise testing. An RPE scale of 1 to 10 can be used, where 1 is the level of perceived exertion at rest and 10 is the perceived exertion at maximal exercise effort. Low-intensity activities would keep a person's RPE below 5, intermediate activities would result in an RPE between 5 and 7, and high-intensity activities would result in an RPE of 7 or greater.

The most straightforward and practical way of prescribing the intensity of activity is to use known levels of intensity and energy expenditure that have been measured for specific activities. For example, it is known from measuring a person's $\dot{V}o_2$ during various activities that certain activities are of low intensity (require less than 4 MET of energy expenditure, where one MET is the energy expended at rest, equivalent to 3.5 mL $\dot{V}o_2$/kg per minute), some are of intermediate intensity (4 to 8 MET) and others are of high intensity (8 MET and above) (46). Using this method, a patient who is cleared for low-intensity activities can be given a list of sports activities in which they could participate. Table 21.4 lists various types of exercise activities by their level of intensity as well as by their static and dynamic demands. Patients with atherosclerotic cardiovascular disease often benefit most from dynamic exercise, particularly intermittent dynamic exercise, but they may also benefit from static exercises, such as low- to intermediate-intensity cir-

cuit weight training (47). In other patients, such as those with mild aortic stenosis, exercise activities with relatively lower dynamic and higher static demands are recommended. Table 21.5 lists activities that have a high risk of bodily collision, activities which are particularly dangerous for persons with certain forms of CVD such as Marfan's syndrome and surgically corrected coarctation of the aorta. For a more comprehensive list of physical activities and their corresponding energy requirement (intensity) the reader is referred to work published previously by Ainsworth and coworkers (46).

For optimal cardiopulmonary conditioning and other health benefits, the prescribed frequency and duration of physical activity for most people should be 3 to 5 days per week for 15 to 60 minutes at a time, although health benefits are likely to accrue even with less frequent and shorter bouts of exercise (48,49). Furthermore, shorter and more frequent bouts of exercise (10–15 minutes, twice a day, for example) may bring about similar health benefits as longer and less frequent regimens (20–30 minutes, once a day) (50).

EXERCISE IN PERSONS WITH SPECIFIC TYPES OF CARDIOVASCULAR DISEASE

The following section has been condensed and adapted from the information and landmark recommendations developed by an expert panel that participated in the 16th Bethesda Conference on cardiovascular abnormalities in the athlete. For the complete details of those recommendations the reader is referred to the previous publication of the panel's work (36).

Table 21.4. Type of Sports Activities by Static Demands, Dynamic
Demands, and Level of Intensity

	Moderate-to-High Static Demands	Low Static Demands
Moderate-to-High Dynamic Demands	Group 1: High Intensity	Group 2: Intermediate Intensity
	Boxing	Badmitton
	Crew (rowing)	Baseball
	Cross-country skiing	Basketball
	Cycling	Field hockey
	Downhill skiing	Lacrosse
	Fencing	Ping pong
	Football	Race-walking
	Ice hockey	Racquetball
	Rugby	Running/jogging
	Running (sprint)	Soccer
	Speed skating	Squash
	Water polo	Swimming
	Wrestling	Tennis
		Volleyball
		Walking (brisk)
Low Dynamic Demands	Group 3: Intermediate Intensity	Group 4: Low Intensity
	Archery	Bowling
	Diving	Cricket
	Equestrian	Curling
	Field events	Fishing
	Gymnastics	Golf
	Karate or judo	Housework
	Rodeo	Riflery
	Sailing	Walking (leisurely)
	Ski jumping	Yardwork
	Water skiing	
	Weight lifting	

SOURCE: Modified from JH Mitchell. J Am Coll Cardiol 1985;6:1198–1199.

Table 21.5. Sports Activities with a High Risk of Body Collision

Bicycling
Boxing
Diving
Downhill skiing
Equestrian
Football
Gymnastics
Ice hockey
Karate or judo
Lacrosse
Rugby
Ski jumping
Soccer
Water polo
Water skiing
Weight lifting
Wrestling

SOURCE: Modified from JH Mitchell. J Am Coll Cardiol 1985;6:1198–1199.

Congenital Heart Disease

Atrial Septal Defect

The majority of children with an atrial septal defect (ASD) are asymptomatic, although, when severe, an ASD can be associated with pulmonary hypertension (accentuated P_2 on physical examination), right ventricular hypertrophy (by ECG or echocardiography), MVP, mitral regurgitation, or tachyarrhythmias.

Activity Recommendations. Patients with severe pulmonary hypertension should be limited to participation in only low-intensity sports (group 4 in Table 21.4). Patients with no pulmonary hypertension, with or without MVP, can participate in sports without restriction. In patients with MVP with associated mitral regurgitation or ventricular arrhythmias, limitations to activity should follow the recommenda-

tions given for patients with MVP (see below).

For patients in whom successful surgical repair of the ASD has been performed, no restrictions should be placed on sports participation once they have recuperated from the surgery, unless any of the following conditions are present: pulmonary hypertension (pulmonary artery mean pressure >20 mmHg), bradycardia-tachycardia syndrome, complete atrioventricular (AV) conduction block, or cardiomegaly on chest x-ray (cardiothoracic ratio >0.55). When any of these conditions are present, patients should be limited to low-intensity activities.

Ventricular Septal Defect

The presence of a small ventricular septal defect (VSD) can generally be detected by clinical findings alone, including a harsh, holosystolic murmur with a normal diastolic phase, S_2, chest x-ray, and ECG.

Activity Recommendations. No restrictions on activity are warranted for persons with a small VSD. Patients with a moderately severe VSD and exceptional patients with a severe VSD should be limited to low-intensity sports (group 4 in Table 21.4). Patients with a surgically corrected VSD who have recuperated from the surgery should not be restricted from any sporting activity, provided that all of the following conditions are met:

1. Normal pulmonary artery pressure by cardiac catheterization
2. Normal 24-hour ambulatory ECG (low-grade, nonsustained supraventricular and ventricular arrhythmias are acceptable)
3. Normal exercise ECG
4. No more than mild ventricular hypertrophy by ECG

Patent Ductus Arteriosus

Patients with a small patent ductus arteriosus are usually asymptomatic, but will typically have a characteristic apical diastolic flow rumble. Persons with a more severe patent ductus arteriosus will, in addition to the murmur, have cardiomegaly and ventricular hypertrophy (left or biventricular) by ECG.

Activity Recommendations. Patients with a small patent ductus can participate in all types of sports activities. Patients with a larger defect should be limited to low-intensity sports (group 4 in Table 21.4) until the defect is ligated, after which full participation in all sports can be recommended.

Coarctation of the Aorta

Elevations in arm blood pressures (sometimes unilateral) in comparison with blood pressure in the legs are characteristically seen in patients with coarctation of the aorta. The greater the ratio of arm-to-leg blood pressures, the more severe the coarctation. In severe cases patients have a history of very limited exercise capacity and perform poorly on exercise tolerance testing. Coarctation often occurs in association with other congenital heart defects, including septal and valvular defects.

Activity Recommendations. Only patients with mild coarctation can participate in low-to-moderate intensity (groups 2, 3, and 4 in Table 21.4), noncollision sports activities (see Table 21.5), provided that they have a normal exercise test, have no evidence of aortic root dilatation by echocardiography or angiography, and have no resting or exertional hypertension. Patients who undergo the successful surgical correction of the coarctation can undertake participation in all sports, although participation in colli-

sion sports should be avoided for approximately 1 year to avoid the possibility of traumatic rupture of the aorta.

Eisenmenger Syndrome

Cyanosis, dyspnea, distended neck veins, and complex ventricular arrhythmias are often seen in Eisenmenger syndrome. This syndrome, which involves pulmonary hypertension and a right to left shunt, is relatively rare, but the risk of sudden death is high in affected patients.

Activity Recommendations. Persons with pulmonary vascular congestion related to either Eisenmenger syndrome or primary pulmonary hypertension should be restricted from participating in all sports activities.

Tetralogy of Fallot

Despite advances in the surgical correction of tetralogy of Fallot, and associated improvements in symptoms, two significant problems emerge when considering sports participation for such patients. First of all, persistent physiologic defects, including a fibrotic right ventricle, right ventricular hypertension, or a persistent VSD, can be present after surgery despite improvements in symptoms. Secondly, patients with surgically repaired tetralogy of Fallot are at high risk for sudden death (51). Generally speaking, such patients must undergo extensive medical evaluation before a decision can be made about participation in sports. This evaluation would typically include a thorough physical examination, a chest x-ray, ECG, exercise test, ambulatory ECG, and cardiac catheterization.

Activity Recommendations. Postoperative patients can be cleared for participation in all sports if the following criteria are met:

1. Normal right heart pressures (systolic pressure ≤40 mmHg or less, remaining <70 mmHg during intermediate-intensity supine exercise, and end-diastolic pressure ≤8 mmHg or less)
2. No right to left shunt and no persistent septal defect
3. No cardiomegaly by chest x-ray (cardiothoracic ratio <0.55)
4. Normal ventricular function (by echocardiography, cardiac catheterization, or nuclear imaging)
5. No significant ventricular arrhythmias (low grade, uniform, and nonsustained) at rest, during ambulatory ECG monitoring, or during exercise testing

Patients with a mildly abnormal right ventricle (mild right ventricular dysfunction or enlargement) may participate in low-intensity sports. If such patients have normal exercise tolerance testing and no significant ventricular arrhythmias they may be considered for sports activities of intermediate intensity (groups 2 and 3 in Table 21.4). Periodic reexamination of these athletes should be the rule, with particular attention paid to ventricular function and arrhythmias.

Transposition of the Great Vessels

The activity levels of most patients with transposition are usually quite limited, both before and after surgical correction. In the Senning or Mustard operation the right ventricle serves as the systemic "pump," which results in an improved although limited cardiac output. Supraventricular arrhythmias and deterioration in right ventricular function may occur with training in this group, conditions that increase the risk of sudden death.

An extensive evaluation is needed before a patient with surgically corrected transposition can be considered for exercise partici-

pation, including a physical examination, chest x-ray, ECG (resting and ambulatory), and cardiac catheterization. Special attention should be given to supraventricular as well as ventricular arrhythmias. In patients who have had the Senning or Mustard operation, careful evaluation and periodic re-evaluation should be made of right ventricular function because it may deteriorate with exercise training.

Activity Recommendations. Patients who have undergone a successful Senning or Mustard operation can participate in low-intensity sports and can participate in intermediate-intensity sports with low static demands (group 2 in Table 21.4) if the following conditions are met:

1. No cardiomegaly on chest x-ray
2. Normal resting ECG (right ventricular hypertrophy and P waves of low voltage are acceptable) and ambulatory ECG (no tachyarrhythmias or bradyarrhythmias)
3. Normal right ventricular size and function
4. Normal exercise test

Patients who are cleared for sports participation should be reexamined and retested periodically (approximately once a year).

Anomalous Coronary Arteries

Although people with an anomalous coronary artery may be asymptomatic, they will occasionally give a history consistent with myocardial ischemia (i.e., exercise-related chest pain and dyspnea). Exercise testing will usually be abnormal, but a definitive diagnosis requires coronary angiography. In cases where coronary bypass surgery can be performed to provide a more normal coronary circulation, an evaluation by coronary angiography and exercise testing is recommended prior to clearance for sports participation.

Activity Recommendations. Patients who have recuperated from successful surgical treatment of anomalous coronary arteries and have a normal exercise test can participate in sports activities, but should avoid collision sports for approximately 1 year following surgery to avoid the risk of injury to the healing sternectomy site.

Marfan's Syndrome

Marfan's syndrome is an inherited disorder of connective tissues that affects the cardiovascular, skeletal, and ocular systems. A family history of Marfan's syndrome or sudden unexpected cardiac death is seen in most cases of Marfan's syndrome involving the cardiovascular system. On physical examination, several findings are characteristic (52):

1. *Cardiovascular abnormalities.* Dilation of the ascending aorta is the most worrisome cardiovascular defect in Marfan's syndrome, one that is associated with dissection of the aorta and subsequent sudden death (53). Echocardiography is the most effective way of screening for a dilated aorta and should be performed on all patients with suspected Marfan's syndrome. Mitral valve defects are relatively common, including mitral valve prolapse and regurgitation. Aortic regurgitation can be seen in association with a dilated aortic root.

2. *Skeletal abnormalities.* Long extremities are common and the arm span is usually greater than the height. The ratio of upper body length to lower body length is less than usual (less than the normal values of 0.88 in whites and 0.82 in blacks). Kyphoscoliosis and pectus excavatum are also common, as are a high arching palate and flat feet. Arachnodactyly (long thin fingers) is characteristic of the syndrome and can

be detected by two signs, the thumb sign and the wrist sign. The thumb sign is tested by closing the fingers of one hand down over the thumb. The sign is positive if the tip of the thumb protrudes beyond the edge of the little finger. The wrist sign is tested by having the patient encircle the wrist with the thumb and little finger from the opposite hand. If the thumb and little finger overlap, the wrist sign is positive.

3. *Ocular abnormalities.* Myopia is commonly observed in patients with Marfan's syndrome as is dislocation or subluxation of the lens. A flat cornea and retinal detachment can also be present. Visual acuity is usually diminished due to myopia, but may not always occur after a dislocated lens.

Activity Recommendations. Patients with Marfan's syndrome can participate in noncollision low-intensity sports provided no evidence of dilation of the aortic root or mitral regurgitation is found. Patients cleared for athletic participation should be re-evaluated at least yearly to check for changes in aortic root dimensions and valvular competence.

Valvular Heart Disease

Aortic Stenosis

The identification of aortic valve stenosis, whether congenital or acquired in origin, can be made by the patient's history and physical examination. Patients with aortic stenosis often report exertional fatigue, chest pain, dizziness, or syncope and usually have a characteristic holosystolic murmur heard best at the right upper sternal border. The severity of the disorder can also be estimated from the patient's history and examination along with additional information from ECG and echocardiography.

In the case of a congenital bicuspid aortic valve, detected by a click alone or in combination with a soft (grade 1) murmur, the patient can be cleared for sports participation without a cardiac catheterization. Otherwise, echocardiography can be used to estimate and cardiac catheterization can be used to definitively assess stenosis severity before a recommendation can be given regarding sports participation. *Mild stenosis* is defined as a systolic pressure gradient of 20 mmHg or less; *moderate stenosis* as a gradient of 21 to 39 mmHg; and *severe stenosis* as a gradient of 40 mmHg or greater.

Activity Recommendations. Patients with mild aortic valve stenosis can be cleared for participation in all sports activities if ECG, exercise testing, echocardiography, and chest x-ray reveal no other significant abnormalities (arrhythmias, ventricular hypertrophy, or ventricular dysfunction). Patients with moderate stenosis who are asymptomatic can participate in low-intensity sports. Such patients who have a normal exercise test can also participate in sports of intermediate intensity with low dynamic demands (group 3 in Table 21.4). Patients with mild or moderate aortic stenosis who have exercise-related ventricular arrhythmias should participate only in low-intensity activities. Symptomatic patients with moderate stenosis and patients with severe stenosis should not participate in any sports activities.

Aortic Regurgitation

Aortic valve regurgitation can be caused by congenital (e.g., bicuspid aortic valve, Marfan's syndrome) as well as acquired conditions (e.g., secondary to rheumatic heart disease, infective endocarditis, or aortic aneurysms). It can be identified from the patient history and physical examination.

Symptoms can include angina pectoris, syncope, and palpitations. In severe cases, symptoms and signs of left ventricular failure can be detected (e.g., shortness of breath, orthopnea, ventricular gallop [S_3], or rales). The murmur is usually high pitched, decrescendo, and blowing in character, heard best with the diaphragm of the stethoscope after the patient has exhaled and is leaning forward.

Several other characteristic signs are often noted (54), including "pistol-shot" arterial sounds, Corrigan pulse (bounding, due to high pulse pressures), pulsus bisferiens (dicrotic pulse), Mayne's sign (decrease of >15 mmHg in diastolic blood pressure when the arm is lifted above the head), and Duroziez's sign (femoral artery systolic to-and-fro murmur with intermediate pressure with the stethoscope).

The severity of the regurgitation can be judged by the associated physical signs in addition to the measurement of left ventricular volume and function by echocardiography or nuclear imaging. Exercise testing can also be of help in assessing the patient's level of exercise tolerance. *Mild regurgitation* is defined when the left ventricle is normal in size and when there are few if any "peripheral" physical signs of regurgitation. *Moderate regurgitation* is when peripheral signs are noted, left ventricular size is mildly to moderately increased, and ventricular function is normal. *Severe regurgitation* is when peripheral signs are noted and left ventricular function is impaired.

Activity Recommendations. Asymptomatic patients with mild or moderate regurgitation can be cleared for participation in low-intensity sports, and in some cases, for participation in intermediate-intensity sports with low static demands. All patients with severe regurgitation, severe dilatation of the aortic root, or symptomatic patients with even mild regurgitation should not participate in any sports activities.

Mitral Valve Prolapse

Although MVP occurs commonly in the general population (5% to 10%), it is an infrequent cause of ERSD. Findings consistent with prolapse include a midsystolic click and a late systolic murmur. The significance of echocardiographic evidence of physiologic prolapse in patients without any ascultatory findings is unclear. Certain echocardiographic findings, such as redundancy or thickness of the mitral valve leaflets, may signify those at highest risk of serious events (e.g., sudden death and systemic embolization) (55).

Activity Recommendations. Patients with MVP can participate in all sports activities, provided that none of the following conditions are present:

1. Sustained tachyarrhythmias, particularly those that worsen with exercise
2. Moderate to severe mitral regurgitation
3. Dilation of the aortic root in patients with mitral valve prolapse and Marfan's syndrome

Low-intensity exercise is recommended when the above are present. Family history of sudden death, chest pain, and exertional syncope in the presence of MVP should be verified and evaluated. These issues may be serious enough to recommend low-intensity exercise.

Mitral Regurgitation

The murmur of mitral valve regurgitation is typically apical, high pitched, and holosystolic. The clinical severity of regurgitation can be judged by heart size (on chest x-ray, ECG, and echocardiogram) and by ventricular function (on echo-cardiogram, cardiac catheterization, or nuclear imaging). Dynamic exercise does not appear to worsen regurgitant flow, but it may slightly worsen left ventricular function. Static exercise, on the other hand, can worsen regurgitant flow by increasing systemic vascular resistance.

Activity Recommendations. Patients can participate in all sports activities provided that they are free from symptoms, are in sinus rhythm, and have normal left ventricular size and function. Patients who are asymptomatic but have mildly enlarged left ventricular dimensions, with or without atrial fibrillation, can participate in low-intensity sports and selectively in sports of intermediate intensity with low static demands (group 3 in Table 21.4). Patients with any degree of left ventricular dysfunction at rest should be restricted from participating in any sports activities.

Mitral Valve Stenosis

Mitral stenosis, usually caused by rheumatic heart disease, can be identified by an apical, low-pitched rumble that is heard best in the supine position and disappears when the patient is in the left lateral position. The first heart sound is usually accentuated. The patient history is somewhat unreliable although most patients with severe stenosis experience significant symptomatic limitations. Although mitral stenosis is not a common cause of ERSD, it can lead to serious conditions, including pulmonary hypertension, right ventricular failure, atrial fibrillation, and systemic embolization. Echocardiography and cardiac catheterization are required before a recommendation can be made regarding sports participation. Exercise testing is also helpful in assessing the work capacity and safety of exercise for patients with mitral stenosis.

Mitral stenosis is classified as either mild, moderate, or severe by measuring mitral valve area, pulmonary wedge pressure, and pulmonary systolic pressure.

Activity Recommendations. Patients with mild mitral stenosis can participate in all sports provided that the patient is asymptomatic and in sinus rhythm. Patients with mild stenosis who have symptoms or are in atrial fibrillation, as well as patients with moderate stenosis, can participate in low-intensity sports. In exceptional cases, such patients can participate in intermediate-intensity sports with low dynamic demands (group 3 in Table 21.4). Patients with severe stenosis should not be cleared for participation in any sports activities.

Pulmonary Valve Stenosis

Pulmonary valve (pulmonic) stenosis is characterized by a systolic ejection murmur, right ventricular hypertrophy by ECG, and pulmonary artery engorgement on chest x-ray. Cardiac catheterization and echocardiography can quantify the severity of the stenosis.

Activity Recommendations. Patients with normal right ventricular function whose peak systolic pressure gradient is less than 50 mmHg can be cleared for participation in all sports activities. Patients whose gradient is greater than 50 mmHg or whose right ventricular function is impaired should be limited to low-intensity sports only. Such patients who have recuperated from successful repair of their stenosis (valvuloplasty or surgical repair) can participate in all sports.

Tricuspid Regurgitation

Primary tricuspid regurgitation (i.e., regurgitation that is not secondary to such conditions as pulmonary hypertension) can be associated with symptoms of right ventricular failure. The condition is relatively rare and has not been associated with sudden death in athletes.

Activity Recommendations. Patients who are asymptomatic and have a right atrial pressure below 20 mmHg with normal right ventricular pressure and function can participate in all sports activities.

Myopericardial Disease

Hypertrophic Cardiomyopathy (Idiopathic Hypertrophic Subaortic Stenosis)

Hypertrophic cardiomyopathy, one of the leading causes of ERSD, should be suspected and looked for in patients who have any of the following symptoms or signs:

1. A family history of HCM (usually inherited in an autosomal dominant pattern, but can also occur in a sporadic, nongenetic form)
2. Exertional syncope
3. Bifid carotid pulse
4. A harsh systolic ejection murmur at the left lower sternal border that may vary from beat to beat, increase on standing, and decrease on squatting
5. An abnormal ECG, with left ventricular hypertrophy or inferior lead Q waves

In addition, some patients with HCM have significant exertional dyspnea, chest pain, or fatigue and may notice frequent episodes of palpitations. The murmur of HCM is not present in all affected patients and may be confused with the murmur of aortic valve stenosis, although the latter is usually loudest at the right upper sternal border and is associated with a "plateau" carotid pulse rather than the bifid pulse of HCM. Most athletes who die from HCM have previous abnormal ECGs, but the best predictor of sudden death is nonsustained ventricular tachycardia (56). Echocardiography reveals several findings, including asymmetrical septal hypertrophy and left ventricular outflow obstruction. Outflow obstruction is usually associated with systolic anterior motion of the anterior and occasionally the posterior mitral valve leaflet. Although the degree of outflow obstruction correlates with symptoms in HCM, it is not generally correlated with a patient's risk of sudden death (57).

Activity Recommendations. Patients with HCM should be restricted from participation in all sports activities. Select patients can be cleared for low-intensity sports provided that the following conditions are *not* present:

1. Severe left ventricular hypertrophy (wall thickness ≥20 mm)
2. Significant outflow obstruction (peak systolic pressure gradient ≥50 mmHg)
3. Significant tachyarrhythmias
4. Family history of sudden death associated with HCM
5. History of syncope

It is unclear whether or not patients who have undergone medical or surgical treatments for any of these disorders are at decreased risk of ERSD. It should be remembered that ERSD is always a risk in patients with HCM, even those with only mild outflow obstruction.

Other Myopericardial Diseases

Patients with *myocarditis* or *pericarditis* should be restricted from participation in sports activities until after a recuperation period of approximately 6 months. An assessment of ventricular function before and after exercise is essential before such patients can be cleared for athletic participation. Those who have recovered with normal ventricular function who are free from significant arrhythmias can participate in all sports activities.

Less common disorders, including *primary dilated cardiomyopathy*, *restrictive nondilated cardiomyopathy*, and *right ventricular dysplasia*, generally require the restriction of all sports activities in affected patients.

Hypertension

Hypertension is one of the most common cardiovascular disorders encountered in the adult population (58), affecting as many as 50 million adults in the United States. Hypertension is defined in adults as a diastolic blood pressure 90 mmHg or greater or a systolic blood pressure of 140 mmHg or greater (or both). In children hypertension is defined as a blood pressure above the 95th percentile for children of that age (Table 21.6).

The ECG and blood pressure responses to exercise testing are also important to consider when formulating exercise recom-

Table 21.6. Definition of Hypertension in Children and Adolescents

Age (yr)	Definition of Hypertension (>95th percentile of blood pressure for age [mm Hg])
3–5	Systolic ≥116
	Diastolic ≥76
6–9	Systolic ≥122
	Diastolic ≥78
10–12	Systolic ≥126
	Diastolic ≥82
13–15	Systolic ≥136
	Diastolic ≥86
16–18	Systolic ≥142
	Diastolic ≥92

SOURCE: The fifth report of the Joint National Committee on Detection, Evaluation, and Treatment of High Blood Pressure. NIH Publication no. 93-1088, 1993.

mendations. Systolic blood pressure normally increases with exertion. However, certain people have an exaggerated blood pressure response to exercise (systolic blood pressure >200 mmHg). Such people, whether or not they have resting hypertension, should exercise below the intensity at which the blood pressure surpassed 200 mmHg. Habitual dynamic exercise can be beneficial for people with hypertension by helping to normalize blood pressure, particularly in overweight patients who are on a low-sodium, alcohol-restricted, and prudent hypocaloric diet (59,60).

Activity Recommendations. Patients with mild or moderate hypertension who are under successful therapy and have no end organ damage (cardiac, renal, or eye damage) can participate in sports of intermediate intensity with low static demands (group 2 in Table 21.4). Occasionally, such patients can be cleared for participation in sports of higher intensity with greater static demands (groups 1 and 3 in Table 21.4), if under close direction of the health care provider. Patients with poorly controlled hypertension should participate only in low-intensity activities. Patients who have a history of previously severe hypertension (diastolic >115 mmHg), who do not have end organ damage and whose hypertension is under adequate control can participate in low- to intermediate-intensity exercise with low static demands. Patients with evidence of end organ damage whose blood pressure is adequately controlled can be permitted to participate in low-intensity activities. Patients with secondary hypertension (secondary to conditions such as renal disease) can participate in low-intensity sports activities but should avoid sports with a high likelihood of collision. Exercise testing is helpful in patients with well-controlled hypertension who wish to exercise because

it allows the physician to monitor the patient's blood pressure response to gradually increasing intensities of exercise to ensure that the exercise intensity prescibed is safe.

Arrhythmias

Atrial Arrhythmias

Patients with *atrial premature complexes* can participate in all sports activities. Patients with *atrial fibrillation* or *atrial flutter* can participate in low-intensity sports provided that their ventricular rate is adequately controlled by medical therapy (i.e., controlled such that the maximum ventricular rate does not exceed that of sinus tachycardia). Patients with recurrent *supraventricular tachycardia*, both with or without a history of syncope, can participate in all sports activities if under successful therapy (i.e., no recurrent episodes for at least 6 months).

Ventricular Arrhythmias

Patients with *ventricular pre-excitation syndromes* (e.g., Wolff-Parkinson-White syndrome, Long-Ganong-Lown) require extensive evaluation for structural and electrical heart disease, including echocardiography and electrophysiologic testing of the heart. Patients who have asymptomatic evidence of a short PR interval (<120 msec) or a delta wave and who have no structural heart disease can participate in all sports. Patients with RR intervals exceeding 300 msec during atrial fibrillation or with an accessory pathway refractory period of more than 220 msec with isoproterenol infusion can participate in all sports provided that the ventricular rate is controlled by therapy (i.e., does not exceed 200 beats per minute). Patients with RR intervals less than 300 msec during atrial fibrillation or whose accessory pathway refractory period is less than 200 msec are at very high risk of rapid ventricular rates and should not participate in any sports activities. Patients in whom drug therapy prolongs these times can participate in low intensity activities.

Isolated, uniform, and nonsustained *ventricular premature complexes* are relatively common and are not associated with an increased risk of sudden cardiac death. Complexes that are multiform and sustained complexes (two or more complexes in succession) may increase the risk of sudden cardiac death, particularly in people with structural heart disease (61). Such patients require thorough evaluation and may not be able to exercise.

In patients with structural heart disease and medically suppressed ventricular premature complexes, low-intensity activities can be approved. Patients with frequent premature complexes that increase with exercise, in whom there is no structural abnormalities of the heart, can participate in low-intensity activities and in some cases in intermediate- to high-intensity sports under proper supervision. Patients who have no structural heart disease and premature complexes that do not increase during exercise can participate in all sports activities. Exercise may decrease or eliminate premature complexes.

Ventricular tachycardia, defined as three or more ventricular premature complexes lasting for at least 120 msec, is potentially lethal and nearly always requires an extensive evaluation of heart structure and function. In asymptomatic patients with nonsustained monomorphic ventricular tachycardia (less than three consecutive ventricular premature complexes) that does not exceed 150 beats per minute during exercise can be cautiously cleared for participation in all sports activities.

Patients who are symptomatic (i.e., syncope or presyncope), have structural heart disease, have sustained ventricular tachycardia at rates greater than 150 beats per minute during exercise, or who have the long QT interval syndrome should be prohibited from all sports activity. Patients in whom drug treatment prevents a recurrence of syncope for at least 6 months and keeps the ventricular tachycardia below rates of 150 beats per minute can participate in low-intensity activities. All patients with the *long QT syndrome* and ventricular tachycardia should be restricted from all athletic activities.

Conduction Disturbances

Disorders of sinus node function are numerous, including *sinus bradycardia*, *sinus arrhythmia*, *sinus pause or arrest*, *sinoatrial exit block*, *wandering pacemaker*, and *sick sinus syndrome*. Patients may participate in all sports activities if there is no associated symptoms or structural heart disease. Careful follow-up of patients should be done periodically to watch for worsening of sinus node function with exercise. Patients who are symptomatic with syncope or near syncope can participate in all sports if they are successfully treated and asymptomatic for at least 6 months. All patients with pacemakers should be restricted from participating in collision sports.

Patients with *first-degree AV conduction block* or *type 1 second-degree AV block* (*Wenckebach*) may participate in all sports provided they are asymptomatic, they have no structural heart disease and the heart block does not worsen with exercise. Such patients who have structural heart disease may be cautiously cleared to participate in all sports if there is no worsening of the heart block with exercise.

Patients with *type 2 second-degree AV block* (*Mobitz*) and *acquired complete heart block* should generally be treated with a permanent AV synchronous pacemaker. They may participate in low-intensity, noncollision sports if there are no uncontrolled ventricular arrhythmias. Patients with *congenital complete heart block* can compete in all sports if the following conditions are met:

1. No structural heart disease
2. No history of syncope or near-syncope
3. A ventricular rate greater than 40 beats per minute at rest that increases to at least 70 beats per minute with exercise
4. No ventricular premature complexes during exercise

Patients with type 2 second-degree AV block, acquired complete heart block, or congenital complete heart block require a permanent AV synchronous pacemaker prior to their participating in low-intensity, noncollision sports.

Patients with *right bundle branch block* or *acquired left bundle branch block* can participate in all sports if they have no associated ventricular arrhythmias or structural heart disease. Children with left bundle branch block should be considered for electrophysiologic testing. Those with abnormal responses to pacing should receive a pacemaker before participating in noncollision sports.

Coronary Artery Disease

The risk of serious cardiovascular events in patients with known CAD is related to the presence or absence of three important factors: 1) myocardial ischemia at rest or during exercise, 2) left ventricular dysfunction, and 3) complex ventricular arrhythmias. The patient history can give valuable information regarding these factors, but the exercise test is the standard test used to evaluate the risk status of a patient with CAD. Low-risk patients are those who have no evidence of ischemia, left ventricular dysfunction, or complex ventricular arrhythmias. They have a functional capacity of at least 8 metabolic equivalents on an exercise test. Such patients may have a recent history of an uncomplicated myocardial infarction or coronary revascularization.

Intermediate-risk patients are those who have evidence of moderate exercise-induced ischemia (<2 mm of ST-segment depression), a recent history of cardiac shock or heart failure (withing the past 6 months), or moderately impaired functional capacity (4–8 metabolic equivalents).

High-risk patients have severe exercise-induced ischemia (>2 mm of ST depression), severely depressed left ventricular function (ejection fraction below 30% or evidence of exertional hypotension), high-grade ventricular arrhythmias (e.g., ventricular premature complexes that increase with exercise, sustained ventricular tachycardia, or history of cardiac arrest), or severely impaired exercise capacity (<3 metabolic equivalents) (62).

Activity Recommendations

Low-risk patients can be cleared to participate in low-intensity sports activities or in intermediate- to high-intensity activities if under medical supervision (see section on Cardiac Rehabilitation). Intermediate-risk patients may participate in low- to intermediate-intensity activities if under close medical supervision and should be re-evaluated at least once a year with exercise testing to assess changes in risk status. High-risk patients should be cleared only for medically supervised low-intensity exercise and should be re-evaluated frequently for possible worsening of clinical risk status. Results of a study from England suggest that home-based exercise of low intensity can be safe and beneficial for patients with chronic heart failure (63). Such a practice is not currently the standard in the United States, however.

These guidelines were developed from information on adults with CAD. This should be considered when applying them in the rare children and adolescents who have CAD, in whom such guidelines may be appropriate, but have not been validated.

CARDIAC REHABILITATION

Cardiac rehabilitation is a relatively new activity that has grown in popularity and application since its birth in the 1950s. It was then that researchers noted the relative superiority of low-intensity physical activity to the traditional bed rest regimen patients received after a myocardial infarction. Today research has uncovered numerous benefits of cardiac rehabilitation in patients with CVD. These are similar to the benefits of exercise in healthy individuals, mentioned earlier in this chapter. They include improvements in physiologic factors (e.g., exercise capacity, blood pressure, and fibrinolytic activity), symptomatic factors (e.g., decreased angina threshold, dyspnea, and fatigue) and psychologic factors (decreased levels of anxiety and depression) (16–26).

The risk of serious cardiac events is relatively small in cardiac rehabilitation programs, especially when taking into consideration the high-risk status of many of its participants (7,8). Such events tend to occur in those patients with exercise-induced ischemia who tended to exceed their prescribed exercise heart rate limits (64).

Intermediate- and high-risk patients with CAD and low functional capacity probably benefit most from cardiac rehabilitation programs. However, cardiac rehabilitation can benefit several groups of patients, namely those with chronic angina pectoris, recent myocardial infarction, recent coronary bypass surgery, recent coronary angioplasty, recent valve replacement surgery, and recent heart transplant. In fact, the use of cardiac rehabilitation in such patients has been strongly endorsed by several national organizations (65–67). Particularly noteworthy are two policy statements by the Agency for Health Care Policy and Research (68,69), which support the use of cardiac rehabilitation in these six groups of patients. Cardiac rehabilitation services are also used by non-CAD patients who have multiple risk factors for developing CAD. The use of cardiac rehabilitation programs by children and young adults with CVD is less common, but a limited number of pediatric programs do exist that provide medically supervised exercise programs for high-risk patients with congenital heart disease (70).

Contraindications to cardiac rehabilitation (47) include:

1. Unstable angina pectoris
2. Severe aortic stenosis
3. Active thrombophlebitis
4. Recent pulmonary embolus
5. Severe hypertension (systolic >200 mmHg or diastolic >110 mmHg)
6. Uncontrolled complex ventricular arrhythmias
7. High degrees of heart block
8. Active pericarditis, myocarditis, or systemic illness
9. Resting or exertional hypotension
10. Poorly controlled diabetes
11. Other health problems that may preclude exercise training (e.g., orthopedic or psychiatric problems)

Cardiac rehabilitation is generally classified into three distinct phases. In the phase I, patients are seen in the hospital following a qualifying cardiac event (e.g., myocardial infarction or bypass surgery). The rehabilitation nurse gives the patient basic instructions regarding CVD risk factors and typically recommends low-level physical activity appropriate to the individual patient as he or she recuperates in the hospital. The patient is also encouraged to discuss with the physician the possibility of participating in an outpatient cardiac rehabilitation program. In phase II, patients with a recent qualifying cardiac event who are referred by their primary physician, undergo an initial evaluation of risk status, which includes an exercise test. Based on the patient's history and exercise test results, an individualized exercise program is prescribed that will optimize a patient's fitness and encourage a safe return to their "normal" life (i.e., work and family responsibilities). Patients begin this program at relatively low intensity to enhance patient acceptability and are usually under continuous ECG and periodic blood pressure monitoring to ensure patient safety. The patient is usually monitored by continuous ECG for the first six to eight exercise sessions after which ECG monitoring is used periodically at the discretion of the supervising physician. Patients gradually increase their exercise intensity and duration during phase II sessions, which are typically held for 45 to 60 minutes, 3 days a week for up to 12 weeks. Patients are also instructed about improving other CVD risk factors besides physical activity, including smoking, obesity, hypertension, and hypercholesterolemia.

Phase III is recommended for those who have successfully and safely completed phase II. In addition, some people with chronic stable angina or multiple CAD risk factors may not require the close monitoring and added expense of phase II sessions, but may begin the program in phase III. In phase III exercise sessions are held 3 days a week for 45 to 60 minutes. Patients continue to gradually increase the exercise intensity and duration until reaching a level at which they have reached an optimal yet practical level of fitness. Patients can choose to participate in a group-based phase III program indefinitely, usually at their own expense. Most health insurance policies cover only the cost of phase I and phase II sessions. Some will cover the cost of phase III sessions for patients who have not achieved acceptable benefit during phase II and who will likely gain additional improvement in functional capacity with additional cardiac rehabilitation.

Home-based rehabilitation is a relatively new concept that appears to be a safe and effective alternative for low-risk patients with CAD, for both phase II and phase III rehabilitation (71). Such programs may represent a less expensive way of providing rehabilitation services to the large number of eligible patients each year who do not enroll in cardiac rehabilitation. In fact, a recent national survey indicates that less than 10% of patients who are eligible for cardiac rehabilitation enrolled in programs in 1990 (R. Thomas, unpublished data).

The key to the proper use of cardiac rehabilitation services lies in the hands of primary care physicians. One recent study found, in fact, that the primary care physician's recommendation was the most important determining factor that led to a patient's participation in cardiac rehabilitation (72).

References

1. Powell KE, Caspersen CJ, Koplan JP, Ford ES. Physical activity and chronic diseases. Am J Clin Nutr 1989;49:999–1006.

2. Paffenbarger RS, Hyde RT, Wing AL, Hsieh C. Physical activity, all-cause mortality, and longevity of college alumni. N Engl J Med 1986;314:605–613.

3. Berlin JA, Colditz GA. A meta-analysis of physical activity in the prevention of coronary heart disease. Am J Epidemiol 1990;132:612–628.

4. Sternfeld B. Cancer and the protective effect of physical activity: the epidemiological evidence. Med Sci Sports Exerc 1992;24:1195–1209.

5. Larson EB, Bruce RA. Health benefits of exercise in an aging society. Arch Intern Med 1987;147:353–356.

6. Morris CD, Menashe VD. 25-Year mortality after surgical repair of congenital heart defect in childhood. JAMA 1991;266:3447–3452.

7. Haskell WL. Cardiovascular complication during exercise training of cardiac patients. Circulation 1978;57:920–924.

8. Van Camp SP, Peterson RA. Cardiovascular complications of outpatient cardiac rehabilitation programs. JAMA 1986;256:1160–1163.

9. Thompson PD, Funk EJ, Carleton RA, Sturner WQ. Incidence of death during jogging in Rhode Island from 1975 through 1980. JAMA 1982;247:2535–2538.

10. Kohl HW, Powell KE, Gordon NF, Blair SN, Paffenbarger RS Jr. Physical activity, physical fitness, and sudden cardiac death. Epidemiol Rev 1992;14:37–58.

11. Driscoll DJ, Edwards WD. Sudden unexpected death in children and adolescents. J Am Coll Cardiol 1985;5:118B–121B.

12. Mueller FO, Cantu RC. Catastrophic injuries and fatalities in high school and college sports, fall 1982–spring 1988. Med Sci Sports Exerc 1990;22:737–741.

13. Kennedy JL, Whitlock JA. Sports related sudden death in young persons. J Am Coll Cardiol 1982;3:622. Abstract.

14. Maron BJ, Roberts WC, McAllister HA, Rosing DR, Epstein SE. Sudden death in young athletes. Circulation 1980;62:218–229.

15. Neuspiel DR, Kuller LH. Sudden and unexpected natural death in childhood and adolescence. JAMA 1985;254:1321–1325.

16. Brownell KD, Bachorik PS, Ayerle RS. Changes in plasma lipid and lipoprotein levels in men and women after a program of moderate exercise. Circulation 1982;65:477–483.

17. Leighton RF, Repks FJ, Birk TJ, et al. The Toledo exercise and diet study. Arch Intern Med 1990;150:1016–1020.

18. Arroll B, Beaglehole R. Does physical activity lower blood pressure; a critical review of the clinical trials. J Clin Epidemiol 1992;45:439–447.

19. Eriksson K-F, Lindgarde F. Prevention of type 2 (non–insulin-dependent) diabetes mellitus by diet and physical exercise: the 6-year Malmo feasibility study. Diabetologia 1991;34:891–898.

20. Williams RS, Logue EE, Lewis JL, et al. Physical conditioning augments the fibrinolytic response to venous occlusion in healthy adults. N Engl J Med 1980;302:987–991.

21. Oldridge NB, Guyall GH, Fisher ME, Rimm AA. Cardiac rehabilitation after myocardial infarction: combined experience of randomized clinical trials. JAMA 1988;260:945–950.

22. Lau J, Antman EM, Jimenez-Silva J, Kupelnick, et al. Cumulative meta-analysis of therapeutic trials for myocardial infarction. N Engl J Med 1992;327:248–254.

23. O'Connor FT, Buring JE, Ysuf S, et al. An overview of randomized trials of rehabilitation with exercise after myocardial infarction. Circulation 1989;80:234–244.

24. DeBusk RF, Houston N, Haskell WL, et al. Exercise training soon after myocardial infarction. Am J Cardiol 1979;44:1223–1229.

25. Houston-Miller N, Taylor CB, Davidson DM, et al. The efficacy of risk factor intervention and psychosocial aspects of cardiac rehabilitation: position paper of the American Association of Cardiovascular and Pulmonary Rehabilitation. J Cardiopulm Rehab 1990;10:198–209.

26. Dennis CA, Houston-Miller N, Schwartz RG, et al. Early return to work after uncomplicated myocardial infarction: results of a randomized trial. JAMA 1988;260:214–220.

27. Lambert EC, Menon VA, Wagner H, Vlad P. Sudden unexpected death from cardiovascular disease in children. Am J Cardiol 1974;34:89–96.

28. Maron BJ, Epstein SE, Roberts WC. Causes of sudden death in competitive athletes. J Am

Coll Cardiol 1986;7:204–214.

29. Waller BF. What causes sudden cardiac death in athletes? Cardiovasc Rev Rep 1988;7:39–44.

30. Cannistra LB, Balady GJ, O'Malley CJ, et al. Comparison of the clinical profile and outcome of women and men in cardiac rehabilitation. Am J Cardiol 1992;69:1274–1279.

31. Smith ML, Mitchell JH. Cardiorespiratory adaptations to training. In: American College of Sports Medicine, resource manual for guidelines for exercise testing and prescription. Philadelphia: Lea & Febiger, 1988:62–65.

32. Haskell WL. Cardiovascular benefits and risks of exercise: the scientific evidence. In: Strauss RH, ed. Sports medicine. Philadelphia: WB Saunders, 1984:57–75.

33. Clausen JP. Circulatory adjustments to dynamic exercise and effect of physical training in normal subjects and in patients with coronary artery disease. Prog Cardiovasc Dis 1976;28:459–495.

34. Todd IC, Bradnam MS, Cooke MBD, Ballantyne D. Effect of daily high-intensity exercise on myocardial perfusion in angina pectoris. Am J Cardiol 1991;68:1593–1599.

35. Gordon NF, Scott CB. The role of exercise in the primary and secondary prevention of coronary artery disease. Clin Sports Med 1991;10:87–103.

36. 16th Bethesda conference on cardiovascular abnormalities in the athlete. J Am Coll Cardiol 1985;6:1186–1232.

37. Coelho A, Palileo E, Ashley W, et al. Tachyarrhythmias in young athletes. J Am Coll Cardiol 1986;7:237–243.

38. Sharkey BJ. Specificity of exercise. In: American College of Sports Medicine, resource manual for guidelines for exercise testing and prescription. Philadelphia: Lea & Febiger, 1988:55–62.

39. Balady GJ, Weiner DA. Physiology of exercise in normal individuals and patients with coronary heart disease. In: Wenger NK, Hellerstein HK, eds. Rehabilitation of the coronary patient. New York: Churchill Livingstone, 1992:103–122.

40. Epstein SE, Maron BJ. Sudden death and the competitive athletes: perspectives on preparticipation screening studies. J Am Coll Cardiol 1986;7:220–230.

41. Cobb LA, Weaver WD. Exercise: a risk for sudden death in patients with coronary heart disease. J Am Coll Cardiol 1986;7:215–219.

42. Frank MJ, Alvarez-Mena SC, Abdulla AM. Innocent murmurs. In: Cardiovascular physical diagnosis, 2nd ed. Chicago: Year Book Medical Publishers, 1983:242–249.

43. Epstein SE, Maron BJ. Sudden death and the competitive athlete: perspectives on preparticipation screening studies. J Am Coll Cardiol 1986;7:220–230.

44. American College of Sports Medicine. Health appraisal, risk assessment and safety of exercise. In: Guidelines for exercise testing and prescription, 4th ed. Philadelphia: Lea & Febiger, 1991:1–10.

45. American College of Sports Medicine. Principles of exercise prescription. In: Guidelines for exercise testing and prescription, 4th ed. Philadelphia: Lea & Febiger, 1991:93–119.

46. Ainsworth BE, Haskell WL, Leon AS, et al. Compendium of physical activities: classification of energy costs of human physical activities. Med Sci Sports Exerc 1993;25:71–80.

47. American College of Sports Medicine. Exercise prescription for cardiac patients. In: Guidelines for exercise testing and prescription, 4th ed. Philadelphia: Lea & Febiger, 1991:121–159.

48. Blair SN, Kohl HW III, Paffenbarger RS, et al. Physical fitness and all-cause mortality: a prospective study of healthy men and women. JAMA 1989;262:2395–2401.

49. Fletcher GF, Blair SN, Blumenthal J, et al. Statement on exercise: benefits and recommendations for physical activity programs for all Americans. A statement for health professionals by the Committee on Exercise and Cardiac Rehabilitation of the Council on Clinical Cardiology, American Heart Association. Circulation 1992;86:340–344.

50. DeBusk RF, Stenestrand U, Sheehan M, Haskell WL. Training effects of long versus short bouts of exercise in healthy subjects. Am J Cardiol 1990;65:1010–1013.

51. Garson A, Gillette PC, Gutgesell HP, McNamara DG. Stress-induced ventricular

arrhythmia after repair of tetralogy of Fallot. Am J Cardiol 1980;46:1006–1012.

52. Pyeritz RE, McKusick VA. The Marfan syndrome: diagnosis and management. N Engl J Med 1979;300:772–777.

53. Marsalese DL, Moodie DS, Vacante M, et al. Marfan syndrome: natural history and long-term follow-up of cardiovascular involvement. J Am Coll Cardiol 1989;14:422–428.

54. DeGowin EL, DeGowin RL. Bedside diagnostic examination, 4th ed. New York: Macmillan, 1981:402–407.

55. Nishimura RA, McGoon MD, Shub C, et al. Echocardiographically documented mitral-valve prolapse. Long-term follow-up of 237 patients. N Engl J Med 1985;313:1305–1309.

56. McKenna WJ, Camm AJ. Sudden death in hypertrophic cardiomyopathy. Assessment of patients at high risk. Circulation 1989;80:1489–1492.

57. Maron BJ, Roberts WC, Epstein SE. Sudden death in hypertrophic cardiomyopathy: a profile of 78 patients. Circulation 1982;65:1388–1394.

58. The fifth report of the Joint National Committee on Detection, Evaluation, and Treatment of High Blood Pressure. NIH Publication no. 93-1088, 1993.

59. Gordon NF, Scott CB, Wilkinson WJ, et al. Exercise and mild essential hypertension. Recommendations for adults. Sports Med 1990; 10:390–404.

60. Stamler R, Stamler J, Gosch FC, et al. Primary prevention of hypertension by nutritional-hygenic means. JAMA 1989;262:1801–1807.

61. Cheitlin MD. Finding the high-risk patient with coronary artery disease. JAMA 1988; 259:2271–2277.

62. Health and Public Policy Committee, American College of Physicians. Cardiac rehabilitation services. Ann Intern Med 1988;15:671–673.

63. Coats AJS, Adamopoulos S, Radaelli A, et al. Controlled trial of physical training in chronic heart failure: exercise performance, hemodynamics, ventilation, and autonomic function. Circulation 1992;85:2119–2131.

64. Hossack KF, Hartwig R. Cardiac arrest associated with supervised cardiac rehabilitation. J Card Rehab 1982;2:402–408.

65. American College of Cardiology. Position paper on cardiac rehabilitation: recommendations of the American College of Cardiology. J Am Coll Cardiol 1986;7:451–453.

66. Cardiac rehabilitation services. Health and Public Policy Committee, American College of Physicians. Ann Intern Med 1988;109:671–673.

67. AMA Council Report: Physician-supervised exercise programs and rehabilitation of patients with coronary heart disease. JAMA 1981;245:1463–1466.

68. Cardiac Rehabilitation Services. AHCPR Health Technology Assessment Reports, Number 6, 1987. Rockville, MD: Department of Health and Human Services, Publication no. 88-3427, 1987.

69. Cardiac Rehabilitation Services. AHCPR Health Technology Assessment Reports, Number 3, 1991. Rockville, MD: Department of Health and Human Services, Publication no. 92-0015, 1992.

70. Donovan EF, Matthews RA, Nixon PA, et al. An exercise program for pediatric patients with congenital heart disease: psychosocial aspects. J Cardiac Rehabil 1983;3:476–480.

71. DeBusk RF, Haskell WL, Miller NH, et al. Medically directed at-home rehabilitation soon after clinically uncomplicated acute myocardial infarction: a new model for patient care. Am J Cardiol 1985;55:251–257.

72. Ades PA, Waldmann ML, McCann WJ, Weaver SO. Predictors of cardiac rehabilitation participation in older coronary patients. Arch Intern Med 1992;152:1033–1035.

NUTRITIONAL CONCERNS IN SPORTS MEDICINE

JUDY GOFFI
JOHANNA DWYER
MIRIAM NELSON

Reasons for Concern
Body Composition
Dietary Recommendations
Heat Stress, Sweating, and Dehydration
Weight Gain
Dietary Ergogenic Aids

22

REASONS FOR CONCERN

There are two good reasons for being concerned about nutrition in sports. First, diet, physical activity, and exercise are important in health promotion and disease risk reduction. Diet and physical activity act synergistically to affect many health-related bodily functions and events. For example, individuals are more likely to maintain optimal weights for health over the long term, and those who diet to lose weight are more likely to keep weight off if they stay physically active. An optimal weight and a diet low in fat, saturated fat, and cholesterol, coupled with regular physical activity, are all critical for cardiovascular health. Dietary factors, leanness, and physical activity appear to decrease risks for some cancers such as those of the colon, breast, and prostate. Moderation in use of alcohol, fat, salt, and smoked foods and high intakes of fruits and vegetables and dietary fiber minimize risks of certain cancers and heart disease. Finally, adequate intakes of vitamin D and calcium along with weight-bearing exercise are among the factors that reduce the risk of osteoporosis.

Second, good nutrition can support and maintain optimal performance. Improvements in athletic performance can result from reduction of body fat, increased fat-free body mass, maintenance of healthy weights, and adequate intakes of water and food.

The eating patterns of athletes are often closer to the recommendations in the Dietary Guidelines for Americans than are those of nonathletes, but some athletes have diets that are suboptimal in fluid, carbohydrate, fat, and vitamins and minerals for optimal performance. Thus there is much room for improvement of their diets (1–9).

BODY COMPOSITION

Body Weight

A healthy weight optimizes physiologic function and good health. Attaining and maintaining it involves balancing energy intakes and outputs. The concept of what constitutes a desirable body weight has recently changed. It is now recognized that gains in fatness and weight after young adulthood are neither healthy nor inevitable. Today desirable body weight is defined as a body mass index (BMI) between 18 and 25 at age 21 years, with gains of no more than 5 kg later in life (10). BMI is calculated as follows:

$$BMI = weight (kg)/height (m^2)$$

Weight standards based on BMI are close to the 1983 Metropolitan Height and Weight tables for minimal mortality among insured persons (11). Weight for height is often specified for different frame sizes in desirable weight tables. However, this implies an exactitude that is missing in the actual data because the persons examined did not actually have their frames measured. Therefore such refinements are approximations at best and should be used cautiously, especially for athletes.

Currently available weight-for-height charts provide weight ranges that are inappropriate for many athletes because the components of body composition and weight of athletes differ from nonathletes. Therefore, competitive athletes should have their body composition estimated, as described below. They should strive to achieve and maintain body fat levels and weights for height that are ideal for the type of competition they engage in. Specific sports and athletic events favor different body types and weights for maximal per-

formance. For example a 95-lb (43-kg) gymnast and a 300-lb (136-kg) lineman differ in
their optimal body composition and body
weight for optimal performance.

Body weights for female athletes typically range from 52 to 66 kg for aerobic
sports and 56 to 88 kg for anaerobic sports.
Body weights for young, elite male athletes
typically range from 61–88 kg for aerobic
sports and 76–109 kg for anaerobic sports.
Excess weight over these desirable levels is
associated with increased risks, especially
when other risk factors such as high
blood pressure, smoking, high serum cholesterol, and high serum glucose are present
(12).

Weight, Body Composition, Fatness, and Performance

Table 22.1 describes usual body fat levels
for adults of various ages, derived from
a wide range of studies on normal
nonathletic individuals. Table 22.2 de-

Table 22.1. Average Percent Body Fat by
Age for Nonathletes

	Age (yr)	Body Fat (%)	Reference
Men	6–22	10–15	a
	23–44	11–24	b
	45–54	26	c
	55–64	25	c
	65–78	30	c
Women	6–22	16–26	a
	23–44	25–33	d
	45–54	34	c
	55–64	42	c
	65–78	43	c

a. Lohman TG. JOPERD Nov–Dec 1987:98–102.
b. Myhre LG, Kessler WV. J Appl Physiol 1966;21:
1251.
c. Frontera WR, et al. J Appl Physiol 1991;71:644–650.
d. Chen KP. J Formosan Med Assoc 1953;52:271.

Table 22.2. Average Percent Body Fat of
Athletes

	Age (yr)	Aerobic (%)	Anaerobic (%)
Male	<40	8–13	10–17
Female	<40	13–27	21–29

SOURCE: Economos C, Bortz M, Nelson M.
Nutritional practices of elite athletes. Sports Med
1993; 16(6): 381–394.

scribes usual body fat levels for athletes.
Both body fat levels and fat-free mass levels
influence fitness and performance. Standard measures of body weight and BMI can
be misleading about the actual body composition of athletes. Because their fat-free
body mass is often greater than normal,
stocky, muscular, athletic individuals may
be misclassified as obese when they are
really simply overweight because of their
large bones and muscles.

Neither male nor female athletes should
be emaciated because performance may be
affected. Among U.S. Army Rangers who
engage in a variety of vigorous training activities, health and performance are improved by providing enough energy during
training to minimize loss of fat-free body
mass and weight (13). Female athletes'
body fat should not fall below recommended levels because very low body fat is
associated with menstrual dysfunction and
this may cause demineralization of bone
even when sufficient dietary calcium is ingested (1,14–16).

Grossly excessive body weight diminishes performance in endurance exercise
and lower weight enhances it (17–19). Excess weight decreases performance in running and in sit-ups, push-ups, or other tasks
that involve lifting the body because the
greater the body weight, the more energy
that must be expended. Smaller, lighter
weight individuals do best on such tasks of

muscle strength and endurance, all other things being equal. For example, a runner who is 5% lighter in body fat has a 5.6-minute advantage in a marathon (20).

Adjustments may be needed for juvenile athletes who have not yet reached their full growth (21). There are also no solid data on which to base recommendations on optimal body composition for older (>40 years of age) elite athletes at present. Conventional wisdom is that fat mass may have to increase in the older athlete to keep fat-free mass at optimal levels. If so, body weights would need to increase with age. Research on this issue is needed.

Fat-Free Body Mass

The best correlations between body composition and physical performance are with fat-free body mass, especially on tasks for which strength rather than endurance alone is required. Fat-free body mass is also a good predictor of maximal aerobic capacity, treadmill run times, and short distance runs with a weight pack as a measure of performance (18,19). When individuals are fat, times to carry loads over a given distance increase; as fat-free body mass increases, times decrease. The best predictor of load carrying and lifting ability is fat-free body mass. Very obese people are significantly impaired in their performance during running, sit-ups, and push-ups. However, overweight persons usually perform adequately on tasks involving the ability to push loads and produce torque, whereas underweight persons do not, possibly because of the differences between the fat and lean in fat-free body mass. The correlations between BMI, fatness, and injury are also high among U.S. Army military trainees. As obesity increases, poor fitness also increases. As fitness decreases, injury rates rise (22). Both low-weight athletes

(who have low fat-free mass) and obese athletes are therefore at a disadvantage in load-carrying tests of performance.

Since fat-free body mass is the best predictor of performance for many military activities, ultimately it is probably best for the military to have fat-free body mass standards rather than maximum percentage body fat standards to maximize physical performance among military personnel, as was recently suggested (13). The main concerns in sports are about fat-free mass and body fat mass because these variables relate most directly to performance. Athletes performing activities similar to those assessed in military standards, such as football, hockey, and lacrosse, may be most fit when they meet standards for both minimum body fat and maximum fat-free body mass, taking age and sex into consideration.

Assessment of Body Composition for Athletes

The assessment of body composition is important in setting weight goals. In assessing body composition it is important to determine the individual's relative proportion of both fat-free and body fat mass. Fat-free mass can be subdivided into muscle mass, nonmuscle lean tissue, body water, and bone mass. Each component differs between individuals and within individuals over time.

In most persons, anthropometric techniques such as circumferences and skinfolds are sufficient to assess the body fat burden. The usual measures are height, weight, skinfold thicknesses at the triceps and subscapular sites, body diameters, and body circumference measurements (abdomen). These must be taken in a standardized fashion, and the errors in estimation need to be recognized.

Underwater weighing, body volume measurements, body water measurements, or total potassium (40 K) measurements may also be taken to determine the components of body weight more precisely for research purposes. Underwater weighing to determine body density is probably the most common research technique. The problem is that standards for body density are nonexistent for most groups by race, age, gender, or ethnic group, let alone by various sports. Also, this is difficult, costly, and time-consuming measurement to take.

New tools, such as bioelectrical impedance, are becoming more popular because they are portable and easy to use. The principle behind bioelectrical impedance analysis is that lean tissue conducts electricity better than does fat tissue. Electrodes are placed on the arms and legs, a low-level electrical current is turned on, and impedance or resistance to the flow is measured. Total body water is then measured and from that measurement body fat can be estimated by use of a formula. The problem is that it depends on the hydration status of the individual and its performance is not always better than anthropometry (23), although in some studies it is (24,25).

DIETARY RECOMMENDATIONS

Energy

In general, athletes who engage in moderate exercise require 32 kcal/kg desirable body weight. Those who exercise strenuously need 44 kcal/kg (21). For athletes exercising longer than 90 minutes, energy needs may be as high as 50 kcal/kg (26).

Athletes who train about 1 hour per day should follow the Dietary Guidelines for Americans (9) to promote good nutrition, reduce health risks, and maximize their performance. Athletes who train more vigorously may need to make further modifications to this basic pattern such as increasing intakes of carbohydrate, calories, and fluids. These are described later in the chapter.

The Dietary Guidelines for Americans recommend a moderate low-fat, moderate high-carbohydrate diet for the general population. The USDA's Food Guide Pyramid graphically depicts them and provides guidelines on serving sizes for each of the food groups (Figure 22.1). Total calorie intakes for eating the servings suggested in the Food Pyramid range from 1600 to 2800 calories (kcal) daily. These energy levels are too low to meet the needs of most athletes. Therefore they should eat more of the food groups, especially those groups (breads, cereals, fruits, and vegetables) at the base of the pyramid, to meet their energy needs.

Attention to energy intake is critical if athletes are to achieve and maintain desirable levels of weight and body composition. Women have less fat-free body mass per unit body weight and therefore lower resting energy needs than do men. Recommended energy intakes are usually about 1000 calories (kcal) higher for males than females due to sex differences in fat-free mass. Variations in weight and height further affect caloric needs for resting metabolism and the cost of physical activity. Energy needs also depend on physical activity levels, including the duration, frequency, and type of physical activity or exercise. Energy needs decrease with age, largely because of age-associated declines in physical activity and consequent declines in fat-free mass. Fat-free mass decreases with age, especially in sedentary individuals, and it accounts for most of the decline in resting metabolic rates with aging. Probably most of these age-associated changes in body composition are not inevitable and

Food Guide Pyramid

A Guide to Daily Food Choices

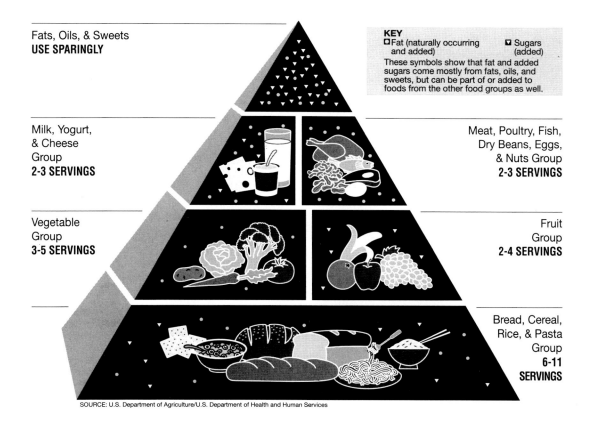

Fats, Oils, & Sweets
USE SPARINGLY

KEY
☐ Fat (naturally occurring and added) ▨ Sugars (added)
These symbols show that fat and added sugars come mostly from fats, oils, and sweets, but can be part of or added to foods from the other food groups as well.

Milk, Yogurt, & Cheese Group
2-3 SERVINGS

Meat, Poultry, Fish, Dry Beans, Eggs, & Nuts Group
2-3 SERVINGS

Vegetable Group
3-5 SERVINGS

Fruit Group
2-4 SERVINGS

Bread, Cereal, Rice, & Pasta Group
6-11 SERVINGS

SOURCE: U.S. Department of Agriculture/U.S. Department of Health and Human Services

Use the Food Guide Pyramid to help you eat better every day. . .the Dietary Guidelines way. Start with plenty of Breads, Cereals, Rice, and Pasta; Vegetables; and Fruits. Add two to three servings from the Milk group and two to three servings from the Meat group.

Each of these food groups provides some, but not all, of the nutrients you need. No one food group is more important than another — for good health you need them all. Go easy on fats, oils, and sweets, the foods in the small tip of the Pyramid.

To order a copy of "The Food Guide Pyramid" booklet, send a $1.00 check or money order made out to the Superintendent of Documents to: Consumer Information Center, Department 159-Y, Pueblo, Colorado 81009.

U.S. Department of Agriculture, Human Nutrition Information Service, August 1992, Leaflet No. 572

Figure 22.1.   Food guide pyramid.

can be slowed by alterations in life-styles such as sustained physical activity throughout life.

Carbohydrate Recommendations: Simple and Complex Sources

For those who exercise less than 1 hour per day, 55% of daily energy needs should come from carbohydrates (12). The carbohydrate intakes of athletes engaged in both aerobic and anaerobic events who exercise more than 1 hour per day should be higher, 55% to 70% of total calories. At least 45% of calories should come from complex carbohydrate (e.g., 6–10 gm complex carbohydrate/kg body weight) (27–29). The other 10% or more of carbohydrate calories may come from sugars.

Both simple and complex carbohydrates can replenish glycogen stores. However, foods rich in complex carbohydrate usually contain more vitamins and minerals. Also, they are more slowly absorbed, possibly facilitating maintenance of blood sugar levels (30–32). Therefore, they should be emphasized.

Foods high in complex carbohydrates include breads, cereals, pastas, rice and other grains, as well as starchy vegetables such as potatoes, corn, squash, and legumes. Whole grains, legumes, and starchy vegetables also contain relatively large amounts of fiber. Large amounts of high-fiber foods may be difficult for some athletes to tolerate as their primary carbohydrate source simply because of their sheer bulk and gastric fullness. Therefore, mixtures of high- and low-fiber foods are usually best tolerated. Vegetables are important as sources of vitamins and minerals, and also as carbohydrate energy sources, but they also have a high fiber-to-carbohydrate ratio and large amounts may not be tolerated.

Fruits, fruit juices, milk, and yogurt supply mostly simple sugars and also provide significant vitamins and minerals. Fruits contain simple sugars (mostly fructose). Their soluble fiber content helps to slow absorption and blunt blood sugar response, and the fructose does not require insulin for its metabolism. Thus they provide good energy sources for athletes.

Sugars like table sugar or candy provide few nutrients other than calories. Other high-sugar foods include soda, fruit and punch drinks, sugar, honey, candy and other sweets, sports drinks, and sports bars. They may be used for 9% to 14% of carbohydrate intake or even in higher amounts for very active individuals (27,28).

Some athletes who are lactose intolerant may benefit from lactose-reduced milk, use of lactaid enzymes before eating, or low-lactose yogurt. Low-fat cheeses are good sources of vitamins and minerals; they contain less lactose and less carbohydrates than other milk products.

Carbohydrate Metabolism and Intake in Exercise

Serum glucose is the primary substrate for muscle functions during short bouts of exercise. Exercise of high intensity but short duration such as sprinting depends on anaerobic metabolism and uses carbohydrate. The likely causes of fatigue in activities lasting less than 1 hour results from lactate and hydrogen ion buildup (33). As the duration of exercise increases and its intensity decreases, a mix of carbohydrate and fat is preferentially used as fuel (26). About 8% of the fuel used in long-lasting exercise is derived from muscle glycogen, with about 30% coming from blood glucose. Liver glycogen stores supply less energy in long exercise bouts than does muscle glycogen. The other 60% to 70% of energy needs under such circumstances are derived from fat and are mostly from muscle triglyceride with some from blood free fatty acids (34–

37). *A well-trained athlete uses more fat in endurance events than does a less fit individual.* A small amount of energy is also derived from branched chain amino acids in muscle during long-sustained exercise (33). Glycogen stores virtually disappear in events lasting more than 3 hours (26).

High-carbohydrate ingestion ensures that glycogen stores are maximal prior to exercise. Carbohydrate ingestion also facilitates the replacement of both liver and muscle glycogen after exercise and during training and the competition event. Therefore, athletes need to make sure that their diets are high in carbohydrate (37–42). A diet of 40% carbohydrate failed to replenish glycogen stores even after 3 days of daily 2-hour heavy aerobic exercise, but a 70% carbohydrate diet did so. With adequate rest and consumption of such high-carbohydrate diets, glycogen stores can increase between training bouts even beyond initial levels (33). Factors such as exercise intensity, physical conditioning, mode of exercise, environmental temperature, and pre-exercise diet all influence rates of muscle glycogen depletion (33).

During prolonged exercise, carbohydrate supplementation can delay fatigue by as much as 30 to 60 minutes (40–42). Athletes in "ultra" endurance events lasting 10 or more hours such as ironman triathlons, 50- to 100-mile runs, and 200-mile bike races need a total of 12–13 gm carbohydrate/kg body weight per day or about 3650 calories (kcal) from carbohydrates; since energy outputs are very high even these high intakes are not excessive (46–48).

When foods containing protein as well as carbohydrate are fed, recovery from exercise may improve because glycogen stores are replenished more quickly than with high-carbohydrate foods alone (49). Insulin levels are elevated more from a carbohydrate and protein feeding, but the plasma blood glucose response is higher with the carbohydrate only feeding. Because insulin increases glycogen synthesis by stimulating glucose transport and glycogen synthase, its increase may result in higher stores of glycogen (49).

Precompetition Diet: Carbohydrate Loading

During the 3 days prior to competition in an aerobic event lasting more than 90 minutes, carbohydrates should contribute 65% to 70% of total calories or 550 gm/day, whichever is greater (27). This high-carbohydrate diet is used for "modified carbohydrate loading." It is coupled with a tapered training regimen and adequate fluid to maximize glycogen stores in well-trained athletes (29,38).

The day of competition, athletes should eat a meal about 3 to 4 hours before the event to minimize gastrointestinal discomfort. The meal can be a mixture of complex carbohydrates and simple carbohydrates, and high-fat foods should be avoided. Athletes should consume 1–5 gm carbohydrate per kg up to 4 hours before exercising in an endurance event (28). For some individuals, consuming carbohydrates 30 to 60 minutes before an event may produce a rapid fall in blood glucose (50) and adversely affect performance (30,51,52). Athletes should experiment with prerace meals during training sessions to see what is best for them. They should avoid new foods or eating regimens during race days. Table 22.3 presents a sample precompetition meal.

Protein: High-Protein Supplements Are Usually Not Needed

Dietary protein needs as described in the Recommended Dietary Allowance (RDA) for the reference adult and older adolescent are 0.8 gm protein per kg desirable body

Table 22.3. Sample Precompetition Meal

Precompetition Breakfast: 434 kcal,
88% carbohydrate (95 gm)
½ cup orange juice
1 cup 1% milk
1 oz wheat cereal
1 slice bread with 2 tsp jam
1 banana

Precompetition Lunch or Dinner: 586 kcal,
66% carbohydrate (96 gm)
2 slices bread
2 slices lean ham
1 slice cheese
2 tsp mustard
1 apple
1½ cup orange juice

weight per day (53). Protein needs for younger adolescent athletes aged 11 to 14 years are 1 gm/kg. Those aged 7 to 10 years need 1.2 gm protein per kg. Some studies have suggested that there is an increased need for protein among endurance athletes with 1.0–1.4 gm/kg being recommended (27,54–57). However, experts do not agree on the necessity of these higher values. In any event, for most athletes this is not an issue because they already consume large amounts of protein. Most Americans consume 1 gm/kg per day, and many athletes consume 1.2–2.0 gm/kg per day (12% to 26% of calories) because their energy needs are higher and therefore their food intakes are higher as well (27–29).

Extra dietary protein from either food sources or amino acid supplements and protein drinks does not increase muscle mass or strength nor does it improve performance (57–59). Amino acid supplements in tablet form do not significantly contribute to protein intake because they generally contain less than 1 gm of protein. Also, they are extremely expensive. Single

amino acid supplements do not supply the eight amino acids that are essential building blocks of human protein. Very high-protein intakes (e.g., >200 gm/day) may lead to dehydration. High intakes of high-protein, high-fat foods such as red meats also increase calories, saturated fat, and cholesterol intakes.

Protein supplements in the form of drinks or bars usually contain an average of 10–18 gm protein per 8 oz or per bar (Table 22.4). The source of protein in these supplements may be soy, casein, whey, or albumin. When eaten with a mixed plant-based diet these supplements only aid the very few athletes who may have difficulties meeting their protein needs from other sources. They are a pleasant but neither necessary nor inexpensive source of food energy for snacks.

Vegetarian athletes who consume diets low or devoid in all animal protein (milk, cheese, chicken, eggs, fish, or meat) or those who restrict their energy intakes may be at risk for inadequate protein intakes if their diets are not carefully planned (5,60–62). However this is rarely a problem. Lacto or lacto-ovo vegetarians (those who consume only milk products or milk and eggs) or vegan vegetarians (those who consume no animal products) and who eat a variety of protein sources and get enough energy are not at risk for protein deficiency (63–65).

Fat and Cholesterol Recommendations for Health and Performance

Fat is an important energy source for athletes, and it is usually present in diets in ample amounts. Body fat stores and usual dietary intakes provide adequate energy from fatty acid and supplementation with essential fatty acids is unnecessary (66). With physical conditioning there is increased oxidation of fat and fatty acid mobi-

Table 22.4. Sports Drinks and Bars*

PART 1: During Event
Sports Drinks (per 1 cup–8 oz)

Sports Drink	Carbohydrate (%)	Sodium (mg)	Potassium (mg)	Kcal
10-K	6	55	30	60
All Sport	8	55	55	70
All Sport Lite	0	40	50	2
Body fuel 100	0.3	28	none	5
Body fuel 450	4	80	20	40
Carbo plus	16	5	100	170
Daily's 1st Ade	7	55	25	60
Exceed	7.2	66	56	68
Gatorade	6	110	25	50
Gatorade Light	3	80	25	25
Gookinaid ERG	5.7	70	100	45
Hydra Fuel	7	25	50	66
Max	7.5	15	none	70
Nautilus Plus	7	93	87	60
PowerAde	8	73	33	67
R.P.M.	7.6	0	70	70
Snapple Snap-Up	8	58	49	80

PART 2: During Event or After Event
Sports Bar

Sports Bar	Carbohydrates (gm)	Fat (gm)	Protein (gm)	Kcal
BTU Stoker	50	3	10	252
Clif Bar	50	3	5–6	250
Cross Turner	46	<2	11	245
CytoBar	42	2	12	235
EdgeBar	46	<2	10	240
Exceed	53	2	12	280
FinHalsa	28	2	11	170
PowerBar	42	2	10	225
PR Bar	19	6	14	190
Pro-Sports	40	<2	15	240
PurePower	42	3	12	240
Time Bar	40	<2	8	235
Ultra Fuel	100	3	15	490

Table 22.4. *Continued*

PART 3: After Event
High-Calorie, High-Carbohydrate Supplements

Product Name	Carbohydrate (gm)	Fat (gm)	Protein (gm)	Kcal
Great Gains mixed with milk	133	29	18	864
GatorLode	53	0	0	210
Gator Pro	44	5	13	270
Pro-Optibol: 2 scoops	45	2*	18	266

*Contains MCT oil (medium chain triglyceride).

lization with glycogen sparing (67). Table 22.5 provides a sample of a high-carbohydrate, low-fat, adequate protein meal plan that is adequate in all nutrients.

Currently American adults consume about 37% of total calories from fat (with 12% from saturated fat, 10% from monounsaturated fat, and 14% from polyunsaturated fat), 400 mg cholesterol, 15% to 20% calories from protein, and 43% to 48% of calories from carbohydrates.

Current recommendations for most adults, adolescents, and children over the age of 2 years are for an eating pattern moderate in cholesterol and saturated fat to maximize heart health. The National Cholesterol Education Program recommends that a moderate low-fat, low-saturated fat, low-cholesterol diet contain no more than 30% of total calories from fat with 10% or less of the calories from saturated fat, 10% from monounsaturated fat, and 10% from polyunsaturated fat. Less than 300 mg of cholesterol is desirable for healthy persons; even lower intakes of fat and saturated fat may be optimal (68). Elite male athletes probably consume slightly less fat than other Americans, although their intakes vary widely. Aerobic sport participants in-

gest 20% to 40% of calories from fat and athletes engaged in anaerobic sports ingest 18% to 47% calories from fat, according to various studies (1–8).

Moderate aerobic exercise and a physically active life along with a heart healthy dietary pattern and weight control further improve serum lipids (69). More data are needed to assess the independent contributions of exercise, diet, and weight loss on serum lipid and lipoprotein levels (37). However, very high-fat diets appear to have negative effects on performance as well as on general health. For example, an experimental diet, consisting of 70% calories from fat with only 20 gm carbohydrate, greatly reduced muscle glycogen stores in trained athletes. Athletes were able to exercise even at these deficient carbohydrate intakes because their muscles adapted to oxidizing more lipids (70). However, there is no reason to consider that this practice should be recommended. High-fat diets may have adverse effects even on highly trained athletes. In one study athletes who were fed diets high in saturated fat exhibited significant increases in serum cholesterol (71). Also for athletes trying to control their weight, a high-fat diet greatly limits

Table 22.5. Sample Meal Plan for Training

SAMPLE MENU #1 (2600 calories, 63% carbohydrate, 18% fat, 19% protein)	SAMPLE MENU #2 (3800 calories, 63% carbohydrate, 19% fat, 18% protein)
BREAKFAST	*BREAKFAST*
4 oz orange juice	8 oz orange juice
8 oz skim milk	8 oz skim milk
1 oz cereal	2 oz cereal
1 piece toast with 2 tsp jam	2 pieces toast with 4 tsp jam
1 banana	1 banana
coffee/cream/sugar	coffee/cream/sugar
SNACK 1	*SNACK 1*
1 blueberry muffin	1 blueberry muffin
8 oz skim milk	8 oz skim milk
LUNCH	*LUNCH*
1 chicken salad sandwich/ lettuce/tomato	2 chicken salad sandwiches/ lettuce/tomato
4 oz cranberry juice	8 oz cranberry juice
1 apple	1 apple
$\frac{1}{2}$ cup carrot sticks	$\frac{1}{2}$ cup carrot sticks
SNACK 2	*SNACK 2*
2 tbsp peanut butter	3 tbsp peanut butter
12 crackers, no fat added	15 crackers, no added fat
8 oz apple juice	16 oz apple juice
8 oz frozen yogurt	8 oz frozen yogurt
DINNER	*DINNER*
$\frac{2}{3}$ C lentil soup	$1\frac{1}{2}$ C lentil soup
6 oz broiled fish, no fat used in cooking	6 oz broiled fish, no fat used in cooking
8 oz skim milk	16 oz skim milk
$\frac{3}{4}$ C broccoli, steamed	$\frac{3}{4}$ C broccoli, steamed
$1\frac{1}{2}$ C rice, boiled	2 C rice, boiled
1 dinner roll	2 dinner rolls
1 pat butter or margarine	2 pats butter or margarine
4 small cookies	5 small cookies

SOURCE: Information on food values from Pennington JAT. Bowes and Church's food values of portions commonly used, 15th ed. Philadelphia: JB Lippincott, 1989.

the quantity of food they can consume while meeting their energy needs. Finally, high-fat diets are not necessarily adequate in vitamins and minerals. For all of these reasons high-fat diets are to be discouraged.

Athletes should therefore consume no more than 25% to 30% of their calories from fat (27,28). During a hypocaloric diet for weight loss it may be necessary to reduce fat to 20% of total calories to meet carbohydrate and protein needs. Diets less than 20% fat are difficult to adhere to and provide no additional performance benefit.

Vitamin and Mineral Recommendations

The RDA for vitamins and minerals are levels that meet the needs of almost all persons in the population (Table 22.6) (27,28,53). The body needs vitamins and minerals for metabolism, oxygen transport, muscle contraction, health, and maintenance of tissues. The B complex vitamins such as thiamin, riboflavin, niacin, and pantothenic acid function as coenzymes in glycolysis and for this reason they have been popular as supplements among athletes (72). Evidence indicates that the need for riboflavin increases with physical activity. Because these needs are only slightly elevated, consumption of high-carbohydrate diets easily meets them, making supplements unnecessary (73). Riboflavin is abundant in milk and meat products. Thiamin is found in whole grain or enriched bread, cereals, and grains. There is currently no evidence that supplementation with vitamins or minerals improves athletic performance (8,74–77). Therefore, supplements in excess of the RDA are not recommended, and a balanced diet should be stressed.

Iron deficiency can reduce exercise performance during exercise (78–82). Iron deficiency may ensue due to increased

Table 22.6A. Recommended Dietary Allowances[a]

Category	Age (years) or Condition	Weight[b] (kg)	(lb)	Height[b] (cm)	(in)	Protein (g)	Fat-Soluble Vitamins Vitamin A (µg RE)[c]	Vitamin D (µg)[d]	Vitamin E (mg α-TE)[e]	Vitamin K (µg)	Water-Soluble Vitamins Vitamin C (mg)	Thiamin (mg)	Riboflavin (mg)	Niacin (mg NE)[f]	Vitamin B6 (mg)	Folate (µg)	Vitamin B12 (µg)	Minerals Calcium (mg)	Phosphorus (mg)	Magnesium (mg)	Iron (mg)	Zinc (mg)	Iodine (µg)	Selenium (µg)
Infants	0.0–0.5	6	13	60	24	13	375	7.5	3	5	30	0.3	0.4	5	0.3	25	0.3	400	300	40	6	5	40	10
	0.5–1.0	9	20	71	28	14	375	10	4	10	35	0.4	0.5	6	0.6	35	0.5	600	500	60	10	5	50	15
Children	1–3	13	29	90	35	16	400	10	6	15	40	0.7	0.8	9	1.0	50	0.7	800	800	80	10	10	70	20
	4–6	20	44	112	44	24	500	10	7	20	45	0.9	1.1	12	1.1	75	1.0	800	800	120	10	10	90	20
	7–10	28	62	132	52	28	700	10	7	30	45	1.0	1.2	13	1.4	100	1.4	800	800	170	10	10	120	30
Males	11–14	45	99	157	62	45	1000	10	10	45	50	1.3	1.5	17	1.7	150	2.0	1200	1200	270	12	15	150	40
	15–18	66	145	176	69	59	1000	10	10	65	60	1.5	1.8	20	2.0	200	2.0	1200	1200	400	12	15	150	50
	19–21	72	160	177	70	58	1000	10	10	70	60	1.5	1.7	19	2.0	200	2.0	1200	1200	350	10	15	150	70
	25–50	79	174	176	70	63	1000	5	10	80	60	1.5	1.7	19	2.0	200	2.0	800	800	350	10	15	150	70
	51+	77	170	173	68	63	1000	5	10	80	60	1.2	1.4	15	2.0	200	2.0	800	800	350	10	15	150	70
Females	11–14	46	101	157	62	46	800	10	8	45	50	1.1	1.3	15	1.4	150	2.0	1200	1200	280	15	12	150	45
	15–18	55	120	163	64	44	800	10	8	55	60	1.1	1.3	15	1.5	180	2.0	1200	1200	300	15	12	150	50
	19–24	58	128	164	65	46	800	10	8	60	60	1.1	1.3	15	1.6	180	2.0	1200	1200	280	15	12	150	55
	25–50	63	138	163	64	50	800	5	8	65	60	1.1	1.3	15	1.6	180	2.0	800	800	280	15	12	150	55
	51+	65	143	160	63	50	800	5	8	65	60	1.0	1.2	13	1.6	180	2.0	800	800	280	10	12	150	55
Pregnant						60	800	10	10	65	70	1.5	1.6	17	2.2	400	2.2	1200	1200	320	30	15	175	65
Lactating	First 6 months					65	1300	10	12	65	95	1.6	1.8	20	2.1	280	2.6	1200	1200	355	15	19	200	75
	Second 6 months					62	1200	10	11	65	90	1.6	1.7	20	2.1	260	2.6	1200	1200	340	15	16	200	75

[a] The allowances, expressed as average daily intakes over time, are intended to provide for individual variations among the normal persons as they live in the United States under usual environmental stresses. Diets should be based on a variety of common foods in order to provide other nutrients for which human requirements have been less well defined.

[b] Weights and heights of Reference Adults are actual for the U.S. population of the designated age, as reported by NHANES II. The median weights and heights of those under 19 years of age were taken from Hamill et al (1979). The use of these figures does not imply that the height-to-weight ratios are ideal.

[c] Retinol equivalent: 1 retinol equivalent = 1 µg retinol or 6 µg β-carotene.

[d] Cholecalciferol equivalent: 10 µg cholecalciferol = 400 IU of Vitamin D.

[e] α-Tocopherol equivalent (TE): 1 mg of α-tocopherol = 1 α-TE.

[f] Niacin equivalent (NE): = 1 mg of niacin or 60 mg of dietary tryptophan.

SOURCE: Reprinted with permission from Recommended Dietary Allowances, 10th ed. Copyright © 1989 by the National Academy of Sciences. Courtesy of the National Academy Press, Washington, DC

Table 22.6B. Estimated Safe and Adequate Daily Dietary Intakes of Selected Vitamins and Minerals[a]

Category	Age (yr)	Vitamins	
		Biotin (µg)	Pantothenic Acid (mg)
Infants	0–0.5	10	2
	0.5–1	15	3
Children and	1–3	20	3
adolescents	4–6	25	3–4
	7–10	30	4–5
	11+	30–100	4–7
Adults		30–100	4–7

Category	Age (yr)	Trace Elements[b]				
		Copper (mg)	Manganese (mg)	Fluoride (mg)	Chromium (µg)	Molybdenum (µg)
Infants	0–0.5	0.4–0.6	0.3–0.6	0.1–0.5	10–40	15–30
	0.5–1	0.6–0.7	0.6–1.0	0.2–1.0	20–60	20–40
Children and	1–3	0.7–1.0	1.0–1.5	0.5–1.5	20–80	25–50
adolescents	4–6	1.0–1.5	1.5–2.0	1.0–2.5	30–120	30–75
	7–10	1.0–2.0	2.0–3.0	1.5–2.5	50–200	50–150
	11+	1.5–2.5	2.0–5.0	1.5–2.5	50–200	75–250
Adults		1.5–3.0	2.0–5.0	1.5–4.0	50–200	75–250

[a] Because there is less information on which to base allowances, these figures are not given in the main table of RDA and are provided here in the form of ranges of recommended intakes.
[b] Since the toxic levels for many trace elements may be only several times usual intakes, the upper levels for the trace elements given in this table should not be habitually exceeded.

hemolysis, decreased iron absorption, increased iron losses in sweat, feces and urine, or from low dietary intakes (83–86). Low hemoglobin concentrations may also be due to expanded plasma volume; this is often the cause of the condition referred to as "sports anemia" rather than a true iron deficiency (87,88). Other athletes may have low dietary intakes of iron, or high losses of iron due to occult gastrointestinal blood loss. Iron supplementation may be needed for those who do not respond to dietary treatment.

Vitamin E is important in the maintenance of muscle tissue. During endurance exercise to exhaustion it has been asserted that the need for vitamin E may increase because free radicals formed are neutralized by the antioxidant and this in turn acts to preserve muscle structures. However, definitive studies are lacking and deficiencies of vitamin E are rare, so RDA levels suffice given present evidence. Food sources rich in vitamin E include wheat germ, green leafy vegetables, egg yolks, and nuts (89).

For body building and strength sports the mineral chromium has been promoted as a muscle and strength builder. Chromium functions with insulin to aid in amino acid uptake in muscles. Deficiency is very rare. There is no conclusive evidence on the need for supplementation with this nutrient either (90). Rich food sources of chromium include whole wheat, molasses, and brewer's yeast. Fruits and vegetables contain small amounts, and the chromium in drinking water is variable (91).

HEAT STRESS, SWEATING, AND DEHYDRATION

During exercise, heat produced within the working skeletal muscle is carried to the body core and as a result the central temperature rises. In response, cutaneous blood flow increases to transport heat from the core to the skin and sweating begins. Depending on a number of factors, sweat rates can rise as high as 2–3 L/hr and create 1080 kcal of heat in the process (94,95). In athletics, the ability to defend body temperature against heat stress depends on the level of activity, acclimatization, aerobic fitness, and hydration level. Factors other than hydration level are outside the scope of this chapter.

When exercise is heavy and temperatures in the outside environment are high, heat loss declines by radiation and convection, and only sweating is left to rid the body of heat. If humidity is high, the process is further impaired and less heat is lost. The danger of excess sweating in exercise is that dehydration and the sequelae such as reduced blood volume and cardiac filling may ensue. Eventually, if compensation in the circulation and heart are insufficient, skin and muscle blood flow will be impaired, and both heat loss and physical performance will be affected.

With heat stress, gastric emptying and intestinal motility decrease as core temperature rises; they also decrease in hypohydration. Among marathon runners, heat stress and exercise are often associated with cramps, disorientation, dizziness, gastrointestinal reflux, flatulence, bloody stools, nausea and the like, as well as vomiting and diarrhea and loss of coordination (58,96). Usually, these subside when the physical activity decreases.

Fluids

Hydration is critical in sports, but fluid intake is often forgotten during exercise and competition. If athletes wait until after exercise to replenish their fluid losses, they run the risk of suffering from dehydration (see above). What is ingested during recovery, especially in the first 2 hours, can also markedly influence the rate of recovery and performance in a subsequent athletic event.

Guidelines for Optimal Fluid Replacement Beverages for Athletic Events

Fluid, electrolyte, and energy supplementation is desirable during exercise to support normal circulatory, metabolic, and thermoregulatory functions and to maintain plasma volume. Although excessive sweating depletes water reserves the most, electrolytes are also lost. In addition, prolonged exercise can result in hypoglycemia and glycogen depletion, both of which contribute to the onset of fatigue.

Sufficient fluids and electrolytes cannot be stored in the body prior to vigorous exercise in sufficient amounts to meet needs so attention to their repletion during and after exercise is warranted. Glycogen supercompensation is possible, but carbohydrate supplementation during long, continued exercise improves performance (41,50).

Fluid needs increase with the duration of the event. Middle distance events are defined as those exercise bouts lasting less than 1 hour; long distance events are those lasting 1 to 3 hours, and ultra-long distance events are those lasting greater than 3 hours. The recommendations listed in Table 22.7 should satisfy fluid requirements for most competitive athletes.

Weight Loss

When weight loss is recommended, the first task is to determine if the athlete actually needs to lose fat weight for health or performance reasons. If there is such a need, the next step is to devise a sensible weight control plan because rapid weight loss can adversely affect performance. Weight losses greater than 1 kg/wk (about 2 lb) in the nonobese person suggest exces-

Table 22.7. Fluid Replacement Guidelines

	Event Time (hr)			
	<1	1–3	>3	Recovery
Examples	Most team sports, many cycling and virtually all track events	Soccer, elite marathoners, some cycling events	Triatholons and all other forms of ultra marathons	N/A
Intensity ($\dot{V}o_2$max)	75–130%	60–90%	30–70%	N/A
Concerns	Limited time to drink, lack of desire to drink, decreased gastric emptying due to high intensity	Potential for hyperglycemia, hypovolemia, hyperthermia, dehydration, glycogen depletion	Same as previous plus hyponatremia	Glycogen resynthesis, fluid and electrolyte replacement
Recommendations	Ingest 300–500 mL of 6–10% CHO beverage 0–15 min before event	300–500 mL water before event, 800–1600 mL/hr of a cool (5–15°C), 6–8% CHO drink during event with 10–20 mg of both Na and Cl	300–500 mL water before event, 500–1000 mL/hr of cool (5–15°C) 6–8% CHO drink with 20–30 mg Na and Cl	Drink beverage with 30–50 mg of Na and Cl and ingest CHO at a rate of 50 g/hr

CHO, carbohydrate; $\dot{V}o_2$max, maximum oxygen consumption.
SOURCE: This is a summary of an excellent review by Gissotfi C, Duchman S. Guidelines for optimal replacement beverages for different athletic events. Med Sci Sports Exerc 1992;24:679–687.

sive fluid losses and dehydration or very
rapid losses of fat-free mass. Therefore they
should be avoided.

Dehydration as a Weight Loss Method

Wrestlers often fast or ingest very little
food and restrict their fluid intake for
several days prior to a competition. For example, many wrestlers lose 5% to 10% of
their body weight to qualify for a lower
weight class (97). Dehydration causes reduced endurance due to decreased glycogen stores, increased body temperature,
and decreased plasma volume, among
other factors. These behaviors, especially
when combined with exercising in rubber
sweat suits, sitting in saunas, and using
laxatives, diuretics or self-induced vomiting to reduce weight, greatly increase risks
of dehydration (97–100). Such practices also
result in an inadequae intake of calories,
protein, carbohydrate, vitamins, and minerals. Finally they can cause dehydration and
decreased fat-free mass rather than fat loss.
It is possible for wrestlers who indulge in
these weight loss techniques to replace
much of the fluid loss if there is a 5-hour
time period between weigh-in and competition. However, glycogen and fat-free mass
take longer to replace. Repeated bouts of
rapid weight loss with weight regain can
result in chronic glycogen depletion, continued fat-free mass loss, lowered resting
metabolic rate (although this may be temporary), and increased body fat if the athlete does not eat enough carbohydrate- and
protein-rich foods between competitions.
Aerobic performance is impaired in some
studies of wrestlers, whereas anaerobic
performance is not if at least 5 hours of
rehydration are allowed (97,101). However,
weight cycling may be as frequent as 15
times in a season or 100 times in a wrestler's
career. Thus, the long-term health effects
are not known (101).

Other Inappropriate Weight Control Practices (Anorexia Nervosa and Bulimia)

Wrestlers are not alone in having weight
reduction habits that sometimes compromise performance. Female dancers, runners, gymnasts, swimmers, and cyclists are
all at high risk for anorexia nervosa (102–
111). *Anorexia nervosa* is defined as persistent, intentional weight loss of 15% to 25%
below normal body weight, and in females,
amenorrhea of at least 3 months' duration
(112). Anorectics have a distorted body image and an intense fear of becoming obese
although they are underweight. They may
also develop a rigid exercise program to
burn calories to lose weight. The prevalence
of anorexia in athletes may range from 4%
to 14%; in the general population the range
is 3% to 5% (113,114).

Female gymnasts, synchronized swimmers, runners, rowers, swimmers, and
divers as well as male wrestlers are all
likely to be at risk of bulimia (115). *Bulimia*
is characterized by cycles of eating large
amounts of food in a relatively short
amount of time (called binge eating), followed by purging to avoid weight gain to
rid the body of most of the calories eaten.
The binge phases can involve intakes over
4000 calories in one episode. The purging
phase can consist of self-induced vomiting,
laxative or diuretic abuse, excessive exercise to burn calories, or restrictive eating.
Bulimia is reportedly found in 5% to 20% of
college age women (116) and in athletes it
ranges from 14% of males to 39% of females
(113). Both bulimia and anorexia are eating
disorders that require psychotherapy. It is
important for the coach, trainer, nutritionist, and physician working with athletes to
be familiar with these diseases to assist the
athletes to obtain the proper treatment.
Anorectics are easier to identify because of
their drastically reduced weight, whereas

bulimics are generally around average weight. Consequences of bulimia include electrolyte imbalances that can cause cardiac arrhythmia and cardiac arrest and anorexia nervosa can result in starvation and death. Many of these athletes need continued encouragement to receive help for their eating disorder.

Sensible Weight Control: Exercise and Dietary Recommendations

It is possible to combine a moderate to strenuous aerobic exercise program with a balanced hypocaloric diet with deficits of about 500 calories daily while achieving body fat loss (117). A balanced deficit diet is one with a composition of 30% or less of calories from fat, 15% to 20% of calories from protein, and 55% or more for the calories from carbohydrate. With a weight training program and a low-fat, isocaloric diet it is possible to build fat-free mass and reduce body fat while keeping weight constant (118).

Athletes who need to lower their body fatness should decrease their intakes by approximately 500 calories a day, especially from high-fat foods and alcohol. This will achieve a weight loss of approximately 0.5 kg/wk, assuming energy outputs stay constant (119). Reductions in dietary fat may aid in weight loss by allowing the athlete to consume larger quantities of lower calorie foods possibly increasing satiety, but a reduction of total calorie intake is still necessary to lose body fat (117). Weight losses higher than 0.5–1 kg/wk are not recommended; they require reductions in intakes of greater than 500–1000 calories and are difficult to achieve, especially if energy outputs stay high. Drastic reductions in energy intakes also decrease resting energy expenditure and can induce metabolic changes, including diuresis and loss of fat-free body mass, which are undesirable and

which may decrease strength and endurance. Very low calorie diets (e.g., 800 calories or less) are also low in carbohydrate and can cause excessive losses of nitrogen and fat-free mass and failure to replenish glycogen stores and thus are not recommended.

WEIGHT GAIN

The athlete who wishes to gain weight and increase muscle strength and endurance should add approximately 500 calories daily to his or her current dietary intake using a food guide (Table 22.8) while continuing training. It is extremely difficult to increase muscle mass more than a pound per month (120). Further increases in calories may be necessary to reach goal weights—these are best done gradually while maintaining the training regimen to ensure gains in muscle and not fat.

Many athletes have difficulty eating enough food to keep their weights constant because their energy needs are so high. Adolescent and young adult males who train an hour or more per day often need as many as 5000 to 6000 calories each day. Snacks and minimeals help to meet their high energy (and fluid) needs. Table 22.4 lists some common sport drinks and sport bars. Nutritional supplements such as sport

Table 22.8.   Weight Gain Boosters

2 slices whole wheat bread with 2 tbsp peanut butter, 2 tbsp jam and 8 oz orange juice
8 oz fruit low-fat yogurt and 12 crackers with 2 slices cheese
4 fig cookies with 1 cup 1% milk
2 cups whole grain cereal, 1 cup 1% milk, 1 banana, 2 tbsp raisins

These snacks contain approximately 500 calories.

drinks can supply needed fluids, carbohydrates, and energy along with some
protein, vitamins, and minerals. These
products range from 50 to 800 calories per
8 oz. Low-fat milk, homemade milk shakes,
and juice provide similar nutrient contributions at a much lower cost. Special sport or
candy bars are increasing in popularity.
They are high in carbohydrate content and
energy and come packaged conveniently.
The bars range from 200 to 500 calories
each. Triathletes and distance cyclers often
stick or wrap the sport bars around their
bike frames so they can eat them during
rides lasting several hours.

DIETARY ERGOGENIC AIDS

Many substances have been proposed to
enhance energy, strength, or endurance.
Carnitine, for example, transports long
chain fatty acids into the mitochondria for
oxidation. Skeletal muscle contains 90% of
the body's total carnitine stores. Carnitine
supplementation does not seem to enhance
endurance exercise (120).

A vitamin-like compound, coenzyme Q_{10},
is involved in energy metabolism and is
also produced endogenously. In one study
it was shown to enhance exercise tolerance
in cardiac patients and sedentary young
men, but the study had many flaws. It is not
viewed as effective. Coenzyme Q_{10} has been
a recent addition to the long list of vitamin
supplements athletes take. No level of safe
intake has been established. More research
is needed on this vitamin-like substance to
establish safety and effectiveness (120).

Caffeine consumed before exercising has
been shown to have an ergogenic effect in
enhancing performance in endurance exercisers, but effects are lacking in others
(121,122). Caffeine spares glycogen and
increases utilization of free fatty acids

(61,121,123). Some athletes may experience
gastrointestinal problems or nervousness if
they ingest very large doses. The International Olympic Committee established an
acceptable level of caffeine at 12 µg/mL. An
intake of 800 mg of caffeine or 5 to 6 cups of
coffee consumed in a short amount of time
could exceed this level (79,123).

SUMMARY

Exercise can augment good nutrition for
health and good nutrition can enhance
performance. Exercise itself can improve
the nutritional status of an individual. Exercise improves body composition, glucose
metabolism, and serum lipids, and may
decrease an individual's risks of some
cancers.

Athletes generally consume slightly more
carbohydrates, less fat, and about the same
percentage of protein as nonathletes. Their
diets can still be suboptimal for meeting
the recommendations for best health and
risk reduction as well as for performance.
Athletes wishing to improve their performance should rely on a balanced diet, high in
carbohydrates, low in fat, with plenty of
water and energy to maintain healthy
weights to enhance their training and
talent. Overdosing with vitamin and mineral supplements, especially fat-soluble
vitamins, can be toxic and results in no
significant gains in physical ability.

Acknowledgment

Partial support was provided from the
U.S. Department of Agriculture, Agricul-
tural Research Service, under contract
number 53 K06-01. The contents of this
publication do not necessarily reflect the
views or policies of the U.S. Department of
Agriculture, nor do members of trade

names, commercial products, or organizations imply endorsement by the U.S. government.

References

1. Burke L, Read R. Diet patterns of elite Australian male triathletes. Physician Sports Med 1987;15:140–155.

2. Duester P, Moser P, Vigerdky R, Singh A. Nutritional survey of highly trained women runners. Am J Clin Nutr 1986;44:954–962.

3. Hickson J, Johnson T, Lee W, Sidor D. Nutrition and the precontest preparations of male bodybuilder. J Am Diet Assoc 1990;90:264–267.

4. Kleiner S, Bazzarre T, Litchford M. Metabolic profiles, diet and health practices of championship male and female bodybuilders. J Am Diet Assoc 1990;90:962–967.

5. Neiman D, Bulter J, Pollett L, Dietrich S, Lutz R. Nutrient intake of marathon runners. J Am Diet Assoc 1989;89:1273–1278.

6. Schulz L, Alger S, Harper I, Wilmore J, Ravussin E. Energy expenditure of elite female runners measured by respiratory chamber and doubly labeled water. J Appl Physiol 1992;72:23–28.

7. Van Erp-Baart A, Saris W, Binkhorst R, Elevers J. Nationwide survey on nutritional habits in elite athletes, part I. Energy, carbohydrate, protein, and fat intake. Int J Sports Med 1989;10(suppl 1):S3–S10.

8. Weight L, Noakes T, Labadarios D, et al. Vitamin and mineral status of trained athletes including the effects of supplementation. Am J Clin Nutr 1988;47:186–191.

9. US Senate Select Committee on Nutrition and Human Needs. Dietary goals for the United States, 2nd ed. Washington, DC: Government Printing Office, 1977.

10. Consensus Panel addresses obesity question. JAMA 1985;254:1878.

11. Metropolitan height and weight tables. Stat Bull Metrop Insur Co. Jan–June 1983;64:3.

12. Committee on Diet and Health. Diet and health implications for reducing chronic disease risks. Washington, DC: National Academy Press, 1989.

13. Committee on Military Nutrition. Research review of the results of nutritional intervention, Ranger Training class, 11/92 (Ranger II). Washington, DC: National Academy Press, 1992.

14. Davies K, Pearson P, Huseman C, Greger N, Kimmel D. Reduced bone mineral in patients with eating disorders. Bone 1990;11:143–147.

15. Nelson M, Fisher E, Catsos P, Meredith C, Turksoy R, Evans W. Diet and bone status in amenorrheic runners. Am J Clin Nutr 1986;43:910.

16. Snow R, Barbieri R, Frisch R. Estrogen 2-hydroxylase oxidation and menstrual function among elite oarswomen. J Clin Endocrinol Metab 1989;69:369–376.

17. Vogel J, Freidl K. Army data: body composition and physical capacity. In: Marrott BM, Grunstrup SJ, eds. Body composition and physical performance. Washington, DC: National Academy Press, 1992:89–103.

18. Harman E, Frykman P. The relationship of body size and composition to the performance of physically demanding military tasks. In: Marrott BM, Grunstrup SJ, eds. Body composition and physical performance. Washington, DC: National Academy Press, 1992:105–118.

19. Cureton KJ, Sparling PB, Evans BW, Johnson SM, Kong WD, Purvis JW. Effect of experimental alterations in excess weight on aerobic capacity and distance running performance. Med Sci Sports Exerc 1978;10:194–199.

20. Williams M. Nutritional aspects of human physiology and athletic performance. Springfield, IL: CC Thomas, 1985.

21. American Dietetic Association (ADA) and SCAN, Marcus J, eds. Sports nutrition: a guide for the professional working with active people. Chicago: American Dietetic Association, 1986.

22. Jones BH, Bovee MW, Knapik JJ. Associations among body composition, physical fitness and injury in men and women Army trainees. In: Marrott BM, Grunstrup SJ, eds. Body composition and physical performance. Washington, DC: National Academy Press, 1992:141–173.

23. Grinker JA. Body composition measurements. In: Marrott BM, Grunstrup SJ, eds. Body composition and physical performance. Wash-

ington, DC: National Academy Press, 1992:223–235.

24. Lukaski HC. Methods for the assessment of human body composition: traditional and new. Am J Clin Nutr 1987;46:5347–5356.

25. Forbes GB. Body composition: influence of nutrition, disease, growth and aging. In: Shils ME, Olson JA, Shike M, eds. Modern nutrition in health and disease, 8th ed. Philadelphia: Lea & Febiger, 1993:781–805.

26. Brotherhood J. Nutrition and sports performance. Sports Med 1984;1:350–389.

27. American Dietetic Association (ADA). Position of the American Dietetic Association: nutrition for physical fitness and athletic performance for adults. J Am Diet Assoc 1987;87:933–939.

28. Hoffman C, Coleman E. An eating plan and update on recommended dietary practices for the endurance athlete. J Am Diet Assoc 1991;91:325–330.

29. Neiman D. An introduction. In: Fitness and sports medicine. Palo Alto, CA: Bull Publishers, 1990:221–270.

30. Foster C, Costill D, Fink J. Effects of pre-exercise feeding on endurance performance. Med Sci Sports Exerc 1979;11:1–5.

31. Lohman D, Liebold F, Hilman W, Senger H, Pohl A. Diminished insulin response in highly trained athletes. Metabolism 1978;27:521–526.

32. Mann J. Complex carbohydrates: replacement energy for fat or useful in their own right? Am J Clin Nutr 1981;45:1202–1206.

33. Costill D. Carbohydrates for exercise: dietary demands for optimal performance. Int J Sports Med 1988;9:1–18.

34. Astrand P, Rodahl K. Textbook of work physiology. New York: McGraw-Hill, 1977:556.

35. Fox E. Sports physiology. New York: Saunders College, 1984.

36. Gollnick P. Metabolism of substrates: energy substrate metabolism during exercise and as modified by training. Fed Proc 1985;44:353–357.

37. Miller G, Massaro E. Carbohydrate in ultra-endurance performance. In: Hickson J, Wolinsky I, eds. Nutrition in exercise and sport. Boca Raton, FL: CRC Press, 1990:51.

38. Costill D, Sherman W, Fink W, Moresh C, Witten M. The role of dietary carbohydrates in muscle glycogen resynthesis after strenuous running. Am J Clin Nutr 1981;34:1831–1836.

39. Costill D, Miller J. Nutrition for endurance sports: carbohydrate and fluid balance. Int J Sports Med 1980;1:2–14.

40. Coggan A, Coyle E. Reversal of fatigue during prolonged exercise by carbohydrate infusion or ingestion. J Appl Physiol 1987;63:2388–2395.

41. Coyle E, Ar C, Hemmert M, Ivy J. Muscle glycogen utilization during prolonged strenuous exercise when fed carbohydrate. J Appl Physiol 1986;61:165–172.

42. Coyle E, Hagberg J, Hurley B, Martin W, Ehsani A. Carbohydrate feedings during prolonged strenuous exercise can delay fatigue. J Appl Physiol 1983;55:230–235.

43. Fallowfield J, Williams C. Carbohydrate intake and recovery from prolonged exercise. Int J Sport Med 1993;3:150–164.

44. Sherman W, Costill D, Fink W, Miller J. The effect of exercise and diet manipulation of muscle glycogen and its subsequent utilization during performance. Int J Sports Med 1981;2:114.

45. Sherman W, Wright D. Prevention nutrition for prolonged exercise. The theory and practice of athletic nutrition: bridging the gap. Report of the Ross Symposium. Columbus, OH: Ross Laboratories, 1989.

46. Brouns F, Saris W, Stroecken J, Beckers E, Thijssen R. Eating, drinking, and cycling: a controlled Tour de France simulation study, part I. Int J Sports Med 1989;10(suppl 1):S32–S40.

47. Brouns F, Saris W, Stroecken J, Beckers E, Thijssen R. Eating, drinking, and cycling: a controlled Tour de France simulation study, part II. Effect of diet manipulation. Int J Sports Med 1989;10(suppl 1):S41–S48.

48. Sherman W. Carbohydrates, muscle glycogen and muscle glycogen supercompensation. In: Williams MH, ed. Ergogenic aids in sports. Champaign, IL: Human Kinetic Publishers 3, 1983.

49. Zawadzki K, Yaspelkis B, Ivy J. Carbohydrate-protein complex increase the rate of muscle glycogen storage after exercise. J Appl Physiol 1992;72:1854–1859.

50. Hargreaves M, Costill D, Katz A, Fink W. Effect of fructose ingestion on muscle glycogen usage during exercise. Med Sci Sports Exerc 1985;17:360–363.

51. Costill D, Coyle E, Dalsky G, Evans W, Fink W. Effects of elevated plasma FFA and insulin on muscle glycogen usage during exercise. J Appl Physiol 1977;43:695–699.

52. DeFronzo R, Sato Y, Felig P, Wahren J. Synergistic interaction between exercise and insulin on peripheral glucose uptake. J Clin Invest 1981;68:1468–1474.

53. Food and Nutrition Board. Recommended dietary allowances, 10th rev. ed. Washington, DC: National Academy of Sciences, 1989.

54. Tarnopolsky M, MacDougall J, Atkinson S. Influence of protein intake and training status on nitrogen balance and lean body mass. J Appl Physiol 1988;64:187–193.

55. Gontzea I, Stuzescw P, Domitrache S. The influence of adaptation to physical effort on nitrogen balance in man. Nutr Rep Int 1971;11:233.

56. Short S, Short W. Four-year study of university athletes' dietary intake. J Am Diet Assoc 1983;82:632.

57. Zackin M, Meredith C, Frontera W, Evans W. The effect of chronic exercise on protein requirements in middle-aged men. Abstract for the Sixth International Symposium on the Biochemistry of Exercise, 1985.

58. Ahlman V, Karoven M. Weight reduction by sweating in wrestlers and its effect on physical fitness. J Sports Med Phys Fitness 1962;1:58.

59. Lemon P, Proctor D. Protein intake and athletic performance. Sports Med 1991;12:313–325.

60. Brooks S, Sanborn C, Albrecht B, Wagner W. Diet in athletic amenorrhea. Lancet 1984;1:559–560.

61. Slavin J, Lutter J, Cushman S. Amenorrhea in vegetarian athletes. Lancet 1984;1:1475.

62. Zierath J, Kaiserauer S, Snyder A. Dietary patterns of amenorrheic and regularly menstruating runners. Med Sci Sports Exerc 1986;18:S55.

63. Hardinge M, Crooks H, Stare F. Nutritional studies of vegetarians: proteins and essential amino acids. J Am Diet Assoc 1966;48:25–27.

64. Register U, Inano M, Thurston C. Nitrogen balance studies in human subjects on various diets. Am J Clin Nutr 1967;20:753–759.

65. Sanchez A, Scharffenberg J, Register U. Nutritive value of selected proteins and protein combinations. Am J Clin Nutr 1963;13:243–249.

66. Bjorntorp P. Importance of fat as a support nutrient for energy: metabolism of athletes. J Sports Sci 1991;9:71–76.

67. Hurley B, Nemeth P, Martin W, Hagberg J, Dalsky GM. Muscle triglyceride utilization during exercise: effects on training. J Appl Physiol 1986;60:582–587.

68. National Cholesterol Education Program. Report of the expert panel on detection, evaluation and treatment of high blood cholesterol in adults. US Department Health and Human Services, NIH Publication no. 89-2925, January 1989.

69. Wood PD, Stefanick ML, Williams PT, Haskell WL. The effect on plasma lipoproteins of a prudent weight-reducing diet with or without exercise in overweight men and women. N Engl J Med 1991;325:461–466.

70. Phinney SD, Bisttian B, Evans WJ, Gervino E, Blackburn GL. The human metabolic response to chronic ketosis without caloric restriction: preservation of submaximal exercise capability with reduced carbohydrate oxidation. Metabolism 1983;32:769–776.

71. Thompson PD, Cullinane EM, Eshleman R, Kantor MA, Herbert PN. The effects of high-carbohydrate and high-fat diets on the serum lipid and lipoprotein concentrations of endurance athletes. Metabolism 1984;33:1003–1010.

72. Economos C, Bortz M, Nelson M. Nutritional practices of elite athletes. Sports Med 1993;16:381–389.

73. Belko A, Meredith M, Kalkwarf H, et al. Effects of exercise on riboflavin requirements: biological validation in weight reducing women. Am J Clin Nutr 1985;41:270–277.

74. Barnett D, Conlee R. The effects of commercial dietary supplementation of human performance. Am J Clin Nutr 1985;40:586–590.

75. Matter M, Stittfall T, Graves J. The effect of iron and folate therapy on maximal exercise per-

formance in iron- and folate-deficient female marathon runners. Clin Sci 1987;72:415–422.

76. Van Der Beek E. Vitamin supplementation and physical exercise performance. J Sports Sci 1991;9:77–89.

77. Williams M. Nutritional ergogenic aids and athletic performance. Nutr Today 1989;Jan/Feb:7–14.

78. Anderson H, Barkve H. Iron deficiency and muscular work performance: an evaluation of cardio-respiratory function of iron deficient subjects with and without anemia. Scand J Lab Invest 1970;25(suppl 144):1–39.

79. Beutler E, Larsh S, Tanzi F. Iron enzymes in iron deficiency: VII. Oxygen consumption measurements in iron-deficient subjects. Am J Med Sci 1960;239:759–765.

80. Edgerton V, Ohira Y, Hettiarachchi J, Senewiratne B, Gardner G. Elevation of hemoglobin and work tolerance in iron-deficient subjects. J Nutr Sci Vitaminol 1981;27:77–86.

81. Finch C, Gollnick P, Hlastala M, Miller L, Dillmann E. Lactic acidosis as a result of iron deficiency. J Clin Invest 1979;64:129–137.

82. McDonald R, Keen C. Iron, zinc and magnesium nutrition and athletic performance. Sports Med 1988;5:171–184.

83. Pauley P, Jordal R, Strandberg Pederson R. Dermal excretion of iron in intensely training athletes. Clin Chem Acta 1983;127:19.

84. Stewart J, Ahlquist D, McGill D, Ilstrup D, Schwartz S. Gastrointestinal blood losses and anemia in runners. Ann Intern Med 1984;100:843.

85. Pate R, Miller B, Davis J, Slentz C, Klingshirn L. Iron status of female runners. Int J Sport Nutr 1993;3:222–231.

86. Siegel A, Hennekens C, Solomon H, Van Boeckel B. Exercise-related hematuria: findings in a group of marathon runners. JAMA 1979;241:391.

87. Buskirk E. Some nutritional considerations in the conditioning of athletes. Annu Rev Nutr 1981;1:319.

88. Clement D, Sawchuk L. Iron status and sports performance. Sports Med 1984;1:65.

89. Krause MV, Mahan LK. Vitamins. In: Food, nutrition and diet therapy, 6th ed. Philadelphia: WB Saunders, 1979:157–159.

90. Clarkson P. Nutritional ergogenic aids: chromium, exercise, and muscle mass. Int J Sport Nutr 1991;1:289–293.

91. Krause MV, Mahan LK. Minerals. In: revised by Food, nutrition and diet therapy, 6th ed. Philadelphia: WB Saunders, 1979:141.

92. Shephard RJ. Body composition and performance in relation to environment. In: Marrott BM, Grunstrup SJ, eds. Body composition and physical performance. Washington, DC: National Academy Press, 1992:195–206.

93. Pacy PJ, Webster N, Garrow JS. Exercise and obesity. Sports Med 1986;3:89–113.

94. Gisotfi C, Duchman S. Guidelines for optimal replacement beverages for different athletic events. Med Sci Sports Exerc 1992;24:679–687.

95. Klinzing J, Karpowicz W. The effects of rapid weight loss and rehydration on a wrestling performance test. J Sports Med 1986;26:149–156.

96. Tipon C. Commentary. Physician Sports Med 1987;15:160–165.

97. Steen S, McKinney S. Nutrition assessment of college wrestlers. Physician Sports Med 1986;14:100–116.

98. Houston M, Green H, Thomas J. The effects of rapid weight loss on physiological functions in wrestlers. Physician Sports Med 1981;9:73.

99. Horswill C. Weight loss and weight cycling in amateur wrestlers: implications for performance and resting metabolic rate. Int J Sports Med 1993;3:245–261.

100. Cohen J, Kim C, May P, Ertel N. Exercise, body weight, and amenorrhea in professional ballet dancers. Physician Sports Med 1982;10:92–101.

101. Dale E, Gerlach D, Wilhite A. Menstrual dysfunction in distance runners. Obstet Gynecol 1979;54:47–53.

102. Frisch R, Wyshak G, Vincent L. Delayed menarche and amenorrhea in ballet dancers. N Engl J Med 1980;303:17–19.

103. Lutter J, Cusman S. Menstrual patterns in female runners. Physician Sports Med 1982;10:60–72.

104. Schwartz B, Cumming D, Riordan E, Selye M, Yen S. Exercise-associated amenorrhea:

a distinct entity? Am J Obstet Gynecol 1981;141:662–670.

105. Shangold M, Levine H. The effect of marathon training upon menstrual function. Am J Obstet Gynecol 1982;143:862–869.

106. Speroff L, Redwine D. Exercise and menstrual function. Physician Sports Med 1980;8:41–52.

107. Wilmore J, Brown C, Davis J. Body physique and composition of the female distance runner. Ann NY Acad Sci 1977;301:764–776.

108. Dummer G, et al. Pathogenic weight-control behaviors of young competitive swimmers. Physician Sports Med 1987;15:75–84.

109. Sundgot-Borgen J. Prevalence of eating disorders in elite female athletes. Int J Sport Nutr 1993;3:29–40.

110. Schocken D, Holloway J, Powers P. Weight loss and the heart: effects of anorexia nervosa and starvation. Arch Intern Med 1989;149:877–881.

111. Burkes-Miller M, Black D. Male and female college athletes: prevalence of anorexia nervosa and bulimia nervosa. Athletic Training 1988;23:137–140.

112. Weight L, Noakes T. Is running an analog of anorexia? A survey of the incidence of eating disorders in female distance runners. Med Sci Sports Exerc 1987;19:213–217.

113. Guthrie S. Prevalence of eating disorders among intercollegiate athletes: contributing factors and preventative measures. In: Black D, ed. Eating disorders among athletes. Reston, VA: American Alliance for Health Physical Education and Dance, 1991.

114. Kirkley B. Bulimia: clinical characteristics, development and etiology. J Am Diet Assoc 1986;86:468–475.

115. Pavlou K, Steffee W, Lerman R, Burrows B. Effects of dieting and exercise on lean body mass, oxygen uptake, and strength. Med Sci in Sports and Exercise 1985;17:466–471.

116. Manore M, Thompson J, Russo M. Diet and exercise strategies of a world-class bodybuilder. Int J Sport Nutr 1993;3:76–86.

117. Weltman A, Stamford B. Safe and effective weight loss. Physician Sports Med 1982;10:141–145.

118. Bucci L. Nutritional ergogenic aids. In: Hickson J, Wolinsky I, eds. Nutrition in exercise and sport. Boca Raton, FL: CRC Press, 1990:107–136.

119. Ivy J, Costill D, Fink W, Lower R. Influence of caffeine and carbohydrate feedings of endurance performance. Med Sci Sports Exerc 1979;11:6.

120. Clarkson P. Nutritional ergogenic aids: caffeine. Int J Sport Nutr 1993;3:103–111.

121. Essig D, Costill D, VanHandel P. Effects of caffeine ingestion on utilization of muscle glycogen and lipids during leg ergometer cycling. Int J Sports Med 1980;1:86.

122. Voy R. Ergogenic aids. In: A.a.S. Grandjean J, eds. The theory and practice of athletic nutrition: bridging the gap. Report of the Ross Symposium. Columbia, OH: Ross Laboratories, 1989.

123. Slavin J, Joehsen D. Caffeine and sports performance. Physician Sports Med. 1985;13:191.

WOMEN ATHLETES: UNIQUE ISSUES

DONNA I. MELTZER

23

Physiology
Injury Patterns
The Breasts
Genitourinary System
Gynecologic Concerns
The Female Athlete Triad
Osteoporosis
Contraception
Pregnancy

In the last decade or so, more females of all ages have dramatically increased their participation in athletic activities. This growth in athletic performance is evident at both recreational and competitive levels. Today women exercise regularly and participate in many of the same sports as men (1). This increased interest in fitness and sports has provoked concerns about gender differences (2), injury patterns (3–6), gynecologic matters (7–9), and reproductive function (10,11). As a result, physicians need to enhance their understanding of sports and exercise-related issues unique to women.

PHYSIOLOGY

Several important skeletal and physiologic differences exist between males and females, which are important for the physician to recognize to optimize performance and maintain the health and safety of the athletic performer. Appreciation and awareness of musculoskeletal gender differences may also enable the physician to better counsel females in the area of exercise prescription (Table 23.1).

Girls have a shorter period of growth than boys; thus the average female is shorter and weighs less. A shorter stature results in a lower center of gravity, which has different ramifications depending on the athletic activity. Females also tend to have shorter limbs (3), especially the upper extremities, which supply less leverage and consequently less power. In general, the adult female has narrower shoulders and is wider in the hips than her male counterpart, who tends to have the reversed shoulder-hip pattern (3,12). The wider pelvic area in females probably enhances stability but may account for some females experiencing patellofemoral syndrome and knee prob-

lems. In addition, the narrower shoulder may create a mechanical disadvantage for muscles acting on the shoulder joint.

Not only do females have a greater percentage of body fat (2,12) (average 24%) compared to males (average 13%), but the distribution of body fat is different. Body fat is concentrated more in the hips and thighs in females and less in the abdomen and upper body parts, as in males. Hormonal differences account for a greater muscle mass in males, but no significant difference in the percentage of slow and fast twitching muscle fibers has been recognized. Heredity or athletic activity, and not gender, seem to determine which muscle fibers are slow or fast twitch (2,13). The larger muscle mass in males (40% to 50% versus 35% to 40% in females) is a reflection of the increased size of various muscle fibers. Females are about one half (54%) as strong as males in the upper body and about two thirds (68%) as strong in the lower body (14,15). However, when strength is expressed relative to lean body weight, this difference is less detectable (16). Although studies indicate that males have greater strength and a greater absolute endurance, females tend to have more relative endurance.

When females undergo a strength training program, they experience a decrease in fat-free body mass and body fat, but less muscle hypertrophy (2,3,13) compared to males. There is also variation in the amount of muscle hypertrophy that women undergo with training and this seems to be genetically determined.

Heart size (12), stroke volume, and maximum cardiac output (3) are smaller in females than in males, even when differences in body size are considered. Females tend to have a lower vital capacity and residual volume secondary to their smaller thoracic cavity. Women also have a lower maximum oxygen concentration ($\dot{V}o_2max$) (3) and de-

Table 23.1. Differences Between Males and Females

Females
- are shorter and weigh less, which gives them a lower center of gravity
- have shorter limbs especially the upper extremities
- have narrower shoulders and wider hips
- have a greater percentage of body fat (average 24% compared to males 13%) and the body fat is concentrated in the thighs and hips, not abdomen and upper body like males
- have less muscle mass (40% versus 50% in males)
- are 54% as strong in the upper body and 68% as strong in the lower body
- have smaller heart size, stroke volume, and maximum cardiac output
- have lower vital capacity and $\dot{V}O_2$max
- have higher heart rates, shortened conduction times, prolonged repolarization time, and lower ST-segment elevation

creased hemoglobin concentration, which subsequently limit oxygen-carrying capacity (2). This gender difference in $\dot{V}O_2$max is less pronounced when contrasted in terms of muscle mass rather than in terms of total body weight (2).

Although athletes who are matched for gender and age have been shown to have lower heart rates, longer conduction times, and increased voltages on electrocardiograms (ECGs) compared to sedentary controls, gender differences have also been noted in ECG parameters. Specifically, healthy young females, whether trained or not, were noted to have significantly higher heart rates, shortened conduction times (PQ, Q, QRS), prolonged repolarization time, decreased P, Q, and T amplitudes and lower ST-segment elevation (17).

INJURY PATTERNS

Over the last two decades, as females have increased their participation in sports and exercise programs, there has been a heightened interest in the numbers and types of injuries and in medical concerns unique to women. The types of injury that females sustain seem to be more sports specific and not gender related (18,19). Studies of injury patterns in male and female athletes are controversial. Many studies on athletic injury patterns were generated after women were admitted to the U.S. Air Force Academy in 1976. At that time, the female injury rate of 10% surpassed the male rate of 4% in coed intramural activities, but 21% versus 40% in sports initially considered female or male only (20). Some data support a higher injury rate for female athletes, whereas another study (6) comparing adult male and adult female sports injury rates in matched intercollegiate sports, controlling for exposure time to injury, found no evidence for gender differences except in gymnasts. It has also been demonstrated that female athletes experienced the same relative number and types of injuries as their male counterparts, except for an increased number of patellar injuries occurring in the female (5). When gender-specific injury patterns are examined, it may be important to differentiate preadolescent from adult athletic injuries (21) and to recognize that not all sporting activities are technically equivalent.

Although earlier studies reported a higher incidence of injuries in female athletes, it remains to be determined whether this was due to a lack of adequate conditioning and preparation in the female, a predisposition to injury, or to true physiologic weakness (15). Differences in anatomy, conditioning, and socialization may also account for some of these differences. Females may also become more vulnerable to certain injuries as they enter new sports and develop more aggressive playing styles. More recent studies fail to confirm an increased injury rate among conditioned athletes and seem to suggest that injury patterns may be more sport specific than sex specific.

Of the injuries that affect female athletes, many are overuse syndromes (3,18). Overuse syndromes, while often secondary to recurrent microtrauma, seem to have a multifactorial etiology. Overuse injuries in females may be anatomically related to bone and joint misalignments or to muscular-tendon imbalances (15). Training errors, increases in cardiovascular fitness that supersede musculoskeletal strength increases (3), or improper athletic equipment and apparel are other factors that may play a role in overuse injuries.

Anterior knee pain is a common complaint and is secondary to different etiologic factors, especially biomechanical abnormalities that stress the patellofemoral joint: femoral anteversion, patella alta, genu valgum (19) with tibia varus or pes planus. The increased Q angle (18,19,22–24) noted in females (approximately 15° compared to 10° in the male) helps to demonstrate how the patella is predisposed to excessive lateral tracking and potential subluxation or dislocation (24), even though the angle is not always a clinically useful measurement. Quadriceps strengthening, especially of the vastus medialis oblique muscle (18,19, 24), is helpful in reducing and preventing knee injuries in females. Although stair climbing has been advocated in males, it is not advisable for the female athlete because such repetitive high patellofemoral forces may actually aggravate the problem (18). Instead, the female athlete with patellofemoral syndrome should perform re-

petitive short arch extensions with minimal weight (23). A patella stabilization brace with a lateral buttress may help if the patella subluxates laterally with gentle medial pressures. Additionally, arch supports (19,22) may lessen foot pronation and help to reduce knee valgus. (See Chapter 15 for further discussion.)

Although the female athlete does not seem predisposed to collateral ligament injuries or meniscal injuries of the knee, there is an increased risk of anterior cruciate ligament injury in both soccer and basketball. There have been several hypotheses proposed to explain this, but no conclusive evidence to explain this increased injury rate. Because the hip and pelvis account for only 5% of overuse injuries (25), there are currently limited data on whether there is any gender predisposition. Sacroiliitis has been more commonly encountered in females (15.6%) than in males (6.4%), whereas osteoarthritis of the hip and osteitis pubis were two times more common in men (25). It remains to be researched whether this is secondary to any structural or functional anatomic gender differences.

Both females and males involved in jumping and running sports experience a higher rate of ankle injuries, especially sprains. More recent statistics do not support any increased frequency of such sprains among females compared to male athletes. However, ankle impingement syndromes are more commonly seen in gymnasts, ice skaters, ballerinas, and divers. The gymnast often suffers more anterior capsule impingement with repeated landings on a hyperflexed ankle (18). Conversely, ballet dancers may get impingement of the posterior capsule due to hyperextension exercises required for pointe work. Females may also be predisposed to bunions (26), corns, calluses, and retrocalcaneal bursitis (18). Modifying footwear may help prevent or alleviate these problems.

Past military studies demonstrated that females have less upper body strength than their male counterparts. Shoulder pain, especially in female swimmers, may be secondary to impingement or subluxation (18,27). The crawl and butterfly strokes have been implicated as a cause of impingement syndrome in swimmers. Female swimmers may be at an increased risk secondary to the increased stroke turnover rate required to cover the same distance (18,19). Increased ligament laxity has also been blamed for some of the shoulder complaints in female athletes, but this association requires further study because some propose that there is no increased ligament laxity except during pregnancy (28). Women athletes who have generalized laxity of the glenohumeral joint or weak external rotators and supraspinatus musculature should engage in a rotator cuff strengthening program.

It is not uncommon for female cyclists to experience neck and back pain after long rides. The problem is compounded when female cyclists ride bicycles built for the male athlete, that is, with a long top tube (29), which forces the female to lean forward excessively, especially if she is short waisted. The problem of back and neck strain can be remedied by using a bicycle of proper design for the female: shorter top tube, adjusted stem, and handlebars with less drop. Repetitive hyperextension of the spine in conjunction with rotation frequently causes back injuries in gymnasts and may result in symptomatic spondylolysis. Such back injuries may be prevented by avoiding forced hyperextension on layouts and landing and by an exercise regimen emphasizing abdominal and paravertebral muscle strengthening (19).

THE BREASTS

The consistency of breast tissue varies among individuals and within the same individual at different times of the menstrual cycle. With aging, breast tissue and anatomy undergo change. Breasts are not composed of muscular tissue but are mostly fat (8). Therefore, breast size is proportionate to the fatty tissue component and does not correlate with musculature. Suspensory structures or Cooper's ligaments are not truly ligamentous but maintain breasts in position. With activity, breasts swing in a pendulum-like motion, which may affect athletic performance. For example, swimmers may note increased drag that slows performance. It is a myth that breasts will droop after exercising without support. The use of a brassiere and the degree of support are issues of individual preference.

Breast soreness (30) after exercise has been reported by some female athletes and is probably underreported due to a paucity of studies. Although breast pain is often associated with the onset of menses or with cold weather, there are probably many other causes. Breast pain during or after exercise could be secondary to structural tissue damage or to overstretching of the connective tissue fibers (31). Large-breasted women may also suffer more discomfort because of size and lack of support.

Both males and females may complain of "jogger's nipples" (32) or "bicyclists nipples" (3), which is nipple irritation produced by chafing against a shirt or bra. The problem is often remedied by an application of a lubricant (e.g., Vaseline) (19) or talcum powder to decrease friction or by applying adhesive tape to the nipple or breast to break the chafing interface. Similarly, wearing silk or synthetic undergarments may help to alleviate this problem.

Only a minimal number of sports-related breast injuries have been reported. Serious breast injuries occurring during athletic activities are rare. However, forceful blows to the breast may result in contusions (31) and hematomas and would be treated similarly to corresponding injuries in other parts of the body. Adverse sequelae include fat necrosis or scar tissue formation. Female athletes need to understand and can be reassured by their physicians that there is no known association between breast trauma and a predilection toward the development of breast cancer.

Over the last decade or so, several brands of sports bras have been marketed. Just as footwear is designed for certain athletic activities, the same concept needs to be applied to sports bras. Small-, medium-, and large-breasted females require different biomechanical breast support and this support may be contingent on the type of athletic activity. A well-fitted bra should help minimize extreme vertical and lateral breast excursions in addition to providing proper and firm support (31). The female athlete needs to consider cup size, fabric, protective needs, design, construction, and the sports activity. A rigidly constructed bra may be more compatible with a large-breasted female, whereas a small-breasted female might find a stretchable bra gives adequate support and is more comfortable. Different activities also require varying amounts of arm involvement and range of motion. A bra that is firm with nonelastic straps may be more suitable for an activity that has less arm and shoulder motion (i.e., running, jogging) versus sports that involve a great deal of arm and shoulder stretching (i.e., volleyball, basketball), in which a stretchable strap may be less irritating. Choice of fiber and fabric weight is influenced by personal preference, sensitivity, and climatic and seasonal conditions, in addition to the intensity of the exercise. Some athletes may prefer bras that have a hook or clasp in the front as opposed to the back, to avoid irritation when diving or rolling on the floor. Quality items to search for include absorbent materials, seamless cups, and nonirritating clasps to reduce the risk of abrasions and chafing. Bras that are easy to launder, durable, inexpensive, and available in a variety of sizes and styles are other features to bear in mind (33). Although breast trauma seems to be rare or underreported, breast protection or padding, especially for the athlete involved in contact or collision sports, should be considered. Lastly, in addition to the above, a sports bra should always be comfortable, both at rest and with activity (34).

Breasts undergo many changes during pregnancy with engorgement occurring 2 to 4 days postpartum. Although little information is available regarding breast support during pregnancy, it is probably prudent for the pregnant female athlete to wear a comfortable and supportive bra that minimizes vertical and lateral excursions. During the postpartum period, an underwire bra should be avoided because it could place pressure on milk ducts and lead to plugging.

The effect of exercise on lactation has recently generated interest and research. Moderate aerobic exercise has been shown to have little effect on the quality or quantity (35) of a mother's milk or on infant growth (36). Even vigorous exercise has been shown not to affect the lipid, protein, or lactose content of breast milk when compared to a sedentary control lactating population. In fact, a higher milk volume and higher caloric content have been noted in physically active lactating groups (35). One potentially negative side effect of exercise is the accumulation of lactic acid in breast milk following exercise (36). As lactation places an additional 500 cal/day energy demand on the breast-feeding females, the lactating female athlete should be counseled to pay proper attention to nutritional needs, including caloric and fluid requirements. It is also important for the lactating athlete to avoid fatigue and to moderate the frequency, duration, and intensity of exercise to an individually comfortable level and one that ensures an adequate weight gain in the newborn infant.

GENITOURINARY SYSTEM

Female sex organs seem to be relatively better protected from injury than those of males. In fact, injury to the uterus or ovaries is extremely rare (15). However, straddle injuries may induce a wide variety of vulvar trauma. These include superficial abrasions, lacerations, contusions, and hematomas. There have been a limited number of case reports of vaginal lacerations due to jet ski (37) or waterskiing injuries. As vaginal lacerations can extend into the broad ligament or involve the bladder and or rectum, a thorough physical examination is often necessary to avoid overlooking occult injury to these sites. Vaginal or urethral injuries sustained in high-speed water sports may often be prevented with adequate protective clothing (37).

In contrast to the male urethra, the female urethra is shorter and is not rigidly fixed to the pubic bone (no puboprostatic ligament). These anatomic properties of the female urethra tend to be protective (38). Another anatomic difference between male and females is the steepness of the pubic arch. Consequently, it is not uncommon for female cyclists to experience saddle problems. The female's shallower pubic arch means that the soft tissue of the anterior perineum presses against the nose of the bicycle saddle (29). There are now bicycle saddles that have shortened noses and wider rears (39), which accommodate the female anatomy better. Although there are case reports (40) of men with chronic prostatitis and erectile dysfunction, presumably secondary to pudendal neuritis, data are lacking on female perineal discomfort. Some female cyclists sit more upright in an attempt to redistribute weight and alleviate perineal discomfort secondary to ill-fitting or inadequately designed saddle seats. Female cyclists can be advised to wear protective clothing, have a bike seat of proper design, keep the bike seat level, and use padding if uncomfortable.

GYNECOLOGIC CONCERNS

The relationship between menstruation and athletic activity can be viewed from two perspectives: 1) the effect of training on the menstrual cycle and 2) how exercise performance is affected by the menstrual cycle. Approximately 80% of competitive athletes and 10% to 20% of recreational athletes experience some type of menstrual dysfunction (11). Luteal phase deficiency, oligomenorrhea, amenorrhea, and menstrual delay are known to be more common among athletes than nonathletes (8,9). Other common menstrual complaints include dysmenorrhea and premenstrual syndrome.

By definition, the normal menstrual cycle has an interval ranging from 21 to 36 days and can be viewed from various perspectives: pituitary (follicle-stimulating hormone [FSH], luteinizing hormone [LH] levels), endometrial (proliferative and secretory phases), and ovarian (follicular, ovulatory and luteal phases). The follicular or preovulatory phase begins with the first day of bleeding and lasts approximately 14 days. It is characterized by an initial slight increase in FSH resulting in follicular maturation and a slow rise in LH. A preovulatory surge in estradiol leads to a midcycle increase in LH that results in release of an ovum. The luteal or postovulatory phase of the cycle averages 14 days in length and ends with the onset of menses. The duration of menstrual flow is approximately 3 to 7 days with an average menstrual blood loss between 30 and 40 mL. This phase represents the life span of the corpus luteum, which produces progesterone. The luteal phase is also associated with high levels of estrogen, while circulating LH and FSH levels decline and remain low throughout this phase. It is the rising progesterone level that promotes secretory changes in the endometrium to make it appropriate for implantation. Without fertilization, the corpus luteum involutes and the endometrium sloughs (menses). This results in the release of prostaglandins with subsequent vasoconstriction and myometrial contraction.

Luteal Phase Deficiency

A luteal phase deficiency of progesterone has been associated with recurrent abortions and possibly with reduced fertility or infertility. Although abnormal luteal phase function is common among female athletes, the defect is frequently unrecognized as the total cycle length is often undisturbed. Consistently low serum progesterone levels in the luteal phase may correlate with the severity of the luteal phase progesterone deficit. While plotting a basal body temperature curve and home measuring of the urinary LH surge (7,9) can assist in the diagnosis of a luteal phase deficiency (monophasic basal body temperature pattern or menses occurring <10 days after the LH surge),

endometrial sampling is often required for confirmation (9). The evaluation may also include a serum prolactin level, as elevated values may cause a luteal phase deficiency. Treatment may be conservative and noninterventional unless fertility is desired (11). If so, reduction of exercise, the administration of progesterone (suppositories or intramuscular injections) or clomiphene citrate (Clomid) may remedy the problem (7,9).

Oligomenorrhea/Amenorrhea/Delayed Menarche

Not only do many professional female athletes report menstrual irregularities, but it is also reported in recreational athletes as well. Amenorrhea, delayed menarche, and oligomenorrhea are the menstrual cycle irregularities commonly noted by athletic women. *Amenorrhea* is the absence of menstruation and is classified as primary (failure to begin menstruation, usually by age 16 years) or secondary (discontinuance of menstruation for approximately 6 months at some time after menarche has occurred). *Oligomenorrhea* is defined as intervals of 35 days to 6 months between menstrual cycles.

Although the true incidence of athletic amenorrhea has not been firmly established, estimates vary between 2% and 37% (41) depending on the definitions and research methodologies. It is fairly well established that as the intensity of an exercise program increases, so does the risk of menstrual irregularities (3). Menstrual irregularities are probably underreported because they are mild or of recent onset or because athletes do not want to stop exercising. It should not be automatically assumed that a menstrual disturbance is secondary to exercise, but certain athletic activities such as long distance running and ballet dancing are associated with a higher incidence of menstrual irregularities (7). The topic of menstrual irregularity has only recently generated more interest and study and perhaps is not as benign as previously thought. Also, many females are unaware of the osteoporotic risks and some may prefer the convenience of not menstruating. Newer evidence supports an increased risk of scoliosis, decreased bone density, and increased stress fractures in females with menstrual irregularities (9).

During training, many factors such as lowered body weight, decreased body fat, nutrient imbalance, physical and emotional stressors, and alterations in hormone concentrations and secretory patterns probably act synergistically or contribute in some fashion to athletic menstrual irregularity or dysfunction. Other proposed but not proven factors include the effects of elevated body temperature, ovarian function, modified endorphin levels, and changes in energy levels.

It is clinically important to differentiate between primary amenorrhea and delayed menarche. Menarche usually occurs at 12.8 years, with a range of 10 to 16 years. If menstruation has not occurred by age 16 years (11), it is considered delayed and requires an evaluation because it is a diagnosis of exclusion. It is important to appreciate that the time of onset and the tempo of development during puberty has individual variability. In females, the earliest but most subtle hint of puberty is an increase in height with breast development (thelarche) beginning shortly thereafter. The degree of breast budding is often a reflection of fluctuating estrogen secretion, which may wax and wane. Menarche usually occurs 2 years after thelarche and is often nonvovulatory for the first year or so.

Investigation should probably begin by age 13 or 14 years (8,9), if no secondary sexual characteristics are apparent. It may be clinically useful to approach this work-up based on the presence or absence of secondary sexual characteristics such as breast development, pubic and axillary hair, and normal female reproductive organs. Although menarche and thelarche may be delayed in the adolescent athlete, the growth of pubic hair should appear without delay. The work-up for delayed menarche without thelarche includes FSH, LH, and prolactin levels, thyroid studies (thyrotropin) and radiographic studies for bone age (9). Serum estradiol values may also provide an indication of estrogen levels. If FSH or LH is elevated, a blood karyotype should be obtained to rule out mosaicism or gonadal dysgenesis. Similarly, absent breast and uterine development (as evidenced by pelvic ultrasound) should prompt karyotyping and biochemical studies searching for an enzyme deficiency.

Primary Amenorrhea

Treatment for delayed menarche needs to be individualized. If hormonal and structural abnormalities are excluded, the young teen with delayed menarche should be so informed and reassured to try to avoid conflicts with sexuality and self-image. Teens may also be more vulnerable because of the higher incidence of eating disorders and stress; hence, these issues need to be addressed. A delay in menarche associated with prepubertal exercise, which promotes thinness and postpones critical body composition, may be managed with a reduction in activity and attempts to increase body weight. If the latter approach is not acceptable, optional treatment consists of hormone replacement (11) (oral contraceptive pills [OCPs] or cyclic estrogen and progesterone), especially if estrogen levels are low and the athlete has attained her full height.

This may retard bone loss associated with hypoestrogenism.

Secondary Amenorrhea

A thorough history and physical examination are the initial diagnostic steps to evaluate secondary amenorrhea. The history should detail prior menstrual history, nutritional status, weight changes, sexual activity, and medications. It is also important to gather information on exercise specifics including the intensity, frequency, and duration of training. Additionally, a thorough psychosocial evaluation should not be overlooked. The physical examination should include a pelvic examination, Tanner staging, and evaluation of any signs of pregnancy, androgen excess (acne, hirsutism), and hypoestrogenism (vaginal dryness). If the physical and history exclude nutritional, exercise, or weight changes, a progestin challenge test (7,42) is in order to determine the patient's estrogen status. Medroxyprogesterone acetate (Provera) 5 to 10 mg is administered daily for 5 to 10 days. Withdrawal bleeding, including spotting after a course of progestin suggests an adequate level of estrogen. Lack of withdrawal bleeding suggests that the female has low levels of estrogen and further laboratory tests are warranted. The laboratory investigation should begin with a pregnancy test. Other diagnostic tests include serum prolactin to rule out a pituitary adenoma, FSH and LH levels to rule out ovarian failure, and thyroid function tests (42). Some authorities advise measurements of serum testosterone and dehydroepiandrosterone sulfate (7) because some athletes develop menstrual dysfunction in the absence of or before hirsutism develops.

Treatment options depend on etiology. Athletes may be given an option of reducing activity level or increasing body weight and waiting to see if menses return. It is understandable if this approach is not an acceptable alternative to the elite athlete. It has been proposed that females who have hypoestrogenic amenorrhea may suffer significant loss of bone density (11) similar to that seen in menopausal females. Several hormonal management (7) options are available and probably should be initiated if amenorrhea persists well beyond 6 months. These include cyclic estrogen and progesterone therapy, OCPs, or clomiphene (if pregnancy is desired) to induce ovulation. It is currently unknown if the same doses of estrogen and progesterone prescribed to prevent bone loss in postmenopausal women will have the same affect on amenorrheic athletes. Cyclic estrogen and progesterone with conjugated estrogen (Premarin) 0.625 mg daily on days 1 to 25 and medroxyprogesterone acetate (Provera) 5–10 mg daily on days 16–25 of each calendar month should result in resumption of bleeding. For the hypoestrogenic amenorrheic female who does not desire pregnancy, OCPs will probably help to reduce bone loss. The stimulation of ovulation with clomiphene in the amenorrheic athlete may be tried, especially if pregnancy is desired. Health care providers should be aware that both cyclic hormone replacement and OCPs may have side effects that the female athlete finds unacceptable. It is also not known whether hypoestrogenic athletes, who continue with weight-bearing exercise in conjunction with calcium supplementation can retard bone loss without hormonal therapy.

Dysmenorrhea

There is anecdotal evidence that women who exercise experience less dysmenorrhea. Other studies dispute this and have indicated that women involved in exercise training programs have more or greater awareness of dysmenorrhea, presumably because training and injuries release prostaglandins, which may increase uterine contractions. Dysmenorrheic symptoms include local symptoms of painful cramping in the lower abdomen, which may radiate to the back and anterior thigh. Systemic symptoms such as nausea, vomiting, fatigue, headache, diarrhea, and dizziness are also very common before or during menses. The term *primary dysmenorrhea* is used to describe the condition in which there is no recognizable gynecologic pathology. *Secondary dysmenorrhea* is associated with organic pelvic disease, such as endometriosis, ovarian cysts, or uterine tumors.

Athletic women who experience primary dysmenorrhea are treated similarly to nonathletic women, with prostaglandin synthetase inhibitors or nonsteroidal anti-inflammatory drugs being the mainstay of treatment. The classes of prostaglandin synthetase inhibitors that are useful include the propionic acids such as ibuprofen, naproxen and naproxen sodium, and the fenamates such as mefenamic acid (43). Medications should be initiated with the onset of dysmenorrheic symptoms and are usually required for 1 to 2 days. If one preparation fails to alleviate symptoms, another formulation should be tried. If pain is not responsive to the above medications and there is also a concomitant need for contraception, oral contraceptives may be prescribed. Additionally, it is important for the health care provider to reassure and educate the patient to dispel any lingering myths or misunderstandings.

THE FEMALE ATHLETE TRIAD

Although the symptoms have been observed for years, the term *female athlete triad*
was recently coined and is defined as consisting of an eating disorder, amenorrhea, and osteoporosis (44,45). Although the exact prevalence of this triad is not known, there is probably an increased incidence of these disorders in females participating in endurance and appearance-based sports. Pressure to succeed in athletics by maintaining an unrealistically low body weight or a prescribed weight through food restriction and exercise may lead some women to develop an eating disorder, amenorrhea, or osteoporosis. It is now conceptualized that a restricted food intake and subsequent loss of weight is associated with hypoestrogenic amenorrhea, which may lead to premature osteoporosis.

The term *eating disorder* is now recognized as a constellation of abnormal eating behaviors with poor nutritional habits at one extreme and anorexia and bulimia at the other end (44,46). In the past, the former was not necessarily considered an eating disorder. Over the course of an eating disorder, it is not uncommon to alternate between anorexia nervosa and bulimia. Many females who do not meet the criteria of the *Diagnostic and Statistical Manual of Mental Disorders-IV* (DSM-IV) nevertheless experience some symptoms of eating disorders, such as preoccupations with food and weight. It is not known if females with eating disorders select certain sports to maintain weight control or whether the pressure to succeed in certain sports stresses low body fat and fosters the eating disorder.

The diagnosis may be facilitated by screening for the triad and maintaining a high index of suspicion, which may prompt a more thorough history and examination. Specifically, one should ask about use of laxatives, diuretics, diet pills, purging, weight changes, and conception of ideal body weight (27). A 24-hour dietary recall is often a helpful tool. Details of menstrual history (age of menarche, timing and regularity of cycles) (44) and athletic activities (training schedules, injuries) can help to identify this triad (45). An athlete presenting with body weight less than 85% ideal for height and hyperactivity coexisting with elements of denial (46) should create a high index of suspicion. Stress fractures, particularly if multiple, may also be a clue to identify the athlete with an eating disorder. Always consider the problems of amenorrhea and eating disorders when treating an athlete with a stress fracture. Physical sequelae can include hypothermia, bradycardia, dependent edema, hypotension, erosion of tooth enamel, and lanugo. Starvation can also lead to sleep disturbances, impaired concentration, indecisiveness, mood lability, irritability, anxiety, and depression.

The treatment of the female athletic triad is multidisciplinary with emphasis on psychosocial and nutritional counseling. Optimizing nutrition may by itself normalize menstruation. Hormonal manipulation (45) may be necessary in athletes unwilling to reduce training or those who do not resume menstruation. This multidisciplinary team (46) approach also means educating parents, athletes, trainers, and health care workers. Increased awareness is not only the key to diagnosis but aids prevention and early identification (45). It is also important to dispel any myths that optimal athletic performance is associated with very low body fat. Data on prognosis is currently not available; however, it is important for the health care team to arrange long-term follow-up plans.

Although many athletes have felt that their athletic performance is impaired during certain phases of the menstrual cycle, there have been too few controlled studies researching the effect of the menses on exercise response. In one study (47), there was no significant difference in strength performance in female weight lifting and no significant differences in sprint swimming speed during the premenstrual, menstrual, and postmenstrual cycles; however, this was a limited short-term study. Further research is warranted and should evaluate the phase of the menstrual cycle and perceived versus actual athletic performances. It remains to be determined if and to what degree different athletic activities are influenced by menstruation.

OSTEOPOROSIS

The true incidence of osteoporosis among female athletes is not known. Osteoporosis, which is characterized by low bone mass, represents a major health hazard to women (48,49). Although both sexes may lose bone mass, men rarely develop symptoms before 70 years of age. The mechanisms are not completely understood, but the problem is that bone is not reformed once lost. It is also now being realized that conditions other than aging can lead to osteoporosis. Women who have low body weight, smoke, and remain sedentary seem to be at a higher risk. Other risk factors for osteoporosis include white or Asian heritage, delayed puberty, nulliparity, early menopause, excessive alcohol intake, and possibly low calcium intake (48,49). Estrogen deficiency, whether secondary to exercise or to an eating disorder, seems to place athletes at higher risk. Although postmenopausal females lose most bone 4 to 6 years after menopause, it remains to be proven whether young amenorrheic female athletes follow a similar pattern. If so, athletic amenorrhea is probably not nearly as benign as previously thought.

A goal in the management of osteoporosis is to minimize bone loss and thus reduce the risk of fracture. Estrogen replacement (50) in the peri- and post-menopausal state may help decrease bone loss. Regular exercise and adequate calcium intake (1500 mg daily in amenorrheic athletes as well as in adolescent and young females and 1000–1500 mg/day in adult females) (7,44,45,50) are also important parts of the regimen. In particular, weight-bearing exercise such as walking has been shown to at least retard the rate of bone loss or possibly increase bone density (51). Oral contraceptives may give adequate hormone replacement, but it remains to be seen if bone density losses are stabilized in the athlete at risk for osteoporosis.

Different recipes of hormone replacement are in vogue. Estrogen administration may be cyclic or continuous (48) and if the patient has a uterus, progesterone is added to the regimen for its endometrial protective effect. Cyclic sequential hormone replacement may be advised to help minimize side effects. One such schedule consists of 0.625 mg conjugated estrogen (Premarin) on calendar days 1 to 25 and Provera 5–10 mg daily for days 13 to 25. The continuous sequential regimen consists of a similar daily dose of estrogen on days 1 to 30 with progesterone added on days 1 to 13. This method may be advised for women who experience menopausal symptoms on the estrogen-free days at the end of each month. Withdrawal bleeding is considered a normal consequence of cyclic administration of hormones and is generally light. Additionally, the physician may prescribe combination therapy in which estrogen is given continuously with low-dose progestin (2.5 mg Provera), resulting in the subsequent development of amenorrhea, a side effect preferred by many women (50). Also, combination therapy may be continuous (both estrogen and progesterone on every calendar day) or cyclic (estrogen and

progesterone usage on days 1 to 25). With the latter method, there is often less breakthrough bleeding. Alternately, estrogen may be delivered with a transdermal patch (49). It is currently not known whether one method is superior to another method. The selection of dosing regimen and hormone products should be tailored to the individual. The physician should help explain to each patient the risks and benefits of the various options based on data currently available.

CONTRACEPTION

Forms of contraception for the sexually active athlete are generally similar to those used by nonathletic women. Counseling about relative or absolute contradictions to available contraception methods is no different for the athlete or the nonathlete (52). These measures include natural family planning and reversible methods such as OCPs, spermicides, and barrier methods (condoms, diaphragm, sponge, cervical cap). Long-term reversible contraceptive measures such as subdermal levonorgestrel implants (Norplant), intrauterine devices (IUDs), and intramuscular Depo-Provera injections are also available. Tubal ligation or vasectomy of the partner are two means of permanent surgical contraception. As with any patient population, there is no ideal method and contraceptive choices need to be individualized. Counseling should incorporate nonjudgmental information about efficacy, side effects, risks, benefits, disadvantages, and advantages of each of the various methods.

The currently available low-dose OCPs have minimized some of the side effects associated with the older higher-dose pill preparations. In addition, the newly approved progestins (i.e., desogestrel, norgestimate) are good choices for some women (especially those in the premenopausal age group) due to their selective progestogenic activity.

Although there are no firm conclusions on how OCPs affect athletic performance and endurance capacity, there may be certain beneficial side effects. OCPs may decrease the amount of menstrual flow, thus reducing the risk of anemia, and they have also been used successfully to alleviate dysmenorrhea (53). Additionally, athletes might manipulate menstrual cycles around competitive events by stopping oral contraceptives 10 days before the event and anticipating a withdrawal bleed in approximately 3 days (53). The pill is then resumed after completion of the competitive event or after menses. The onset of a menstrual period may also be delayed for up to 10 days with the administration of a high-dose monophasic contraceptive pill. On the other hand, women using OCPs occasionally experience breakthrough bleeding during the first few months of use (54).

Although the IUD may be a convenient contraceptive method for some women, it has also been associated with increased dysmenorrhea and heavier menstrual periods (8), which may cause an adverse effect on athletic performance. Some consider the diaphragm fairly easy to use; however, it must remain in place for several hours after intercourse. This may pose a problem for athletes who find it uncomfortable to exercise while wearing a diaphragm. Under these circumstances one authority (8) has suggested fitting the patient with a smaller sized diaphragm. No data are currently available regarding the effect of high-impact aerobics or contact sports on women who have had Norplant capsules implanted in the arm. On the other hand there is a case

report of uterine perforation by an IUD secondary to trauma (3).

PREGNANCY

With the emergence of more females of childbearing age engaged in recreational and competitive athletics, several fundamental issues have been raised. There are concerns about how pregnancy may effect one's ability to perform exercise and more importantly, what the effect of exercise might be on the course and outcome of the pregnancy, the labor, and the fetus. Not surprisingly, women are now turning to their health care providers for more specific exercise prescription guidelines.

There are several physiologic and anatomic adaptations to pregnancy. Early in pregnancy there is an increase in maternal blood volume, heart rate, and cardiac stroke volume, which in turn results in raised cardiac output (10,28), which peaks in midpregnancy (55). Some females report improved exercise tolerance in early pregnancy as a result of this increased cardiac reserve. Later in pregnancy when fetal needs increase, the maternal cardiovascular reserve decreases. As the uterus enlarges and pushes upward on the diaphragm, the maternal vertical chest height may be decreased by 4 cm. To compensate, chest diameter can increase by approximately 10 cm (55). Vital capacity (28) is essentially unchanged during pregnancy, but functional residual volume decreases in late pregnancy, resulting in a decrease in oxygen reserve.

It has been proposed that there is increased relaxation of joints and ligaments secondary to raised estrogen and relaxin levels during pregnancy (55). Joints (especially interspinous, sacroiliac, pubic symphysis, knees, and ankles) may then possibly become less stable and more susceptible to injury, but this remains to be proven. No actual studies document that increased joint laxity occurring normally during pregnancy predisposes to soft tissue injuries such as sprains.

A displaced center of gravity, especially as the pregnancy advances, is associated with increased lumbar lordosis (28) and back complaints (56). Lumbosacral pain can be treated with restriction of activity, performance of abdominal strengthening exercises, wearing a corset, and sleeping on a firm mattress. In particular, anterior pelvic tilt can be lessened by strengthening the abdominal and hip extensor (hamstrings) muscles in conjunction with relaxation or stretching of the erector spinae (iliopsoas) and hip flexors (rectus femoris) (56). The physician can also counsel the pregnant female with low back pain to avoid wearing high-heeled shoes and to refrain from sitting with the knees lower than the hips, actions that tend to accentuate lordotic curves (56). Partial or complete pubic symphysial separation and symphysitis due to ligament laxity may be remedied by restricting activity or by use of a pelvic girdle.

The average weight gain during pregnancy is approximately 12.5 kg (27.5 lb) or a 20% increase in body weight (28) for most women. It has been estimated that an extra 300 cal/day (28) is required to provide for the increased metabolic needs of pregnancy. Unfortunately, the nutritional needs of women who exercise are not well defined. Due to this paucity of data, physicians should simply counsel pregnant patients to eat a well-balanced diet and one that sufficiently attempts to approximate her additional metabolic needs.

Many studies have evaluated exercise and pregnancy and the results are conflicting and inconclusive. The literature is problematic from different perspectives. Animal models may not apply to human beings and caution is advised in extrapolating animal data to human beings. Also, many studies have been conducted on females with average aerobic fitness levels or on unconditioned models and may not be appropriate for the athlete who exercised regularly and vigorously before pregnancy. Many of the recommendations concerning exercise during pregnancy are based on the American College of Obstetricians and Gynecologists (ACOG) guidelines (57) that were developed to help counsel the average female seeking to improve her level of physical fitness through exercise without incurring excessive risk of injury. This document is controversial because some of the guidelines are not supported by hard data and the recommendations may not apply to the endurance-trained pregnant female who achieved a high level of performance before becoming pregnant. *More recent studies on aerobically fit women who continued to exercise throughout pregnancy have documented that most are able to maintain similar exercise routines throughout pregnancy* (58).

The major hemodynamic response to exercise is to redistribute blood flow away from the splanchnic organs such as the uterus and toward working muscles. However, the increase in cardiac output and blood volume during pregnancy tends to minimize the risk of reduced uterine blood flow. In the conditioned female athlete, physiologic adaptations may also occur that further lessen the decreased uterine flow (1).

Maternal hyperthermia secondary to exercise has caused some concern because of the risk of fetal abnormalities. The increase in maternal blood volume (40%) (28,59) that occurs during pregnancy may help to transfer heat away from the fetus. However, it is probably reasonable to advise pregnant women not to become overheated by modifying the intensity and duration of the workout (3,55).

Transient fetal bradycardia has been noted in 15% of pregnant females after performing vigorous exercise (60). The importance of this transient change in fetal heart rate is unknown and may be of little clinical significance. Others have reported increased fetal movement with exercise but no sustained tachycardia or bradycardia (59). Doppler studies have also demonstrated increased uterine arterial resistance with exercise but no change in umbilical artery flow, which led some researchers to conclude that the fetal splanchnic blood flow is not adversely affected.

In the second and third trimesters, the enlarging uterus can compress the vena cava and block venous return, which in turn reduces cardiac output and interferes with uterine circulation. This risk of orthostatic hypotension which occurs in the supine position promoted the ACOG guidelines recommending that no reclining exercise be performed after 4 months' gestation (57). More recently, critics have questioned this advice, especially because the dorsal position is very common childbirth position.

Well-conditioned pregnant athletes who continued aerobic exercise at or above minimal training levels have been observed to give birth to newborns of lower birth weight, that is newborns who had a decreased fat mass (61)—lean like the mother. These infants are normal in all other aspects and have no increased incidence of fetal abnormalities. This asymmetric pattern of growth restriction confirms the multifaceted interaction between physiologic adaptation to exercise and physical adaptation to pregnancy.

Another problem with past research is that there are many different parameters to follow to see how mother and fetus respond to exercise. When two groups of well-conditioned athletes were divided into one group who continued to exercise and a control group that stopped training, there was no difference in the occurrence of preterm labor (62). More importantly, the exercising group had earlier labor (by 5 days), shorter active labor, decreased fetal stress (as measured by fetal heart patterns, Apgar scores, and meconium), and less obstetric intervention (decreased number of episiotomies, less use of epidural anesthesia, lower incidence of vaginal and abdominal operative deliveries) (62). Some authorities believe that exercise may stiffen the pelvic floor and perineum and make for a more difficult labor, whereas others believe that strengthened pelvic and abdominal musculature is an asset during the second stage of labor (pushing). More research is in order before definitive advice can be given to pregnant athletes.

The advantage to exercise during pregnancy includes enhanced self-esteem (11), increased energy, relief of tension, less backache (55), and maintenance of ideal body weight (51,59). Additional benefits to exercise during pregnancy are supported by a study finding increased plasma β-endorphin levels and decreased pain perception during labor in multiparous women who performed aerobic exercising during pregnancy (63).

Although much of the data are new, it is important for pregnant females to have some guidelines to follow regarding an exercise program. Counseling for an exercise program should be personalized and should consider the individual's previous level of conditioning, as well as the type, intensity, and duration of exercise. Exercise prescription should encourage activities that accentuate potential benefits and minimize possible fetal or maternal risks. ACOG guidelines suggest a maximum maternal heart rate of 140 beats per minute and a core body temperature less than 38°C (57). Other authorities recommend that heart rate should be less than or equal to 70% predicted maximum (predicted maximum = 220 bpm – age in years) and that body temperature should never exceed 40°C. Both these parameters should normalize 15 minutes after exercise has stopped (59).

Exercise should probably be avoided if the pregnancy is complicated by uterine bleeding, severe maternal hypertension, renal disease, or hemodynamically significant anemia or cardiac disease. Although no one type of exercise is recommended during pregnancy, the following suggestions may help a physician counsel his or her patients. These are simply guidelines and will probably be challenged when more data on exercise during pregnancy are collected and analyzed.

The following is a list of sport-specific recommendations during pregnancy.

Walking/Jogging/Running

Recommendations vary regarding a jogging program during pregnancy. One meta-analysis (64) did not demonstrate any adverse effects to this form of exercise. The key is to gradually commence a program especially because walking may be beneficial for the beginner or unconditioned pregnant female. The trained athlete may want to consider modifying the frequency, intensity, and duration of any workouts, especially as pregnancy progresses.

Bicycling

Bicycling requires coordination and balance. Some serious cyclists might consider changing to a bike with wider tires and saddles and without dropped handlebars, especially later in the pregnancy. The use of a stationary bike (59) may minimize any risk of falling and this form of exercise can probably be initiated at any time during pregnancy.

Swimming

Swimming is an excellent aerobic exercise that can be safely started during pregnancy. Extremes in water temperature should be avoided. Swimming is an ideal activity for most pregnant women because of the buoyant (52) and thermal regulatory properties of water (60), which help to decrease joint stress and accelerate heat transfer. Immersion in water may help to decrease edema by mobilizing extravascular fluid, which will result in diuresis (65). Also, patients may wish to refrain from water sports for approximately 3 weeks postpartum or until bleeding subsides (3,8) to minimize any risk of endometrial infection.

Weight Lifting

It is best to avoid lifting heavy weights that stress the lower back and cause Valsalva maneuvers that may divert blood flow away from internal organs. If an athlete who previously participated in weight lifting insists on continuing the activity, a low-weight, high-repetition (56) exercise program is preferable. Overhead lifts, dead lifting, and squatting should be avoided (57). More studies are warranted before weight lifting can be safely endorsed.

Racquet Sports

Racquet sports such as tennis (56), squash, or racquetball are probably reasonably safe (55). The pregnant female may wish to modify the intensity of play as her pregnancy continues.

Contact Sports

Due to the potential of abdominal trauma, contact and collision sports are probably best avoided. Specifically, this includes field hockey, football, basketball, gymnastics, and volleyball (55,56).

Waterskiing

This activity should probably be avoided due to risk of a high-speed fall causing a forceful water douche.

Scuba

Scuba diving is controversial and considered taboo or inadvisable by some authorities. However, others feel it should not necessarily be prohibited if the pregnant female is an experienced diver. However, she should probably avoid dives exceeding one atmosphere (33 feet) or lasting longer than one half hour (55).

Snow Skiing

Downhill and cross-country skiing should be avoided by inexperienced individuals. A pregnant female may continue to ski with caution if she is experienced (55). Cross-country skiing inherently probably carries less risk of abdominal trauma than downhill skiing.

Ice Skating

This is not an activity recommended for the neophyte due to the potential risk of falling and abdominal trauma. Ice skating should be pursued with extreme caution even by the experienced skater (55).

Aerobics

The ACOG guidelines recommend that ballistic movements be avoided (57). However, low-impact aerobics and stretching activities are usually well tolerated. High-impact aerobics and bouncing activities should be approached with caution. The level of exertion might be modified with advanced stages of pregnancy.

Pregnancy should not be a 40-week period of confinement. There are many physical benefits to exercising during pregnancy. In addition to the sense of well-being and self-mastery that a female experiences as a result of being fit, more recent studies have demonstrated that moderate exercise is probably safe in the uncomplicated pregnancy.

Recent surveys have indicated that recovery from childbirth often requires more than the 6 weeks traditionally allotted (66). Little specific data are available regarding exercise prescription in the postpartum period. An exercise program in the postpartum period should be individualized with activities tailored to each woman's comfort level.

In summary, pregnant females should avoid activities that may cause trauma such as contact or collision sports or activities where there is a risk of falling. Regular exercise is advised and should incorporate warm-up and cool-down periods. It is important to maintain adequate hydration and appropriate caloric intake and to avoid extreme elevations in core body temperature. One should probably avoid strenuous activities greater than 30 minutes in duration. With a few exceptions, physical activities should be confined to activities to which the female is accustomed, except for brisk walking and exercises geared toward strengthening back and abdominal musculature. Hopefully, with more studies and new data, there will be less guesswork and more informed options available for pregnant women and their physicians to select an appropriate exercise program and athletic activity level.

References

1. Corbitt RW, et al. Female athletes. JAMA 1974;228:1266–1267.

2. Lewis DA, Kamon E, Hodgson JL. Physiologic differences between genders. Sports Med 1986;3:357–369.

3. Fardy HJ. Women in sport. Aust Fam Physician 1988;17:183–186.

4. Ferretti A, et al. Knee ligament injuries in volleyball players. Am J Sports Med 1992; 20:203–207.

5. Haycock CE, Gillette J. Susceptibility of women athletes to injury. JAMA 1976;236:163–165.

6. Lanese RR, et al. Injury and disability in matched men's and women's intercollegiate sports. Am J Public Health 1990;80:1459–1462.

7. Peterson DM. Menstrual abnormalities in women athletes. Fam Pract Recertification 1994;16:13–32.

8. Shangold M. Gynecologic concerns in the women athlete. Clin Sports Med 1984;3:869–875.

9. Shagold M, et al. Evaluation and management of menstrual dysfunction in athletes. JAMA 1990;263:1665–1669.

10. Leaf DA. Exercise during pregnancy. Postgrad Med 1989;85:233–238.

11. Ratts VS. Women and exercise effects on the reproductive system. The Female Patient 1993;18:59–68.

12. Good JE, Klein KM. Women in the military academies: US Navy (part 1 of 3) Physician Sports Med 1989;17:99–106.

13. Cinque C. Women's strength training. Physician Sports Med 1990;18:123–127.

14. Heyward VH, Johannes-Ellis SM, Romer JF. Gender differences in strength. Res Q Exerc Sport 1986;57:154–159.

15. Micheli LJ. Injuries to female athletes. Surg Rounds 1979;2:44–55.

16. Giel D. Women's weight lifting: elevating a sport to world-class status. Physician Sports Med 1988;16:163–170.

17. Storstein L, et al. Electrocardiographic findings according to sex in athletes and controls. Cardiology 1991;79:223–236.

18. Hunter LY. Women's athletics: the orthopedic surgeon's viewpoint. Clin Sports Med 1984;3:809–827.

19. Rubin CJ. Sports injuries in the female athlete. NJ Med 1991;88:643–645.

20. Petosa S. Women in the military academies: US Air Force Academy (part 2 of 3). Physician Sports Med 1989;17:133–142.

21. Zillmer DA, Powell JW, Albright JP. Gender specific injury patterns in high school varsity basketball. J Women's Health 1992;1:69–76.

22. Davidson K. Patellofemoral pain syndrome. AAFP 1993;48:1254–1262.

23. Potera C. Women in sports: the price of participation. Physician Sports Med 1986;14:149–153.

24. Ruffin MJ, Kiningham RB. Anterior knee pain: the challenge of patellofemoral syndrome. Am Fam Physician 1993;47:185–194.

25. Lloyd-Smith R, et al. A survey of overuse and traumatic hip and pelvic injuries in athletes. Physician Sports Med 1985;13:131–141.

26. Reynolds JW. Common foot problems in women. The Female Patient 1991;16:31–36.

27. Knortz KA, Reinhart RS. Women athletes: the athletic trainer's viewpoint. Clin Sports Med 1984;3:851–868.

28. Artal R. Exercise and pregnancy. Clin Sports Med 1992;11:363–377.

29. Cohen EC. Cycling injuries. Can Fam Physician 1993;39:628–632.

30. Schuster K. Equipment update: jogging bras hit the streets. Physician Sports Med 1979;7:125–128.

31. Gehlsen G, Albohm M. Evaluation of sports bras. Physician Sports Med 1980;8:89–95.

32. Levit, F. Jogger's nipples. N Engl J Med 1977;297:1127.

33. Hunter L, Torgan C. The bra controversy: are sports bras a necessity? Physician Sports Med 1982;10:75–76.

34. Lorentzen D, Lawson L. Selected sports bras: a biomechanical analysis of breast motion. Physician Sports Med 1987;5:128–139.

35. Lovelady CA, Lonnerdal B, Dewey KG. Lactation performance of exercising women. Am J Clin Nutr 1990;52:103–109.

36. Schelkun PM. Exercise and breastfeeding mothers. Physician Sports Med 1991;19:109–116.

37. Wein P, Thompson DJ. Vaginal perforation due to jet ski accident. Aust NZ J Obstet Gynecol 1990;30:384–385.

38. Diekmann-Guiroy B, Young DH. Female urethral injury secondary to blunt pelvic trauma. Ann Emerg Med 1991;20:1376–1378.

39. Dickson TB. Preventing overuse and cycling injuries. Physician Sports Med 1985; 13:116–123.

40. Desai KM, Gingell JC. Hazards of long distance cycling. Br Med J 1989;298:1072–1073.

41. Munnings F. Exercise and estrogen in women's health: getting a clearer picture. Physician Sports Med 1988;16:152–170.

42. Bergfeld JA, et al. Women in athletics: five management problems. Patient Care 1987;21: 60–82.

43. Sanfillipo JS. Dysmenorrhea in adolescents. The Female Patient 1994;19:27–28, 49–55.

44. Skolnick AJ. Female athlete triad risk for women. JAMA 1993;270:921–923.

45. Nattiv A, Lynch L. The female athlete triad. Physician Sports Med 1994;22:60–68.

46. Haller E. Eating disorders. West J Med 1992;157:658–662.

47. Quadagno D, et al. The menstrual cycle: does it affect athletic performance? Physician Sports Med 1991;19:121–124.

48. Gambrell RD Jr. Update on hormone replacement therapy. Am Fam Pract (suppl) 1992;46:87–95S.

49. Filer WD, Filer RB. Transdermal estrogen and prevention of osteoporosis. AAFP 1994; 49:1639–1642.

50. Miller V. Postmenopausal hormone replacement: picking up where nature leaves off. Mod Med 1994;62:34–40.

51. Carlucci D, et al. Exercise: not just for the healthy. Physician Sports Med 1991;19:46–52.

52. American College of Obstetricians and Gynecologists (ACOG) Technical Bulletin. Women and Exercise 173, October 1992.

53. Schelkun PH. Exercise and "the pill." Physician Sports Med 1991;3:143–152.

54. Fowler GC, et al. Menstrual irregularities: a focused evaluation. Patient Care 1994;28:155–164.

55. Paisley JE, Mellion MB. Exercise during pregnancy. Am Fam Phys 1988;38:143–150.

56. Artal R, Friedman MJ, Mcnitt-Gray, JL. Orthopedic problems in pregnancy. Physician Sports Med 1990;18:93–105.

57. American College of Obstetricians and Gynecologists (ACOG) Technical Bulletin. Exercise during pregnancy and the postnatal period. Washington DC: 1985.

58. Pivarnick JM, et al. Effects of maternal aeorobic fitness on cardiorespiratory response to exercise. Med Sci Sports Exerc 1993;25:993–998.

59. Jarski RW, Trippett DL. The risks and benefits of exercise during pregnancy. J Fam Pract 1990;30:185–189.

60. Watson WJ, et al. Fetal responses to maximal swimming and cycling exercise during pregnancy. Obstet Gynecol 1991;77:382–386.

61. Clapp JF, Capeless EL. Neonatal morphometrics after endurance exercise during pregnancy. Am J Obstet Gynecol 1990;163:1805–1811.

62. Clapp JF. The course of labor after endurance exercise during pregnancy. Am J Obstet Gynecol 1990;163:1799–1805.

63. Varrassi G, Bazzano C, Edwards WT. Effects of physical activity on maternal plasma β-endorphin levels and perception of labor pain. Am J Obstet Gynecol 1989;160:707–712.

64. Lokey EA, et al. Effects of physical exercise on pregnancy outcomes: a meta-analysis review. Med Sci Sports Exerc 1991;23:1234–1235.

65. Katz VL, et al. A comparison of bed rest and immersion for treating edema of pregnancy. Obstet Gynecol 1990;75:147–151.

66. Gjerdingen DK, et al. Changes in women's physical health during the first postpartum year. Arch Fam Med 1993;2:277–283.

WILDERNESS MEDICINE

24

JAMES S. KRAMER
RICHARD R. EHINGER

Acute High-Altitude Illness
Cold-related Illness
Plant Dermatitis
Lightning
Venomous Arthropods
Venomous Reptiles
Infectious Disease and Field Water
Wilderness Medical Kit

The great outdoors—a source of beauty, sport, and adventure—offers a diverse array of readily accessible recreational opportunities. This being the case, participation in wilderness activities is becoming more popular. However, the rewards of many outdoor activities does not come without undue risk. When problems arise in the wilderness, the complex interplay of man and environment creates unique and specialized medical concerns. Wilderness medicine is a rapidly growing area that attempts to synthesize those medical problems encountered in the environment. Primary care physicians taking care of active individuals are likely to encounter wilderness medicine issues and need be aware of their unique nature. This chapter discusses high-altitude illness, cold-related injury, plant dermatitis, lightning strikes, insect bites, snake bites, and diarrhea.

ACUTE HIGH-ALTITUDE ILLNESS

High-altitude illness is the body's dysfunctional adjustment to acute hypoxia and occurs when the rate of ascent exceeds the rate of acclimation (1,2). *High altitude* is generally defined as elevation greater than 8000 ft (2400 m), the height at which most people's arterial oxygen saturation falls below 90% (3,4). Each year about 40 million people travel to high-altitude locales for recreation (5), which has increased interest in the prevention and treatment of high-altitude medical problems. The number of active mountain climbers in the United States has escalated in recent years. Each year millions of people ski at elevations of 8200 to 11,500 ft (2460 to 3450 m) and thousands of tourists scale Pike's Peak in Colorado (most by automobile) to an elevation of 14,764 ft (4429 m). As high altitude becomes more accessible,

the chance of going too high, too quickly increases.

Acute high-altitude illness encompasses a spectrum of disorders which, although different, possess similar features and a common underlying pathogenesis (6,7). These illnesses include acute mountain sickness (AMS), high-altitude pulmonary edema (HAPE), high-altitude retinal hemorrhages (HARH), and high-altitude cerebral edema (HACE). Despite advances in this area, high-altitude illnesses incapacitate large numbers of wilderness users and significant morbidity and mortality still persists. Because most altitude illness is preventable, better education of the population at risk is needed. Acclimation, recognition, and appropriate treatment are the key factors.

To reduce the incidence and severity of high-altitude illness the following measures should be followed:

1. *Staged ascent*. Acclimation to the hypoxia of higher elevations is important. Climbers need to allow 1 day to ascend 1000 ft (300 m) from elevations of 10,000 to 14,000 ft (3000 to 4200 m) and 2 days to ascend 1000 ft (300 m) at elevations above 14,000 ft (4200 m) (3,8). Climbers should also proceed higher during the day and return to a lower elevation to sleep "climb high—sleep low." Although this is slower, a staged ascent can help prevent altitude sickness.

2. *High-carbohydrate diet*. A diet of at least 70% carbohydrates reduces symptoms of AMS.

3. *Exercise level*. Until acclimated exercise should not exceed moderate exertion in the first 24 hours.

4. *Minimize alcohol consumption.*

5. *Stay well hydrated and avoid sedatives.*

6. *Drug prophylaxis*. Although not recommended as routine, acetazolamide use can lessen the symptoms of high-altitude illness (9,10). The indications for acetazolamide prophylaxis are: 1) a forced rapid ascent or 2) history of recurrent AMS despite reasonable rates of ascent. Acetazolamide has been approved by the United States Food and Drug Administration for the prophylaxis of this disorder. The dose for adults is 250 mg twice daily, or a 500-mg sustained-release capsule once a day, starting 24 hours prior to ascent and continuing for 24 to 48 hours while at altitude (11). Dexamethasone, 4 mg every 6 hours starting 48 hours before ascent has also been claimed to be an effective prophylactic medication as well (12–14).

Acute mountain sickness is the most common of the high-altitude illnesses and occurs in poorly acclimated individuals. AMS is rare at elevations below 8000 ft (2400 m) and is directly related to the rate of ascent, the elevation achieved, the duration of stay at altitude, and the degree of acclimation. AMS is divided into two types. Mild AMS symptoms include headache, anorexia, nausea, malaise, insomnia, and Cheyne-Stokes respirations. Headache is the most common symptom, characteristically bitemporal, throbbing, and aggravated by exercise (7). Symptoms begin about 6 hours after arrival, peak 24 to 36 hours after ascent and resolve over 1 to 4 days. The syndrome resembles "feeling hungover." Usually a self-limited disorder, most cases of AMS are benign and transient. Basic treatment is to descend or stop ascent and wait for improvement before proceeding. Mild or moderate symptoms can be treated with rest, oxygen, fluids, analgesics, antiemetics, and acetazolamide 250 mg every 8 hours (3). Approximately

7.5% of AMS cases become potentially life-threatening (15). Ataxia is the most useful sign for recognizing the progression of AMS into its severe form. Severe AMS is characterized by altered consciousness, unsteady gait, dyspnea at rest, and vomiting. At this stage traits of both HACE and HAPE are present although the clinical distinction among them is blurred. Treatment consists of mandatory descent, continued supplemental aid, and dexamethasone 4 mg every 6 hours until symptoms resolve (16,17).

High-altitude cerebral edema is a life-threatening form of altitude illness that occurs at elevations above 12,000 ft (3600 m). Unlike other altitude illnesses it can result in permanent injury. Neurologic features are hallmark with severe headache, marked ataxia, and altered mental status. It is accompanied by several symptoms including impaired judgment, hallucinations, and focal neurologic deficits, which may progress to stupor, coma, and death (17). Treatment is immediate descent with use of supplemental oxygen. If not treated promptly, HACE can rapidly result in death. Advanced treatment consists of airway control, intravenous fluids, and dexamethasone 4–8 mg every 6 hours. Diuretics have not been shown to be useful.

High-altitude pulmonary edema can present in mild, moderate, or severe forms and develops in approximately 1% of those who venture above 12,000 ft (3600 m). Although uncommon, it is the most common cause of death related to high altitude (18). HAPE, a unique pulmonary edema of noncardiac origin, is reversible and need not be fatal if recognized early and treated promptly. Without descent or supplemental oxygen, the death rate is 44% (19). Symptoms develop 1 to 4 days after ascent to high altitude. Mild HAPE presents with dyspnea on exertion only, dry cough, fatigue, and localized rales. Monitored closely, descent is not always necessary if strict bed rest and oxygen are used. In the moderate to severe form, symptoms include dyspnea at rest, marked weakness and fatigue, productive cough, cyanosis, orthopnea, and diffuse rales (17). Neurologic signs and symptoms may also be present. Immediate descent is essential; 2000 to 4000 ft (600 to 1200 m) is usually adequate. In addition to oxygen, acetazolamide 250 mg may be given every 8 hours as well as dexamethasone, although its effectiveness has not been proved. In addition, nifedipine may be helpful in this disorder (18).

High-altitude retinal hemorrhages can occur at elevations above 12,000 ft (4000 m) and are common above 18,000 ft (6000 m), especially with rapid ascent and strenuous exertion. Usually benign and asymptomatic, the hemorrhages resolve spontaneously in 7 to 14 days without any visual impairment. Rarely, macular hemorrhages affecting vision may occur and require immediate descent to prevent permanent vision loss (11).

In summary, the treatment of acute mountain sickness is based on six principles:

1. Prevention by acclimation.
2. Recognition of the clinical manifestations of acute high-altitude illness.
3. Stop ascent if symptoms occur.
4. Immediate descent if HAPE, loss of coordination, or changes in consciousness are present.
5. Descent if no improvement or condition worsens.
6. Never leave ill companions alone.

COLD-RELATED ILLNESS

Cold-induced injuries are the most preventable and treatable exposure-related conditions. These injuries include hypothermia, frostbite, frostnip, trench foot, and chilblains.

Hypothermia

Hypothermia is classified as mild (core temperature >90°F [32.2°C]) or severe (core temperature <90°F [32.2°C]). Clinical signs of mild hypothermia include shivering to generate body heat, thick or slurred speech, difficulty keeping up with a group, and incoordination. Victims of severe hypothermia will have stopped shivering because of exhaustion and depletion of energy stores. The body may then cool quite rapidly and the victim may demonstrate confusion, lassitude or apathy, an inability to walk, or paradoxical undressing or inappropriate behavior. It is helpful to think of these categories as representing the progression of illness rather than distinct diseases although treatment regimens depend on the severity of hypothermia.

A distinction can be made between chronic or subacute hypothermia, which is a gradual drop in body temperature over hours to days, and acute hypothermia which occurs over minutes to hours and is often associated with immersion.

In addition to respiration, body heat is lost via direct transfer to another object (conduction), air or liquid movement at the body surface (convection), energy emission (radiation), and conversion of body sweat or surface water to a gas (evaporation). Damp or wet clothing decreases insulation and causes increased evaporative, conductive, and convective heat loss. Wind increases the rate of heat loss by convection as reflected in the wind chill factor. Immersion causes a profound increase in conductive heat loss.

Most hypothermia deaths occur between 30° and 50°F (−1.1° and 10°C) rather than at subfreezing temperatures, and one can become hypothermic in 77° (25°C) water. Hypothermia is not easily recognizable; therefore the primary care physician must be alert to the variety of conditions under which it can happen.

Once hypothermia is diagnosed, immediate treatment is imperative. Treatment strategies must be tailored to the individual patient and situation, some general principles can be followed.

Therapy for chronic hypothermia depends on its severity. *Mild chronic hypothermia* can be treated with rewarming in the field by simply limiting further exposure to environment. Wet clothing must be removed and replaced with dry insulating clothing, and the victim placed in a sleeping bag insulated from the ground with head and neck covered to prevent further heat loss. Oral rehydration with a glucose containing solution should begin, and no alcohol should be given. A fire is helpful for initial rewarming but if rewarming is not possible, evacuation should be attempted.

Severe chronic hypothermia is a medical emergency and the victim must be handled with the utmost care. Any physical exertion can cause cold, acidotic blood from the outer tissues to flow to the heart and cause ventricular fibrillation. Clothing should be removed gently, and the victim must not ambulate. After initial steps are initiated to reverse heat loss, evacuation is the first priority.

If evacuation is not possible, field rewarming should consist of hot packs, hot water bottles, and radiant heat from a fire. *Hot baths are contraindicated.* Sudden peripheral vasodilatation pulls warm blood from core protected organs. With an already compromised blood volume, rapid rewarming causes a "rewarming shock" as

the low total intravascular volume is dispersed from core organs to the entire vasculature. Also, as noted above cold acidotic blood flowing to the heart can cause ventricular fibrillation.

For extreme cases, cardiopulmonary resuscitation (CPR) may be needed to maintain the patient until advanced medical care is available. In determining whether CPR is to be initiated, more time than usual should be used to determine pulselessness and a central pulse should be sought. CPR should not be given if the victim has a lethal injury, is moving or breathing, the chest is frozen, or if performing CPR places the rescuers in danger. If the respiratory rate is less than 6 to 7 breaths per minute, rescue breathing should be given. For a severely hypothermic person, the decision not to administer CPR should not preclude immediate evacuation to more advanced medical attention. *Remember, no one is dead until warm and dead.*

As with a victim of severe chronic hypothermia, victims of *acute hypothermia* or immersion hypothermia must be handled very gently. General principles regarding rewarming are similar for these two types of cases with one notable exception. Although hot baths are not recommended for the chronic severely hypothermic, they may be beneficial for the victim of acute immersion hypothermia. Rapid rewarming in hot water (104° to 110°F [40° to 43.3°C]) can avoid the so-called "afterdrop" phenomenon. Afterdrop is the further lowering of core body temperature after rewarming. It is dependent on the rate of cooling and not the rate or method of rewarming. The core temperature of acutely hypothermic patients is initially near normal, but it will drop quickly as their core heat stores equilibrate with their very cold periphery. For this reason rapid rewarming in a hot bath or shower may be necessary. If this is not possible, naked huddling with the victim by one or two rescuers should be done similar to the case of initial field rewarming of the chronic hypothermic.

Several factors aid in preventing hypothermia. A good level of physical fitness will allow for longer maintenance of body heat. Adequate hydration and nutrition are imperative during a wilderness trip. During a strenuous outing, an intake of 3–4 L of fluid a day is appropriate—more in arid or low humidity conditions. Ingesting snow can worsen hypothermia. Carbohydrates are best for quick calorie sources and frequent (up to every 2 hours) snacking helps maintain energy levels.

The correct clothing can significantly lessen conductive and convective heat losses. Multiple layers of clothing trap air and are more effective as insulation. Layering allows easy adjustment for overheating, perspiration, and overcooling. Wool and several of today's synthetic fibers are excellent for cold or damp weather because they are lightweight and warm, and maintain their insulating powers when wet. Cotton, in contrast, is a poor insulator and accelerates cooling by its wicking action especially when it becomes wet.

Frostbite

Frostbite is tissue injury or death caused by freezing of tissues. The most susceptible body parts are those furthest from the core with large surface-to-volume ratios—the feet, hands, ears, and nose. Some factors predisposing a person to frostbite are:

1. Low ambient temperature (especially <20°F [–6.6°C])
2. Wind chill, humidity and wetness
3. High altitude (above 8000 ft [2400 m])
4. Poor circulation from various causes (in-

trinsic vascular disease, previous frostbite, smoking, alcohol intake and vasodilatation, tight-fitting boots or clothing)
5. Fatigue and overexertion
6. Deep snow (temperatures are lower deeper in the snow)

The severity of frostbite has historically been classified in stages:

First degree—numbness, erythema, edema, a whitish or yellowish firm plaque may form at the center of the injury. There is very little tissue loss.
Second degree—superficial blisters form with a clear or milky fluid.
Third degree—deeper blisters form, which can appear purple and contain blood.
Fourth degree—involvement to subdermal tissues frequently including muscle and bone.

In superficial injury the skin feels firm but underlying soft tissue is still soft. Deep injury causes skin to feel hard because it may be frozen solid. Numbness is the most frequent initial symptom of frostbite. A numb sensation followed by a prickling or tingling sensation after rewarming does not represent true frostbite because even in its mildest forms, frostbite does some damage to affected tissues (see Frostnip section below). Practically speaking, the early staging of frostbite is often academic because 1) it is difficult initially to predict the extent of damage, and 2) the treatment for all stages is the same—rapid rewarming.

Superficial frostbite may be treated in the field with immediate thawing. However, it is extremely important that *frostbite is not thawed if the affected part will soon be again exposed to cold or possible refreezing.* Refreezing results in tissue damage far greater than the initial frostbite damage.

Even partial thawing or rewarming should be avoided while the patient is transported to a site for rapid rewarming. It is much better to hike out several miles with frostbitten toes than to thaw them and risk refreezing. Vigorous rubbing can cause tissue damage and should be avoided, but all *constricting and wet clothing should be removed and replaced.* Blisters should be left intact and protected with gauze.

Rapid rewarming is accomplished by placing the frostbitten body part in water heated to 104° to 108°F (40° to 42.2°C). Monitor water temperature frequently because immersion can quickly cool the bath. Thawing usually takes no more than 30 minutes and is complete when the skin is pliable and erythematous and sensation has returned. Extreme pain may accompany thawing and should be treated appropriately. Postthaw care involves application of aloe vera, loose bandaging between digits, elevation, splinting as necessary, and analgesia. Ibuprofen 400 mg or aspirin 650 mg two to four times daily may improve microcirculation and healing.

Prevention of frostbite involves wearing properly fitted boots and clothing, covering exposed body parts, and keeping dry. Also, keep shaving and washing of susceptible parts to a minimum because these can remove skin oils and protective skin cell layers. Lastly, do not touch metal with bare skin in cold weather, rather some form of insulation or wrapping should be used.

Frostnip

Frostnip is reversible, superficial ice-crystal formation distinguished from frostbite by the lack of tissue damage. The intense vasoconstriction can be painful but the condition is easily treated. Covering or blowing on the involved part may affect total rewarming. Although obviously not as serious as frostbite, frostnip should alert the individual that extra skin protection is required.

Trench Foot (Immersion Foot)

Prolonged exposure of wet feet to cool temperatures (68°F [20°C] down to freezing) can result in *trench foot*. Early symptoms can be similar to frostbite (tingling and numbness) but trench foot develops over hours to days and does not result in tissue freezing. During the first stage of this illness, which can last up to a week, the skin appearance progresses from hyperemic to pale and swollen. Painful paresthesias and cramps can ensue.

The second stage lasts several weeks and frequently involves blister formation, infection, and occasionally gangrene. The pathophysiology of trench foot is related to sympathetic vasomotor instability and hypersensitivity to cold with microvascular stasis and thrombosis.

In addition to supportive care and pain management, therapy can include ibuprofen or aspirin up to four times a day to inhibit platelets and clotting. Although cold sensitivity can persist for years, prognosis is generally better for trench foot than for frostbite.

Chilblains (Pernio)

Chilblains result from chronic exposure of dry skin to cold, harsh, wet weather conditions. It is characterized by skin that is locally erythematous, swollen, tender, and pruritic. Frequent sites of involvement are the arms, hands, lower legs, toes, ears, and cheeks. The chilblain syndrome—thought to have a pathophysiology similar to that of trench foot—is a mild form of cold injury and no tissue loss results. Treatment is essentially preventive with the mainstay being the use of protective clothing and ointments (such as petrolatum) on exposed parts.

PLANT DERMATITIS

Plants of the genus *Toxicodendron*—poison ivy, poison oak, and poison sumac—are responsible for most allergic contact dermatitis suffered by wilderness outdoorsmen. Recognition and avoidance of these plants are key to preventing this type of dermatitis.

Poison ivy is found throughout the United States. Poison oak grows primarily along the Pacific coast and has a bushlike appearance. Its leaves tend to have a more rounded lobelike appearance. The leaves of both plants are pinnate with three leaflets, giving rise to the saying "leaves three, let them be." Typically the leaves of poison ivy cluster together in groups of three but may be seen in groups of five, seven, or nine. Poison ivy may also grow as a vine or shrub; thus, its recognition may not always be easy. Poison sumac is found primarily in swampy areas of the eastern United States. It has seven to 13 leaflets with white "berries at the base," unlike benign sumacs, which produce flowers and berries at the tip of each branch. Plant morphology and habits vary greatly from area to area. Hence, these plants' appearance in different parts of the country must be known to be able to avoid them (Figure 24.1).

Urushiol is the active allergenic factor found in poison ivy and poison oak. The blister fluid of the patient with poison ivy dermatitis does not contain urushiol and is not contagious. Plant contact dermatitis is a type 4 cell-mediated delayed hypersensitivity reaction to the urushiol oleoresin (20). The process of initial sensitization to

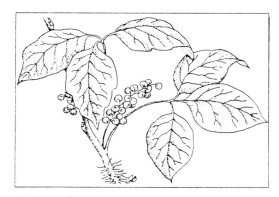

Poison Ivy

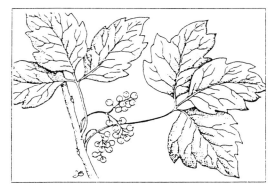

Poison Oak

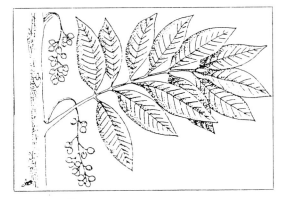

Poison Sumac

Figure 24.1. Poisonous plants. (Reproduced by permission from Guin JD, Kligman AM, Maibach HI. Managing the poison plant rashes. Patient Care 1992;30:63–78.)

the chemical requires 1 to 2 weeks. Subsequent exposure to the allergen will usually induce a skin eruption within 1 to 2 days. After skin exposure, common findings are itching, erythema, swelling, and blisters, which may be vesicular or bullous distinguishing this kind of contact dermatitis from almost any other. Many initial home remedies are ineffective, although immediate irrigation with water or wiping with alcohol may be helpful. The severity of lesions, discomfort of the patient, and disabling effects of the dermatitis guide therapy. Treatment is similar to other allergic contact dermatitis. In general, the greater the skin involvement, the greater the need for aggressive therapy. Oral antihistamines may provide relief from the pruritus. High-potency topical corticosteroids are the drugs of choice for all but severe skin reactions. Over-the-counter hydrocortisone creams in strengths of 0.5% and 1.0% offer little benefit. Avoidance of creams or ointments like topical antihistamines that might be sensitizing is important as they may compound the problem. Topical corticosteroids need to be applied twice or three times a day for at least a week with gradual tapering to once a day after resolution of the rash. Systemic corticosteroids should be used in patients who have major areas of involvement (face, genitalia, multiple patches of vesicles and bullae) (21). High-dose oral corticosteroid therapy should be continued for 14 days. Patients treated for less than this period are at risk for return of their dermatitis (22).

Avoidance is the best prevention. The only prophylaxis is oral or intramuscular administration of urushiol, a long and difficult procedure that results in limited hyposensitivity and is generally not recommended. One barrier compound that shows some promise is Stokogard, but there is no known topical agent that can totally prevent urushiol-induced dermatitis.

LIGHTNING

Injuries due to lightning are uncommon, yet lightning accounts for more weather-related deaths than any other natural phenomenon (23), including nearly 300 deaths per year in the United States (24). Most fatalities occur among young, active people engaged in outdoor activities. Seventy percent of lightning strikes occur during the summer months. Lightning can strike people in three ways: 1) direct strike, associated with high morbidity; 2) side flash, striking secondarily after a primary object has been hit; or 3) ground or "step" current. Of the three, side flash is the most common event (25). Victims can also suffer significant blunt trauma as a result of the implosive or explosive shock wave effects of lightning. Despite the awesome electrical force lightning holds, it is estimated that several thousand victims are injured each year but survive (26). This is most likely due to the flashover effect of lightning in which the majority of electrical energy flows over the victim's body rather than into or through it.

The initial treatment of a lightning victim should always begin with assessment and stabilization of the airway, breathing, and circulation. The major cause of death in lightning injuries is cardiopulmonary arrest. Lightning acts as a massive DC countershock, sending the heart into asystole (27). Prolonged and aggressive resuscitation is the key to the management of lightning strike victims. There are multiple accounts of successful revival of persons thought to be "dead," as in patients who have what is believed to be an unresuscitative cardiac arrhythmia. Artificial respiration may have to be continued for hours, but the result of such treatment is often good. Open chest CPR has been successful and should be considered.

The clinical manifestations of lightning injury are diverse. Lightning strike victims should be thoroughly evaluated for multiple organ injury, especially the cardiopulmonary and central nervous systems, as well as for secondary injuries. Hospitalization may be required, especially in the case of severe burn injury although it is rare that full-thickness, entry/exit burns are found. Rather, victims typically experience linear, punctate, feathering and thermal burns (24), which are superficial in nature and require little therapy. In the absence of cardiac arrest or serious secondary injury, care for the lightning strike victim is generally supportive in nature. For patients who do not warrant hospitalization appropriate follow-up evaluation is mandatory. Ophthalmologic evaluation several days after injury is recommended because of the potential for development of cataracts. More than 50% of lightning strike victims have ruptured tympanic membranes and temporary deafness is common (28). Neurologic deficits such as paralysis or paresthesias demand follow-up to determine if any permanent sequelae are present. Initial neuropsychiatric complications typically clear rapidly, whereas late-appearing defects tend to be more persistent or permanent (28).

Precautions for avoiding lightning injury should be taken when outdoors and thunderstorms are imminent. If caught in the open, individuals should lie down on a plastic liner with their limbs tucked under their torso. To lessen the chance of a lightning strike, high areas, isolated trees, and metal objects should be avoided; groups should spread out and if caught in the water, get out.

VENOMOUS ARTHROPODS

Arachnids, Ticks

Tick bites are painless, and people are usually not aware of them until days afterward when itching begins or an engorged tick is found. Ticks should be removed from the skin with tweezers using gentle force to remove the imbedded head completely. The cause for concern is not the local skin reaction, but rather that ticks are vectors of diseases including Rocky Mountain spotted fever, Lyme disease, and tick paralysis.

Rocky Mountain spotted fever is caused by *Rickettsia rickettsii* and transmitted by Ixodid (hard-shelled) ticks. The peak incidence is from May to September most commonly reported in the Middle Atlantic states. The clinical syndrome includes severe headache, fever, and a maculopapular rash arising on the wrists, palms, ankles, and soles of the feet. Antibiotic therapy should be started immediately, especially in children, if the characteristic triad is noted and there is history of tick exposure. The most sensitive and specific serologic tests currently available are the indirect fluorescent antibody and indirect hemagglutination tests. The antibiotic of choice is a 2-week course of tetracycline (2 gm/day in adults). When used early, the mortality rate is decreased significantly (29).

Lyme disease is caused by a treponema-like spirochete *Borrelia burgdorferi*. It is transmitted to humans by Ixodid ticks as well. Not discovered until 1975, it is now the most common vector-borne disease in the United States (30). The common manifestation of Lyme disease is erythema chronicum migrans (ECM) observed in more than half the cases. It appears as an expanding, red, annular lesion with a clear center resembling a target. Symptoms suggestive of a viral illness may accompany the rash. This is the first of three stages of Lyme disease. Disseminated infection (stage II) can cause a host of signs and symptoms; the most common presentation is frank neurologic (cranial neuropathy) or cardiac (atrioventricular block) abnormalities. If untreated, 60% go on to stage III months or even years later marked by persistent arthritis (29). There is no definitive laboratory test to make the diagnosis, but the enzyme-linked immunosorbent assay is best. Early use of antibiotics is helpful in shortening the duration of ECM with its associated symptoms and in avoiding the more serious problems of recurrent arthritis, meningo-encephalitis, and myocarditis seen in the chronic aspect of the disease. Doxycycline is the most effective antibiotic, 100 mg twice daily for 2 to 3 weeks. Treatment of choice for stage II and III Lyme disease is with high-dose penicillin G (20 million units intravenously daily for 10 days) (31).

Tick paralysis is caused by an unknown tick neurotoxin and occurs only after prolonged tick attachment to its human host (5–7 days). The acute ataxia and paralysis seen in the disease resolves spontaneously within 48 hours after removal of the tick.

Scorpions

There are some 650 species of scorpions with approximately 40 inhabiting the United States (32). Scorpions inject venom, which is primarily neurotoxic, through a stinger at the tip of their tail. Few, however, are considered dangerous to human beings. The venomous scorpions belong to the family Buthidae. In the United States the one

deadly scorpion is *Centruroides sculpturatus* (also known as *Centruroides exilicaude*). This scorpion inhabits Arizona and parts of California, Texas, and New Mexico.

Although the appearance of these arachnids can be both intimidating and frightening, envenomation, albeit painful, rarely is fatal to human beings. Most scorpion stings produce minor, localized wheal and flare reactions requiring only local wound care. Centruroides stings are acutely painful with numbness and a hypersensitive zone soon developing around the site. Severe reactions may cause hypertension, salivation, diaphoresis, incontinence, paresthesias, visual symptoms, seizures, respiratory impairment, and coma (33). Therapy depends on the symptoms. Most serious envenomations are seen in small children, the elderly, and hypertensive adults. Nonlethal symptoms typically last less than 4 hours. Antivenin, only available in the United States in Arizona, is reserved solely for cases of severe poisoning (32).

Spiders

There are two venomous spiders of significance in the United States: *Latrodectus mactans* (black widow), and *Loxosceles reclusa* (brown recluse). The black widow is found throughout the continental United States. The female spider is aggressive and venomous. The trademark red hourglass on the globular abdomen makes it readily identifiable. The black widow spider bite is painful, with subsequent erythema and swelling, which subsides quickly. Thereafter, systemic symptoms become paramount due to the release of the neurotransmitters acetylcholine and norepinephrine (34). Symptoms begin within 30 minutes after the bite and over several hours crampy, muscular pain occurs in the victim's thigh, chest, and back. A boardlike abdomen, often simulating an acute abdomen, may occur. Generalized neurologic hyperstimulation is present to make the distinction. Occasionally, patients appear and demonstrate a flushed, contorted face giving rise to the term fascies latrodectismica. These symptoms usually resolve in 24 hours but, unfortunately, may recur for weeks to months later. Treatment is supportive and management revolves around correct diagnosis. Calcium gluconate and methocarbamol and intravenous morphine are used to control muscle spasm and pain. A fatal outcome is rare; antivenin (derived from horse serum) is available but should be reserved only for what appears to be a potentially life-threatening reaction.

The brown recluse is found in the Missouri, Ohio, and Mississippi river valleys. Loxosceles spiders are identified by their delicate body habitus, tan to brown color, and a violin-shaped marking on their thorax; thus the common name "fiddle-back" spider. Secretive creatures, the brown recluse never bites unless threatened or accidentally disturbed. Most human encounters occur indoors; for example, the spiders like dark crannies, cardboard boxes, and stored clothes or shoes. Their bite is relatively painless. Several hours later the red bite site will turn into a blister surrounded by a blue-white halo. This may be further encircled by a ring of ecchymosis, creating a characteristic "bull's eye" lesion. Most lesions will resolve; fewer than 10% worsen and become deeply ulcerated and necrotic. Local cell and tissue injury is caused by direct action of sphingomyelinase found in Loxosceles venom (35). Systemic symptoms are minimal, as compared to *Latrodectus* envenomation, but may include flulike symptoms. The most significant systemic reaction that can occur is hemolysis, a rare complication almost always seen in children. Loxosceles bites should be treated with local wound care. Excision of the bite wound and skin grafting are rarely required. The efficacy of oral dapsone in the treatment of brown recluse spider bites has been seriously questioned.

Hymenoptera

Insects of four families make up the order Hymenoptera. These include 1) Apidae—honeybee, which accounts for most stings, and in doing so the stinger is retained; 2) Bombidae—bumblebee; 3) Vespidae—hornets, wasps, and yellowjackets; and 4) Formicidae—fire ant. Anaphylaxis to Hymenoptera venom accounts for more deaths in the United States than does any other envenomation: up to 40 to 45 deaths are reported annually (36). It is estimated that 1% of the population is hypersensitive to the complex venom of bee stings with these severe reactions being more common in adults than children.

Venom in many *Hymenoptera* species is used for both defense and subjugation of prey. They contain histamines and other vasoactive substances lending them their hemolytic and neurotoxic properties. Venom is also an effective hypersensitizing agent in human beings. The normal reaction to the stings of bees, wasps, and hornets is an immediate, intense burning pain followed rapidly by erythema, swelling, and itching at the sting site. These symptoms usually subside in 1 to 2 hours. On the other hand, most large local reactions evolve slowly and peak 6 to 12 hours after the sting, to then disappear by 36 to 48 hours. Immediate systemic reactions (anaphylaxis) are apparent within the first 15 to 30 minutes of a sting, and nearly all occur within 6 hours. Only a single sting is necessary to produce serious anaphylaxis in the hypersensitive victim. Nearly 70% of fatal cases are due to edematous airway obstruction and subsequent respiratory failure (37).

Treatment of bee stings requires removal of the stinger if retained (i.e., honeybee) and local supportive care. Commercial "sting-sticks" containing a topical anesthetic or an oral antihistamine may be helpful. Therapy for anaphylaxis follows conventional lines for the treatment of acute allergic emergencies. Aqueous epinephrine 1:1000 should be given subcutaneously at the first indication of serious hypersensitivity. The dosage is 0.3 to 0.5 mL in adults and 0.01 mL/kg in children. Anyone stung by large numbers of *Hymenoptera* needs to be observed for 12 to 24 hours to watch for a delayed reaction.

For hypersensitive patients, immunotherapy provides complete protection in 70% of treated individuals (37). Desensitization with purified insect venom rather than whole body extracts need to be used. Patients known to be allergic to insect stings should carry an epinephrine self-injector such as the Ana-Kit (Hollister-Stier) or Epi-Pen (Center Laboratories) and be instructed in its use. Allergic individuals should also wear medical identification badges.

VENOMOUS REPTILES

Snakes

Each year in the United States poisonous snakes inflict about 8000 snakebites that result in around 15 fatalities; therefore, despite the fear of snake envenomation, the case fatality ratio is less than 0.5% (38). The highest snakebite rates are found in the southern and southwestern states. Only four types of venomous species are indigenous to the United States. Of these, three are of the family known as pit vipers (Crotalidae): rattlesnakes, which include 16

species; cottonmouth or water moccasin; and the copperhead. The fourth venomous species is the coral snake, which is a member of the Elapidae family. This snake is brightly colored with a black nose and black-yellow-red banding pattern. Rattlesnakes are responsible for approximately 65% of all venomous snakebites in the United States each year. Most fatal bites result from the eastern diamondback (*Crotalus adamenteus*) or the western diamondback (*Crotalus atrox*) (39).

In treating snake envenomation, medical personnel must be able to distinguish between poisonous and harmless snakes. Vipers can be differentiated from harmless snakes by the presence of fangs, a triangular-shaped head, and the elliptical shape of their pupils. They also exhibit only a single row of subcaudal plates on the underside of their tails, whereas harmless snakes will have a double row (Figure 24.2).

Pit Viper

Pit viper venom contains enzymatic proteins that provoke proteolysis and hemolysis. Up to 30% of poisonous snakebites, however, do not result in envenomation and require no further treatment. Distinct localized findings of pit viper envenomation are fang puncture(s), pain, edema, and ecchymosis of the bite site and adjacent tissues. If local signs and symptoms have not manifested within 4 hours after a snakebite, it is generally safe to assume that the patient did not suffer from pit viper envenomation. When evident, the degree of toxicity of a poisonous snake bite depends on the size and species of snake, location of the bite, the potency of the venom and amount injected, and the size of the person bitten. Edema, associated with hemorrhagic blebs, can be massive and will slowly progress up the bitten extremity. Systemic symptoms such as nausea, vomit-

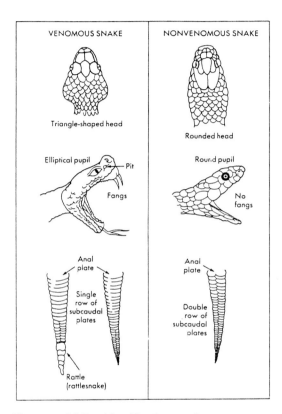

VENOMOUS SNAKE	NONVENOMOUS SNAKE
Triangle-shaped head	Rounded head
Elliptical pupil — Pit — Fangs	Round pupil — No fangs
Anal plate — Single row of subcaudal plates — Rattle (rattlesnake)	Anal plate — Double row of subcaudal plates

Figure 24.2. Identification of venomous snakes. (Reproduced by permission from Otten EJ. Venomous animal injuries. In: Rosen P, Barkin RM, eds. Emergency medicine: concepts and clinical practice, 3rd ed. St. Louis: CV Mosby, 1989:563–587.)

ing, diaphoresis, fever, weakness, and paresthesias may then develop. Hemorrhagins in crotalid venom commonly cause petechia, bleeding of the gums, and hematemesis.

Treatment of pit viper bites is, unfortunately, surrounded by controversy and based on tradition. The hysteria a snakebite creates compounds the problem. First aid measures such as wound cleansing and application of a dressing needs to begin in the field. However, time honored therapy such

as incision and suction, pressure dressings, tourniquets, and field snakebite kits are no longer acceptable. The proper procedures are: 1) avoid panic; 2) locate and identify the snake; 3) immobilize and elevate the bitten extremity; 4) never apply ice; and 5) obtain medical assistance (40). For victims alone in the wilderness, walking out is a necessity. Severe manifestations of snake envenomation may not occur for hours after the bite, so travel is usually possible. If the victim is many hours away from medical care, the use of a constricting band—not a tourniquet—2 to 4 inches proximal to the bite may be applied. It should be applied loosely (barely indenting the skin) in an attempt to occlude lymphatic drainage.

Definitive treatment is focused on either medical or surgical management. Medical therapy concentrates on the use of intrave-

Table 24.1. Envenomation Severity Grading System

Grade	Signs and Symptoms
0	No envenomation, fang punctures present, no local or systemic signs
I	Mild envenomation, fang punctures present, local pain and swelling only
II	Moderate envenomation, fang punctures present, severe pain, swelling <12 inches from site, mild systemic symptoms
III	Severe envenomation, fang punctures present, severe pain, swelling >12 inches from site, petechiae and bullae present, severe systemic symptoms, bleeding and/or disseminated intravascular coagulation, markedly abnormal laboratory findings
IV	Multiple envenomations, severe signs and symptoms in all categories, life-threatening

SOURCE: Christopher DG, Rodning CB. Crotalidae envenomation. South Med J 1986;79:159–162.

nous polyvalent Crotalidae antivenin. This substance is effective for all native pit viper bites. Rapid treatment, ideally within 4 hours, is important for preventing absorption of venom and neutralizing it at the bite site. Guide to dosage includes symptoms, signs, and laboratory tests (Table 24.1). Because antivenin is a horse serum product, its use carries risk of serum sickness and anaphylaxis. Before its administration, antivenin sensitivity should be tested and be prepared for allergic reactions. Field use of antivenin is not recommended. Remember, most Crotalidae envenomations can survive without antivenin treatment.

Surgical management consists of excision or incision, with or without fasciotomy (41). This approach is now not considered favorable. Fasciotomy need only be performed in instances of true compartment syndrome. Despite the presence of massive tissue swelling typically seen in pit viper bites, vascular compromise is rare.

Coral Snake

Elapidae snakes, such as the cobra, sea snake, and coral snake have venom that is primarily neurotoxic. There will be minimal local signs following coral snake envenomation. Fang marks may not be evident and there will be no local swelling. Systemic symptoms such as euphoria, paresthesias in the bitten part, nausea, vomiting, and excessive salivation develop several hours later. Rapid progression to such signs of bulbar paralysis as ptosis, myosis, and diplopia along with generalized paralysis and respiratory depression are indicative of a life-threatening reaction. Eastern coral snake (*Micrurus fulvius*) antivenin is available and is recommended in this situation. Death, if it occurs, is usually within 24 hours. Deaths are rare, however, and coral snakebites account for less than 2% of all snakebites in the United States (42).

The best treatment for snakebite is prevention. Those who traverse wilderness areas with care are rarely bitten by snakes. Snakebites can be avoided by staying away from snake-infested areas, not hiking during times of snake activity, wearing protective shoes and clothing, and never stepping or reaching into concealed areas where snakes are common.

Gila Monster

The Gila monster (*Heloderma suspectum*) is a venomous reptile of the lizard family found in the Great Sonoran Desert. A slow-moving but extremely powerful reptile, evenomation is rare. Heloderm wounds are usually puncture type, although teeth may be shed during the bite and remain in the wound. After biting, the Gila monster will either drop off or retain its strong grasp and chew. In the latter case, mechanical means such as using a crowbar or pliers, may be required to loosen the tenacious grip on the victim. The victim will experience severe, burning pain at the bite site along with localized swelling and ecchymosis. Systemic symptoms of diaphoresis, nausea, and weakness are short-lived. Treatment is relatively simple focusing on irrigation, antiseptic solution soaks, and local wound care. Always explore the wound for shed or broken teeth.

INFECTIOUS DISEASE AND FIELD WATER

Giardia lamblia is the number one enteric pathogen encountered in the outdoors (43). Human beings are the major carriers of *Giardia* infection ("backpacker's diarrhea"), but many animals including beavers ("beaver fever") and deer act as reservoirs of the parasite. The life-cycle of

Giardia is well known. Drinking surface water infected with the *Giardia* cysts leads to profound gastrointestinal upset and diarrhea. Flagyl is the antibiotic of choice for treatment with a repeat stool test 1 to 2 weeks after therapy to be certain cysts are no longer being expelled. The use of antidiarrheals is controversial, but they can provide symptomatic relief.

When diarrhea occurs in the wilderness, rehydration is critical. Large fluid losses need to be replenished with 4 to 5 quarts every 24 hours. One method is to use an oral solution recommended by the Centers for Disease Control and Prevention. It consists of alternating glasses of the following two fluid mixtures:

Glass #1: 8 oz fruit juice; $\frac{1}{2}$ tsp honey or corn syrup; one pinch of salt

Glass #2: 8 oz water (boiled or treated); $\frac{1}{4}$ tsp baking soda

Gatorade, available in a powdered form, is more practical and may be used to replace glass #1, except that the water must be boiled or treated. It should also be diluted with twice the volume of fluid recommended by the manufacturer.

The only sure way to prevent giardiasis in the wilderness is to stay away from surface water (even toothbrushing). If the water must be used it must first be disinfected by using either physical or chemical methods. To be most effective, start with the clearest water available. Cloudy, muddy water can be treated by using sedimentation, mechanical filters, or granular activated charcoal purifiers. However, these purifiers used alone are not adequate for disinfection; they do remove bad tastes and odors by absorbing dissolved chemicals. In this sense, they are most useful for removing chlorine and iodine from water after chemical disinfection. The simplest way to disinfect water is to boil it. Any water brought to a boil, even at altitude, is safe to drink.

Chemical methods using halogens (chlorine and iodine) are effective disinfectants for viruses, bacteria, and protozoan cysts. There are several factors to consider when treating potable wilderness surface water. Contact time and the concentration of halogens are inversely related. Thus, the larger the contact time the lower the concentration of halogen required to disinfect the water. Also, cold decreases the action of halogens; in cold water, prolong the contact time for effective disinfection (44). Although effective, a negative to halogen use is the bad taste it imparts to treated water. Taste may be improved by several means:

1. Decrease the amount of halogen while increasing the contact time.
2. Add flavored drink mix after the appropriate contact time.
3. Filter the treated water with granular activated charcoal after the contact time.
4. Use a chlorination/dechlorination purifying system.

Examples of specific halogen doses and techniques are available.

WILDERNESS MEDICAL KIT

The first thing to remember when putting together a wilderness medical kit is that there is no one perfect kit. You cannot carry the local emergency room on your back, but neither should you be caught unprepared. Variations are made for each separate trip based on several parameters.

1. *Pretrip physical fitness and experience.* It is likely that "out of shape" and inexperi-

---

*This list was adapted from the Wilderness Medical Society, Position Statements, 1989:14–15.

enced wilderness explorers will have more medical problems. Pretrip conditioning and planning help avert problems.

2. *The purpose of the trip.* Medical needs for a day hike will differ from those for an extended backpacking trip, or a mountain climbing excursion, or a scuba tour.

3. *The environment or destination.* Terrain, weather, physical activity, endemic diseases, and specific local snakes, arthropods, or plants will all help determine medical needs. Remote trips may place demands on supplies if local people request assistance or medical attention.

4. *Length of the trip.* Although it may seem that longer trips would require a great deal more gear, this may not be the case. Specific supplies may only be needed at certain times (e.g., blister treatment early in a trip), and restocking along the way is frequently possible.

5. *Distance from medical care.* This may not be simply physical distance, but also length of time to outside care. For instance, evacuation from a raft trip through a canyon may be much more time consuming than a rescue from a lengthy mountain hike.

6. *Size of the group.* Larger parties might need more of some supplies but not more of everything. If a kit is larger to serve more people, the extra weight can be distributed to more people, making each person's load lighter.

7. *Preexisting medical conditions.* In addition to regularly prescribed medicines, group members should also take drugs to treat potential exacerbations. Pay attention to physical limitations caused by chronic illnesses.

8. *Level of medical training.* A medical kit should only include equipment that can be safely used given the group members' levels of medical training. It is inappropriate to carry prescription or parenteral medications if no member of the expedition is trained in their use. If necessary, pretrip training can be given for more advanced medical equipment.

Whenever possible, medications and supplies should be chosen so as to have several applications. With these guidelines in mind, Tables 24.2 through 24.5 provide a list of supplies for the wilderness medical kit.

Table 24.2. Basic Medical Supplies

Medical guidebook	Pen or pencil and
First aid report forms	paper
Adhesive bandages	Biodegradable soap,
(Band-Aid),	bar or liquid
various sizes	Steri-Strips or
Sterile gauze pads	coverstrip
(2 × 2″ and 4 × 4″)	closures
Gauze roll (2″ and 4″)	Sterile eye patches
Tape, cloth and	Elastic wrap (2″ and
plastic (1″)	4″)
Mole skin or spenco	Bandana or cravat
2nd skin	cloth
Tincture of benzoin	Cotton-tipped
Thermometer (low-	swabs
reading type)	Sterile eyewash
Scissors, bandage and	Forceps
iris	Scalpel blade and
Tongue blades	handle
Paper clips	Safety pins
Isopropyl alcohol	Tegaderm
(swabs or 70% liquid)	Petrolatum jelly
Penlight	Bulb syringe

Table 24.3. Basic Medications

Disinfectant solution (Betadine or Hibiclens)	Topical antifungal cream
Sunscreen SPF 15 or higher	Oral nonsteroidal anti-inflammatory
Topical antibiotic cream	Codeine 30 mg
Acetaminophen 325 or 500 mg	Prednisone 10 mg
Antacid tablets	Antidiarrheal (Imodium or Lomotil)
Diphenhydramine 25 or 50 mg	Ophthalmic antibiotic
Nasal decongestant	Allergy kit (Ana-Kit or Epi-Pen)
Otic antibiotic	Laxative (Senekot or bisacodyl 5 mg)
Acetazolamide 250 mg	Oral antibiotic (take 2 or 3)
Temporary dental filling (Cavit)	Bactrim DS/Septra DS
Oral sedative (lorazepam or triazolam)	Doxycycline 100 mg
Oral rehydration solution	Ciprofloxacin 500 or 750 mg
Topical steroid cream	Amoxicillin 250 or 500 mg
	Dicloxacillin 250 or 500 mg
	Cephalexin 250 or 500 mg

Antiemetic (promethazine suppositories or pills 25 mg)
Motion sickness medicine (transdermal scopolamine or meclizine 25 mg)

Table 24.4. Advanced Medical Supplies

Oral and nasal airways	Angiocaths
Sterile needles and	Otoscope
syringes	Stethoscope
Ophthalmoscope	Nylon suture
Sphygmomanometer	(3-0 and/or 5-0)
Needle holder	
Hemostats	Splint material
Foley catheter	

Table 24.5. Parenteral Medications

Ceftriaxone (1-gm vials)
Lidocaine 1% (local anesthetic in multiuse vials)
Narcotic analgesic (morphine or meperidine)
Sterile water for irrigation
Hydroxyzine (50 mg/mL multiuse vials)
Corticosteroid (Decadron, Solu-Medrol, Kenalog)

References

1. Meehan RT, Zavala DC. The pathophysiology of acute high-altitude illness. Am J Med 1982;73:395–403.

2. Hackett PH, Hornbein TF. Disorders of high altitude. In: Nadel J, Murray J, eds. Textbook of respiratory medicine. Philadelphia: WB Saunders, 1989:1646–1663.

3. Jacobson ND. Acute high altitude illness. Am Fam Physician 1988;38:135–144.

4. Hackett PH. High altitude medical problems. In: Tintinalli JE, Krome RL, Ruiz E, eds. Emergency medicine: a comprehensive study guide, 3rd ed. New York: McGraw-Hill, 1992:670–677.

5. Moore LG. Altitude-aggravated illness: examples from pregnancy and prenatal life. Ann Emerg Med 1987;16:965–973.

6. Hackett PH, Rennie D, Grover RF, et al. Acute mountain sickness and the edemas of high altitude: a common pathogenesis. Respir Physiol 1981;46:383–390.

7. Johnson TS, Rock PB. Acute mountain sickness. N Engl J Med 1988;319:841–845.

8. Houston CS, Dickinson J. Cerebral form of high-altitude illness. Lancet 1975;2:758–761.

9. Hultgren HN. High altitude medical problems. West J Med 1979;131:8–23.

10. Hackett PH, Roach RC. Medical therapy of altitude illness. Ann Emerg Med 1987;16:980–986.

11. Abramowicz M, ed. High altitude sickness. Med Lett 1988;30:89–91.

12. Zell SC, Goodman PH. Acetazolamide and dexamethasone in the prevention of acute mountain sickness. West J Med 1988;148:541–545.

13. Johnson TS, Rock PB, Fuko CS, et al. Prevention of acute mountain sickness by dexamethasone. N Engl J Med 1984;310:683–686.

14. Levine BD, Yoshimura K, Kobayashi T, et al. Dexamethasone in the treatment of acute mountain sickness. N Engl J Med 1989;321:1707–1713.

15. Hackett PH, Rennie D, Levine HD. The incidence, importance and prophylaxis of acute mountain sickness. Lancet 1976;2:1149–1154.

16. Ferrazini G, Maggiorini M, Kriemler S, et al. Successful treatment of acute mountain sickness with dexamethasone. Br Med J 1987;294:1380–1382.

17. Hackett PH, Roach RC, Sutton JR. High altitude medicine. In: Auerbach PS, Geehr EC, eds. Management of wilderness and environmental emergencies, 2nd ed. St. Louis: CV Mosby, 1989:1–34.

18. Oelz O, Ritter M, Jenni R. Nifedipine for high altitude pulmonary edema. Lancet 1989;2:1241–1244.

19. Schoene RB. High altitude pulmonary edema: pathophysiology and clinical review. Ann Emerg Med 1987;16:987–992.

20. Kalish RS, Johnson KL. Enrichment and function of uroshil (poison-ivy) specific T lymphocytes in lesions of allergic contact dermatitis to uroshiol. J Immunol 1990;145:3706–3713.

21. Guin JD, Kligman AM, Maibach HI. Managing the poison plant rashes. Patient Care 1992;30:63–78.

22. Ives TJ, Tepper RS. Failure of a tapering dose of oral methylprednisolone to treat reactions to poison ivy. JAMA 1991;226:1362. Letter.

23. Wiegel E. Lightning, the underrated killer. NOAA 1976;6:2.

24. Cooper MA. Lightning injuries. In: Auerbach PS, Geehr EC, eds. Management of wilderness and environmental emergencies, 2nd ed. St. Louis: CV Mosby, 1989:173–193.

25. Epperly TD, Stewart JR. The physical effects of lightning injury. J Fam Pract 1989;29:267–272.

26. Craig SR. When lightning strikes: pathophysiology and treatment of lightning injuries. Postgrad Med J 1986;79:109–124.

27. Taussig HB. "Death" from lightning and the possibility of living again. Ann Intern Med 1968;68:1345–1353.

28. Cooper MA. Lightning injuries: prognostic signs for death. Ann Emerg Med 1980;9:134.

29. Gentile DA. Tick-bone diseases. In: Auerbach PS, Geehr EC, eds. Management of wilderness and environmental emergencies, 2nd ed. St. Louis: CV Mosby, 1989:563–587.

30. Centers for Disease Control. Update: Lyme disease and cases occurring during pregnancy—United States. MMWR 1985;34:376.

31. Rahn DW, Malavista SE. Lyme disease: recommendations for diagnosis and treatment. Ann Intern Med 1991;114:472–481.

32. Bonner W Jr. Scorpion envenomation. In: Auerbach PS, Geehr EC, eds. Management of wilderness and environmental emergencies, 2nd ed. St. Louis: CV Mosby, 1989:603–616.

33. Likes K, Bonner W Jr, Chavez M. *Centruroides exilicauda* envenomation in Arizona. West J Med 1984;141:634.

34. Miller TA. Latrodectism: bite of the black widow spider. Am Fam Physician 1992;45:181–187.

35. Rees R, Campbell D, Reiger E, et al. The diagnosis and treatment of brown recluse spider bites. Ann Emerg Med 1987;16:945.

36. Valentine MD. Insect venom allergy: diagnosis and treatment. J Allergy Clin Immunol 1984;73:299.

37. Minton SA, Bechtel HB. Arthropod envenomation and parasitism. In: Auerbach PS, Geehr EC, eds. Management of wilderness and environmental emergencies, 2nd ed. St. Louis: CV Mosby, 1989:513–541.

38. Otten EJ. Venomous animal injuries. In: Rosen P, Barkin RM, eds. Emergency medicine: concepts and clinical practice, 3rd ed. St. Louis: Mosby-Year Book, 1992:875–893.

39. Gold BS, Barish RA. Venomous snake bites: current concepts in diagnosis, treatment and management. Emerg Med Clin North Am 1992;10:249–267.

40. Kunkel DB. Treating snake bites sensibly. Emerg Med 1991;15:161–171.

41. Glass TG Jr. Early debridement of pit viper bites. JAMA 1976;235:2513–2516.

42. Johnson CA. Management of snake bite. Am Fam Physician 1991;44:174–180.

43. Backer HD. Infectious diarrhea from wilderness and foreign travel. In: Auerbach PS, Geehr EC, eds. Management of wilderness and environmental emergencies, 2nd ed. St. Louis: CV Mosby, 1989:759–803.

44. Backer HD. Field water disinfection. In: Auerbach PS, Geehr EC, eds. Management of wilderness and environmental emergencies, 2nd ed. St. Louis: CV Mosby, 1989:805–827.

Bibliography

There are many more unique and exciting areas that are a part of wilderness and outdoor medicine. Physicians interested in obtaining more information in this field are directed to the resources listed below, or contact the Wilderness Medical Society, P.O. Box 460635, Aurora, CO 80046.

Auerbach PS. Medicine for the outdoors. Boston: Little, Brown, 1986.

Auerbach PS, Geehr EC, eds. Management of wilderness and environmental emergencies, 2nd ed. St. Louis: CV Mosby, 1989.

Christopher DG, Rodning CB. Crotalidae envenomation. South Med J 1986;79:159–162.

Forgey WW. Wilderness medicine, 3rd ed. Merrillville, IN: Indiana Camp Supply Books, 1987.

Gill PG Jr. Simon and Schuster's pocket guide to wilderness medicine. New York: Simon and Schuster, 1991.

Iserson KV, ed. Wilderness Medical Society Position Statements. Aurora, CO: Wilderness Medical Society, 1989.

Kizer KW. Wilderness emergencies—be prepared. Emerg Med 30 April 1991:89–102.

Olshaker JS, Tek D, eds. Environmental emergencies. Emerg Med Clin North Am 1992;2:211.

Ravitch MM, et al. Lightning stroke. N Engl J Med 1961;264:36–58.

DRUG ABUSE IN SPORTS

WILLIAM E. MOATS

25

History
Classification
Drug Testing

The illegal use of drugs to enhance athletic ability has an impact on all primary care physicians. Drug abuse in sports is no longer limited to the elite or professional athlete. For the past several years, illicit drug usage has been reported at the junior high and high school levels (1). Vitamins, amino acids, and protein supplements guaranteeing anabolic success abound on shelves of health stores and other commercial establishments. In this environment, the step to illegal performance-enhancing drugs may be easy for the athlete. Anabolic/androgenic steroids, clenbuterol, human growth hormone (HGH), insulin, recombinant erythropoietin (rEPO), blood doping, and amphetamines are at present the common ergogenic drugs available to athletes of all ages, competitive or noncompetitive.

Primary care physicians have an advantage in the prevention, recognition, and treatment of drug abuse in athletes because they provide ongoing care of young patients who become involved in sports. Knowledge of the drug problem, insight into the athlete's goals, and the ability to recognize the subtle physical and emotional changes caused by drug abuse give the physician credibility and rapport with these athletes.

Alcohol remains the drug most universally abused by athletes. This should not be surprising given American culture and the permissive attitude of parents toward alcohol being consumed by teenagers in the home. The various media frequently extol the qualities of alcoholic beverages preferred by both professional and recreational athletes. Anderson and colleagues compared alcohol usage by varsity athletes with the general population of college students at 11 NCAA schools and found almost identical utilization in these two groups (2). Alcohol abuse deserves significant atten-

tion, but it is not unique to athletes and therefore will not be discussed in detail. This chapter on drug abuse in sports provides an understanding of the various classifications of drugs, adverse effects, sources of supply, costs, and a reference table for the more common drugs being abused.

HISTORY

The present dilemma of drug abuse in sports has roots as remote as the third century BC when the Greeks used ground animal bones boiled in oil and roses as "speed." In the 1904 Olympics, a marathoner collapsed, requiring resuscitation after drinking an unlikely combination of brandy and strychnine. Anabolic steroids were reportedly given to Hitler's troops in World War II to increase aggression and were first used in athletic competition by Russian athletes in 1954 (3). In the 1960 Olympic games, a cyclist using amphetamines collapsed during a race and later died (4). In the 1976 Olympics, the East German female swimmers performed magnificently, triggering many accusations concerning anabolic steroid usage, and in the 1988 Olympics, Ben Johnson became the world's fastest human being, aided not by the wind at his back, but by the use of illegal drugs. In 1992 in Barcelona, an American entered in field events tested positive for clenbuterol and was disqualified.

The nature of drugs used by athletes and methods employed to avoid detection continually change. Elite athletes using anabolic/androgenic steroids are training in remote unspecified countries and, prior to returning to competition, are discontinuing the drugs. Physicians dealing with athletes need to 1) accumulate sound information about all forms of drugs being used by athletes; 2) develop a close professional rapport with their athlete patients (the primary care physician should excel in this aspect); 3) be able to recognize symptoms and signs of potential drug abuse (i.e., development of gynecomastia or severe acne); 4) be able to communicate the potential health risks intelligently without dictating to the athlete suspected of drug usage; and 5) not abandon the health care of the athlete who refuses to cease usage. The health of the athlete remains the major concern of all physicians practicing sports medicine, and the primary care physician should be at the forefront of the ongoing battle with drug abuse.

CLASSIFICATION

Medical professionals, coaches, and school officials are often asked to respond to issues concerning drug abuse and drug testing. Responses are diverse but the striking outcome is that the media is asking about "apples" and the interviewee is frequently responding in "oranges" and neither can recognize the discrepancy. A response to the question of "Should our athletes be drug tested?" cannot be a simple "yes" or "no" due to several factors. What kind of drugs will be assayed? Anabolic steroids? Speed? Marijuana? Cocaine? Alcohol? Which athletes will be tested? How often? How expensive will it be? Will the entire student body be tested? Can we single out athletes for certain drugs? Why? What will be done with the results? When will the athletes be tested?

Drugs used in sports fall into three categories: performance continuance, performance enhancement, and recreational, of which the last two are illegal.

Performance Continuance Drugs

The one accepted class is that of performance continuance drugs, which includes: 1) nonsteroidal anti-inflammatory drugs (NSAIDs) such as aspirin, ibuprofen, piroxicam, diclofenac, and naprosyn; 2) asthma preparations such as albuterol and chromolyn sodium; and 3) corticosteroids. Athletes frequently do not recognize the difference between corticosteroids and anabolic steroids and often berate physicians for speaking against anabolic/androgenic steroids while prescribing corticosteroids. Side effects can occur with all of these medications, and judicious usage is imperative when treating athletes. Continued as needed usage of any of these drugs, although legal, is unwise.

Performance Enhancement Drugs

Anabolic/androgenic steroids, amphetamines, HGH, clenbuterol, blood doping, and its synthetic successor, rEPO, are the major agents used to improve performance.

Anabolic/Androgenic Steroids

Anabolic/androgenic steroids are analogues of the male hormone testosterone and were developed to separate the anabolic from the androgenic effects of testosterone. This has been only partially accomplished (5,6). There are two accepted uses for these drugs currently: stimulation of erythropoiesis and promoting sexual development in hypogonadal males (6).

Several theories have been proposed concerning the mechanism of performance enhancement of anabolic/androgenic steroids. Haupt reports that size and strength gains are accomplished via anticatabolic, anabolic, and motivational effects on the athlete (7). The anticatabolic effects are a result of the action of higher levels of cortisol produced by stress or high levels of training (8). The anabolic effects are related to protein synthesis as well as to the stimulation of endogenous HGH release (7). The motivational effects of anabolic/androgenic steroids include aggressive behavior and the ability to endure very intense and demanding workouts (9).

Anecdotal reports of the ramifications of this aggression abound. Athletes report excessive needs to train vigorously, using heavier weights, for longer periods of time per workout. An excellent resource for physicians, coaches, and parents dealing with violence associated with anabolic/androgenic steroid abuse can be found in an article in the October 24, 1988 issue of *Sports Illustrated* entitled "The Nightmare of Steroids," by Tommy Chaiken with Rick Telander. This article chronicles the case history of a Division I college football player trapped in the world of illicit drug usage.

To the contrary, data compiled by Bahrke and colleagues, who used standardized and well-accepted psychological inventories, suggest that while perceived or actual psychological changes possibly occur in anabolic/androgenic steroid users, the study inventories were insensitive to these changes or the effects may have been too subtle to detect (10).

Does the use of anabolic/androgenic steroids actually produce significant muscle mass and strength gains? Studies by Haupt and Rovere suggest a definite increase in the above parameters if the following criteria are met: 1) a strength-training program prior to steroid usage, 2) a continuous strength-training program during steroid usage, 3) adequate dietary protein intake, and 4) measurement of strength gains using free weights as op-

posed to isometric weight-training devices (11,12).

Adverse Effects. The prevalence of adverse effects of anabolic steroids is difficult to ascertain because of underreporting. Some of the adverse effects are known to athletes, so they will discontinue usage, and if symptoms are reversed then no reporting will occur. The fear of disqualification and criminal charges are also deterrents to reporting symptoms.

Adverse effects from anabolic/androgenic steroid usage are known to occur in the cardiovascular, hepatic, reproductive, musculoskeletal, psychological, and endocrine systems. The transmission of hepatitis and the human immunodeficiency virus (HIV) and the development of acquired immunodeficiency syndrome (AIDS) via the use of infected needles must also receive consideration as a side effect. Table 25.1 lists the side effects and reversibility if the drugs are discontinued.

Anabolic/androgenic steroids are used by power lifters and body builders, both male and female, and by shotputters and discus throwers (13). However, it is not uncommon to see these drugs being used by athletes in other sports, as well as by noncompetitors wishing to increase muscle definition, mass, and strength.

Anabolic/androgenic steroids are available in three forms: oral, injectable water based, and injectable oil based. To avoid detection, athletes will frequently use oral or water-based anabolic/androgenic steroids because they are cleared from the system in 3 to 4 weeks. Injectable oil-based drugs are detectable for months. Athletes frequently avoid this last group due to the higher risk of detection. Unfortunately, the oil-based anabolic/androgenic steroids are the safest and produce fewer

Table 25.1. Adverse Effects and Reversibility of Anabolic/Androgenic Steroid Usage

System	Adverse Effect	Reversibility
Cardiovascular	Increased LDL cholesterol	Yes
	Decreased HDL cholesterol	Yes
	Hypertension	Yes
	Elevated triglycerides	Yes
	Arteriosclerotic heart disease	No
Reproductive—male	Testicular atrophy	Yes
	Gynecomastia	Possible
	Impaired spermatogenesis	Yes
	Altered libido	Yes
	Male pattern baldness	No
Reproductive—female	Menstrual dysfunction	Yes
	Altered libido	Yes
	Clitoral enlargement	No
	Hirsutism	No
	Deepening voice	No
	Male pattern baldness	No
Hepatic	Elevated liver enzymes	Yes
	Jaundice	Yes
	Hepatic tumors	No
	Peliosis hepatis	No
Endocrine	Altered glucose tolerance	Yes
	Decreased FSH, LH	Yes
	Acne	Yes
Musculoskeletal	Premature epiphyseal closure	No
	Tendon degeneration	?
Psychological	Mood swings	Yes
	Violent behavior	Yes
	Depression	Yes
	Psychoses	Yes

FSH = follicle-stimulating hormone; HDL = high-density lipoprotein; LDL = low-density lipoprotein; LH = luteinizing hormone.

adverse effects due to the slow rate of absorption.

At present, most of the anabolic/androgenic steroids are obtained via the black market. Due to increased policing by the Drug Enforcement Agency far fewer prescriptions are being written. The majority are being imported from Mexico with correspondingly high black market prices. Table 25.2 compares prescription versus black market prices for some of the more common drugs. A less common source is Europe where these drugs can be purchased over the counter in some countries. There is great concern as to the purity of the product being purchased. Black market drugs are

Table 25.2. Prices of Commonly Abused Drugs

Drug	Retail Price (Approx)	Black Market
Anadrol (Oxymetholone)	$90 for 100 tablets	$300 for 100 tablets
Depo-testosterone (Testosterone cypionate)	$35 for 10 mL	$150–200 for 10 mL
Winstrol V (Stanazolol)	$250 for 30 mL	$300–450 for 30 mL
Equipoise (Boldenone)	$150 for 30 mL	$350–450 for 30 mL
Dianabol (Methandrostenolone)	$100 for 100 tablets	$125–225 for 100 tablets
Anavar (Oxandrolone)	$75 for 100 tablets	$150 for 100 tablets

more likely to be altered, diluted, or substituted for and this may be an increasing problem in the future for drug users due to the difficulty of obtaining anabolic/androgenic steroids legally.

Athletes using anabolic/androgenic steroids do so in everchanging patterns. Hough states users will cycle, spending 6 to 8 weeks taking the drugs followed by a drug-free period of 6 weeks to several months. This cycle is then repeated. Amounts taken frequently are 10 to 40 times higher than therapeutic dosages (12). A common practice is the "stacking" of drugs whereby the athlete will simultaneously take two or more anabolic/androgenic steroids. Stacking seems to be more common than substituting, suggesting that these athletes believe "more of a good thing is better." The drug-free period between cycles in some users has become significantly shortened with continued use suggesting the possibility of an increase in adverse effects and psychological dependence.

Table 25.3 lists many of the more common anabolic/androgenic steroids being used and route of administration.

Clenbuterol

Performance enhancement is not restricted to anabolic/androgenic steroids. In recent years an unlikely class of drugs has been utilized to enhance muscle mass—the β agonists. Clenbuterol, in particular, has been the most widely abused of this group. In the 1992 Olympics, clenbuterol was detected in the urine of an American hammer thrower who was subsequently disqualified. Usage of β agonists as anabolic agents can be traced to veterinary research that suggests that this class of drug appears to enhance lean muscle mass and possibly reduce body fat (14). The logical conclusion that clenbuterol will be utilized in the meat industry is warranted. The Department of Agriculture has condemned the use of meat contaminated with clenbuterol after a reported 156 individuals in France and Spain reported illness due to clenbuterol found in meat they had consumed (14).

The mechanism of action of β agonists may be its direct binding to skeletal muscle membrane receptors, which activates a sequence of events leading to protein accretion, or an indirect route by its action on other target anabolic hormones such as insulin, HGH, and thyroxin. This indirect action may also be a result of vasodilatation that increases blood flow to skeletal muscles and provides substrates for muscle growth (15).

Side effects are those characteristic of β agonists and include headaches, myalgias, dizziness, palpitations, epistaxis, nausea, vomiting, sweating, muscle cramps, and

Table 25.3. Anabolic/Androgenic Steroids Commonly Used by Athletes

Name	Drug Strength	Dosage Used	Route of Administration	Clearance Time
Dianabol (Methandrostenolone)	5 mg	10–150 mg/day	Oral	3–4 wk
Anavar (Oxandrolone)	2.5 mg	10–75 mg/day	Oral	3–4 wk
Anadrol (Oxymetholone)	50 mg	125–200 mg/day	Oral	3–4 wk
Maxibolin (Ethylestrenol)	2 mg	10–20 mg/day	Oral	3–4 wk
Winstrol (Stanazolol)	2 mg 5 mg	20–25 mg/day	Oral	3–4 wk
Halotestin (Fluoxymesterone)	5 mg	10–20 mg/day	Oral	3–4 wk
Primobolan (Methenolone)	2.5 mg	20–25 mg/day	Oral	3–4 wk
Testosterone aqueous	100 mg/mL	300–400 mg/wk	IM (water)	3–4 wk
Primobolan (Methenolone)	50 mg/mL	100 mg/3 days	IM (oil)	3–4 mo
Durabolin (Nandrolone phenpropionate)	50 mg/mL	200 mg/wk	IM (oil)	8–9 mo
Deca-durabolin (Nandrolone decanoate)	50 mg/mL	200–400 mg/wk	IM (oil)	8–9 mo
Testosterone propionate	100 mg/mL	200–300 mg/wk	IM (oil)	3–4 mo
Depo-Testosterone (Testosterone cypianate)	100–200 mg/mL	200 mg/wk	IM (oil)	2–3 mo
Dianabol (Methandrostenolone)	50 mg/mL	100–150 mg/wk	IM (oil)	3–4 mo
Equipoise-Veterinarian (Boldenone)	50 mg/mL	100 mg/wk	IM (oil)	3–4 mo
Finajet (Trenbolone)	50 mg/mL	100 mg/wk	IM (oil)	3–4 mo
Sustanon (Testosterone esters)	250 mg/mL	250–750 mg/wk	IM (oil)	8–9 mo
Winstrol V-Veterinarian Stanazolol	50 mg/mL	150–300 mg/wk	IM (emulsion)	3–4 mo

severe cardiovascular events of myocardial infarction or cerebrovascular accidents.

Clenbuterol is available orally and can be detected in the urine up to 3 weeks after discontinuation. Because of availability and legitimate usage in asthmatics, β agonists have the potential to be the illicit drugs of choice in the future as anabolic agents.

Human Growth Hormone

Human growth hormone has been used by athletes since the early 1980s. HGH is produced in the anterior pituitary gland. A lack of HGH results in the syndrome of dwarfism, but an overabundance as a result of hypersecretion from a pituitary tumor in adults results in acromegaly. Legitimate usage is essentially limited to the treatment of dwarfism. HGH historically has been harvested from human cadavers and therefore limits availability. To complicate matters several fatal cases of Creutzfeldt-Jakob disease were reported in the mid 1980s attributed to the use of HGH (7). This latent appearance of a viral disease is similar to what can be expected if the donors are infected with the AIDS virus. HGH is now becoming available in synthetic form and athletes have been willing to pay exorbitant prices for the drug. Reports range from $1000–$1500 for a 2-month supply to over $10,000 yearly.

Not only does HGH produce significant anabolic changes, it is also virtually undetectable by urine testing. This is an obvious positive benefit to the athlete using HGH. Cowart reports that HGH, in conjunction with somatomedins, inhibits glucose uptake in muscles while increasing amino acid uptake and protein synthesis (16). HGH also stimulates lipid mobilization from fatty tissue, increasing their oxidation and sparing muscle glycogen (17). This may benefit endurance athletes and increase performance as well as strength.

The adverse effects of HGH are those of acromegaly—increased frontal bones and other facial bones, osteoporosis, large hands and fingers, diabetes mellitus, cardiovascular disease, and sexual dysfunction.

The prescribing of HGH as an anabolic agent for athletes is a federal offense, which contributes significantly to its black market acquisition by athletes with the inherent risks of nonhuman (animal) sources, HIV-infected donors, and impure or bogus drugs.

Blood Doping and Recombinant Erythropoietin

Blood doping is the transfusion of red blood cells into athletes to improve the oxygen-carrying capability of their circulation and subsequently improve endurance. The usual methodology requires the removal and freezing of the athlete's blood, usually 2 pints, several weeks or months prior to the planned competition, and then reinfusion shortly before the event. Blood doping was declared illegal in 1985, first by the International Olympic Committee (IOC) and later by the United States Olympic Committee (USOC). Training at high altitudes may produce similar effects and is not illegal, but studies suggest this technique does not work (18). A major difference exists. Blood doping via rapid transfusion is illegal and is more likely to produce side effects than the gradual increase in hemoglobin or hematocrit produced by high altitude training.

Endurance athletes, particularly cyclists, are most likely to blood dope. Marathon runners have also used this method of gaining an advantage. Assuming that blood doping improves performance is logical. However, most of the literature is anecdotal and positive laboratory findings are not necessarily supported in field studies (18).

Detection is difficult and athletes have been unafraid to use blood doping in an attempt to obtain ergogenic effects. The cost is minimal because it involves only needles, intravenous tubing, and freezing capabilities.

In recent years the use of rEPO has become the primary method of blood doping. This drug is readily available to the athlete. Human erythropoietin is produced by the kidneys and stimulates red blood cell production as a response to a decrease in hemoglobin or hypoxia. With the development of the DNA recombinant form (rEPO), availability has not been a problem and it apparently is as effective as natural erythropoietin. The primary legitimate use of rEPO is in the patient with chronic renal disease whose normal production of erythropoietin is compromised.

The use of rEPO in endurance athletes, cyclists in particular, is not without significant potential adverse effects. In a recent 3-year period, 19 cyclists from Belgium and Holland have died and suspicions are high that rEPO may have been used. The likelihood that these highly trained young athletes died from natural causes is questionable. Autopsy findings have been difficult to obtain and official reports have not been helpful. The use of rEPO ablates the normal feedback mechanism resulting in continued production of red blood cells. Not only will the hematocrit rise significantly, but a dramatic increase in blood viscosity ensues once the hematocrit rises to 55% to 60% or greater (19). This sludging effect may cause angina or frank infarction, headaches, transient ischemic attacks, and intermittent claudication. Berglund and Ekblom studied 15 healthy males and found significant elevations in hemoglobin concentrations, hematocrit levels, and submaximal exercise systolic blood pressures after 6 weeks of rEPO treatment (20).

Adding a drug that significantly increases the hematocrit and viscosity of blood in an already naturally dehydrated state that occurs during endurance events is dangerous. This complex picture darkens with the knowledge that a subcutaneous injection of rEPO a few days prior to an event will continue to stimulate erythropoiesis after the race, raising the hematocrit and viscosity levels even higher.

Detection is virtually impossible. At present, using hematocrit levels is being considered as the test of choice with levels over a yet to be decided percent resulting in disqualification of the athlete. Wholesale costs of rEPO run from $24.00 to $120.00 per dose depending on the strength. Retail and black market prices will be significantly higher.

Amphetamines

Amphetamines, commonly known as speed, are also ergogenic. Usage of these psychomotor stimulants appears to be on the decline. Anderson and coworkers reported a significant decrease in usage at the college level between 1985 and 1989 (2). Amphetamines remain illegal to use in athletic competition.

Amphetamines are felt to obscure the athlete's physiologic fatigue level and may also allow the ignoring of pain potentiating further injury. Aggression, as in anabolic/androgenic steroid usage, is possible and psychotic states have been known to occur. Detectability of this class is not as difficult as many of the others, which may deter usage by athletes.

Recreational (Destructive) Drugs

The use of drugs in this classification by athletes or nonathletes signifies abuse in most cases. Describing cocaine, crack, marijuana, heroin, and other psychogenic drugs as "recreational" is oxymoronic. Destructive may be a more fitting title. These drugs are abused equally by athletes and nonathletes. The problem is more societal than sports related.

Use of recreational drugs by athletes is illegal. However, the use of alcohol, the most abused of this recreational class, is not. Until alcohol consumption becomes a problem affecting the athlete's performance, little is said or done.

Smokeless tobacco has been used primarily by baseball players over the years. In 1993, the use of smokeless tobacco was banned in the minor leagues. It is not yet a policy for the major leagues.

Although cocaine is not considered ergogenic, the effects experienced by athletes suggest a psychological performance enhancement. Self-confidence, mental alertness, and well-being increase. Perceived strength and endurance increase, and decreased pain sensation can result. Because the effects are short-lived, usually up to 40 minutes, it is not inconceivable for an athlete to use cocaine on more than one occasion per event. Cocaine has resulted in the deaths of athletes due to the production of ventricular arrhythmias or myocardial infarctions. The sudden death of healthy athletes can no longer be assumed to be due to natural causes, and the use of cocaine/crack must be considered.

DRUG TESTING

As long as illicit drugs are available to athletes striving for a competitive edge, drug testing will be necessary in an attempt to curb such usage. Drug testing is a complex issue. It has been estimated that less than 5% of drug users are detected by present testing techniques. Athletes use drugs such as diuretics to dilute the urine to block detection. Laboratories exist which, for a significant fee, will perform urinalyses for athletes to determine doses of anabolic/androgenic steroids that can be taken without appearing in the urine. While collecting samples, unless absolute direct visualization of both the male and female athletes

urinating is accomplished, the possibility of bogus specimens exists.

The cost of comprehensive drug testing is enormous. The National Football League (NFL) spends over $1,000,000 per year on its testing program. The number of athletes involved in high school and college football is greater than the number of athletes in the NFL. Testing each high school football player once a year would cost over $100 million. To test all high school and college athletes would be cost prohibitive.

The collective cheers of Olympic officials, competing athletes, medical personnel, and the public in general were heard worldwide when Canadian Ben Johnson, the world's fastest human being, was stripped of his title because anabolic/androgenic steroids were detected in his urine. His postdrug performances have been significantly slower, suggesting that anabolic/androgenic steroids contributed significantly to his prior successes.

Johnson's accomplishments impressed high school sprinters. They recognize that anabolic/androgenic steroids assisted Johnson in achieving his records. They know that they can use illicit drugs, perhaps enhancing their chance of college scholarships, and that they will not be drug tested at the high school level. Until affordable testing is available, few school districts will be able to provide monies for drug testing; presently, such affordable testing remains remote. The measurement of total cholesterol and high-density lipoprotein (HDL) cholesterol levels may evolve as a relatively inexpensive screening tool for potential anabolic/androgenic steroid users. A high total cholesterol and a very low HDL cholesterol in an active high school athlete would suggest anabolic/androgenic steroid abuse and could warrant more expensive studies.

Finally, if drug testing is accomplished at any level of competition, it must be clearly defined as to which classification of drugs is being tested. Assaying for performance enhancement (ergogenic) drugs is more expensive than testing for the recreational (destructive) class but, in this author's opinion, it is far more important to detect the former class than the latter.

The use of ergogenic drugs elevates the level of performance of the users establishing a very uneven playing field. This is illegal, unfair, and hopefully one day will cease. The use or abuse of recreational drugs may or may not affect the level of performance of the athlete, and if so, a below par performance may result. It would seem as important, or perhaps more so, to drug test bus drivers, pilots, physicians, and governmental leaders for these recreational (destructive) drugs because their impact on the health and safety of the average citizen far surpasses that of the athlete on the field of play.

What does the future hold? Drug abuse in athletes has become common. It is a certainty that educating athletes stressing the illegality, immorality, and danger of illicit drug usage will not convince 100% of these competitors to remain drug free. Economical drug testing must be pursued and will, unfortunately, remain the most viable method to deter anabolic/androgenic steroid usage.

The primary care physician must be willing to educate athlete patients on the side effects of illicit drug usage. Primary care physicians should attempt to guide potential abusers and continue to establish the rapport necessary to counsel these athletes.

The logical treatment of the drug abuse problem is prevention. Ideally, educational programs to honestly and scientifically present data to athletes concerning chemical abuse are necessary. Attempts should be made to deter usage by stressing the illegality and the adverse effects and emphasizing that many of these drugs used chronically will ultimately shorten careers. Well-designed antidrug campaigns may also be of benefit. Unfortunately, drug testing, or the threat of testing, is the primary deterrent and even though this may exist at all levels of competition in the future, drug abuse will be a continuing problem the medical profession must face.

The role of primary care physicians is paramount and knowledge of these drugs will enable them to care for their athletic family of patients. An athlete must be able to approach the physician without fear of reprisal. Armed with current knowledge the physician will be better prepared to render advice and treatment.

References

1. Yesalis CE, Kennedy NJ, Kopstein AN, Bahrke MS. Anabolic-androgenic steroid use in the United States. JAMA 1993;270:1217–1221.

2. Anderson WA, Albrecht RR, McKeag DB, Hough DO, McGrew CA. A national survey of alcohol and drug use by college athletes. Physician Sports Med 1991;19:91–104.

3. Wade N. Anabolic steroids: doctors denounce them, but athletes aren't listening. Science 1972;176:1399–1403.

4. Prokop C. The struggle against doping and its history. J Sports Med Phys Fitness 1970;10:45–48.

5. Lamb DR. Androgens and exercise. Med Sci Sports Exerc 1975;7:1–5.

6. Goodman LS, Gilman A. The pharmacological basis of therapeutics, 5th ed. New York: MacMillan, 1975:1451–1471.

7. Haupt HA. Anabolic steroids and growth hormone. Am J Sports Med 1993;21:468–474.

8. Barron JL, Noakes TD, Levy W, et al. Hypothalmic dysfunction in overtrained athletes. J Clin Endocrinol Metabol 1985;60:803–806.

9. Haupt HA. Drugs in athletics. Clin Sports Med 1989;8:561–582.

10. Bahrke MS, Wright JE, Strauss RH, Catlin DH. Psychological moods and subjectively perceived behavioral and somatic changes accompanying anabolic-androgenic steroid use. Am J Sports Med 1992;20:717–723.

11. Haupt HA, Rovere GD. Anabolic steroids: a review of the literature. Am J Sports Med 1984;12:469–484.

12. Hough DO. Anabolic steroids and ergogenic aids. Am Fam Physician 1990;41:1157–1164.

13. Loughton SJ, Ruhling RO. Human strength and endurance responses to anabolic steroids and training. J Sports Med Phys Fitness 1977;17:285–296.

14. Goldman B. Clenbuterol the dangers of a new growth drug. Prof J Sports Fitness 1992;Fall:6.

15. Yang YT, McElligott MA. Review article: multiple actions of beta adrenergic agonists on skeletal muscle and adipose tissue. Biochem J 1989;261:1–10.

16. Cowart VS. Human growth hormone: the latest ergogenic aid. Physician Sports Med 1988;16:175–185.

17. MacIntyre JG. Growth hormone and athletes. Sports Med 1987;4:129–142.

18. Eichner ER. Blood doping: results and consequences from the laboratory and the field. Physician Sports Med 1987;15:121–129.

19. Coward VS. Erythropoietin: a dangerous new form of blood doping? Physician Sports Med 1989;17:115–118.

20. Berglund B, Ekblom B. Effect of recombinant human erythropoietin treatment on blood pressure and some haematological parameters in healthy men. J Intern Med 1991;229:125–130.

SPORTS PSYCHOLOGY AND THE INJURED ATHLETE

26

R. KELLY CRACE
CHARLES J. HARDY

When the Injury Occurs
Coping with Injury
Facilitating Psychological Recovery
   During Rehabilitation
Predicting Injury and Injury Proneness

Athletes confront many challenges within the competitive environment that require their use of mental and emotional resources as well as physical talent. One of the most common and stressful challenges is dealing with injury. It is estimated that 17 million sport injuries occur yearly among American athletes (1). This figure indicates that individuals are at significant risk each time they engage in a sport activity and that injuries may be an unavoidable consequence of participation in sport.

Much attention has been given to the causes and rehabilitation of injury in sport. For example, an enormous amount of time and money has been devoted to the design and development of athletic equipment, uniforms, footwear, and playing surfaces. In addition, the field of sports medicine has developed more effective treatment programs to facilitate the rehabilitation process. Although such efforts have yielded positive results, the environmental and physical factors are only part of the story. That is, there is a psychological side of injury as well. Injury may force athletes to accept a new definition of their abilities, redefine their role on the team, withdraw from or change one's current level of involvement, and redirect future career opportunities, both within and outside of sport (2,3). This chapter examines the psychological dimensions of sport injury and the role physicians may play in psychological recovery during rehabilitation.

WHEN THE INJURY OCCURS

Personal Reactions to Injury

Generally athletes view injury as a negative experience to be avoided at all costs (4). But athletes may react to injury in many different ways. Some athletes are com-pletely devastated; others may see injury as an opportunity to assume a new and respected role, such as the "hero," by trying to play through the pain. One of the most important factors that influences athletes' reactions to injury is the degree their identity is invested in being an athlete. Those whose athletic role is a strong anchor for them will experience a much greater reaction than others. Examples include those athletes whose self-worth is dictated by their athletic accomplishments, who pour themselves into athletics to cope with conflict or stress in other roles, or when given the chance to describe themselves focus almost exclusively on their athletic role. That is not to say these attitudes are not valid, but it is an indication that injury will be perceived as much more threatening to athletes with a single role identity.

Nideffer (5) has suggested that the following personal characteristics influence reactions to injury:

- *Perceived control*—Although some athletes perceive that they control their rehabilitation, others prefer to be controlled by an "expert."
- *Self-confidence*—Athletes with low self-confidence may find the injury as well as the rehabilitation process extremely threatening to their self-worth. Those with high levels of self-confidence may bounce back rather quickly, adjust to life without sport more favorably, or find it rather difficult to follow the advice or rehabilitation program that the "experts" have devised.
- *Interpersonal style*—Introverted athletes may withdraw from others, setting up their own private world, whereas the extrovert may try to deny or seek refuge in the social world.
- *Decision-making*—The manner in which athletes prefer to take in information as

well as how they prefer to make decisions is a strong influence on rehabilitation. Whereas the "sensing" athlete may focus on the here and now ("Let's fix this thing and get on with it"), the more "intuitive" athlete may tend to prefer to occupy himself or herself with the possibilities of the injury and rehabilitation ("Will I ever be as good as I was? What are the long range consequences of the injury?"). The "feeling" athlete may make decisions based on emotions and how others will react, whereas the "thinking" athlete may prefer to act on the facts.

* *Patience*—Most athletes desire and are expected to return from injury rather quickly. Perhaps the most important personal characteristic of the athlete, as well as others (e.g., coaches, teammates, parents, trainers), is patience. If the athlete returns to action before he or she is ready, both physically and psychologically, the results can be damaging.

These personal characteristics interact with *environmental factors* such as the athlete's role or status on the team, the practice and competitive environments, the nature of the injury, the time and context of injury, the type of sport, and the expectations of significant others to yield unique reactions to injury.

COPING WITH INJURY

Although reactions to injury do vary based on personal and environmental characteristics, it has been suggested that athletes experience a sequence of predictable psychological reactions following an injury. Rotella and Heyman (6) maintain

that the reaction to injury is similar to responding to loss. Using Kubler-Ross' (7) stage model of reacting to loss, they indicate the following forms of responses through which athletes may progress:

* *Denial*—Downplaying or ignoring the reality of the injury, injured athletes may appear to be in a state of disbelief.
* *Anger*—Expressing anger toward the perceived cause of the injury, athletes may lash out at themselves or others.
* *Bargaining*—Attempting to rationalize or work a deal to avoid dealing with the reality of the trauma, athletes may guarantee good behavior or extra rehabilitation work in hopes of being able to compete sooner than is suggested.
* *Depression*—As the reality of the injury and its consequences become evident, injured athletes may sense a loss of control. They may perceive that they have lost their capabilities and no matter how much effort they expend, they may never attain their preinjury status. Such a perception may cause them to psychologically give up.
* *Acceptance*—Accepting and resigning themselves to the reality of the injury, athletes begin to feel more hopeful of the eventual return to participation and accepting of the rehabilitation process.

Other models have been proposed such as Brown and Stoudemine's (8) stages of shock, preoccupation with the injury, and reorganization. Research by McDonald and Hardy (9) supported a two-stage model involving a *reactive phase*, characterized by shock and negative emotions such as denial, anger and depression. This phase is eventually replaced by an *adaptive phase*, characterized by positive emotions such as acceptance, hope, confidence and vigor.

FACILITATING PSYCHOLOGICAL RECOVERY DURING REHABILITATION

Initial Injury

Crisis Intervention

Because of the intense reactions that can occur from injury, a crisis intervention model has been suggested to deal with the initial injury (6,10). Physicians should take immediate action to direct the process, state limited goals, provide hope and expectations, offer support, provide focused problem-solving, and involve the athlete in the process. The purpose of the crisis intervention model is to restore equilibrium, emotional control, and decrease their sense of helplessness.

Assessment and Communication

Heil (11) has noted that successful rehabilitation and recovery depend on the relative balance of the positive and negative factors associated with athletic injury. On the positive side, athletes typically possess a high level of motivation and strong goal orientation. They typically have good physical training habits and may have had to build up a certain degree of pain tolerance associated with training and competition. The negative factors that may counterbalance the positive are the sense of loss athletes may feel, a threat to their self-esteem, the high demands of sport performance that require more than a return to normal daily functioning, and pressures and expectations that may exist for a quick recovery. It is important for a physician to assess these factors to gain insight as to how the scale may be initially tipped.

Effective communication skills can be the most important psychological "bandages" physicians can possess (12). This involves

being clear and forthcoming on three principal areas:

1. Information about the injury
2. The prescribed program of treatment and rehabilitation
3. Expectations for pain, mobility and recovery

In addition, they should be *active listeners* by expressing empathy for the athlete's situation and offering positive encouragement and reinforcement for progress made. When dealing with an injured athlete it is important to be aware of the stages of emotional reactions, but it is most important for physicians to be *accepting* of these stages. It is one thing to be aware, it is quite another to be accepting of an athlete who is biting your head off or uncooperative because of anger about the injury. Although coaches play a vital role in maintaining an athlete's sense of team membership, the physician plays a vital role in keeping the athlete informed and motivated toward recovery.

Feedback about the rehabilitation process should be delivered in a sincere and personalized manner using the sandwich principle (13–16). In this approach, the primary information to be communicated is sandwiched between affirming and encouraging statement. In general, the process begins by commenting on the progress they have made or the effort they are expending, communicating the primary message, and then ending with encouraging comments as to what the positive consequences will be if they comply with the information. For example, "I can see that you have been putting a lot of effort into your exercises. Over the next few weeks I want you to focus on getting a full range of motion so that your strength and flexibility will be even more effectively increased." This method has the effect of increasing the likelihood that your message is received properly by the athlete without being tuned out because it may have a negative connotation.

Motivation

Injured athletes may have to adjust to a slow recovery process that has very subtle indicators of improvement. Couple this with the emotional difficulties associated with injury and athletes often face motivational problems. Two effective ways of maintaining or increasing motivation during the rehabilitation process are through goal setting and social support (17,18).

Goal Setting

An effective goal-setting program should be developed with close collaboration among the physician and athlete. It is crucial for the physician to get input from the athlete regarding goals and anticipations about recovery. Goals should incorporate every dimension of the recovery process, both psychologically and physically. *They should include short- and long-term goals, be specific and measurable, challenging but realistic, and flexible enough to change if necessary* (17). Physicians play an important role in the reinforcement and feedback of achieved goals. Every accomplished goal, no matter how small, should be reinforced and shown how each step leads the athlete closer to the final goal of full recovery. It is equally important to monitor how realistic the goals are. Athletes may have unrealistically high expectations about the length of recovery and should be shown in clear terms what is a realistic time-table.

Social Support

When an athlete is injured, loss can be experienced as a loss of identity, independence, social mobility, and capacity to per-

form (19). During this period athletes will often seek the support of others to help them cope with the injury (20). It has been reported that the treatment and recovery process is often enhanced by social support (3,18,21–24). But social support refers to much more than being there for someone emotionally as is often the connotation we have with this term. Based upon the work of Pines, Aronson, and Kafry (25), eight distinguishable types of social support have been proposed (22,26,27).

- *Listening support*—Behaviors that indicate people listen to you without giving advice or being judgmental. Listening for how an injury is unique and personal to an athlete rather than rushing into a quick diagnosis can go a long way in making an athlete feel understood and supported.
- *Emotional support*—Behaviors that comfort you and indicate that people are on your side and care for you. Taking a couple of extra minutes to assess how they are reacting to the injury reflects another level of care and support for the athlete.
- *Emotional challenge*—Behaviors that challenge you to evaluate your attitudes, values, and feelings. Those involved in the rehabilitation process who can serve as a sounding board and facilitator for athletes to examine their thoughts and feelings about injury and recovery provide a necessary form of emotional challenge.
- *Task appreciation*—Behaviors that acknowledge your efforts and express appreciation for the work you do. This may come in the form of acknowledging their progress during rehabilitation.
- *Task challenge*—Behaviors that challenge your way of thinking about your work

to stretch you, motivate you, and lead you to greater creativity, excitement, and involvement in your work. As a physician acknowledges an athlete's progress, it can be helpful to explain a next step for which to strive.

- *Reality confirmation*—Behaviors that indicate that people are similar to you—see things the way you do—help you confirm your perceptions and perspectives of the world and help you keep things in focus. A peer modeling network for athletes to talk to athletes who have recovered from similar injuries provides a very effective form of reality confirmation.
- *Material assistance*—Behaviors that provide you with financial assistance, products, or gifts. Something as simple as a brochure or article that helps explain things to injured athletes can be viewed as an important form of support.
- *Personal assistance*—Behaviors that indicate a giving of time, skills, knowledge, or expertise to help you accomplish your tasks. The investment of time and skill into the athlete's injury is most commonly the support athletes believe physicians provide.

These eight dimensions represent three general dimensions of social support: emotional, informational, and tangible social support (22). The degree one feels supported depends on the *availability of people* to whom one can turn in times of need and the *degree of satisfaction* with the support available (22,28). Injured athletes may experience a major change in the availability and satisfaction of support resources. As can be seen, physicians have the ability to provide support in a number of ways and can serve as a facilitator of developing other resources of support.

One of the best ways physicians can facilitate the development of other social support resources is through the use of *peer modeling*. Peer modeling is the process of connecting an injured athlete with another athlete who has had a similar injury and has recovered successfully (24). Talking with other athletes who have "been through it all and lived to tell about it" can fulfill many levels of emotional, informational, and tangible support. Physicians can serve an important function by networking and coordinating peer modeling connections. Physicians may want to ask athletes who are close to recovery if they would be willing to serve as a source of contact for athletes who suffer from similar injuries. An *injury support bank* is then developed for the physician to be able to facilitate communication between athletes to discuss the rehabilitation experience (22). The training room or physical therapy clinic will often function as the injury support bank. Many athletes with similar injuries, at various stages of recovery, may help to provide the injured athlete with the needed social support.

Mental Training Skills

The use of systematic mental training principles have been recognized as important in performance enhancement. The focus on mental training skills during injury rehabilitation not only facilitates the process (18,29) but provides great motivational benefits. Physicians have the opportunity to reframe the injury experience to also be a time to develop a new level of self-regulatory competence that takes their performance to new levels when they return to competition. This is not meant to minimize or disregard the disappointment associated with injury but to allow athletes to see there is some potential future benefit from their

investment in rehabilitation other than
working to return to the same level before
they were injured.

Relaxation

Athletes who are able to relax and maintain a degree of calmness tend to cope better
with the physical and emotional pain of
rehabilitation. Increased muscular tension
or mental overexaggeration of the pain experience can increase one's sensation of
pain. Learning to relax can be as simple as
taking slow deep breaths, scanning the
body for any tension and "letting go" of
any tension in those areas. This facilitates
recovery from injury by reducing pain associated with tension. In addition, relaxation
training allows athletes to regain a sense of
control over their body at a time when they
are feeling at its mercy, facilitates arousal
control, and assists in concentration for
physical or mental training (30). Appendix
F provides a brief relaxation protocol that
can be given to athletes to facilitate their
development of this skill.

Self-talk

Our thoughts and the messages we tell
ourselves play an important role in how we
feel, both physically and emotionally. For
example, athletes during the course of play
may cut themselves or receive a severe skin
abrasion. They may be aware that the injury
to the skin has occurred, but it is not until
after the game when they can focus on the
injury and become concerned about it that
they notice the pain. Appropriate self-
talk can incorporate positive statements
about the reality of the situation and the
confidence in having the ability to deal
with it.

An example is learning how to manage
the pain associated with one of the first recovery stages of knee surgery. In most cases
involving extensive knee surgery, one of

the first tasks for an athlete is to lift the leg
off the bed. This is usually the first step in
physical therapy and a necessary prerequi-
site for being able to leave the hospital. The
very first movement of trying to lift the leg
off the bed is associated with acute pain.
For athletes experiencing this for the first
time, it is common to think that the pain
will continue to increase in intensity as they
raise their leg. This assumption causes them
to begin doubting their ability to cope with
such high degrees of pain and usually results in increased muscular tension, excessive worry, and increased sensitivity to
pain.

A more effective approach would be to
get as much information about the pain that
will be experienced. In this particular situation, the greatest pain is experienced at the
beginning of the movement and does not
increase in intensity. Furthermore, each
time the leg is lifted the pain will gradually
diminish. From this information the athlete
will then be able to say, "Okay, the first time
is the worst. I just have to relax and get over
this first movement. I have already moved
my leg a little and know what to expect
with that first movement. I can take it. Once
I get over this hump I can start the rehabilitation process, go home, and move one step
closer to full recovery." This perspective
allows the athlete to relax and focus on
the task at hand, rather than fearing the
unknown.

Athletes can best cope with pain associated with an injury or rehabilitation by first
fully understanding the nature of the pain
that may be involved, in what circumstances it will occur, how long it will last,
how it will affect mobility, and the difference between pain associated with recovery
and pain that indicates further injury or
nonrecovery. Physicians should be very
clear about these issues throughout the entire recovery process to foster appropriate

self-talk. In other words, coping with pain is associated with reducing the degree an athlete is allowed to wonder about the nature of the pain. You can see this occurring in athletes who have been injured for the first time versus athletes who have undergone the same injury more than once. Athletes injured for the first time tend to exaggerate the senses they are experiencing. Because this is a new experience, they are *less able to differentiate normal pain associated with rehabilitation from pain that indicates further injury.* Athletes who have been through it before, know better what to expect, and allow themselves to remain more calm during rehabilitation (2).

Imagery

Imagery is an invaluable tool for the injured athlete because it can be used to cope with pain, speed up recovery of the injured area, keep physical skills from deteriorating, and improve one's level of preinjury performance (18,29,31). The injured athlete who attends practices and competitions but cannot physically practice should imagine running through all the drills and workouts just as though he or she were actually experiencing them. Vealey (32) notes that imagery can enhance performance and injury recovery by strengthening the neural pathways for certain movements. By systematically practicing sport techniques through imagery, athletes can actually make their body believe they are practicing the skill. Second, imagery may function as a "mental blueprint" to help athletes acquire or understand movement patterns. Third, imagery helps athletes develop a mental set or readiness by focusing their attention on relevant aspects of competition (32).

These explanations have relevance for injury rehabilitation as well. It is important for physicians to encourage athletes to continue visualizing themselves performing in their sport when they are unable to do so physically. Have them create mental practice sessions to maintain skills they have mastered and to work on skills they want to improve. They can also work on issues such as precompetitive anxiety by imagining themselves in situations that normally evoke anxiety and visualizing themselves working through it and coping well. Finally, physicians can use imagery to help athletes cope and manage the rehabilitation process. Creating images for athletes by creatively communicating in detail each stage of the rehabilitation process can allow athletes to visualize the healing process. For example, using metaphors to describe the goals of joint injury rehabilitation, such as ligaments being made up of wound steel and rubber to reflect strength and flexibility (29), may give the athlete a mental anchor to improve motivation and commitment and decrease fear and anxiety. Ievleva and Orlick (18) found the use of such visualization was an important factor in distinguishing between fast and slow recoverers.

Recovery and Re-entry

Typically, returning to athletic participation is a time of high anxiety for athletes. They have been through a long rehabilitation period and are now called on to test how successful it has been. This can be a time of tremendous doubt with athletes questioning the percent of recovery they have made. Obviously if players believe they are only 80% physically recovered instead of 100%, it can have a negative psychological impact on their ability to play at an optimal level. Athletes should recognize that this is a normal reaction and should not become alarmed at this self-doubt.

During this stage, it is crucial for physicians to fully inform the athlete as to what they can expect when they return to practice. Help them understand possible setbacks and obstacles that can occur, as well as positive signs that indicate recovery is progressing well. There also may be cases where 100% recovery will not occur. In these cases, the physicians may be helpful in referring to sports medicine personnel who can assist in the development of performance skills that may compensate for any deficits from the injury or to mental health professionals who can assist in the development of life skills that may facilitate the transition into roles beyond sport (2).

PREDICTING INJURY AND INJURY PRONENESS

Over the past several years, predictive models of injury have been proposed based on personality (33) or the stress-injury relationship (34). The empirical testing of these models is promising but still speculative. The bottom line for physicians is that if an athlete appears to be chronically injured with a variety of injuries or the same injury over and over, consideration should be given to factors that may contribute to their onset. Examination of the situations in which the athlete is injured, understanding aspects of the athlete's personality, or stressful factors associated with elements of the athlete's life outside of sport may help determine whether this is an area of concern (34). Such factors may lead to excessive risk-taking, using injury to avoid a situation with which the athlete feels unable to cope, or using injury to receive greater attention. More extensive psychological evaluation and treatment may be needed.

Referral to a mental health professional for issues related to an injury can be a very sensitive matter and may be responded to with defensiveness by the athlete. This can be minimized by the way in which the athlete is approached. It is recommended that concerns be communicated honestly without accusing the athlete of doing something wrong. The following statement is an example of one way to broach the subject, "Kevin, you have undergone a lot of disappointments with injury over the past 2 to 3 years. It's usually very difficult for athletes to constantly deal with such disappointment when it occurs more than once. Sometimes it can be very helpful to talk with someone about your feelings and thoughts about your injuries. Many times athletes feel more comfortable talking with someone objective who is not associated with the team or your injury. I know of someone who has worked with athletes on helping them deal with the disappointments of injury and develop some skills that may even give you a mental edge when you return to competition. I generally like to encourage athletes to set up an initial appointment with this person to see if it's something in which they might be interested. What do you think?" Such communication demonstrates your concern for the athlete without pointing a finger. It also communicates that this is a normal process and does not indicate that you think there is something wrong with the athlete. We must emphasize, however, that just because an athlete has had more than one injury does not necessarily indicate that there are underlying issues that need to be addressed. Multiple injuries are only small pieces of a total picture that should be considered.

CONCLUSION

The purpose of this chapter was to increase the primary care physician's awareness and understanding of the psychological dimensions of sport injury. In addition, practical suggestions were provided to assist physicians in facilitating the psychological recovery of the injured athlete. Appendix G is provided as a quick reference to the applied principles covered in the chapter. In closing, we would recommend physicians to develop a referral network of mental health professionals that have expertise in dealing with the psychological needs of athletes. Such a network provides the opportunity for periodic consultations, referrals for cases where more extensive counseling is warranted, and being informed of support groups that may develop for injured athletes. Finally, we would encourage physicians to have reading materials related to sport psychology available to their patients. A wide array of publications are targeted toward the athletic population and could be chosen through consultation with a sport psychologist. For a more comprehensive examination of the psychology of sport injury, we recommend two recently published texts: *Psychology of Sport Injury* (Heil, 1993; Human Kinetics); and *Psychological Bases of Sport Injuries* (Pargman, 1993; Fitness Information Technology).

References

1. Booth W. Arthritis Institute tackles sports. Science 1987;237:846–847.

2. Hardy CJ, Crace RK. Dealing with injury. Sport Psychology Training Bulletin 1990;1:1–8.

3. Silva JM, Hardy CJ. The sport psychologist: psychological aspects of injury in sport. In: Mueller FO, Ryan A, eds. The sports medicine team and athlete injury prevention. Philadelphia: FA Davis, 1991.

4. Pargman D. Sport injuries: an overview of psychological perspectives. In: Pargman D, ed. Psychological bases of sport injuries. Morgantown, WV: Fitness Information Technology, 1993:5–13.

5. Nideffer RM. The injured athlete: psychological factors in treatment. Orthop Clin North Am 1983;14:373–385.

6. Rotella RJ, Heyman SR. Stress, injury, and the psychological rehabilitation of athletes. In: Williams JM, ed. Applied sport psychology: personal growth to peak performance. Palo Alto, CA: Mayfield, 1986:343–364.

7. Kubler-Ross E. On death and dying. London: Macmillan, 1969.

8. Brown TJ, Stoudemine AG. Normal and pathological grief. JAMA 1983;250:378–382.

9. McDonald SA, Hardy CJ. Affective response patterns of the injured athlete: an exploratory analysis. Sport Psychologist 1990;4: 261–274.

10. Puryear DA. Helping people in crisis. San Francisco: Jossey-Bass, 1979.

11. Heil J. A framework for psychological assessment. In: Heil J, ed. Psychology of sport injury. Champaign, IL: Human Kinetics, 1993: 73–87.

12. Wiese DM, Weiss MR, Yukelson DP. Sport psychology in the training room: a survey of athletic trainers. Sport Psychologist 1991;5:15–24.

13. Kirkpatrick DL. How to improve performance through appraisal and coaching. New York: AMACOM, 1982.

14. Quick TL. Person to person managing: an executive's guide to working effectively with people. New York: St. Martin's Press, 1977.

15. Quick TL. The Quick motivation method: how to make your employees happier, harder working, and more productive. New York: St. Martin's Press, 1980.

16. Smoll FL, Smith RE. Improving relationship skills in youth sport coaches. East Lansing, MI: Michigan Institute for the Study of Youth Sports, 1979.

17. Heil J. A comprehensive approach to injury management. In: Heil J, ed. Psychology of sport injury. Champaign, IL: Human Kinetics, 1993:137–149.

18. Ievleva L, Orlick T. Mental links to enhanced healing: an exploratory study. Sport Psychologist 1991;5:25–40.

19. Hobfoll SE, Stephens MAP. Social support during extreme stress: consequences and inter-

vention. In: Sarason BR, Sarason IG, Pierce GR, eds. Social support: an interactional view. New York: John Wiley & Sons, 1990:454–481.

20. Hobfoll SE, Stokes JP. The process and mechanics of social support. In: Duck SW, ed. Handbook of personal relationships: theory, research and interventions. New York: John Wiley & Sons, 1988:497–517.

21. Gordon S, Lindgren S. Psycho-physical rehabilitation from a serious sport injury: case study of an elite fast bowler. Aust J Sci Med Sport 1990;22:71–76.

22. Hardy CJ, Crace RK. The dimensions of social support when dealing with sport injuries. In: Pargman D, ed. Psychological bases of sport injuries. Morgantown, WV: Fitness Information Technology, 1993:121–144.

23. Weiss MR, Troxel RK. Psychology of the injured athlete. Athletic Training 1986;21:104–109.

24. Wiese DM, Weiss MR. Psychological rehabilitation and physical injury: implication for the sports medicine team. Sport Psychologist 1987;1:318–330.

25. Pines AM, Aronson E, Kafry D. Burnout. New York: Free Press, 1981.

26. Hardy CJ, Crace RK. Social support within sport. Sport Psychology Training Bulletin 1991;3:1–8.

27. Richman JM, Hardy CJ, Rosenfeld LB, Callanan RAE. Strategies for enhancing social support networks in sport: a brainstorming experience. J Appl Sport Psychol 1989;1:150–159.

28. Sarason IG, Sarason BR, Pierce GR. Social support, personality and performance. J Appl Sport Psychol 1990;2:117–127.

29. Heil J. Mental training in injury management. In: Heil J, ed. Psychology of sport injury. Champaign, IL: Human Kinetics, 1993:151–174.

30. Crace RK, Hardy CJ. Relaxation training. Sport Psychology Training Bulletin 1990;2:1–7.

31. Green LB. The use of imagery in the rehabilitation of injured athletes. In: Pargman D, ed. Psychological bases of sport injuries. Morgantown, WV: Fitness Information Technology, 1993:199–218.

32. Vealey RS. Inner coaching through mental imagery. Sport Psychology Training Bulletin 1990;2:1–7.

33. Sanderson R. Psychology of the injury prone athlete. Br J Sports Med 1977;11:56–57.

34. Andersen MB, Williams JM. A model of stress and athletic injury: prediction and performance. J Sport Exerc Psychol 1988;10:294–306.

APPENDIX F
RELAXATION SCRIPT*

The following script is a relaxation protocol that injured athletes may use during the rehabilitation process. A favorite practice among many athletes is making their own tape utilizing the script presented with combinations of their own favorite music. Most people find it more relaxing to be able to passively listen to script on tape instead of trying to mentally recite it to themselves. Both the music and inflection of the voice should be very soothing to the individual.

As you are getting more comfortable and relaxed in your favorite position, begin slowly bringing your attention inward to focus on your breathing . . . as you do, you may find it easier to slowly allow your eyes to close . . . take some nice, slow deep breaths. With each exhalation, imagine all tension slowly draining from your body . . . feeling very relaxed.

Taking a nice, deep breath, scan the position of your body, and if there are any areas that you would like to make more comfortable by moving them, feel free to spend this time to slowly move yourself into a more comfortable position.

As you take another slow, comfortable breath, focus your attention on your forehead . . . Starting with this area, slowly scan downward over your body and if there are any areas of tension, just focus on these areas and imagine the tension slowly melting and draining down and out of your body and being replaced with a deep sense of relaxation . . . slowly continue scanning your body until all tension has melted away, leaving you completely relaxed.

As you are now feeling relaxed, you can allow yourself to let go completely to a level of even further relaxation . . . Starting with the number 5, count down slowly to 0. Visualize each number in your favorite color . . . with each number, feel yourself getting more and more relaxed and into a deeper state of calm . . . Take a deep breath . . . exhale . . . visualize the number 5 in your favorite color . . . feeling very relaxed . . . 4 . . . going further down, drifting deeper and deeper . . . 3 . . . breathing's getting slower and slower . . . very relaxed . . . 2 . . . going deeper, deeper . . . very peaceful, very calm . . . 1 . . . almost there . . . down . . . down . . . breathing's getting slower . . . deeper . . . 0 . . . very comfortable and relaxed [Allow for several minutes of silence, soft music, or a planned visualization sequence].

[After a few moments] . . . In a moment, begin slowly counting up from 0 to 5 . . . Visualize each number in your favorite color . . . with each number, feel yourself getting more alert and energized. When you reach 5, you will feel refreshed and ready to resume your daily tasks . . . 0 . . . take a deep breath and allow the cleansing oxygen to begin energizing you . . . 1 . . . breathing a little faster . . . becoming more aware of the surroundings around you . . . 2 . . . slowly moving your fingers and toes . . . becoming more alert and aware . . . 3 . . . taking a deep breath . . . coming up . . . more energized . . . 4 . . . slowly moving your arms and legs . . . feeling alert . . . 5 . . . slowly open your eyes and look around (30).

---

* SOURCE: Crace RK, Hardy CJ. Relaxation training. Sport Psychology Training Bulletin 1990;2:1–7.

APPENDIX G
FACILITATING THE PSYCHOLOGICAL RECOVERY OF INJURED ATHLETES—QUICK CHECKLIST FOR PHYSICIANS

Onset of Injury
    Crisis intervention model to restore equilibrium and decrease helplessness
Assessment of Psychological Impact
    To what degree is athletics an anchor role and serves as an important part of their self-worth?
    What has been the nature of previous injuries and what was their recovery history?
    What important environmental factors influence the impact of this injury (e.g., role on team, type of support, expectations of others, time and context of injury)
Facilitating Psychological Rehabilitation
    Effective communication
        Normalize their reactions and empathize
        Genuineness—open, honest, consistent
        Provide information about injury and recovery
        Prescribe program of treatment and rehabilitation

Expectancies for pain, mobility and recovery
        Opportunities for skill development in injury management
        Sandwich principle of feedback
    Motivation
        Goal setting
        Social support
            Assess needed dimensions of social support
            Peer modeling network
    Mental Skills Training for Recovery and Performance Enhancement
        Relaxation training
        Imagery
            Use metaphors to foster rehabilitation images
            Encourage the use of visualization to practice and improve their sport skills
        Self-talk
            Keep athlete fully informed
            Reframe negative thoughts and fears to a more positive focus
    Re-entry
        Normalize anxiety and fears
            Communicate positive signs of progress and possible obstacles

NONSTEROIDAL ANTI-INFLAMMATORY DRUGS

27

TIMOTHY J. IVES

Prescribing Principles
Adverse Drug Events
Selected Drug Interactions
Topically Applied NSAIDs

Nonsteroidal anti-inflammatory drugs (NSAIDs) are one of the most highly prescribed pharmacotherapeutic agents in this country, accounting for over 99 million prescriptions in the United States on an annual basis (1). They are considered to be one of the cornerstones of therapy of the patient with arthritis. NSAIDs have multiple indications for use (Table 27.1), and these agents are available in multiple dosage forms. Table 27.2 provides a listing of the agents, formulations, and pharmacokinetic parameters (e.g., half-life = $t_{1/2}$). Figure 27.1 demonstrates the different chemical classes of NSAIDs.

The primary mechanism of action of the NSAIDs is through inhibition of prostaglandin biosynthesis (2). Prostaglandin H synthetase (also known as cyclooxygenase), is an enzymatic mediator of pain and inflammation that is in the prostaglandin cascade (Figure 27.2) (3). The inhibition of 5-lipoxygenase, the enzyme that produces leukotrienes from arachidonic acid in the prostaglandin cascade, is another mechanism by which pain is diminished. This causes a decrease in the formation of slow reacting substance of anaphylaxis, which has been demonstrated to stimulate peripheral pain receptors. Specific agents that inhibit leukotrienes are under current investigation as a potential therapeutic modality. Leukotrienes have also been implicated in the production of pain. These agents are thought to inhibit both 5-lipoxygenase *and* prostaglandin H synthetase, the enzyme that metabolizes arachidonic acid to prostaglandins. Aspirin has been shown to irreversibly block prostaglandin H synthetase. Interleukin-1, a hormone produced by the immune system in response to injury or infection, serves as an inflammatory mediator to produce pain and swelling (4). It may also be inhibited by these agents, which have the potential to change the course of inflammatory diseases, and not just act as a palliative therapy for pain control. Free oxygen radicals serve as mediators of inflammation, and are inhibited by NSAIDs or acetaminophen.

Table 27.1. Indications for Use of NSAIDs

Acne vulgaris (that is resistant to antibiotic therapy)
Ankylosing spondylitis
Antiplatelet activity
Bartter's syndrome
Bursitis
Cerebrovascular disease (transient ischemic attack, stroke prevention)
Diarrhea (i.e., traveler's, ulcerative colitis, postradiation therapy, or cholera)
Dysmenorrhea
Fever
Glomerulonephritis, acute or chronic
Gout
Hypercalcemia (secondary to malignancy)
Inflammation, acute or chronic
Juvenile rheumatoid arthritis
Menorrhagia
Migraine
Myocardial infarction (secondary prevention)
Ocular inflammation and inhibition of intraoperative miosis during cataract surgery (flurbiprofen sodium and suprofen)
Osteoarthritis
Pain, acute or chronic
Patent ductus arteriosus in premature infants (indomethacin)
Pericardial effusion
Periodontal disease
Polymyalgica rheumatica
Premature labor
Psoriatic arthritis
Premenstrual syndrome
Rheumatoid arthritis
Reiter's syndrome
Sunburn (either orally or topically applied)
Tendinitis

Table 27.2. NSAIDs

Drug	Daily Dosage (mg)	Half-life (hr)
Salicylic Acids		
*Aspirin (various), or Enteric-coated aspirin (Ecotrin, others), or	4000–6000	3
Extended-release aspirin (Easprin, Zorprin, others): 325, 500, 650, 975 mg tablets	4000–6000	4–6
Choline/magnesium salicylate (Trilisate)	3000	
Salsalate (Disalcid)	3000–4000	
Diflunisal (Dolobid, others): 250, 500 mg tablets	500–1500	8–12
Propionic Acids		
Fenoprofen (Nalfon, others): 200, 300 mg capsules and 600 mg tablets	12000–3200	2–3
Flurbiprofen (Ansaid, others): 50, 100 mg tablets	200–300	5.7
*Ibuprofen (Motrin, others): 300, 400, 600, 800 mg tablets; OTC: nuprin, Advil, Motrin IB, Medipren, others (200 mg each); Children's Motrin, Children's Advil: 100 mg/5 mL fruit-flavored suspension for fever (prescription only)	1200–3200	1.8–2.5
*Ketoprofen (Orudis, others): 50, 75 mg capsules; 200 mg extended-release capsule (Oruvail)	150–300	2–5
*Naproxen (Naprosyn, others): 250, 375, 500 mg tablets; 125 mg/5 mL orange-pineapple flavored oral suspension	500–1250	12–15
*Naproxen sodium (Anaprox/Anaprox DS, others Aleve [OTC]): 275 mg (250 mg of naproxen base) and 550 mg (500 mg base) tablets; OTC: 200 mg tablets (182 mg base)	825–1375	12–15
Oxaprozin (Daypro): 600 mg tablets	600–1800	42–50
Indole/phenyl-Acetic Acids		
Diclofenac sodium (Voltaren): 25, 50, 75 mg tablets	50–200	2
Diclofenac potassium (Cataflam): 50 mg tablets	100–225	2
Etodolac (Lodine): 200, 300 mg capsules; 400 mg	600–2400	7
*Indomethacin (Indocin [SR], others): 25 and 50 tablets, 75 (SR) mg capsules; 50 mg suppositories	75–200	4.5–6
Ketorolac tromethamine (Toradol): 10 mg tablets, 15 or 30 mg/mL injections	30–150 30–40 (PO)	3.8–6.3
Nabumetone (Relafen): 500, 750 mg tablets	1500–2000	22.5–30
*Sulindac (Clinoril, others): 150, 200 mg tablets	300–400	8–16
*Tolmetin sodium (Tolectin, others): 200, 600 mg tablets; 400 mg 400 mg DS capsules	600–2000	1–1.5
Oxicams		
*Piroxicam (Feldene, others): 10, 20 mg capsules	10–20	30–86
Anthranilic Acids		
Mefenamic acid (Ponstel): 250 mg capsules	250–1000	2–4
*Meclofenamate sodium (Meclomen, others): 50, 100 mg capsules	200–400	2–3.3
Pyrazolones		
*Phenylbutazone (Butazolidin, others): 100 mg tablets and capsules	100–400	84

* Available generically.

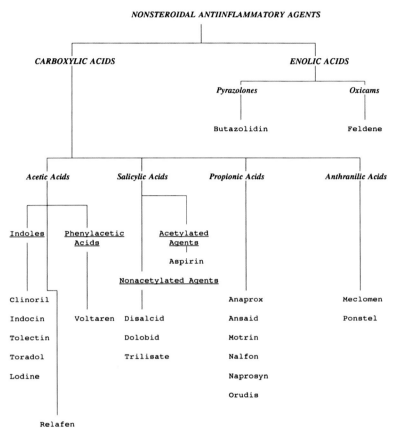

Figure 27.1. Classification of NSAIDs.

In the acidic environment of the gastrointestinal tract, NSAIDs exist in a nonionized state, which contributes to the characteristic adverse events such as nausea, vomiting, diarrhea, or bleeding (5). In the synovial tissue, particularly if inflamed, some NSAIDs in an unionized state (e.g., naproxen) will enter more readily. This may contribute to a longer duration of action than indicated by the $t_{1/2}$ of the drug. The primary route of metabolism for the NSAIDs is via the hepatic system. Alterations in dosage should be considered for patients with altered hepatic function.

Because of its low cost, therapeutic efficacy, and high degree of use, aspirin is still the gold standard by which all NSAIDs are evaluated (6). In general, all of the NSAIDs are at least as effective as aspirin, with less gastrointestinal adverse effects (exception: indomethacin), but at a much higher cost. With once or twice daily dosing regimens with the agents that have longer $t_{1/2}$ (e.g., piroxicam or naproxen), improvement in compliance is also a big factor.

PRESCRIBING PRINCIPLES

The choice of which NSAID to prescribe is based on several factors:

- The relative safety and efficacy for each particular patient
- Adverse event profile

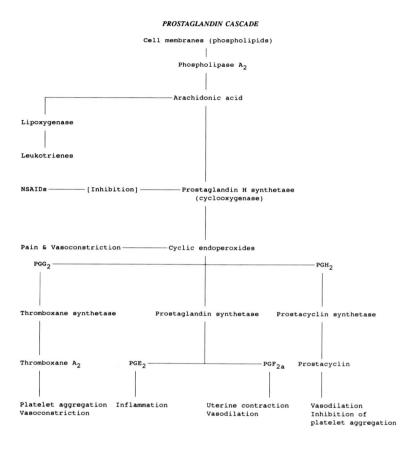

Figure 27.2. Prostaglandin cascade.

- Concomitant disease states
- Other medications used (either acute or chronically)
- Age of the patient
- Personal preference of the prescriber
- Cost (a major factor in the selection of over-the-counter [OTC] products)

No single agent has a predominant role based on its pharmacologic differences. Some of the most common mistakes in prescribing NSAIDs include: prescribing inadequate dosages (usually too low), exceeding the maximum dosage by great amounts, failing to give an adequate trial of efficacy of at least 3 to 4 weeks before making a therapeutic assessment, and using combinations of NSAIDs concomitantly or with aspirin, which may lower NSAID blood levels and therefore, therapeutic efficacy (7,8). In addition, no evidence exists to suggest that a combination of NSAIDs has any greater efficacy over the use of one agent alone.

Individualization of NSAID pharmacotherapy is based on several principles:

1. Similar to the use of any drug, prior to starting treatment (or even new treatments), take a medication history to determine the response to previous NSAID pharmacotherapy. Some patients will respond to one agent (or class of agents) better than others.

2. In older patients, use NSAIDs with shorter half-lives to avoid accumulation and the resulting adverse drug events. Start at lower initial doses in this population. These agents may be best reserved for inflammatory problems such as overuse syndromes, bursitis, tendinitis, or osteoarthritis. Older patients should be given an initial prescription for a limited period and carefully followed for the possible development of gastrointestinal, hepatic, renal, or cutaneous adverse drug effects. Older patients should have renal and hepatic function monitored routinely if chronic use is being considered.

3. Patient response is variable and unpredictable, but some disorders may respond better to one drug than another.

4. Continue the drug for a sufficient time (4 to 10 days for acute problems and at least 3 to 4 weeks for chronic problems) to allow for a full pharmacologic response. If relief is inadequate at this point, increase the dosage. If the higher dosage is still inadequate after another 3 to 4 weeks, then switch to another NSAID with a similar half-life and adverse effect profile, preferably in a different category. To prevent a return of the original symptoms (rebound), overlap the two NSAIDs for 2 to 3 days.

5. If a treatment failure occurs at this point, first consider the dose, frequency of administration, and patient adherence to the drug or its regimen before switching to another agent.

6. Tailor the drug regimen to a patient's life-style to improve compliance.

7. Consider placebo therapy in special cases. Also, consider the placebo effect as a part of the expressed response during the first few days to weeks of therapy, especially when doses are still low. If there is no perceived benefit within the first few days, there probably will not be one at all due to patient bias, and only a 2-week prescription should be filled initially to reduce potential waste. A patient may need several different therapeutic trials before finding a good product and regimen.

8. When a pharmacotherapeutic regimen is successful, decrease the dose to a maintenance level, if possible. Using the lowest effective dosage and instructing patients to take NSAIDs with meals may help to prevent gastrointestinal distress. If it does occur, consider the use of antacids, although they may decrease the absorption of the NSAIDs. Alternatives to antacids include H_2-blockers, sucralfate, and misoprostol.

9. Discontinue pharmacotherapy during remissive periods, if possible.

10. In many cases, a less frequent dosing schedule (e.g., every day or twice a day) may be the most significant factor for adherence to a regimen. In addition, always consider the cost of treatment, based on the monthly price of the selected agent to the patient, and the selected dosing schedule. Generic aspirin is the least expensive NSAID, and generic ibuprofen is the least expensive of the more recent NSAIDs. In comparison, agents such as ketorolac or oxaprozin, both of which are relatively new on the market and do not have a generic substitute, are two of the most expensive NSAIDs available (e.g., monthly cost to the patient: $75 to $130). Based on the success of OTC ibuprofen, several pharmaceutical companies are developing OTC versions of their prescription NSAIDs.

Most recently, naproxen sodium (Aleve) was released.

Nonacetylated salicylates (e.g., diflunisal, salsalate, etc.) have no effect on platelet function, cause no significant gastrointestinal bleeding, and have a less frequent dosing regimen than regular aspirin, and therefore may be a good alternative to aspirin, although they are more expensive. Although it is found as an adjuvant for the provision of analgesia, caffeine, especially in higher doses, can intensify pain. Cutting down or removing the use of nicotine or stimulants may also help in pain relief. NSAIDs should always be considered a good adjunct to opiate agents for pain control.

ADVERSE DRUG EVENTS

The NSAIDs account for just over 20% of all adverse drug events reported to the Food and Drug Administration (FDA) (9). Because of nonlinear (i.e., zero-order) pharmacokinetics, with the use of higher doses of aspirin (e.g., 150 to 300 mg/kg taken acutely, or >100 mg/kg when taken chronically), incremental dosage increases produce large elevations in the serum level due to saturation of the routes of salicylate elimination. Approximately one person in 100 who takes aspirin will develop an allergic reaction, with asthmatic patients experiencing a rate twice that (10). Every patient who is taking NSAIDs should be warned about these potential adverse effects and instructed to stop taking the drug if any symptoms appear (Table 27.3). The American College of Rheumatology has developed a monitoring schedule for patients taking NSAIDs, which includes an initial complete blood count, urinalysis, serum creatinine, potassium, and glutamic-oxaloacetic transaminase tests. These tests

should be repeated every 1 to 3 months until values are stable, and then rechecked every 3 to 12 months, depending on the individual patient.

Safe use in pregnancy is *not* well established in controlled studies. The FDA categorization for assessing risk to the fetus is as follows: Category B (no adequate studies in pregnant women): diclofenac, flurbiprofen, ketoprofen, and naproxen; Category C (no adequate studies in nonpregnant women): etodolac, ketorolac, mefenamic acid, nabumetone, oxaprozin, and tolmetin; and Category D (evidence of human fetal risk): aspirin should *not* be used routinely during pregnancy, unless specifically prescribed during the third trimester for preeclampsia. Because most NSAIDs are excreted in breast milk, use while lactating is not recommended. *If necessary*, only use ibuprofen, and at rec-

Table 27.3. Patient Information on the Use of NSAIDs

1. Avoid aspirin and alcoholic beverages while taking this medication.
2. If gastrointestinal upset occurs, take it with food, milk, or antacids. If these symptoms persist, contact your physician.
3. This drug may cause drowsiness, dizziness, or blurred vision; use caution when driving or performing tasks that require concentration and alertness.
4. Notify your physician if skin rash, itching, visual disturbances, weight gain, edema, black stools, or persistent headache occur.
5. Mefenamic acid: If a rash, diarrhea, or digestive problems occur, discontinue use and contact your physician.
6. Ibuprofen (OTC use): Do not take for more than 3 days for fever or 10 days for pain. If these symptoms persist or worsen or if new symptoms develop, contact your physician or pharmacist.

ommended OTC doses. Acetaminophen is a safe alternative for pain and fever control (11).

In children, avoid the use of mefenamic acid, meclofenamate, or indomethacin in children under age 16. Elevated liver enzymes and hepatotoxicity associated with their use have been reported. Although other agents are under study, tolmetin and naproxen are the only FDA-recognized agents for use in children greater than 2 years of age for juvenile rheumatoid arthritis. The use of aspirin is contraindicated for children under the age of 16 due to numerous reports of Reye syndrome.

The following are selected adverse drug events to consider when prescribing NSAIDs.

- *Gastrointestinal effects*: Nausea, vomiting, diarrhea, occult blood in the stool and constipation. One to 2% of patients taking NSAIDs for more than 3 months will experience gastric ulceration, bleeding, or perforation (12). A confounding variable in this statistic is that although age greater than 60 has classically been considered a risk factor for gastrointestinal problems (13), as people age, there is an increased risk of ulceration, independent of the use of NSAIDs or other ulcerogenic substances. In addition to age, other associated risk factors include: 1) history of peptic ulcer disease, 2) concomitant use of other agents with ulcerogenic potential (e.g., warfarin, prednisone), 3) concurrent use of two or more NSAIDs, and 4) high-dose NSAID use. Although not as clearly defined as risk factors for gastrointestinal problems, the following should also be considered: 1) gender (i.e., female), 2) history of NSAID-induced gastrointestinal adverse drug events, 3) class of NSAID used, and

4) brief duration of use of NSAIDs (thought to be due to gastric mucosal adaptation over time with continued use of the NSAID). Adequate hydration should be ensured to minimize the risk of renal toxicity. Indomethacin has the highest association of ulceration with bleeding. Anthranilic acid products (Ponstel, Meclomen) have a high rate (10% to 33%) of diarrhea when used *longer than* 7 days. In one retrospective study, ibuprofen, salsalate, and enteric-coated (or buffered) aspirin were considered the least toxic, with indomethacin, meclofenamate, and tolmetin having the highest risk of gastrointestinal toxicity. Many athletes experience joint and muscle soreness 8 to 24 hours after strenuous exercise, and in a belief that premedication with aspirin or other NSAIDs before exercise improves postexercise soreness, significant gastrointestinal bleeding has occurred.

- *Central nervous system*: Dizziness (3% to 9%). Frontal headache has been reported in 10% of patients receiving indomethacin and in 3% to 9% taking meclofenamate, tolmetin, naproxen, fenoprofen, and ketoprofen (14).
- *Hepatic*: Elevated liver function tests are found in approximately 15% of patients taking NSAIDs (15). Pancreatitis has been reported in patients taking sulindac.
- *Hematologic*: Prolongation of bleeding time (occurs with both aspirin and NSAIDs). Patients taking chronic aspirin therapy or an NSAID with a long half-life who are preparing to undergo surgery (i.e., either medical or dental) should have the medication discontinued several days to a week prior to the procedure. Bone marrow suppression has been reported with the use of all of

the NSAIDs, but the older agents have much greater risk of producing this adverse effect.

- *Cardiovascular*: Congestive heart failure (CHF). Because NSAIDs are commonly used in patients concomitantly receiving antihypertensive pharmacotherapy, decreased control of blood pressure is often seen (16). This occurs by an NSAID-induced decrease in renal vasodilation (which is mediated by prostaglandins), sodium retention, or changes in the body's response to renin or angiotensin II. Indomethacin is considered to be the agent with the greatest effect on blood pressure because it is the most potent prostaglandin inhibitor, but may be clinically significant in a subset of hypertensive patients (17). As a consequence of this action, peripheral edema and fluid retention (5% to 10%) are also seen.
- *Renal*: Closely monitor patients with CHF, liver disease (especially if ascites is present), impaired renal function (with or without proteinuria), or who are receiving diuretics. Watch for oliguria, increases in serum creatinine and blood urea nitrogen, and fluid retention. In these patients, this may be manifested as weight gain, shortness of breath, peripheral edema, and generalized fatigue (18). Also, acute renal failure may occur, especially in patients with impaired renal function, proteinuria, oliguria, or cystitis that is slow to resolve. Patients with diabetes that take NSAIDs may be at greater risk for renal failure and papillary necrosis.
- *Rheumatologic*: NSAIDs inhibit the synthesis of proteoglycan, leading to cartilage destruction. Although reports have described "indocin hip," the definitive assessment of this effect remains to be determined.

- *Dermatologic*: Piroxicam can produce an erythematous maculopapular rash with pruritus that may progress to vesicular lesions over a variable time period, ranging from several hours to 2 weeks. The use of sulindac or ibuprofen has also been associated with rare photosensitivity reactions. Patients with aspirin sensitivity (e.g., asthma, rhinitis, urticaria, nasal polyps, angioedema, bronchospasm or sensitivity to tartrazine [FDC #5] dye) will exhibit a cross-sensitivity to NSAIDs. Porphyria-like reactions have been reported with all NSAIDs, with naproxen being reported most frequently.
- *Special senses*: Visual disturbances, retinal degeneration, conjunctivitis, facial edema, tinnitus, hearing disturbances or loss, reversible loss of color vision, blurred vision, changes in taste, dizziness, drowsiness.

SELECTED DRUG INTERACTIONS

Due to a high degree of plasma protein binding, NSAIDs can displace other highly protein-bound drugs. The following are some of the clinically significant drug-drug interactions (19).

- *Angiotensin-converting enzyme inhibitors* (e.g., captopril, enalapril): A blunting of the antihypertensive effect is seen when given concurrently with indomethacin, and to a lesser extent, with sulindac.
- *Aspirin*: Decreased activity and blood level of the NSAIDs when used concomitantly. The gastrointestinal adverse events may be increased. The clinical significance is questionable, but if possible, avoid using them together.
- *β Blockers*: Reduction of antihypertensive action in some patients due to NSAID-induced reduction in pros-

taglandin activity. Also, reduction in prostaglandins causes an increase in α-adrenergic receptor sensitivity and receptor tone.

- *Ethanol*: Increased gastritis and gastrointestinal blood loss.
- *Lithium*: Increased plasma lithium levels are seen when taking ibuprofen, indomethacin, or piroxicam.
- *Loop or thiazide diuretics*: Reduced natriuretic and antihypertensive effects seen in some patients also receiving indomethacin through inhibition of plasma renin activity. This effect is also seen with other NSAIDs (e.g., ibuprofen), but the effect is still in question.
- *Oral hypoglycemic agents*: Enhanced hypoglycemic activity due to displacement from albumin binding sites with older agents such as tolbutamide or chlorpropamide. May also be seen with glipizide or glyburide, but to a lesser extent.
- *Phenytoin*: Inhibition of metabolism by aspirin.
- *Probenecid*: Doubling of serum indomethacin levels due to inhibition of renal elimination. Also seen with most other agents.
- *Warfarin*: Increased hypoprothrombinemic effect when given with aspirin because NSAIDs inhibit platelet aggregation. Use with caution with all others.

TOPICALLY APPLIED NSAIDS

Topical OTC products that contain trolamine salicylate (e.g., Aspercreme, Sportscreme, or Myoflex) are thought to act by peripheral inhibition of prostaglandins via topical administration to the dermis or by stimulating sensory nerves, which compete with pain signals from the affected area for transmission to higher centers of the central nervous system, but no definitive explanation of the mechanism of action exists (20). Although data exist to demonstrate that trolamine salicylate is absorbed from the skin, the FDA still does not have sufficient data to demonstrate that the quantity absorbed is sufficient to produce effective analgesia. Trolamine salicylate lacks the odor found in methyl salicylate (Oil of Wintergreen) products (Ben-Gay, Icy Hot, etc). For the most part, any effect that does occur is minor when compared to systemic therapy or may be a placebo effect as many patients using this type of product are taking concurrent NSAIDs or acetaminophen. Penetration of these topical agents has been shown to improve when applied with ultrasound massage. Topical preparations of NSAIDs (e.g., ibuprofen, piroxicam, and others in a cream or gel formulation) are available in Europe, but none have come to the market to date in the United States. These products are thought to exert an effect with the production of therapeutic serum levels of the active ingredient in the affected soft tissue/synovial fluid without production of high serum levels. Data on the efficacy of these agents suggest that 40% to 60% of patients respond to placebo preparations, with 65% to 80% responding to the active agent.

References

1. Kaplan B, Swain RA. NSAIDs: are there any differences? Arch Fam Med 1993;2:1167–1174.

2. Brooks PM, Day RO. Nonsteroidal antiinflammatory drugs—differences and similarities. N Engl J Med 1991;324:1716–1725.

3. Weissmann G. The actions of NSAIDs. Hosp Pract 1991;26:60–76.

4. Ishihara Y, Nishihara T, Maki E, et al. Role of interleukin-1 and prostaglandin in in vitro bone resorption induced by *Actinobacillus*

actinomycetem-comitans lipopolysaccharide. J Periodont Res 1991;26:155–160.

5. Brune K, Graft P. Non-steroid anti-inflammatory drugs: influence of extracellular pH on biodistribution and pharmacological effects. Biochem Pharmacol 1978;27:525–530.

6. Hadler NM. The argument for aspirin as the NSAID of choice in the management of rheumatoid arthritis. Drug Intell Clin Pharm 1984;18:34–38.

7. Miller DR. Combination use of nonsteroidal antiinflammatory drugs. Drug Intell Clin Pharm 1981;15:3–7.

8. Jacobs J, Goldstein AG, Kelly ME, et al. NSAID dosing schedule and compliance. Drug Intell Clin Pharm 1988;22:727–728.

9. Fries JF, Williams CA, Bloch DA. The relative toxicity of nonsteroidal antiinflammatory drugs. Arthritis Rheum 1991;34:1353–1360.

10. Lanza FL, Royer GL, Nelson RS. Endoscopic evaluation of the effects of aspirin, buffered aspirin, and enteric-coated aspirin on gastric and duodenal mucosa. N Engl J Med 1980;303:136–138.

11. Ives TJ, Tepper RS. Drugs in pregnancy and lactation. Primary Care 1990;17:623–645.

12. Gabriel SE, Jaakkimainen L, Bombardier C. Risk of serious gastrointestinal complications related to the use of nonsteroidal anti-inflammatory drugs. A meta-analysis. Ann Intern Med 1991;115:787–796.

13. Langman MJS, Wei J, Wainwright P, et al. Risks of bleeding peptic ulcer associated with individual non-steroidal anti-inflammatory drugs. Lancet 1994;343:1075–1078.

14. Simon LA, Mills JA. Nonsteroidal antiinflammatory drugs. N Engl J Med 1980;302:1179–1185, 1237–1243.

15. Lewis JH. Hepatic toxicity of nonsteroidal anti-inflammatory drugs. Clin Pharmacokinet 1984;3:128–138.

16. Oates JA. Antagonism of antihypertensive drug therapy by nonsteroidal anti-inflammatory drugs. Hypertension 1988;11:114–116.

17. Pope JE, Anderson JJ, Felson DT. A meta-analysis of the effects of nonsteroidal anti-inflammatory drugs on blood pressure. Arch Intern Med 1993;153:477–484.

18. Clive DM, Stoff JS. Renal syndromes associated with nonsteroidal antiinflammatory drugs. N Engl J Med 1984;310:563–572.

19. Shiloul MZ, al-Kiek R, Ivanovich P, et al. Nonsteroidal anti-inflammatory drugs and antihypertensives. Nephron 1990;56:345–352.

20. Editorial. Topical NSAIDs: a gimmick or a godsend? Lancet 1989;2:779–780.

INDEX

A

ABCDE mnemonic, 137

Abdomen, preparticipation
evaluation, 64

Abdominal injuries
anatomy, normal, 151–152
assessment, 160–161
colon and rectum, 166–167
diaphragm, 165
duodenum, jejunum, and ileum,
166
genitourinary system, 167–172
hernias, 167
"hip pointers," 160
hollow viscus, 165–166
initial assessment, 152–155
intra-abdominal, overview, 160–
162
intra-abdominal, specific organs,
162–167
liver, 164
mesentery, 167
muscle, 156–159
pancreas, 164–165
skin, 155–156
solar plexus, blows to, 159–160
spleen, 162–164
stomach, 166
subcutaneous tissue, 156

Abduction, shoulder, 226, 227

Abrasions
chest wall, 143–144
corneal, 131–132

Acclimation, heat, 529–531

Achilles tendinitis, 509–511

Achilles tendon, 452–453

Achilles tendon rupture, 511–512

Acromioclavicular arthritis, 253–
254

Acromioclavicular joint injuries
acute, 247–248
anatomy, normal, 212, 248
history, 248–250
medical clearance, 253
physical examination, 250–251
radiologic evaluation, 233, 251
treatment, 251–253

Acromion fractures, 242

Acupuncture, 204

Acute compartment syndrome,
489–491

Acute epidural hemorrhage, 89–90

Acute high-altitude illness, 633–
635

Acute mountain sickness, 633, 634

Acute subdural hematoma, 90–91

Adduction, shoulder, 226, 227

Adductor longus muscle, 369, 373–
374

Adolescents. *See* Young athletes

Adson's test, 271

Adult recreational leagues, 46

Advanced Trauma Life Support
(ATLS), 137

Aerobics
back injuries, 185
pregnancy and, 627

Aging, exercise and, 14–16

Airway patency, 137–138, 139, 247

Alcohol use, 61, 137, 544, 633, 663

Amenorrhea, 380, 617–619, 620–
621

American Medical Society for
Sports Medicine, 36

Amnesia, 78–79, 84–85, 87

Amphetamines, 662

Anabolic/androgenic steroids, 655,
660

Anaerobic capacity/threshold, 20

Anemia, exercise physiology of,
16–17, 597

Ankle injuries
anatomy, normal, 447–449
biomechanics, 447–449
chronic instability, 457–459
diagnostic tests, 454–455
fractures, 461–464
history, 450, 457
peroneal tendon subluxation/
dislocation, 459–460
peroneal tenosynovitis, 460–461
physical examination, 450–453
preparticipation evaluation, 63
prevention, 456–457
rehabilitation, 464–466
sprains, 449–457
treatment, 455–456, 459

Ankle jerk reflex, 188

Ankylosing spondylitis, 200

Annular flexor pulleys rupture,
344–346

Anomalous coronary arteries, 568–
569

Anorexia nervosa, 600–601

Anterior cord syndrome, 117–118

Anterior cruciate ligament (ACL)
anatomy, normal, 393
assessment, 404

combined injuries, MCL and,
418
injuries, 395–396, 413–416

Anterior drawer test
ankle injuries, 453
knee injuries, 402
shoulder injuries, 255, 257

Anterior glenohumeral instability,
258–264

Anterior knee overuse injuries,
427–434

Anterior subluxations,
glenohumeral, 262–264

Aorta, coarctation of, 567

Aortic regurgitation, 570–571

Aortic rupture, traumatic, 141

Aortic stenosis, 569–570

Apley's grind test, 408, 421

Apprehension test
anterior/posterior shoulder
instability, 231, 256, 257
patellofemoral stability, 406
posterior glenohumeral
instability, 264

Arachnids, 641, 642–643

Arrhythmias, exercise prescription,
574–575

Arthritis
acromioclavicular, 253–254
exercise and, 11–12

Arthrography
knee, 408–409
shoulder, 235

Arthropods, venomous, 641–644

Arthroscopy, shoulder, 237

Asthma
exercise-induced, 59–60, 548–
553
NSAIDs and, 688
performance continuance drugs,
656
sports participation limits of,
59–60

Athletes. *See also* Exercise
physiology; Female athletes;
Preparticipation evaluation
(PPE); Young athletes
cardiovascular dynamics,
changes in, 17–18, 138
head injuries and, 85–86
recreational, 38, 46

Athletic heart syndrome, 17–18

Athletics, community, 45–47. *See
also* School athletics

Atlanto-dens interval, 114
Atrial arrhythmias, 574
Atrial septal defect, 566
Avulsion
    fracture, medial epicondylar, 301
    volar plate, PIP joint, 349–350
Axillary artery occlusion, 277
Axillary nerve injuries, 272–273

B
Back injuries
    anatomy, normal, 180–184
    differential diagnosis, 195–201
    facet syndrome, 201
    fractures/contusions, 197
    history, 186
    intervertebral disk disease, 196–197
    physical examination, 186–195
    radiologic evaluation, 201–202
    risk factors for, 179–180
    spinal abnormalities, 197–201
    sports-specific, 184–186
    treatment, 202–206
"Backpacker's diarrhea," 646
Baker's cysts, 434, 435–436
Bankart lesions, 236
Baseball finger, 336–338
Baseball pitching, shoulder
    kinematics, 217–218
Basilar skull fractures, 83–84
Battle's sign, 83
"Beaver fever," 646
Bee stings, 643–644
Bennett's fracture, 357–358
β-agonists
    asthma, 552
    performance enhancement
        drugs, 659
Biceps muscle rupture, 276
Biceps tendon
    distal, rupture of, 301–302
    subluxation, 277
Bicycling
    genitourinary injuries, females,
        616
    injury prevention, 91
    pregnancy and, 626
"Bicyclist's bladder," 171
"Bicyclist's nipples," 146, 614
Bioelectrical impedance, 588
Biomechanics
    ankle, 447–449
    foot injuries, 501–505

lower leg, abnormal, 475–476
    shoulder, 215–219
Bipartite sesamoid, bilateral, 522
Black widow spiders, 642–643
Blacknail, 523
Bladder injuries, 171
Bleeding. See Hemorrhage
Blood doping, 661–662
Blood pressure. See Hypertension
Blow-out fracture of orbit, 131,
    133
Body composition, 585–588. See
    also Weight, body
Body mass index (BMI), 585
Body temperature. See Cold-
    related illness; Heat illness
Bone scans, 478, 481, 484
Bones. See Musculoskeletal system
Boutonniere injury, 338–341
Boxer's fracture, 355
Boxing injuries, prevention, 91–92
Braces and bracing
    ankles, 456–457
    back, 203
    elbow/wrist, 305
    knees, 441
    lower leg injuries, 488
Brachial plexus
    anatomy, 102, 238
    injury, 59, 103, 116, 272
Brain injuries. See also Head
    injuries
    diffuse, 84–88
    pathophysiology, 75–76
Breast injuries, female athletes,
    143, 614–616
"Breath knocked out, having the,"
    143, 159
Brown recluse spiders, 642, 643
Brown-Séquard syndrome, 117–
    118
Buckled knee, 396, 422, 428
Buddy-taping, fingers, 335, 350,
    355
Bulimia, 600–601
Burners. See Stingers/burners
Bursitis
    greater trochanteric, 377–378
    iliopsoas, 378
    infrapatellar, 432
    knee, 433–434
    olecranon, 313
    prepatellar, 429, 430–431
Burst fracture, 113

C
Caffeine, 602
Carbohydrate loading, 591, 592
Carbohydrates, dietary recommen-
    dations, 590–591
Cardiac rehabilitation, 577–578
Cardiac tamponade, 140
Cardiopulmonary resuscitation
    (CPR), 41, 636
Cardiovascular disease (CVD). See
    also Coronary artery disease;
    Exercise-related sudden death
    (ERSD); Hypertension
    arrhythmias, 574–575
    conduction disturbances, 575–
        576
    congenital, 566–569
    exercise, benefits/risks, 557–558
    exercise physiology, 4–6, 17–18,
        138, 560–561
    exercise prescription, 563–564
    myopericardial, 572–573
    preparticipation evaluation, 62–
        63, 561–563
    sports participation limits of, 57–
        58
    valvular, 569–572
Carnitine, 602
Carpal ligamentous instability, 325
Casting, Achilles tendon rupture,
    512
Cataract, traumatic, 132–133
Cavus deformity, foot, 477
Central cord syndrome, 117–118
Cerebral contusions, 89
Cerebral edema, high-altitude, 633,
    634
Cerebral perfusion pressure (CPP),
    76, 78
Cervical spine injuries
    anatomy, normal, 100–102
    contusions, 110
    diagnosis, overview, 102–110
    dislocations, 110–114
    epidemiology, 97–100, 120
    fractures, 110–114
    history, 103–104
    medical clearance, 119
    neurologic injury with, 116–118
    physical/neurologic
        examination, 103, 104–108
    prevention, 120–121
    radiologic evaluation, 108–110
    rehabilitation, 120

sprains/strains, 110
transient quadriplegia, 118
treatment, overview, 102–110
unstable ligamentous, 114–116
Cervical vertebrae, 100–102
Charley horse, 374
Chest and thorax injuries
aortic rupture, traumatic, 141
cardiac tamponade, 140
esophageal disruption, 141–142
flail chest, 140
fractures, thoracic cage, 145–146
fractures, thoracic vertebrae, 146
hemothorax, 142–143
minor/aggravating conditions,
common, 143–147
myocardial contusion, 140–141
pneumomediastinum/
pneumopericardium, 142
pneumothorax, 142–143
rapid assessment of, 137–138,
152
soft-tissue trauma, neck, 138–
139
tension pneumothorax, 139–140
tracheobronchial tree, 141
Chest expansion, measurement of,
188
Chest wall
contusions and abrasions, 143–
144
strain and costochondral
separation, 144–145
Chilblains (pernio), 638–639
Children. *See* Young athletes
Chiropractors, 203
Cholesterol. *See* Fat/cholesterol,
dietary recommendations
Chondral fractures, 145
Chondromalacia patella, 427, 428,
429
Chronic ankle instability, 457–459
Chronic exertional compartment
syndrome, 491–494
Chronic obstructive pulmonary
disease (COPD), 13–14
Classic cerebral concussion
syndrome, 85
Clavicle
acromioclavicular joint, 247–254
anatomy, normal, 211, 237
distal, osteolysis of, 239–241
fractures, 237–239
sternoclavicular joint, 244–247

Clenbuterol, 659–660
Closed kinetic chain exercises,
436–437
Coaches, education/equipment
for, 41, 42, 49, 534
Coach's finger, 350–352
Coarctation of the aorta, 567
Cocaine, 662, 663
Coenzyme Q$_{10}$, 602
Cold-related illness
chilblains (pernio), 638–639
frostbite, 637–638
frostnip, 638
hypothermia, 635–637
trench foot (immersion foot), 638
College sports. *See* School athletics
Colles' fracture, 331
Colon injuries, 166–167
Coma, defined, 78
Communications
emergency medical
preparedness, 43
psychological aspects, 671–672
Compartment syndrome, acute
and chronic exertional, 489–494
Complete spinal cord injury, 117–
118
Compression and entrapment
neuropathy, elbow, 309–313
Computed tomography (CT)
abdominal injuries, 162
back injuries, 202
head injuries, 80
kidney injuries, 170
shoulder arthrography and,
235–236
sternoclavicular joint, 245
Concentric contractions, defined,
437
Concussion
defined, 75
epidemiology, 59
grading, 84–85, 86
incidence, 85
management, 85–88
Conduction disturbances, exercise
and, 575–576
Congenital heart disease, exercise
and, 566–569
Contact lenses, 130
Contact sports
defined, 98
incidence, cervical spine injuries,
118

pregnancy and, 626–627
Contraception, female athletes,
622–623
Contracoup contusion, cerebral, 89
Contusions
cerebral, 89
cervical spine, 110
chest wall, 143–144
hip pointer, 378
myocardial, 140–141
quadriceps, 374–376
shoulder muscles, 277
thoracic/lumbar spine, 197
Copperhead snakes, 644
Coracoid fractures, 242
Coral snakes, 644, 646
Corneal abrasions, 131–132
Corneal lacerations, 132
Coronary artery disease, exercise
and, 10–11, 568–569,
576–578
Corticosteroids
inhaled, asthma, 551, 552
injection, foot injuries, 511, 514
injection, shoulder injuries, 240,
243–244, 253–254
performance continuance, 656
Costochondral separation, 144–145
Costochondritis, 147
Cottonmouth snakes, 644
Coughing
asthma and, 549
disk disease and, 196–197
Coxsackie virus, 545
Crepitus, defined, 399
Cricket, back injuries and, 185–186
Cricothyrotomy, 139
Cross training, 474, 479, 481, 486
"Crossover" test, 250, 251
Cubital tunnel, 291
Cullen's sign, 154
Cushing's response, 79
Cysts, periarticular, 434–436

D
Dead arm syndrome, 263, 272
Degenerative joint disease, knee,
434
Dehydration. *See also* Fluid intake
prevention, 535–538, 598–599
as weight loss method, 600
Delayed menarche, 617–618
Deltoid muscle, 213, 279
Depressed skull fractures, 81–82

Diabetes, exercise and, 8–9
Diaphragmatic
   injuries, 165
   spasm, 159
Dietary ergogenic aids, 602–603
Dietary Guidelines for Americans, 585
Dietary recommendations
   carbohydrates, 590–591
   during/after events, 593, 594
   energy, 588–590
   fat/cholesterol, 592, 594–595
   protein, 591–592
   vitamins/minerals, 595–598
   weight control, 601
Diffuse axonal injury (DAI), 88
Diffuse brain injuries, 84–88
"Dinged," defined, 87
Diplopia, 131
Disabilities
   exercise and, 13
   resources for young athletes
      with, 49
Dislocations. *See also* Instability
   cervical spine, 110–114
   elbow, 297
   glenohumeral, acute anterior, 258–261
   glenohumeral, recurrent
      anterior, 261–262
   hand and fingers, 346–355
   knee, 418–420
   MCP joint, 353–355
   peroneal tendon, 459–460
   PIP joint, 349–353
   shoulder, voluntary, 255, 262
   sternoclavicular joint, 244–247
   thumb, 346–349
Disposition of the athlete. *See*
   Medical clearance, athletics
Distal biceps tendon rupture, 301–302
Distal clavicle, osteolysis of, 240
Distal humerus physeal fracture, 300–301
Distal interphalangeal joint (DIP)
   extensor injuries, 335–343
   flexor injuries, 343–346
Distal radioulnar joint injuries, 331–332
Distal radius fractures, 328
Distraction test, 188, 192
Diving, cervical spine injuries and, 100

D. J. Morton's syndrome, 521
Dorsal dislocation, PIP joint, 350–352
Dorsal intercalated instability, wrist, 325–326
Double-sheet reduction method, 259–260
Double vision, 131
Drop arm test, 230
Drop finger, 336–338
Drug abuse
   classification, 656–663
   history, 655–656
   preparticipation evaluation, 60
   testing for, 663–664
Drug interactions, NSAIDs and, 690–691
"Duck walking" test, 408
Duodenal injuries, 166
Dysmenorrhea, 619–620

E
Eating disorders, 489, 600–601, 620–621
Eccentric contractions, defined, 437
Education, sports. *See* Coaches;
   Primary care sports medicine
   physicians
Effort thrombosis, 277
Effusion, knee, 399
Eisenmenger syndrome, 567
Elbow injuries
   acute, 292–302
   anatomy, normal, 287–291
   chronic conditions, 302–313
   compression and entrapment
      neuropathy, 309–313
   dislocation, 297
   fractures, 298–301
   history, 291–292
   hyperextended elbow, 296–297
   lateral epicondylitis ("tennis
      elbow"), 302–306
   Little League elbow, 308–309
   medial epicondylitis ("golfer's
      elbow"), 306–307
   medial tension overload
      syndrome, 307–308
   olecranon bursitis, 313
   osteochondritis dissecans, 309
   osteochondrosis, 309
   physical examination, 292–295
   rehabilitation, 313–314
   treatment, acute, 295–302

treatment, chronic, 302–313
   ulnar collateral ligament tears, 295–296
Electrocardiogram (ECG), 65–66, 140–141
Electrolyte balance
   heat illness prevention, 535–538, 598–599
   training, 23–24
Elevation, shoulder, 226
Emergency medical preparedness
   communications for, 43
   equipment, locker room, 41, 42
   equipment, wilderness
      medicine, 647–649
   field care, 41–43
   planning for, 40
Emergency medical technicians
   (EMTs), 37
Emergency room physicians, 35
Energy, dietary recommendations, 588–590
Epidural hemorrhage, acute, 89–90
Epilepsy, 59
Epstein-Barr virus, 546–548
Equestrian injuries, 91
Equipment. *See* Emergency
   medical preparedness;
   Protective equipment/measures
Ergogenic aids
   dietary, 602–603
   drugs, 664
Esophageal disruption, 141–142
Eversion injuries, ankle, 449, 456
Excimer keratotomy, 125
Exercise, benefits of
   aging, 14–16
   arthritis, 11–12
   bones and osteoporosis, 12–13
   cardiovascular disease, 557–558
      COPD, 13–14
   coronary artery disease, 10–11, 576–578
   diabetes, 8–9
   disabilities, 13
   hypertension, 8
   mental health, 14
   obesity, 10
   public education about, 46
Exercise-induced anaphylaxis, 549
Exercise-induced asthma (EIA), 59–60, 548–553
Exercise intensity, 563–564
Exercise physiology

anemia, 16–17
cardiovascular responses, 4–6,
  17–18, 560–561
compared, disease states, 16–18
gastrointestinal tract, 18
immune function, 16
inactivity, 3–4
nutrition, 25–26
pregnancy and, 24–25
pulmonary responses, 6
specific cellular changes, 6
training and, 18–24
Exercise prescription
arrhythmias, 574–575
cardiovascular disease,
  overview, 563–566
conduction disturbances, 575–
  576
congenital heart disease, 566–
  569
hypertension, 573–574
myopericardial disease, 572–573
overview, 6–7
valvular heart disease, 569–572
Exercise-related sudden death
  (ERSD), 57–58, 558–560
Exercises, specific muscles. *See also*
  Rehabilitation; Strength training
back, 204–206
cervical spine, 111
elbow, 313–314
shoulder, 262, 277–282
Extension, shoulder, 226
Extension back exercises, 204
Extensor mechanism, knee, 390–
  391
Extensor tendon injuries
anatomy, normal, 335
boutonniere injury, 338–341
mallet finger, 336–338
rupture, PIP joint, 338–341
sagittal band/hood rupture,
  MCP joint, 341–343
Extra-articular scapular fractures,
  242
Eye, ear, nose, and throat,
  preparticipation evaluation, 64
Eye examination
head injuries, 79–80
instruments for, 126–127
visual acuity, 62, 126
Eye guards, 128–130
Eye injuries
anatomy, normal, 125

ocular examinations, 131–133

F
FABER test, 192
Facet dislocations, cervical, 115
Facet syndrome, 201
Family physicians. *See* Physicians
Fat/cholesterol, dietary
  recommendations, 592, 594–595
Fat-free body mass, 587
Fatness, body, 586–587
Female athletes. *See also* Eating
  disorders
breast injuries, 143, 614–616
contraception, 622–623
exercise-related sudden death
  (ERSD), 559–560
genitourinary injuries, 172, 616
gynecologic concerns, 616–620
injury patterns, 612–614
osteoporosis, 621–622
physiology, 611–612
pregnancy, 623–627
triad of, 620–621
Femoral neck fractures, 380–381
Femoral shaft stress fractures, 382
Field care, school sports, 41–43
Field defects, visual, 130–131
"1500 meter runner's hack," 549
Figure-of-eight dressing, shoulder
  injuries, 246, 247
Figure skater's cough, 549
Finger injuries. *See* Hand and
  finger injuries
Fire ant stings, 643
Fitness level, assessment of, 65
Flail chest, 140
"Flak jacket," 144
"Flank-stripe sign," 161
Flat feet, 433, 477
Flexion, shoulder, 226
Flexion back exercises, 204
Flexion-rotation drawer test, 404
Flexor digitorum superficialis
  rupture, 344
Flexor tendon injuries
annular flexor pulleys rupture,
  344–346
flexor digitorum superficialis
  rupture, 344
Jersey finger, 343–344
Fluid intake
heat illness prevention, 535–538,
  598–599

training, 23–24
Focal injuries, intracranial, 88–91
Foot injuries
Achilles tendon, 509–512
anatomy, normal, 501
biomechanics, 501–505
forefoot, 517–524
heel pain, plantar surface, 512–
  515
hindfoot, 509–516
history, 507–509
ingrown toenails, 523–524
metatarsal stress fractures, 519–
  521
metatarsalgia, 517–519
midfoot, 516–517
Morton's neuroma, 521
physical examination, 507–509
posterior tibial tendinitis/
  rupture, 515
prevention, 505–507
sesamoiditis, sesamoid stress
  fractures, 521–522
turf toe, 522–523
Football injuries
back, 185
cervical spine, 98–99, 118
prevention, 91
"Footballer's migraine," 85
Footwear, athletic, 475, 481, 505–
  507, 511, 514
Forced flexion test, knee, 408
Forefoot injuries, 517–524
Foreign bodies, corneal, 131
Fracture dislocation, PIP joint,
  352–353
Fractures
ankle, 461–464
blow-out of orbit, 133
cervical spine, 110–114
clavicle, 237–239
elbow, 298–301
forefoot, 519–522
hand and finger, 355–357
knee, 424–426
lower leg, 483–489
lumbar spine, 197
metacarpals, 355–357
pelvis, hip, and thigh, 380–382
scapula, 241–243
thoracic cage, 145–146
thoracic spine, 146, 197
thumb, 357–358
Freidberg's infraction, 518

Frostbite, 637–638
Frostnip, 638

G
Gaenslen's extension test, 192
Galeazzi's fracture, 331
Gamekeeper's thumb, 346–349
Gastrocnemius muscle tears, 494–497
Gastrointestinal tract, exercise physiology, 18
Genitourinary injuries
    female genitalia, 172, 616
    kidney, 167–171
    male genitalia, 171–172
    ureters and bladder, 171
Genitourinary system, preparticipation evaluation, 64
Gerdy's tubercle, 433
Giardiasis, 646–647
Gila monster bites, 646
Glasgow coma scale, 77, 78
Glenohumeral joint
    anatomy, normal, 212–213
    instability, anterior, 258–264
    instability, general, 254–258
    instability, impingement syndrome and, 270–271
    instability, inferior, 265–266
    instability, multidirectional, 265
    instability, posterior, 264–265
    internal derangements, 266
Glenoid fractures, 241
Golf injuries
    back, 185–186
    shoulder kinematics, 219
"Golfer's elbow," 306–307
Grashey view, glenohumeral joint films, 233
Greater trochanteric bursitis, 377–378
Groin (adductor longus) strains, 373–374
Growth plate injuries, knee, 425–426
Gymnastics injuries, 100, 184–185

H
Hamate fracture, 330–331
Hammon's sign, 142
Hamstring muscles
    anatomy, 364, 368
    strains, 369–373
Hand and finger injuries

dislocations, 346–355
extensor tendon, 335–343
flexor tendon, 343–346
fractures, 355–358
jammed finger, 335–343
sprains, 346–355
Hangman's fracture, 113
Head injuries
    classification, 81
    concussion, 84–88
    definitions, 75
    diffuse axonal injury (DAI), 88
    evaluation, general, 78
    focal, 88–91
    management, general, 76–77
    neurologic examination, 78–80
    pathology of, 81–91
    pathophysiology, brain injury, 75–76
    radiologic evaluation, 80–81
    statistics, 91–92
    triage scoring, 78
Health issues of exercise. See Exercise physiology
Heat cramps, 531
Heat exhaustion (heat prostration), 532–533
Heat illness
    acclimation process, 529–531
    differential diagnosis, 533
    pathophysiology, 529
    physiology, 527–529
    predisposing factors, 528
    preparticipation evaluation, 60
    prevention, 534–538, 598–599
    spectrum of disease, 531–534
Heat stress index, 534, 535
Heat stroke, 533–534
Heat syncope, 531
Heel pain, plantar surface, 512–515
Heinig view, sternoclavicular joint films, 232
Helmets, 91–92
Hematomas
    abdominal, 157–159
    hip, 160
    subungual, 523
Hematuria, 170, 171
Hemorrhage
    abdominal injuries, 151, 154, 161
    anterior chamber (hyphema), 132
    intracranial, 89–91, 547–548
    retinal, 633, 635

subconjunctival, 132
Hemothorax, 142–143
"Hepatic angle sign," 161
Hernias, 167
Herniated disks, 187, 188, 192, 195, 197
High-altitude illnesses, 633–635
High school sports. See School athletics
Hill-Sachs lesions, 236, 257, 261
Hindfoot injuries, 509–516
Hip injuries. See Pelvis, hip, and thigh injuries
"Hip pointer," 160, 378
History taking, preparticipation evaluation, 61–62
Hobbs view, sternoclavicular joint films, 232
Hollow viscus, 165–166
Hook of the hamate, 321, 322, 326, 330–331
Hornet stings, 643
Hospitals, sports medicine and, 35
Human growth hormone, 661
Hussmaul's sign, 140
Hydration. See Fluid intake
Hymenoptera stings, 643–644
Hyperextended elbow, 296–297
Hypermobility, vertebral spine, 197
Hyperpronation, foot, 476, 477, 479
Hypertension
    exercise and, 8
    exercise prescription, 573–574
    sports participation limits of, 58–59
Hypertrophic mediopatellar plica, 432
Hyphema, 132
Hypothermia, 635–637

I
Ice hockey injuries, 99–100
Ice skating, pregnancy and, 627
Idiopathic hypertrophic subaortic stenosis (IHSS), 572–573
Ileal injuries, 166
Iliac apophysitis, 378–379
Iliac compression test, 192
Iliopsoas bursitis, 378
Iliopsoas muscle, 369
Iliotibial band friction syndrome, 432–433
Immersion foot, 638

Immune function, exercise physiology, 16

Impingement syndrome, rotator cuff, 230, 263, 267–271

Impingement test, 269

Inactivity, exercise physiology, 3–4

Incomplete spinal cord injury, 117

Infectious disease and field water, 646–647

Infectious mononucleosis, 154, 164, 546–548

Inferior glenohumeral instability, 265–266

Inflammatory conditions, spinal, 200–201

Infrapatellar bursitis, 432

Infraspinatus muscle
  anatomy, 214
  exercises for, 279

Ingrown toenails, 523–524

Injuries
  conditions increasing risk of, 61, 676
  female athletes, 612–614

Injury prevention. *See also* Protective equipment/measures
  adult recreational leagues, 46
  ankle sprains, 456–457
  cervical spine, 120–121
  knee, 441
  lower leg injuries, 474–477
  primary care physician's role, 45–46
  psychological aspects, 676
  resources for, 48

Insect bites, 641–644

Instability. *See also* Shoulder instability
  chronic ankle, 457–459
  knee, 401–407
  wrist, 325–328

Internal derangements, glenohumeral joint, 266

Internists. *See* Physicians

Intervertebral disk disease, 196–197

Intra-abdominal injuries. *See* Abdominal injuries

Intra-articular fractures
  base of thumb, 357–358
  scapula, 242–243

Intracranial focal injuries, 88–91

Intracranial hemorrhage, 89–91, 547–548

Intracranial pressure (ICP), 76, 77, 88

Intracranial volume and ICP, 88

Intravenous pyelogram (IVP), 161–162, 170

Inversion injuries, ankle, 449, 451, 462

Inversion stress test, 453

Iron deficiency, 595

Isokinetic exercises, 20–21, 436

Isometric/isotonic exercises
  cervical spine, 111
  knee, 427, 436
  lower leg, 479
  neck, 120
  performance, 20–21

J

Jammed finger, extensor injuries, 335–343

Jefferson fracture, 111–113

Jejunal injuries, 166

Jersey finger, 343–344

Jogging. *See* Running

Joints, shoulder, 212–213

"Jumped facets," unilateral/bilateral, 115

"Jumper's knee," 429

K

Kehr's sign, 154

Kenny Howard splint, 252

Kidney injuries, 167–171

Kinematics, shoulder, 215–219

Knee alignment, 397–398

Knee injuries
  anatomy, normal, 390–393
  articular surface, 422–424
  degenerative joint disease, 434
  dislocations, 418–420
  epidemiology, 389–390
  fractures, 424–426
  history, 393–397, 427
  ligamentous, 410–418
  meniscal, 420–422
  overuse, 426–436
  periarticular cysts, 434–436
  physical examination, 393, 397–408, 427
  preparticipation evaluation, 63
  prevention, 441
  radiologic evaluation, 408–409
  range of motion, 399–400
  rehabilitation, 436–440

  special testing, 407–408
  stability testing, 401–407
  tendon ruptures, 426
  traumatic, 409–426

Knee reflex, 188

Kohler's disease, 517

L

Laboratory testing, preparticipation evaluation, 65–66

Lacerations
  corneal, 132
  eye lid, 131

Lachman test, 401, 402

Lactate, 19–20

Lactose intolerance, 590

Laryngeal trauma/laryngospasm, 138–139

Lateral epicondylitis ("tennis elbow"), 302–306

Lateral (fibular) collateral ligament (LCL)
  anatomy, normal, 392–393
  assessment, 402–403
  injuries, 417–418
  palpation, 398

Lateral patellar compression syndrome, 428

Lateral patellar subluxation, 428

Latissimus dorsi, 213, 281

Leg injuries. *See* Lower leg injuries; Pelvis, hip, and thigh injuries

Legg-Calvé-Perthes disease, 384–385

Lid lacerations, 131

Lift-off test, 229

Ligamentous injuries
  cervical spine, 114–116
  knee, 410–418
  wrist, 325–328

Light projection/perception, 126

Lightning strikes, 640–641

Linear skull fractures, 81

Lipids, exercise and, 9–10

List, spinal, 186, 187

Lister's tubercle, 319, 324

Little League elbow, 308–309

Liver injuries, 164

Locked knee, 396, 400, 421, 422

Locker/training room medical facilities, 40, 41, 42

Log rolling, 76, 104, 138

Long thoracic nerve injuries, 274
Loss of consciousness (LOC)
    assessment, 78–79
    defined, 75
    management, 87–88
Lower leg injuries
    anatomy, normal, 471–474
    compartment syndrome, 489–
        494
    diagnostic studies, 478
    gastrocnemius muscle tears,
        494–497
    history, 474
    medial tibial stress syndrome,
        479–482
    physical examination, 477
    risk factors, 474–477
    stress fractures, 483–489
    treatment, 478–479
Lumbar spine. *See* Back injuries
Luteal phase deficiency, 617

M
Magnetic resonance imaging (MRI)
    back injuries, 202
    head injuries, 81
    knee, 408–409
    knee injuries, 409
    lower leg injuries, 478
    shoulder, 236
Maisonneuve fracture, 452
Male genitalia injuries, 171–172
Mallet finger, 336–338
Mammary souffle murmur, 562
Manipulative therapy, back
    injuries, 203–204
Marfan's syndrome, 569
Maturity, assessment of, 64–65
McMurray's test, 407–408, 421
Medial epicondylar avulsion
    fracture, 301
Medial epicondylitis ("golfer's
    elbow"), 306–307
Medial tension overload
    syndrome, 307–308
Medial (tibial) collateral ligament
    (MCL), 392, 402–403, 411–413,
    418
Medial tibial stress syndrome
    ("shin splints"), 479–482
Median nerve compression
    neuropathy, 312
Medical clearance, athletics
    acromioclavicular joint injuries,

253
    cervical spine injuries, 119
    clavicular fractures, 239
    exercise-induced asthma (EIA),
        548–553
    infectious mononucleosis, 546–
        548
    preparticipation evaluation, 66
    scapular fractures, 243
    sternoclavicular joint injuries,
        247
    viral URIs, 543–545
Menarche, delayed, 617–618
Meniscal cysts, 434, 436
Meniscal injuries, knee, 407–408,
    420–422
Menstruation, athletics and, 616–
    620
Mental health, exercise and, 14
Mesenteric injuries, 167
Metabolic abnormalities, lower leg
    injuries and, 476–477
Metacarpal fractures
    neck, 355–357
    shaft, 357–358
Metacarpophalangeal joint (MCP)
    dislocations, 346–349, 353–355
    extensor injuries, 335–343
    sagittal band/extensor hood
        rupture, 341–343
    sprains, 346–349
Metatarsal stress fractures, 519–
    521
Metatarsalgia, 517–519
Midfoot injuries, 516–517
Minerals, dietary
    recommendations, 595–598
Minor head injury
    defined, 75
    triage scoring, 78
Mitral regurgitation, 571
Mitral valve prolapse, 571
Mitral valve stenosis, 571–572
Moderate head injury, triage
    scoring, 78
Morton's neuroma, 521
Motivation, psychological aspects,
    672–673
"Movie theater sign," 427
Multidirectional glenohumeral
    instability, 265
Murmurs, cardiac, 562
Muscle fatigue, 22–23
Muscle injuries. *See also* Exercises,

specific muscles
    abdominal, 156–159
    biceps rupture, 276
    lower leg, 494–497
    pectoralis major rupture, 275
    pelvis, hip, and thigh, 365–367
    shoulder, 274–277
    subscapularis rupture, 276
Muscle soreness, 22, 367
Musculoskeletal system
    back, 180–183
    elbow, 287–291
    exercise, benefits of, 12–13
    manual testing, shoulder
        muscles, 228–230
    muscle strength grading scale,
        224
    pelvis, hip, and thigh, 364–365
    preparticipation examination,
        63–64
    shoulder, 211–215
Myocardial contusion, 140–141
Myocarditis, 573
Myofascial pain syndrome, 147
Myopericardial disease, 572–573
Myositis ossificans, 376–377

N
Near dislocation, defined, 418
Neck injuries, 138–139. *See also*
    Cervical spine injuries
Needle cricothyrotomy, 139
Neurologic examination
    back injuries, 188
    cervical spine injuries, 103, 104–
        108
    elbow injuries, 293, 295
    head injuries, 78–80
Neurologic injuries. *See also*
    Brachial plexus; Cervical spine
    injuries; Head injuries
    axillary nerve, 272–273
    compression and entrapment,
        elbow, 309–313
    long thoracic nerve, 274
    preparticipation evaluation, 59
    shoulder, 271–274
    spinal accessory nerve, 273–274
    spinal cord, 117–118
    suprascapular nerve, 273
    thoracic outlet syndrome, 271–
        272
Neutral alignment, knees, 397
Neutral elevation, shoulder, 226

Nipple irritation, 146, 614
Non-weight bearing, ankle
 injuries, 456, 464
Noncontact sports
 defined, 98
 medical clearance after cervical
  spine injuries, 119
Nonsteroidal anti-inflammatory
 drugs (NSAIDs)
 adverse drug events, 688–690
 back injuries, 203
 drug interactions, 690–691
 indications, 683
 listed, 684
 mechanism of action, 683, 685
 patient information on use of,
  688
 performance continuance, 656
 prescribing principles, 685–688
 topically applied, 691
Nutrition
 body composition, 585–588
 dehydration/fluid intake, 598–
  599
 dietary recommendations, 588–
  598
 ergogenic aids, 602–603
 exercise physiology, 25–26
 importance of, 585
 weight gain, 601–602
 weight loss, 599–601

O
Obesity, exercise and, 10
"O'Donoghue triad," 418
Odontoid, fracture of, 113
Olecranon bursitis, 313
Oligomenorrhea, 617–618
Olympic athletes, drug abuse and,
 655, 663
Open kinetic chain exercises, 436–
 437
Open skull fractures, 82–83
Orthopedists, 35–36, 37
Orthotics
 chronic exertional compartment
  syndrome, 493
 design/types, 506–507
 heel pain, 514
 hyperpronation, foot, 429, 479
 medial tibial stress syndrome,
  481
Osgood-Schlatter disease, 431–432
Osteitis pubis, 379

Osteoarthritis, 434
Osteochondritis dissecans (OCD),
 422, 423
Osteolysis, distal clavicle, 239–241
Osteopathic physicians, 203
Osteoporosis, 12–13, 620, 621–622
Osteosarcoma, differential
 diagnosis, 377
Overtraining ("staleness"), 19
Overuse injuries
 elbow, 287
 knee, 395, 396–397, 426–436
 pelvis, hip, and thigh, 378–385
 shoulder, 239, 267, 268

P
Pain. *See also* Back injuries;
  Referred pain
 heel, 512–515
 myofascial, 147
 patellofemoral, 427
 shoulder injuries, characteristics
  of, 222–223
 "trigger-point" syndrome, 147,
  157
Pancreatic injuries, 164–165
Panner's disease, 309
Paramedics, 37
Parents, sports education for, 41,
 43, 534
Patella
 anatomy, normal, 390–391
 dislocation, 419
 subluxation, 420
 tendinitis, 429–432
Patella grind (compression) test,
 407
Patella inhibition test, 407
Patella tilt test, 406
Patellofemoral joint
 dislocations, 418
 overuse injuries, 427–429
Patellofemoral pain, 427
Patent ductus arteriosus, 567
Patrick's test, 192
Peak expiratory flow rate (PEFR),
 59–60, 550, 553
Pectoralis major muscle
 anatomy, 213
 exercises, 279–281
 rupture, 275
Pediatricians. *See* Physicians
Pediatrics. *See* Young athletes
Pelvis, hip, and thigh injuries

anatomy, normal, 363–364
 epidemiology, 363
 fractures, 379–382
 greater trochanteric bursitis,
  377–378
 groin (adductor longus) strains,
  373–374
 hamstring strains, 369–373
 hip pointer, 378
 history, 364–367
 iliac apophysitis, 378–379
 iliopsoas bursitis, 378
 Legg-Calvé-Perthes disease,
  384–385
 myositis ossificans, 376–377
 osteitis pubis, 379
 overuse and, 378–385
 physical examination, 367–369
 piriformis syndrome, 382–384
 quadriceps contusions, 374–376
 quadriceps strains, 373
 specific injuries, 369–378
Penetrating injuries, abdomen, 153
Performance continuance drugs,
 656
Performance enhancement drugs,
 656–662
Periarticular cysts, knee, 434–436
Pericarditis, 573
Peritoneal lavage, diagnostic, 162
Pernio, 638–639
Peroneal tendon subluxation/
 dislocation, 459–460
Peroneal tenosynovitis, 460–461
Pes biceps bursa, 433
Pes planus (flat feet), 433, 477
Photophobia, 130
Physical examination. *See*
 Preparticipation evaluation
 (PPE)
Physicians. *See also* Primary care
 sports medicine physicians
 emergency room, 35
 orthopedists, 35–36, 37
 osteopathic, 203
 other specialists, 36
 school sports team, 39–40
Piriformis syndrome, 382–384
Pit vipers, 644–646
"Pivot-shift" phenomenon, 404
Plant dermatitis, 639–640
Plicae, defined, 391
Pneumomediastinum, 142
Pneumopericardium, 142

Pneumothorax, 139–140, 142–143
Poison ivy/poison oak/poison sumac, 639–640
Polycarbonate eye guards, 128–130
Popliteal cysts, 434
Posterior cord syndrome, 117–118
Posterior cruciate ligament (PCL), 393, 416–417
Posterior drawer test
  knee injuries, 402
  shoulder injuries, 255, 257
Posterior glenohumeral instability, 264–265
Posterior tibial tendinitis/rupture, 515
Posttraumatic amnesia, 85
Precompetition diet, 591, 592
Precordial catch syndrome, 147
Pregnancy
  athletics and, 615, 623–627
  exercise physiology, 24–25
  NSAIDs and, 688
Preparticipation evaluation (PPE). See also Medical clearance, athletics
  cardiovascular disease, 561–563
  conditions limiting participation, 57–61
  disposition of the athlete, 66
  fitness level, assessment of, 65
  goals/format for, 55–57
  laboratory/other testing, 65–66
  maturity, assessment of, 64–65
  national/state standards, 55
  physical examination, 40, 61–65
  sample forms for, 68–72
Prepatellar bursitis, 430–431
Primary amenorrhea, 618–619
Primary care sports medicine physicians (PCSMP)
  community contributions, 35–36, 46
  education, 36–38
  orthopedic specialists, 37
  role of, 33–35, 45–46
Proprioception exercises
  ankle injuries, 466
  knee injuries, 439
Prostate examination, 161, 187
Protective equipment/measures. See also Footwear, athletic; Orthotics
  abdomen/genitals, 171, 172–173
  breasts, 143–144, 615

chest shields, 141
eye guards, 128–130
"flak jacket," 144
head, 91–92
proper racquet grip size, 304
thigh, 374–375
Protein, dietary recommendations, 591–592
Protein supplements, 591–592
Proximal humerus, 212
Proximal interphalangeal joint (PIP)
  dislocations, 349–353
  extensor injuries, 335–343
  extensor rupture, 338–341
Proximal radius and ulnar fractures, 301
Psoriatic arthritis, 200
Psychology. See Sports psychology
Pubic rami fractures, 382
Pulmonary edema, high-altitude, 633, 634–635
Pulmonary responses, exercise, 6
Pulmonary valve stenosis, 572
Pupillary assessment, head injuries, 79–80

Q
Q angle, 397–398, 613
Quadriceps femoris muscles
  anatomy, 364
  contusions, 374–376
  strains, 373
Quadriceps tendinitis, 430
Quadriplegia, transient, 118

R
Raccoon eyes, 83
Racquet sports
  elbow injuries with, 287
  pregnancy and, 626
  proper grip size, measurement, 304
Radial fractures, 301, 328
Radial nerve compression neuropathy, 312–313
Range of motion
  knee, 399–400, 437–438
  pelvis, hip, and thigh, 369
  shoulder, 216, 225–228
Rate of perceived exertion (RPE), 564
Rattlesnakes, 644
Recombinant erythropoietin

(rEPO), 661–662
Recreational athletes, 38, 46
Recreational (destructive) drugs, 662–663
Rectal injuries, 166–167
Rectus abdominis muscle rupture, 157–159
Rectus femoris muscle, 368–369, 373
Reduction, glenohumeral dislocations, 259–261
Referred pain
  elbow, 292
  pelvis, hip, and thigh, 365
  shoulder, 154, 221–222
Rehabilitation. See also Exercises, specific muscles
  ankle injuries, 464–466
  cardiac, 577–578
  cervical spine injuries, 120
  facilitating psychological recovery, 671–676
  knee injuries, 436–440
  shoulder injuries, 277–282
Reiter's syndrome, 200
Relaxation techniques, 674, 679
Relocation test, 256, 257
Reptiles, venomous, 644–646
Resistance training, 21–22
Retinal detachment, 133
Retinal hemorrhage, high-altitude, 633, 635
Retrograde amnesia, 85
Return to athletics. See Medical clearance, athletics
Rhomboids, 214, 281
Rib, slipping, 147
Rib fractures, 140, 144, 145–146, 163, 164
RICE treatment principle, 371, 455
"Ring sign," 83
Rolando's fracture, 357–358
Rotator cuff
  anatomy, 214
  baseball pitching, 217–218
  muscle exercises for, 277–279
Rotator cuff injuries. See also Impingement syndrome
  arthrography, 235
  characteristic pain, 222
  MRIs, 236
"Runner's bladder," 171
"Runner's nipples," 146, 614
"Runner's toe," 523

Running
    back injuries, 184
    gait components, 476, 501–503
    lower leg injuries, 480
    pregnancy and, 626

S
Sacral injury, 192
Sacroiliac compression test, 192
Safety, sports
    committees for, 43–45
    resources for, 48
Safety glasses, 128
Sage test, 406
Sagittal band, 341–343
Salt tablets, heat illness and, 531
Scaphoid fractures, 328–330
"Scaphoid view," wrist films, 322, 323
Scapholunate dissociation, 325–328
Scaption, 226
Scapula
    anatomy, normal, 211
    fractures, 241–243
    "snapping," 243–244
Scapular elevation, shoulder, 226
Scapulohumeral rhythm, 215
Scapulothoracic articulation, 213
School athletics. *See also*
    Preparticipation evaluation (PPE)
    conditions increasing injury risk, 61
    conditions limiting participation in, 57–61
    sports medicine programs, 38–43
Sciatic nerve, 188, 192, 382
Scorpion stings, 642
"Scottish terrier" radiograph configuration, 198
Scrotal support, 171, 173
Scuba diving, pregnancy and, 627
Second impact syndrome, head injuries, 86
Secondary amenorrhea, 619
Serratus anterior muscle, 214, 281
Sesamoid stress fractures, 521–522
Sesamoiditis, 521–522
Severe head injury
    defined, 75
    triage scoring, 78
Sever's disease, 510
"Shin splints," 479–482

Shoes. *See* Footwear, athletic
Shoulder injuries
    age and, 223
    anatomy, normal, 211–215
    axillary artery occlusion, 277
    biomechanics, normal, 215–219
    clavicle, 237–241
    diagnosable, but untreatable problems, 221
    diagnostic studies, 222–237
    dislocations. *See* Shoulder instability
    effort thrombosis, 277
    evaluation, 220–222
    history, 222–223
    imaging studies, 232–237
    impingement syndrome, 230, 263, 267–271
    manual muscle testing, 228–230
    muscular, 274–277
    neurologic, 271–274
    physical examination, 223–232
    preparticipation evaluation, 63–64
    provocative tests, 230–232
    range of motion tests, 225–228
    referred pain, 154, 221–222
    rehabilitation, 277–282
    rotator cuff, 230, 263, 267–271
    scapula, 241–244
    sternoclavicular joint, 244–247
    subluxation, biceps tendon, 277
    treatable problems, 220
    undiagnosable problems, 221
Shoulder instability
    anterior glenohumeral, 258–264
    anterior subluxations, 262–264
    classification, 254–255
    history, 255
    impingement syndrome, 230, 263, 270–271
    inferior glenohumeral, 265–266
    multidirectional glenohumeral, 265
    physical examination, 255–257
    posterior glenohumeral, 264–265
    radiologic evaluation, 257
    tests for, 230–232
    treatment, 257–258
    voluntary dislocations, 255, 262
Sinding-Larsen-Johansson disease, 430
Single-leg stand test, 192
Skeletal system. *See*

Musculoskeletal system
Skier's thumb, 346–349
Skin injuries, abdominal, 155–156
Skull fractures, 81–84, 91
SLAP lesions, 266
Sling immobilization, shoulder injuries, 240, 246, 251, 252
Slipped capital femoral epiphysis, 384
Slipping rib syndrome, 147
Slocum test, 404
Snake bites, 644–646
"Snapping" scapula, 243–244
Snow skiing, pregnancy and, 627
"Snuff-box," anatomic, 319, 324, 328–329
Soft-tissue trauma, neck, 138–139
Solar plexus, blows to, 159–160
"Spearing," 98, 99, 120
Speed's test, 230, 269
Spider bites, 642–643
Spinal abnormalities
    bony, 198–200
    hypermobility, 197
    inflammatory conditions, 200–201
Spinal accessory nerve injuries, 273–274
Spinal canal, 102, 180–181
Spinal cord injury, classification, 117–118
Spinal cord neurapraxia, 118
Spleen
    injuries, 162–164
    rupture of, 154, 547
Splinting
    elbow injuries, 305
    fingers, 337, 340–341, 342
    lower leg injuries, 488
    shoulder injuries, 252
    thumb injuries, 348–349
Spondyloarthropathies, seronegative, 200
Spondylolisthesis, 198, 200, 204
Spondylolysis, 198, 204
Sports
    back injuries, sports-specific, 184–186
    cervical spine injuries and, 97–100
    high risk, body collision, 566
    resources on specific, 49–51
    static/dynamic demands, level of intensity, 565

Sports anemia. *See* Anemia
Sports bras, 143–144, 615
Sports medicine, in the community
  athletic facilities, 45
  injury prevention, 45–46
  medical coverage of athletic
    events, 46–47
  paramedics/EMTs and, 37
  physicians and, 33–38
  recreational athletes, 38
  school systems, 38–43
  sports safety committees, 43–45
  youth sports leagues, 37–38
Sports psychology
  coping with injury, 670
  mental training skills, 673–675
  motivation, 672–673
  personal reactions to injury,
    669–670
  rehabilitation/recovery and,
    671–676, 680
Sports safety committees, 43–45
Sprains
  ankle, 449–457
  cervical spine, 110
  defined, 97
  hand and fingers, 346–355
  knee, 410
  thumb, 346–349
  wrist, 322–325
Spurling test, 222
Stable cervical spine fractures, 111
"Stacking" of drugs, 659
"Staleness" (overtraining), 19
Stener lesion, 347
Sternoclavicular joint
  anatomy, normal, 212, 244
  radiologic evaluation, 232
  subluxations and dislocations,
    244–247
Steroids. *See* Anabolic/androgenic
  steroids; Corticosteroids
Stimson's reduction method, 259
Stingers/burners
  brachial plexus injuries, 272
  cervical spine injuries, 103, 116
  defined, 59
"Stitches," 147
Stomach injuries, 166
Straight-leg-raising test, 188
Strains
  cervical spine, 110
  chest wall, 144–145
  defined, 97, 365

groin (adductor longus), 373–
    374
  hamstring, 369–373
  pelvis, hip, and thigh, 365–367
  quadriceps, 373
Strength training
  exercises for, 20–22
  knee muscles, 436–437
  neck muscles, 120
Stress fractures
  lower leg, 483–489
  metatarsal, 519–521
  pelvis, hip, and thigh injuries,
    379–382
  sesamoid, 521–522
Subacromial bursography,
  shoulder, 236
Subacromial space, shoulder, 214–
    215
Subarachnoid hemorrhage, 91
Subconjunctival hemorrhage, 132
Subcutaneous tissue injury,
  abdominal, 156
Subdural hematoma, acute, 90–91
Subluxations. *See also* Instability
  biceps tendon, 277
  peroneal tendon, 459–460
  sternoclavicular joint, 244–247
Subscapularis muscle
  exercises for, 279
  rupture, 276
  testing, 229
Substance abuse. *See* Alcohol use;
  Drug abuse
Subtrochanteric stress fractures,
  381
Subungual hematoma, 523
Sudden death. *See* Exercise-related
  sudden death (ERSD)
Sulcus sign test, 256
Supracondylar humerus fracture,
  300
Suprascapular nerve injuries, 273
Supraspinatus muscle
  exercises for, 279
  testing of, 229
Supraventricular tachycardia, 574
Surfing/surfboarding, cervical
  spine injuries and, 100
Sweating. *See* Dehydration; Heat
  illness
"Swimmer's view", cervical spine
  films, 108
Swimming

pregnancy and, 626
  shoulder kinematics, 218
Syncope, heat, 531
Syndesmophyte, 201
Synovial space, knee, 391
Systolic ejection murmur, 562

T
Tamponade, cardiac, 140
Tanner classifications, maturity, 64
Taping
  ankle injuries, 456
  finger injuries, 335, 350, 355
  thumb injuries, 348–349
Tarsal tunnel syndrome, 513
Team physicians, 39–40
Tendinitis
  Achilles tendon, 509–511
  knee, 434
  patellar, 429–432
  posterior tibial, 515
  quadriceps, 430
Tendon injuries
  ankle, 459–460
  hindfoot, 509–512, 515–516
  knee, 426, 429–432
Tennis, shoulder kinematics, 218–
    219
"Tennis elbow," 302–306
"Tennis leg," 494
Tension pneumothorax, 139–140
Teres minor muscle, 214, 279
Tetralogy of Fallot, 567–568
Thermoregulation, 527
Thigh injuries. *See* Pelvis, hip, and
  thigh injuries
Thompson's test, 453, 512
Thoracic outlet syndrome, 271–272
Thorax. *See* Chest and thorax
  injuries
Thrombosis, effort, 277
Throwing sports. *See* Elbow
  injuries; Shoulder injuries
Thumb. *See also* Hand and finger
  injuries
  dislocations and sprains, 346–
    349
  fractures, 357–358
Tibial plateau fractures, 424–425
Tibial spine fractures, 424
Tibiofemoral articulation, 391–393
Tick bites, 641–642
"Tidemark," defined, 422
Tietze's syndrome, 147

Tinel's sign, 295, 310, 311, 513
Tobacco use, 663
Toes, 515, 517–524
"Too many toes sign," 515
Topically applied NSAIDs, 691
Tracheobronchial tree injuries, 141
Tracheostomy, 139
Training. *See also* Coaches;
  Strength training
  dietary recommendations, 595
  electrolytes and fluids, 23–24
  exercise frequency/intensity/
    duration, 18–19
  improper, 475, 483
  lactate, 19–20
  mental training skills, 673–675
  muscle soreness/fatigue, 22–23
  overtraining/"staleness," 19
  viral URIs and, 543–545
Trampolines, cervical spine
  injuries and, 100
Transchondral talar dome
  fractures, 462–464
Transient quadriplegia, 118
Transient visual loss, 130
Transposition of the great vessels,
  568
Trapezius paralysis, 273
Traumatic aortic rupture, 141
Traumatic cataract, 132–133
Trench foot (immersion foot), 638
Triad, female athlete, 620–621
Triage scoring, head injuries, 78
Triangular fibrocartilage injuries,
  331–332
Tricuspid regurgitation, 572
"Trigger-point" pain syndrome,
  147, 157
Turf toe, 522–523
Turner's sign, 154

U

Ulnar collateral ligament tears,
  295–296
Ulnar fractures, 301
Ulnar nerve compression
  neuropathy, 311–312
Ultrasonography
  abdominal injuries, 163
  shoulder, 236
"Unhappy triad," 418
Unstable cervical spine
  fractures, 111–114
  ligamentous injuries, 114–116

Upper extremity
  innervation, 291
  neurologic examination, 103,
    104–107
Upper respiratory infections
  (URIs), 543–545
Ureteral injuries, 171
Urinary system injuries. *See*
  Genitourinary injuries

V

Valgus extension overload
  syndrome, 307
Valgus (knock-knee) alignment,
  397, 477
Valgus stress test
  elbow, 295
  knee, 403
Valvular heart disease, exercise
  and, 569–572
Varus (bowlegged) alignment, 397,
  477
Varus stress test, knee, 403–404
Vegetarian diet, 592
Venomous
  arthropods, 641–644
  reptiles, 644–646
Venous hum murmur, 562
Ventricular arrhythmias, 574–575
Ventricular septal defect, 566
Vertebral column anatomy,
  normal, 180–181
Visual acuity
  assessment, eye injuries, 126
  preparticipation evaluation, 62
Visual loss, 130
Vital signs, preparticipation
  evaluation, 62
Vitamin E, 597
Vitamins, dietary
  recommendations, 595–598
Volar intercalated instability,
  wrist, 326
Volar plate avulsion, PIP joint,
  349–350

W

Walking, pregnancy and, 626
Wasp stings, 643
Water deficit, calculating, 533
Water moccasin snakes, 644
Water skiing
  injuries, female genital, 172, 616
  pregnancy and, 627

Water supply, infectious disease
  and, 646–647
Weight, body, 585–587
  exercise and, 10
  gain, 601–602
  loss, 599–601
  sensible control, exercise/diet,
    601
Weight lifting, pregnancy and, 626
Wet bulb globe temperature
  (WBGT) index, 535
Wilderness medicine
  acute high-altitude illness, 633–
    635
  cold-related illness, 635–639
  field water, infectious disease
    and, 646–647
  lightning strikes, 640–641
  medical kit for, 647–649
  plant dermatitis, 639–640
  venomous arthropods, 641–644
  venomous reptiles, 644–646
"Winded, being," 143, 159
Women. *See* Female athletes
Wrestlers, weight loss methods,
  600
Wright's test, 271
Wrist injuries
  anatomy, normal, 319–322
  distal radioulnar joint, 331–332
  fractures, 328–331
  ligamentous instabilities, 325–
    328
  radiography, normal, 319–322
  sprains, 322–325
  triangular fibrocartilage, 331–332

Y

Yellowjacket stings, 643
Yergason's test, 230–231, 269
Young athletes. *See also* School
  athletics
  abdominal injuries, 164
  back injuries, 179
  community sports leagues, 37–
    38
  congenital heart disease, 566–569
  CVD, physiologic limitations,
    561
  with disabilities, resources for,
    49
  elbow injuries, 299–301, 308–309
  exercise-related sudden death
    (ERSD), 558–559

growth plate injuries, 425–426
hamstring strains, 372
hypertension, 573
kidney injuries, 168

knee injuries, 389, 416
NSAID use, 689
nutrition, 587, 601
Osgood-Schlatter disease, 431–

432
osteochondritis, 309
patellar tendinitis, 430